Seventeenth Edition

Handbook of
Preventive
and
Social Medicine

Community Health | Community Medicine

for Courses in

Nursing and
Allied Health Sciences

Seventeenth Edition

Handbook of
Preventive and Social Medicine
Community Health | Community Medicine

*for Courses in **Nursing** and **Allied Health Sciences***

Yash Pal Bedi
MBBS (Pb), DOMS (Eng.), DPH (Lond.), LM (Dub.)

Former
Dean, Hygiene and Vaccine Institute, Punjab
Professor of Preventive and Social Medicine
Medical College, Amritsar
Examiner in Hygiene and Public Health, University of Punjab
External Examiner in Universities of Agra, Patna, Bihar, Rajputana and Bombay
Medical Officer of Health, Amritsar

Editor
Pragya Sharma
MBBS, MD

Professor
Department of Preventive and Social Medicine
Maulana Azad Medical College
New Delhi

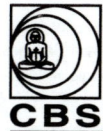

CBS

CBS Publishers & Distributors Pvt Ltd

New Delhi • Bengaluru • Chennai • Kochi • Kolkata • Mumbai
Hyderabad • Jharkhand • Nagpur • Patna • Pune • Uttarakhand

Seventeenth Edition

Handbook of

Preventive
and
Social Medicine

Community Health | Community Medicine

for Courses in Nursing; and Allied Health Sciences

ISBN: 978-93-87085-78-7

Copyright © Publisher

Seventeenth Edition: 2018

First Edition: 1955

Sixteenth Edition: 2003

Published by Satish Kumar Jain and produced by Varun Jain for

CBS Publishers & Distributors Pvt Ltd

4819/XI Prahlad Street, 24 Ansari Road, Daryaganj, New Delhi 110 002, India.
Ph: 23289259, 23266861, 23266867   Website: www.cbspd.com
Fax: 011-23243014   e-mail: delhi@cbspd.com; cbspubs@airtelmail.in.
Corporate Office: 204 FIE, Industrial Area, Patparganj, Delhi 110 092

Ph: 4934 4934   Fax: 4934 4935   e-mail: publishing@cbspd.com; publicity@cbspd.com

Branches

- **Bengaluru:** Seema House 2975, 17th Cross, K.R. Road,
  Banasankari 2nd Stage, Bengaluru 560 070, Karnataka
  Ph: +91-80-26771678/79   Fax: +91-80-26771680   e-mail: bangalore@cbspd.com
- **Chennai:** 7, Subbaraya Street, Shenoy Nagar, Chennai 600 030, Tamil Nadu
  Ph: +91-44-26680620, 26681266   Fax: +91-44-42032115   e-mail: chennai@cbspd.com
- **Kochi:** Ashana House, No. 39/1904, AM Thomas Road, Valanjambalam,
  Ernakulam 682 016, Kochi, Kerala
  Ph: +91-484-4059061-65   Fax: +91-484-4059065   e-mail: kochi@cbspd.com
- **Kolkata:** 6/B, Ground Floor, Rameswar Shaw Road, Kolkata-700 014, West Bengal
  Ph: +91-33-22891126, 22891127, 22891128   e-mail: kolkata@cbspd.com
- **Mumbai:** 83-C, Dr E Moses Road, Worli, Mumbai-400018, Maharashtra
  Ph: +91-22-24902340/41   Fax: +91-22-24902342   e-mail: mumbai@cbspd.com

Representatives

- **Hyderabad**   0-9885175004
- **Jharkhand**   0-9811541605
- **Nagpur**   0-9021734563
- **Patna**   0-9334159340
- **Pune**   0-9623451994
- **Uttarakhand**   0-9716462459

Printed at Mudrak, Delhi, India

Preface
to the Seventeenth Edition

In a vast developing discipline which today claims a large number of textbooks by authors both within and outside India, every textbook will have its own individuality and characteristics. Eleven editions of this book were compiled by the author Dr Yash Pal Bedi himself. Subsequently, three editions were edited, revised and enlarged by Dr SM Marwah, Professor and Head, Department of Preventive and Social Medicine, Benaras Hindu University, Varanasi. This new edition has been further revised and enlarged by me. Certain obsolete portions in the previous edition have been deleted and new ones incorporated without losing original characteristics of the *Handbook*.

All the chapters in the Seventeenth Edition have been thoroughly revised and made up-to-date. It is reasonably hoped that the book in its present form will adequately cover all the requirements of medical, nursing and public health students as well sanitary inspectors, health visitors and other auxiliary health workers, besides being of interest to general readers, as was originally planned by the author. In addition, it will serve the requirements of general practitioners who are today integrating preventive, promotive and national services much more than before.

In a work like this it is not possible to acknowledge cooperation of all those whose direct and indirect interactions get incorporated through an author's write-ups. However, I acknowledge with thanks the most willing assistance of Dr Harsavardhan Nayak and Dr Akanksha, Senior Residents, Department of Community Medicine, Maulana Azad Medical College, New Delhi, for their work in making valuable contribution, repeated revision and proofreading to give this book a final shape.

I would also like to thank Dr S Garg, Director Professor and Head, Dr GK Ingle, Director Professor, and senior colleagues, Department of Community Medicine, Maulana Azad Medical College, New Delhi, for their immense unconditional support and faith, which has been a constant source of motivation behind this mammoth task. Last but not the least, I would also like to acknowledge my family and friends for being a source of constant inspiration in my life.

Besides, I am indebted to the publishers for their general excellence in the production of this edition.

Pragya Sharma
Editor

Foreword
to the First Edition

It was with great pleasure that I have gone through the manuscript of *Handbook of Preventive and Social Medicine* sent to me by Dr Yash Pal Bedi, Professor of Hygiene and Public Health, Medical College, Amritsar. At present more attention is paid to the preventive aspect than before. Sir George Newman rightly observed, "It is not the event of death which we can escape but the incident of avoidable invalidity and premature death", that gives, in a nutshell, the object of studying hygiene.

Health is not merely absence of disease, the conception of health envisages the full development of physical, mental and spiritual powers with which an individual is endowed. In order to attain this ideal attention is now being paid in different countries, especially in England and America, to what is known as "social medicine". The World Health Organization is playing an important part in this respect. Most of the diseases are preventable, specially those caused by some specific organisms, which are carried by different agencies like air, water or through some intermediaries like the insects. It has, therefore, been possible to adopt preventive measures according to the nature and method of spread of the different diseases. Since impure air and water, pollution of soil, bad disposal of refuse and excretal matter, errors in diet and improper cleanliness of the house and its surroundings has an important role in the spread of disease and thus require to be carefully studied. On the other hand, the individual himself, being an important unit of the community, should be properly educated to enable him to appreciate the value of sanitation not for his own health, but also for the community in general.

It is essential that all these different factors should be properly dealt with in a book. And judging from this angle, the handbook which Dr Bedi has written will, I am sure, be of great value in inculating the fundamental principles of hygiene. Apart from environmental hygiene, personal hygiene, village sanitation, sanitation of fairs and melas as also the main principles of prevention of communicable diseases so common in India, have been dealt with succinctly, though nothing of importance has been left out.

I am sure that Dr Bedi's book will meet with all the requirements of the students who, I have no doubt, will read it with interest and profit.

BN Ghosh
Author of
Treatise on Hygiene of Public Health

Contents

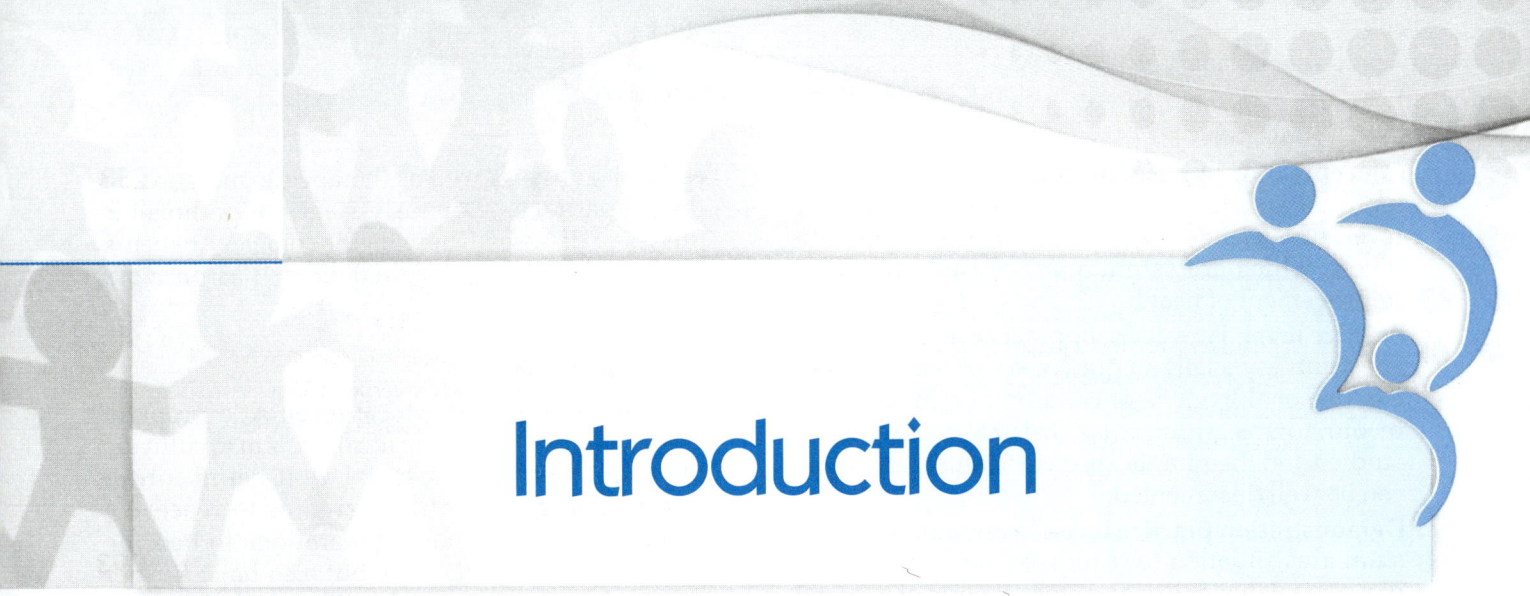

Introduction

To start with, the terms medicine, hygiene, public health, preventive medicine and social medicine may be defined or clarified. There are at least three levels at which any one, two, three or all the above mentioned disciplines exist in any area. The levels are as under:

a. Conceptual or philosophical level
b. Practice level
c. Demonstration level.

a. **Conceptual or philosophical level** may be defined as the unattained (may be also unattainable in the near future) idealistic level of practice for which a scientist may develop the strivings. The conceptual or philosophical level is essential to widen the horizons of the medical profession for ever continued strivings to achieve higher and higher. Without idealistic philosophy, long range scientific achievements are not possible.

b. **Practice level** is the level at which any of the above mentioned disciplines exists in actual practice. Since time immemorial, medical profession has been a practice, a science and an art in the background of the profession's ideals during any phase of human existence.

c. **Demonstration level** may be defined as the scientific effort to demonstrate the raising of the existing practices scientifically towards the conceptual level in a graded manner.

The three levels of the five disciplines, e.g. medicine, hygiene, public health, preventive medicine, and social medicine and community medicine are discussed here under as these concepts provide the guidelines for discussion in the book. Further, each of the five disciplines is a science as well as an art. Each is a science as it is based on scientific knowledge. Each is also an art as it involves the development of skills for systematic application of knowledge for benefits of human beings in their ecological settings.

1. MEDICINE

a. **Conceptual or philosophical level:** The conceptual background for traditional disciplines of medicine are diagnostic and therapeutic services including surgical services of the highest order and quality. The emphasis is mostly on sophisticated and well organised hospital services. In conceptual thinking, the inpatient services have greater emphasis than the outpatient services.

b. **Practice level:** The practice levels of the traditional disciplines are clear in terms of hospital services, both inpatients and outpatients, which are available both on payment and free out of tax or voluntary philanthropic contributions. In addition, diagnostic and therapeutic services are also available in homes on payment only. There is a whole spectrum of the quality of these services.

c. **Demonstration level:** There are, at times, evident scientific efforts to improve the organisational aspects of the hospital services. However, most of these improvements are seen in hospitals with easy resources, especially in developing countries. Scientific strivings to improve the hospital services maximally within available resources are not yet visible in our country.

2. HYGIENE

The word hygiene is derived from the Greek word *Hygeia*—the Goddess of health. Hygiene is defined as the science and art of preserving and improving health. Hygiene deals both with an individual and a community as a whole. Personal hygiene is the term used for improvement of hygiene of an individual or a person. Similarly, other terms like mess hygiene, milk hygiene, hygiene of feeding, hygiene of clothes, hygiene of infant feeding, etc. are self-explanatory.

a. **Conceptual or philosophical level:** For conceptual level, one should strive for attainment of the highest levels of hygiene at personal as well as community levels, which are essential for preservation and improvement of health.

b. **Practice level:** However, the practice level has wide spectrum especially in our socioeconomic setting, e.g. personal hygiene of children in affluent parts of our towns, slum areas or rural areas can be studied and their implications in health and disease can be well documented.

c. **Demonstration practice level:** In any situation, e.g. slum area situation for children, some component of personal hygiene or any other aspects of hygiene can be improved through scientific strivings and health education.

3. PUBLIC HEALTH

a. **Conceptual or philosophical level:** For visualising conceptual level of public health; its definition by Winslow may be quoted. Professor Winslow defined public health as "science and art of (i) preventing diseases, (ii) prolonging life, and (iii) promoting health and efficiency through organised community effort for (a) the sanitation of the environment, (b) the control of communicable diseases, (c) the education of the individual or personal hygiene, (d) the organisation of medical and nursing services for the early diagnosis and preventive treatment of disease, and (e) the development of the social machinery to ensure everyone a standard of living adequate for the maintenance of health, so organising these benefits as to enable every citizen to realise birth right for health and longevity".

b. **Practice level:** The practice level of public health is the traditional public health services, e.g. community water supply, sewage disposal, etc. which exist in a wide-spectrum in various areas.

c. **Demonstration practice level:** All over the world, efforts are being made to provide missing links in the public health services to aim to evolve conceptual level of public health practices.

4. PREVENTIVE MEDICINE

a. **Conceptual or philosophical level:** Idealistically visualising, one may think of prevention of all preventable diseases, communicable as well as non-communicable.

b. **Practice level:** Practice level is constituted by the existing services for eradication and control of diseases, contact tracing, individual immunisations, health examinations, screening, etc.

c. **Demonstration practice level:** Demonstrations in preventive medicine are provided by the methodologies which are being evolved for screening, early diagnosis as well as therapeutic measures in the prepathogenic or early stages of pathogenic phases of diseases. These methodologies are being evolved both on individual as well as on mass basis.

5. SOCIAL MEDICINE

a. **Conceptual or philosophical level:** At conceptual level, social medicine is an idealistic aim to cultivate physical, mental and social well-being for all human beings. Scientific strivings to reach the moon have lasted many generations to become not only a reality of today but also have further widened the borders of scientific strivings to reach even other galaxies in our universe.

b. **Practice level:** Practice level of social medicine in any area is evident in terms of existing medical, public health, developmental and other social welfare services.

c. **Demonstration practice level:** Demonstration practice level efforts are visible all over the world in terms of social security schemes, health insurance schemes, developmental and social welfare activities and efforts at nationalisation as well as socialisation of medicine.

The above mentioned definitions and classifications for the terms medicine, hygiene, public health, preventive medicine and social medicine are given only to provide the background to the discussions. In no case they aim to support, contest, replace or even modify the definitions given in literature. Further, the three levels have been emphasised for (a) meaningful achievements, (b) realistic analysis of existing situations, and (c) objective pursuits for priority based achievements in graded manner towards the idealistic aims. This point may be further illustrated from existing situations. In traditional medical disciplines, the gap between idealistic philosophy and actual practice is very narrow. A physician only aims to diagnose and treat after a disease has occurred in hospital situations. The result is overburdening of the curative services with shortage of resources. On the other hand, there is a lot of emphasis in social medicine on preachings of idealistic philosophies both in training and research without much action/demonstration of graded priority based achievements within the existing situations. The result is that there is a lot of frustration, confusion and resistance to accept the philosophy of social medicine. Philosophical preaching, however, must lead to analysis of existing situations and subsequent scientific actions.

Some other terms may also be explained.

6. PREVENTIVE AND SOCIAL MEDICINE

In India, the terms hygiene and public health have been replaced by preventive and social medicine. In fact, the term incorporates all the concepts discussed under hygiene, public health, preventive medicine and social medicine. In hygiene and public health, there was more emphasis on classical public health. In preventive and social medicine, the emphasis is more on total health care programmes for individuals, families, groups as well as communities through integration of preventive, curative and rehabilitative services.

7. COMMUNITY HEALTH/COMMUNITY MEDICINE

The terms community health and/or community medicine are being used in an interchangeable manner. In fact, the health workers prefer the word community health as the overall emphasis is on health of the entire community. However, the term community health aims at cultivation of community diagnosis and treatment for physical, mental and social well-being in place of traditional individual diagnosis and treatment of an individual's illness. The term community health/community medicine, which is of more recent origin, tends to merely replace the previous terms hygiene and public health or preventive and social medicine.

8. HEALTH

As per the World Health Organization in its preamble, "Health is defined as a state of complete physical, mental and social well-being and not merely absence of disease or infirmity". However, recently 'ability to lead a socially and economically productive life' has been added to it to make it more complete and holistic.

Perfect health is an abstraction which may not be attainable but is essential for an individual family/ group or a community's strivings. Optimum health is the highest level of health attainable by an individual in his/her ecological settings. Positive health means striving for preservation and improvement of health. Negative health means scientific efforts for prevention and cure of diseases. The important factors for cultivation of health are (a) conducive environment for a healthy living, (b) balanced diet, (c) adequate physical activity and rest as per individual needs, (d) promotive, preventive, therapeutic and welfare services, (e) suitable occupation with job satisfaction, (f) proper use of leisure, and (g) wholesome mental attitude to life.

9. ECOLOGY AND HEALTH

The word ecology derived from the Greek word Oikos meaning habitation, and logos meaning study, implies a study of the habitations of organisms. Ernst Haeckel, a German scientist, defined ecology as "the relation of the animal to its organic as well as its inorganic environment, particularly its friendly or hostile relations to those animals or plants with which it comes in contact". The environment of modern man

is partly natural and partly man-made. It consists of physical, mental and social factors which are dynamic and interacting both within themselves and with the life process in the internal environment of man. The important physical factors are air, water, food, buildings, their contents and multiple devices produced by man to adjust the physical environment around him. The important biological factors are pathogens, other micro-organisms as well as living beings, vectors, plants, etc. which have implications on health and disease. The important social factors are customs, beliefs, laws, peculiarities and modes of living of human beings that have their implications on health and disease.

10. ENVIRONMENTAL SANITATION

The word sanitation is derived from the Latin word Sanitas which means a state of health. Environmental sanitation envisages promotion of health of the community by providing clean environment and breaking the cycle of disease. It depends on various factors that include hygiene status of the people, types of resources available, innovative and appropriate technologies according to the requirement of the community, socioeconomic development of the country, cultural factors related to environmental sanitation, political commitment, capacity building of the concerned sectors, social factors including behavioural pattern of the community, legislative measures adopted, and others.

The main goal of the Government of India (GOI) is to eradicate the practice of open defaecation by 2010. A number of innovative approaches to improve water supply and sanitation have been tested in India, in particular in the early 2000s. These include demand-driven approaches in rural water supply since 1999, community-led total sanitation, public–private partnerships to improve the continuity of urban water supply in Karnataka, and the use of microcredit to women in order to improve access to water (discussed in details later).

Total sanitation campaign gives strong emphasis on information, education, and communication (IEC), capacity building and hygiene education for effective behaviour change with involvement of Panchayati Raj Institutions (PRIs), community-based organizations, Non-Governmental Organizations (NGOs), etc. The key intervention areas are individual household latrines (IHHL), school sanitation and hygiene education (SSHE), community sanitary complex, Anganwadi toilets supported by rural sanitary marts (RSMs), and production centres (PCs).

11. PRIMARY HEALTH CARE

Considering the gross inequality in the health status of people particularly between developed and developing countries as well as within countries, the Alma-Ata conference in Sept. 1978 called for provision of Health for All by 2000 AD through primary health care, which was defined as:

"Primary health care is essential health care made universally accessible to individuals and families in the community by means acceptable to them, through their full participation and at a cost that the community and country can afford. It forms an integral part both of country's health system of which it is the nucleus and of the overall social and economic development of the community".

At grassroot levels, especially in the rural areas, primary health care is aimed to be implemented in the realities of human situations and as an integral part of overall socioeconomic development. Further by 2000 AD, it is hoped that this care will be available to all including the poorest billions of the global population. Further, it will be linked with the referral care through a system of regionalisation (discussed subsequently).

12. EVOLUTION OF MEDICINE FROM MAGICO-RELIGIOUS TO PRIMARY HEALTH CARE: GLOBAL SETTINGS

The phases of evolution of medicine from magico-religious to primary health care in the global settings may be summarised as follows:

1. Religions dominated the lives of human beings during primitive and early civilisations, middle ages and periods of cultural revivals, i.e. from 3000 BC to 1800 AD. Attributions of diseases and health seeking was strongly inspired by the religious beliefs. This was the phase of primitive medicine where the causation of diseases was attributed to "Supernatural factors like evil spirits" and thus the treatment was also sought accordingly.

2. The leading phases of evolution of medicine were (a) magico-religious concepts (demonistic, i.e. disease caused by demons; deitistic, i.e. disease caused by deities; and spiritual, i.e. disease caused by a living or dead man), (b) philosophical, i.e. humoral mixed with naturalistic concepts, i.e. natural factors imbibed with divine characteristics (Indian and Greek leading to Roman and Arabic systems of medicine), and (c) scientific concepts in terms of (i) bacterial and associated aetiologies and (ii) in addition to environmental and sociocultural aetiologies.

3. The leading phases of evolution of therapeutics in medicine were (a) drugs as supplements of prayers and incantations (primitive civilizations and dark ages), (b) drugs with or without prayers and incantations (early and Arab civilizations, periods of cultural revival), and (c) drugs especially specifics for treatment as well as prophylaxes and radio-isotopes (scientific periods).

4. Surgery passed through the phases of (a) crude magico-religious surgery like trephining, etc. of primitive cultures, (b) refined surgery of early civilisations and subsequent periods, and (c) antiseptic, aseptic and highly sophisticated surgery of the scientific periods.

5. Public health passed through the phases of (a) taboos, rituals, etc. for groups for protection in primitive civilisations, (b) environmental health and sanitary engineering (i) of early civilisations in developed pockets, (ii) through affluence and industrialization in developed parts of the world, during 1850–1950, and (iii) through community organised efforts in developing parts of the world in the 20th century, (c) various public health acts and creation of local bodies and ministries of health during 1850–1950, (d) formations of state agencies all over the world, (e) global co-operative efforts through international conferences, agencies and global health concepts for control as well as eradication of diseases, and (f) comprehensive health care.

6. Preventive and promotive health concepts passed through the phases of (a) taboos and rituals for individuals in primitive cultures, (b) fitness, personal hygiene and physical culture for aristocrats and soldiers in early civilisations, (c) school health, preventive and promotive services for getting healthy recruits as well as keeping armies feeling fit during 19th and 20th centuries, (d) health as a fundamental right of all citizens during second half of the 20th century, (e) formulations of various health committees to make recommendations to achieve health for all, and (f) setting up of Millennium Development Goals (MDGs) for health and health related socioeconomic factors.

7. Studies of society and its relationship with the individuals have their deep roots in the early civilisations (Egyptian, Indian, Greek and Roman). These studies have gathered phenomenal momentum through (a) industrialisation, (b) revolutionary theories of political and economic ideologies including communist forms of society and democratic rights of individuals, and (c) knowledge explosion in natural and social sciences. Organisation of medical care through private practitioners and state services also have their roots in early civilisations. Hospitals as hospices were started in 400 BC. Dispensaries developed since 1630 and health centre approach developed since 1920. Further sickness insurance started since 1883, has developed into complex systems of health insurance and social security both through socialised and democratic institutions. Further, newer prospectives initially started during Ayurvedic times (physical, mental and spiritual well-being) and now being extensively explored in terms of physical, mental, social and

spiritual well-being have over the centuries led to the present day concepts of social as well as **socialised medicine.**

In short, a medical man today is a scientist for study of problems related to physical, mental and social well-being along with causation of disease in man and in man's ecological settings. The medical education is thus a lifetime learning process that needs to incorporate meaningfully the fundamentals of traditional medical sciences (preclinical, paraclinical and clinical), traditional public health sciences along with social as well as behavioural sciences. The traditional medical disciplines emphasised individual diagnosis and management of disease conditions. The traditional public health disciplines emphasised cultivation of health as well as control of diseases on population basis. The recent discipline of **social medicine** emphasises (a) health and welfare as a part of fundamental right and (b) medicine as a part of overall sociocultural systems through integrated approaches of traditional medical disciplines, traditional public health disciplines and social and behavioural sciences disciplines.

With the evolution of medical science, the emphasis is on primary health care, i.e. care available within homes through health and link workers, through health centres located at commutable distances from home for first contact care in the realities of human situations and referral care, i.e. increasingly skillful care through pyramidal level specific care through a network of health facilities.

1

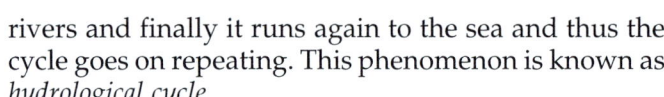

Water

1.1 IMPORTANCE OF WATER

Human body consists of approximately 75% of water and thus it is one of the prime elements responsible for life on earth. Water circulates through the human body, transporting, dissolving, replenishing nutrients and organic matter, while carrying away waste material. It also regulates the activities of fluids, tissues, cells, lymph, blood and glandular secretions.

An average adult body contains 42 litres of water and with just a small loss of 2.7 litres he or she can suffer from dehydration, displaying symptoms of irritability, fatigue, nervousness, dizziness, weakness, headaches and consequently reach a state of pathology. Thus, water intended for human consumption should be both safe and wholesome and for this reason in early times habitation used to be near rivers, lakes and springs.

Sources of water: Rainwater, oceans, rivers, lakes, streams, ponds and springs are natural sources of water. Dams, wells, tube wells, handpumps, canals, etc. are man-made sources of water.

As a matter of fact all water is primarily derived from oceans. Water reaches earth in the form of rain, hail, snow, dew or mist, from water vapour in the atmosphere, derived mainly from evaporation of the sea, from lakes, rivers and other waters of the land. Seawater contains sodium chloride and land water contains lot of dissolved and suspended impurities, but it evaporates in the form of pure distilled water which reaches earth again in the form of rain, snow or hail. This condensed water from the air, which is the ultimate source of all our natural water supply, is pure except for a few impurities that are absorbed from the atmosphere.

A part of rain water on reaching earth is evaporated again into the atmosphere and a part of it percolates into the earth. Some part of it gets collected in the form of lakes, ponds, etc. But a major portion of it runs away at once in the direction of natural slope of ground and gets collected in the form of small streams, which forms rivers and finally it runs again to the sea and thus the cycle goes on repeating. This phenomenon is known as *hydrological cycle.*

1.2 SOURCES OF WATER SUPPLY

The chief sources of water suply are:
  a. Rainwater or snow water.
  b. Surface water, i.e. streams, canals, rivers, lakes, tanks and ponds.
  c. Upland surface water and natural/artificial lakes.
  d. Groundwater, i.e. wells and springs.
  e. Seawater.

a. Rainwater

Rainwater collects on the earth in the form of surface water and underground water. In India, it is used as a source of water supply, where rainfall is heavy and water of springs and wells is brackish. Many countries across the globe are adopting strategies for harvesting rainwater for tapping the natural reservoir to meet the needs of ever larging population and water scarcity.

Rainwater is the purest and cheapest source of water in nature but it receives impurities from the atmosphere such as dust, soot, suspended matter and even microbes, gases like hydrogen sulphide, carbon dioxide, ammonia, nitrogen, oxygen, etc. for initiating 15–20 minutes, then the water becomes (clear) bright and sparkling. But all the same, these impurities are not of much importance, since they are not pathogenic like germs of cholera, enteric fever, etc. The first rain which falls on roofs and other impervious materials is contaminated with dirt, including birds' droppings, eggs of insects, dust, etc. over roofs and other collecting surfaces.

Rainwater can be used for potable water (drinking, cooking, bathing) or non-potable uses such as landscape irrigation, livestock watering and washing. Collecting and using rainwater has numerous benefits, ranging from improved water quality to reduced stress on underground aquifers.

Rainwater can be collected from the impervious surfaces such as rooftops for domestic services other than drinking. Whenever it is to be used for drinking purposes, arrangement should be made to purify the water and make it potable before consumption. The mechanical arrangement such as *"Roberts"* or *"Gibbs" rainwater separator,* were used earlier that used to be fixed to the rainwater pipe to allow first portion of the rainwater to run waste and thus store only pure water. To use rainwater for drinking and potable purposes, it must be filtered before delivery to the distribution tank. For this, one or more sand filters are required in addition to a large storage tank and a smaller one for filtered water.

Rainwater, if properly collected and stored, is a safe water. It is soft, as it contains only traces of dissolved solids. The advantage is that it is suitable for cooking, washing and bathing purposes. However, its one serious drawback is that being soft and slightly acidic, it is liable to corrode lead pipes and thereby cause lead poisoning. In tropics, *Aedes aegypti* breeds in artificial cisterns holding rainwater.

A rainfall of 1" (2.54 cm) in depth corresponds to about 4.67 gallons (21.25 litres) per sq yd (0.836 sq metre) or 22,617 gallons (101 tons) per acre (0.405 hectare) of land. The amount of water that can be collected from a roof in a year is calculated as follows:

The area of the roof in sq feet × half of the amount of rainfall in inches = gallons of water per year.

b. Surface Water

Rainwater on reaching the ground or the melted snow from the hills begins to flow and is seen as a river, canal, stream, lake or a pond and is called *surface water.* These are waters which drain from the surface. In India, many towns like Delhi, Kolkata, Ahmedabad, etc. derive their water supply from rivers.

The great advantage of these sources of water is that they can supply a very large amount of water. The yield of water of a river can be estimated by:

a. Finding out its width over a known distance and its average depth. The product of both these factors gives the sectional area. The mean velocity is 4/5 of the surface velocity. The yield of the river is the product of mean velocity and the sectional area, and

b. Rivulet method. In this case, water is allowed to pass through a channel of known dimensions. The yield of a river is the product of velocity and depth.

The disadvantages are that they represent rain long time after it has fallen, and has travelled a very long distance. The river water is fairly pure and unpolluted at its source but during its course it becomes more or less polluted as most rivers and streams serve as the natural sewer of the region they drain. Consequently, they contain suspended materials, which are harmful mechanically. As a matter of principle, river water is softer than groundwater, but contains sufficiently large amount of organic matter. All rivers are very muddy and turbid during rainy season. They contain much suspended matter. Rivers, streams and canals being open water courses are freely used by the people for washing, bathing and so forth. They get polluted by human and animal excreta either accidentally or through ignorance. Trade affluents are also discharged from the factories. Dead bodies are burnt on the banks of rivers. When places of pilgrimage are situated on the banks of rivers and hundreds of thousands of pilgrims bathe at a time, the river water automatically gets polluted.

However, the running water in rivers, canals and streams is naturally purified to a certain extent since flowing waters possess *auto-* or *self-purifying action:* (a) Where oxidation of impurities occurs by oxygen dissolved in the water, (b) absorption of organic impurities by vegetable and animal life, e.g. fish, etc., (c) settling of solid matter due to gravitation and dilution by the tributaries, etc. Thus, stagnant water in shallow and small rivers, which dry up in summer are dangerous from the sanitary point of view.

The proper remedy is to prevent willful pollution of rivers, streams and canals. For this purpose, the Water (Prevention and Control of Pollution) Act was enacted in 1974 to provide for the prevention and control of water pollution, and for the maintaining or restoring of wholesomeness of water in the country. The Act was amended in 1988. The Water (Prevention and Control of Pollution) Cess Act was enacted in 1977, to provide for the levy and collection of a cess on water consumed by persons operating and carrying on certain types of industrial activities. This cess is collected with a view to augment the resources of the Central Board and the State Boards for the prevention and control of water pollution constituted under the Water (Prevention and Control of Pollution) Act, 1974. The Act was last amended in 2003.

The river water undergoes self-purification in the course of its flow by sedimentation of the solid matter, and also by oxygenation of the organic matter on account of oxygen present in the water. The sun, too, has a purifying action due to its actinic rays and the amount of such purification depends upon depth, magnitude and the rate of flow of the river. However, the ultraviolet rays of sun cannot penetrate through the turbid water.

The caution in drawing water from river can minimize the risk of excretal contamination. The water should be taken from a point of the river from above the spot where sewage and other impurities are discharged into the river. Another precaution to be observed is that water should be taken from the river at least 20–30 ft (6.096 to 9.144 metres) away from the bank, where the contamination is comparatively less. This objective can be achieved by using a pipe attached to a handpump.

Tanks or Ponds

These are important sources of water supply in some villages in India. These are the excavations in which rainwater is collected. These are generally full of silt and colloidal matter, especially after the rains. In these tanks, water undergoes natural purification to some extent.

For an ideal tank or a pond, the following points should be attended to:

1. The soil for excavation should not be made-soil and loose sandy soil having filthy ponds and cesspits. There should be no insanitary or borehole latrines in the vicinity. No surface drain should be allowed to empty into it.
2. The surroundings should be clean with proper fencing. Trees should be planted at a distance around it to keep away the cattle and dirt.
3. It should be fairly deep and large and preferably of a rectangular shape having an area of about an acre. Banks should be properly sloped and planted with grass. The surrounding area should have a low embankment to prevent any outside water getting access into the tank, except the rainwater.
4. All sorts of bathing and washing of utensils or clothes in the tank should be strictly forbidden and a notice to that effect should be displayed at a prominent place near it. Moreover, steps and ghats should not be provided into the tank.
5. Weeds and algae should be removed regularly. Whenever water in the tank or the pond deteriorates, it should be emptied out and re-excavated as growth of algae makes the water unpleasant to taste.
6. Any trade, like jute-steeping, should not be allowed in the tank.
7. Some varieties of fish which thrive on larvae may however, be stocked, if so desired.

Ferrocement tanks are a type of storage tank that consist of an armature (framework) of steel reinforcing, which is then covered with a sand-cement plaster. They offer complete flexibility in shape, have a long life and are cost-competitive when contractor-built, and are owner-buildable in both industrialized and non-industrialized countries.

c. Upland Surface Water

Upland rivers rise in mountaneous regions. It is the water which runs on the sides of hills, slopes and valleys and is taken off as water supply before such water collects to form big streams and rivers. Water may be collected in the form of natural lakes as in the city of Glasgow or in artificially constructed lakes as has been done in cities like Mumbai, Chennai and Darjeeling. The area from which this water is collected, is called the *catchment area*. The water supplied to Simla is an example of this kind of water supply. At a short distance from Simla, there is a ridge of low hills, called the *Mahasu ridge* which drains into a deep *Nala*, between the ridge and Simla. The rainwater flows along the slope of the ridge, which is well wooded and constitutes the catchment area. The water thus collected is called the upland surface water. Similarly, Mumbai city receives its water supply from upland surface water in the form of four artificial lakes *(viz. Tulsi Lake, Tansa Lake, Vihar Lake and Vaitarna Lake)* situated away at great distances from Mumbai proper.

An upland surface water is safe because it is pure rainwater, which has travelled a short distance over the earth. However, the dangers are:

1. Excreta of human beings and animals in catchment area may find its way into the water, and infect it with pathogenic micro-organisms.
2. Freshly collected water is acidic in nature and may corrode lead, thus forming a easily soluble hydrate of lead, which remains on the inner surface of lead pipes, cisterns, etc. and on becoming detached mixes in water. Since the water is acidic in reaction, lead gets dissolved in the water and may cause lead poisoning on consumption.
3. The water may become brownish or yellowish in colour due to the decayed vegetable substance called peat in some catchment areas.

The upland surface water needs purification by filtration and sterilisation by chlorination or it can simply be purified by running the water through a bed of fine sand, before final storage for human consumption.

Yield of the catchment area can be found by E. Pole's formula:

$$Q = 62.15 \, A \, (4/5 \, R - E)$$

$$Q = \text{Gallons per day}$$

Where,

A = Area in acres.

R = Average rainfall for three driest consecutive years.

E = Loss in inches of evaporation.

Lakes

These are simply natural collections of upland surface water in a valley with a high ground at its outlets, which checks all water from escaping at once. When collected from unpopulated hilly districts such water being usually soft and containing a little chlorine, affords an excellent supply. It does not contain ammonia nitrates and nitrites more than the proportion in which they are usually found in rainwater. It, however, contains more dissolved matter than rainwater. Water collected from low land surfaces usually contains much peaty matter as well as phosphates and nitrates, washed from manures of cultivated fields. That is why it becomes yellow or brownish in appearance. The lake water requires filtration and disinfection before drinking. The yield of a lake is based upon the dimensions of catchment area and the annual rainfall.

d. Groundwater

It is superior to surface water, because the ground provides water an effective filtering medium. Water gets filtered and purified, and fills within the void spaces in the rocks below the water table. When a water-bearing rock readily transmits water to wells and springs, it is called an aquifer. Wells and springs thus constitute important sources of groundwater since the wells can be drilled into the aquifers and water can be pumped out.

Wells

These are artificial holes or pits dug into the earth to reach the underground water level. Modern wells are more often drilled by a truck-mounted drill rig, thus the wells can be classified as dug wells, driven wells and drilled wells (Fig. 1.1). However, depending upon the depth of the water table, these can be of three types:

1. *Shallow wells* are those which do not penetrate an impermeable stratum. They simply tap the subsoil water, i.e. groundwater lying between the surface and first impermeable stratum. The water of these wells gets polluted, either from surface water or from contamination of subsoil water. Their water is moderately hard.

2. *Deep wells* are those which tap some water-bearing layer below the first impermeable stratum. They may pass through one or more impermeable layers. They yield comparatively safer water for drinking purposes than shallow wells on account of efficient filtration, because (a) their water travels a greater distance through the earth, and (b) also gets better protection from surface contamination by the impermeable strata above. They yield as a rule, more permanent supplies than shallow wells, however, the water is often hard.

3. *Artesian wells* are a variety of deep wells in which water under great pressure comes out to the surface

automatically. To accomplish this, the strata, which the well penetrates, must be cup-shaped and the upper level of the groundwater tapped between the two impervious strata must be higher than the surface of the earth, where the well lies. Thus, in such a case, the water shoots up. They are named after Artois province in France where they have been in use for a very long time.

4. *Norton's abyssinian tube wells* are really shallow wells which are bored by simply driving iron pipes 1½" to 2" (3.8 to 5 cm) in diameter and 20–25 ft (6.096 to 7.62 metres) deep to tap the ground water. A pump is attached to the pipe to draw the water. Chiefly they were used to supply water in temporary settings like camps, famines, etc. Since water is drawn out by means of pumps, their water is free from most of the dangers manifested in open wells.

5. **Dug wells:** These are commonest types in India. These are of two types in rural India: (i) Unlined *kutcha* well which is a hole dug into the water-bearing stratum, (ii) the masonry or *pucca* well, which is built by bricks or stones.

6. **Step well:** It is a kind of *pucca* well, where steps were used to lead to a pool of water—the water of which was drawn from an adjacent well or through aquifers within the subterranean soil and rock. In these well, there is considerable contact between user and water. Guinea worm disease was quiet a public health problem in areas where step wells were in use.

Cone of filtration of a well: This is an area drained by a well and is regarded as an inverted cone, the apex of which is represented by the bottom of the well. The area drained is about four times the depth of well.

Dangers of shallow wells: Filth on the superficial permeable layer of earth is liable to percolate through, unless special measures are taken to prevent it. Also the cracks and fissures in the soil or nearby rat holes may allow impurities to have an access into the well (Fig. 1.2), if the direction of the flow of groundwater is from the filth towards the well. Therefore, to prevent

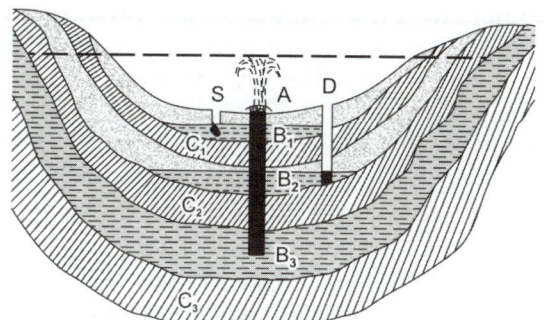

Fig. 1.1: Different varieties of wells. S—shallow well; D—deep well; A—artesian well; B₁, B₂, B₃—water bearing strata; C₁, C₂, C₃—impermeable strata

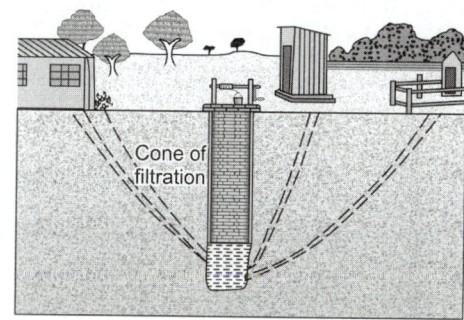

Fig. 1.2: How a well gets infected from surface pollution

contamination of shallow wells, the direction of flow of groundwater should be to and not from the possible sources of pollution and human habitations. Any possible source of contamination like latrines, manure heaps, collection of refuse and burial grounds or disposal of excreta should be prohibited within 200 ft (60.96 metres) of the well and at least 300 ft (91.44 metres) in case the ground is highly porous (Fig. 1.3).

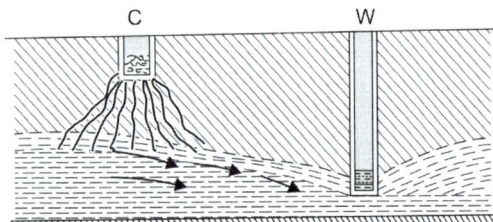

Fig. 1.3: Contamination of well from a cesspool as a result of excessive pumpings. C—Cesspool; W—well

A sanitary well is thus of particular relevance to microbiological quality of water. It is essential to prevent the direct contamination of groundwater at the point of abstraction or resulting from rapid recharge pathways close to the source.

Requirements of a sanitary well (Fig. 1.4)

1. It should be tapped in a good soil and should be at least 50 ft (15.24 metres) away from any possible source of contamination like a leaking cesspool, insanitary privy, etc. However, its distance from the houses of the users should also be kept in view.

2. The site should be sufficiently high to prevent entrance of water from outside into the well.

3. It should be a deep well, i.e. sunk below the first impermeable stratum.

4. It should be properly stained, i.e. built with bricks and lined with cement about 1 inch (2.54 cm) thick or a watertight casting of concrete or bricks set in cement or having a metal wall, reaching below the water level, below which the joints are open to admit the water to the well. The water should only come from the bottom and not through the surface.

5. Roots of trees should not be allowed to sprout from the linings of the wall.

6. The space between the well wall and the lining should be sealed by cement grouting.

7. It should be properly covered to prevent leaves and dust from blowing into it and also to prevent sparrows and pigeons making their nests in the crevices of the well wall.

8. Around the top of the well, a parapet wall, 3 ft (0.91 metre) high should be provided, so as to prevent the surface water entering the well. The top of this well should be sloping and not horizontal to discourage people sitting on it for

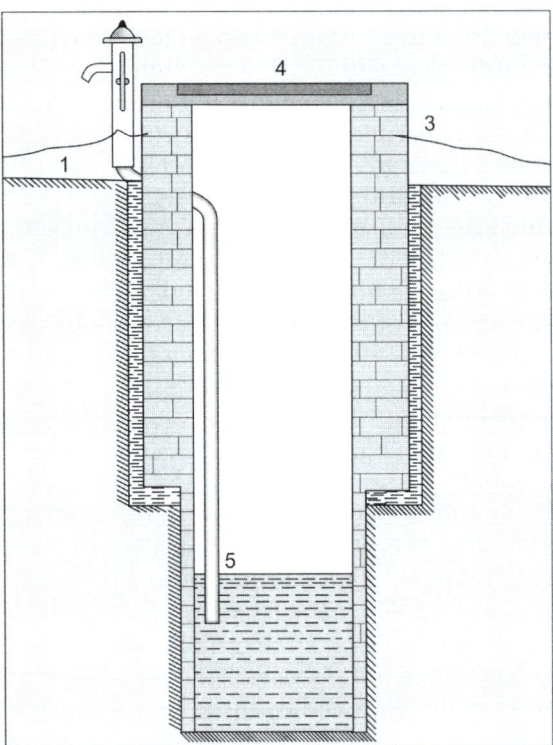

Fig. 1.4: A properly protected well. 1. Cemented brickwork, 2. puddled clay, 3. platform, 4. cover, 5. channelled drain

washing clothes thereupon and thus contaminating the well water.

9. There should be a cemented area at least 6 feet (1.83 metres) with a fall away from the well, so that the surface washings may run away from it and not into it.

10. No washing of clothes, utensils and bathing of persons should be allowed near a well. To ensure this, a proper washing and bathing place at a distance from the well can be made where water can be pumped by means of channels.

11. All hollows, rat burrows, foul tanks, cesspits, etc. near the well should be tilled up and useless trees and vegetation cut down.

12. It is best to have a handpump or any other mechanical contrivance for drawing up the water in a sanitary manner, which should be discharged by a pipe ending at some distance from the well, so that no water after any possible contamination can run back to the well. In the absence of any such provision, it is desirable that a bucket and a chain for public use should be attached to the well permanently.

The well needs periodic cleansing that is usually done at the close of hot weather, when the water becomes turbid, has odour or change in taste, has reduced output and water tests positive for total coliform and/or increased biological activity.

Process of cleansing of well: The wells need to be cleaned for bacteria and encrustations.

There are two basic approaches to well cleaning—mechanical and chemical, with the most effective strategy often being a combination of the two. Within both the chemical and mechanical methods are an array of options. Mechanical processes for loosening debris and/or encrustations and removing them from the well include the use of: (a) Pressurised air or water, (b) wire brushes or scrapers, (c) agitation of water in the well, and (d) sonic waves. Chemical cleaning often involves the use of various acids to loosen or dissolve debris so that it can be pumped out of the well. Depending on the nature of the cleaning job, there are also polymers and "caustic" chemicals (that increase the alkalinity of the water) to remove debris. For chemical cleaning, the well can be chlorinated by treating it with a solution of 1 part of freshly prepared slaked lime to 4 parts of water or bleaching powder or by potassium permanganate solution.

The age of a well may determine which methods are used to clean it. If a well's water intake areas or the well casing have corroded significantly over time, they may be damaged or destroyed by more aggressive cleaning practices.

Examination of wells: The following points should be borne in mind while examining a well:

1. Size and depth of the well.
2. Depth of water in the well.
3. Nature of soil in which the well is sunk.
4. Any possible sources of pollution within 200 to 350 ft (60.96 to 106.68 metres) of the well. Practical aspects are discussed subsequently.
5. Average quantity of water which is daily drawn out.
6. The way in which water is disposed off.
7. Mechanical contrivance with which water is drawn, e.g. pump, rope and bucket, etc.
8. Whether there are cracks and fissures on the sides or not.
9. Whether the mouth of the well is closed or open.

Detection of sources of pollution of a well: If a source of contamination is suspected in the neighbourhood of a well, it is detected by pouring certain chemicals which may be recognised on account of their characteristic smell, taste, colour and other chemical and physical properties into all the pools, drains, etc. which may be regarded as possible sources of pollution. The following methods of examination may be adopted:

1. By adding a strong solution of sodium chloride and detecting the increase in the amount of chlorides in well water by titrating with a standard solution of silver nitrate using potassium dichromate as an indicator.
2. By adding alkaline solution of fluorescein (1 lb or 0.453 kg of fluorescein and 1 lb or 0.453 kg of caustic soda) to 10 gallons (45.5 litres of water) and detecting the fluorescein in well water by means of a fluoroscope.
3. Suspension of *Bacillus prodigiosus* (*viz.* culture of *Chromobacterium prodigiosum*) may be added and subsequently red colonies grown and ultimately isolated from the water.
4. Kerosene oil may be poured and its smell and tinge detected in well water.

Yield of a well: The quantity of water in a well can be measured by the following formula:

Depth of water in feet × square of diameter of the well in feet × 5 = gallons of water.

Tube Wells

These yield water which is bacteriologically safe. These consist of lengths of iron tubing driven deep into ground up to the desired length. Firstly, a hole is made into the soil about 5–6 feet (1.52 to 1.83 metre) deep and first part of the tube having a perforated steel point at its lower end is hammered in. Subsequently, successive lengths of tubes are driven deep into the soil, one length being screwed into the other, till the sub-soil water is reached. In this case, water is drawn by means of a pump. Tube wells form a rapid means of obtaining groundwater and are comparatively more sanitary than dug wells.

Deep tube wells: These are largely used for municipal water supply and also for irrigation purposes. The average yield of a deep tube well of 1 to 1 ½" (2.5 to 3.8 cm) diameter is 200–300 gallons (909.20–1363.80 litres) and of 9" (22.86 cm) diameter is 60,000 gallons (272,760 litres) of water per hour. The yield mainly depends upon the water-bearing strata and a little on the diameter and depth on the tube well.

These are sunk through hard surfaces by boring through rocks with special machines. The depth is between 300–400 ft (91.44 to 121.92 metres) and the characteristics of water are like deep well waters. In many towns, the water supply is now obtained from these tube wells.

The water is hard due to presence of calcium carbonate and sodium chloride in variable quantity, traces of iron, etc., however, is free from bacteria. The greater the depth from which the water is obtained, the more likely is the higher percentage of its mineral contents. While operating, limitation of their working speed must be kept in view, as they silt up, if their rate of pumping exceeds the critical velocity.

Critical velocity: The water flows through the filtering medium of sand outside the strainer of a tube well, without disturbing the sand bed. But if the rate of pumping is rapid or excessive, the water carries sand grains with it and the velocity at which this disturbance starts is called *critical velocity.*

Cone of influence: With the drawing of water the level in the well falls, resulting in a tendency of the water flow into it from surrounding area. The area within which the level is appreciably lowered is called the *circle* or *cone of influence.*

Springs

These are natural outlets of groundwater which is under pressure, due to the approach of the first impermeable stratum of the surface. These can, therefore, be considered as natural wells at places where the geological conditions are favourable. The springs could be **Seepage** or filtration springs (small flow rates in which the source water has filtered into permeable earth), fracture springs (discharge from faults, joints, or fissures in the earth, in which springs have followed a natural course of voids or weaknesses in the bedrock) or tubular springs (underground cave systems formed by underground water).

Varieties of springs

1. *Surface springs or shallow or land springs:* These are outlets of limited collection groundwater resting on the superficial impervious strata. They are of intermittant nature, supplying water when the level of subsoil water is high, as during rains and ceasing to flow in summer season (May-June) and starting again in autumn on commencement of percolation. These are unsatisfactory source of water supply.

2. *Deep or main springs:* They derive their water supply from extensive water-bearing strata. The water of these springs is clear, sparkling and generally safe as it gets filtered while passage through the earth, and the flow is almost constant. The water is often hard. These springs have no surface outlets but issue through fissure or a crack in the soil.

   Ordinarily spring water is pure and less liable to contamination, since there is no mechanical means to draw out the water. It is generally cool and palatable, but is highly charged with carbonic acid gas, which it absorbs from the ground. Moreover, on account of passing under pressure, it dissolves out lime and various other mineral salts contained in the soil through which it passes. Consequently, gets hard and becomes unsuitable for washing and cooking purposes, although it may be valuable from the medicinal point of view.

3. *Hot or thermal springs:* These result from continuance of high internal temperature after a volcanic eruption has ceased. They continue to maintain their heat even for centuries. The springs may arise in places even hundreds of miles away from the actual volcanic event. Examples are Sitakoond (in Chittagong), Rajgir in Bihar, Vajreswari (50 miles, i.e. 80.47 kilometres from Mumbai) in India, springs of Bath and Buxton in England, and Yellowstone Park in USA.

4. *Mineral springs:* The water of mineral springs is highly charged with mineral salts and so used for medicinal or therapeutic purposes. There are also *sulphur springs* which contain sulphuretted hydrogen and various sulphides in solution. Water containing iron or magnesium in solution is known as *chalaybeate* or *magnesia water.*

Yield of a spring: It can be determined by:

1. Finding out the time, which it takes to fill a vessel of known capacity. The output of water in one hour can thus be determined.

2. By leading the entire flow of spring over a V or a rectangular notch and measuring the depth of flow over the side of notch. The yield of a spring can be calculated from charts and different formulae.

Safeguards against pollution of springs: The likely sources of pollution of springs are leaking cesspits, insanitary privies, latrines, stables, etc. Thus, the springs should be protected by a masonry structure, which should extend deep into the ground to protect against surface contamination.

e. Seawater

Distilled seawater is used for drinking purposes, on board ships and in places like Aden, where wells happen to be brackish and rain does not fall even for several years. However, distilled water is unpalatable and flat to taste as all gases are driven out of it by boiling. Thus, to improve its taste, the aeration of distilled water should be done by allowing it to trickle down through a long column of wood charcoal, if it is required for drinking purposes. Seawater acts on lead, copper, zinc and iron, thus none of these metals should be exposed to its action in the condensing apparatus. Silver and tin linings are the best choice for pipes and vessels used in distillation process.

1.3 CLASSIFICATION OF DIFFERENT TYPES OF WATER

These may be classified as follows:

1. *Safe water* in the sanitary sense is one which is free from contamination and is safe for human consumption even when ingested over prolonged periods. From the chemical point of view, absolutely pure water is not available in nature, as it always contains gaseous and solid matters in solution or in suspended form. Standards for safe drinking water are discussed later in the chapter.

2. *Polluted water* is that which has been deteriorated in quality on account of addition of substances, leading to a change in color, taste or odour, e.g. physical qualities of water.

3. *Contaminated water* is one which happens to contain human or animal wastes or other poisonous substances rendering it harmful or injurious to human system. It carries potential infection.

1.4 IMPURITIES OF WATER

These are:

1. *Dissolved impurities*: These may be either gases, like excess of carbonic acid, oxygen, sulphuretted hydrogen or salts as chlorides, calcium, magnesium sulphate, or metals like iron, lead, etc. and other organic matter from the soil.

2. *Suspended impurities*: These may be inorganic like sand, silt, mud and organic, which are derived from vegetable and animal matter, bacteria, ova of worms, etc.

Sources of Impurities

These are classified as follows:

1. *Substances received at the source*: The character of water will depend upon the geological structure through which it has travelled. Thus, chalk wells produce hard water on account of the presence of calcium and water from near the graveyards contains organic impurities. Water obtained from wells in towns or densely populated places often contains calcium, sodium, nitrites, nitrates, sulphates, phosphates, etc.

2. *Impurities derived during transit from source to the reservoir*: Rivers, canals, etc. are liable to be polluted by sewage, house waste water, manufacturing

refuse, etc. But at the same time natural purification also goes on, to some extent by oxidation, absorption of organic impurities by animals and vegetable life, action of ultraviolet rays of sun and settling of solid matter due to force of gravitation.

3. *Impurities during storage.*

4. *Impurities during distribution.*

Classification: Impurities of water may be inorganic or organic in origin. They may be in suspension or in solution form:

1. *Inorganic impurities in suspension*: These consist of more or less minute particles of sand, chalk, clay, silt or other insoluble minerals, which are mixed with water, the drinking of which leads to mechanical irritation of the intestines and may cause gut disturbances. Simple sedimentation in storage tanks may clear up the muddy water. To accelerate such sedimentation on a large scale, 4–6 grains (360 mg) of alum is added to a gallon (4.55 litres) of water. It forms a precipitate of aluminium hydrate, which is gelatinous and while sinking to the bottom carries down the suspended matter along with it.

2. *Inorganic impurities in solution*: These include salts causing hardness of water and other salts of metals such as lead, iron, zinc, etc.

Hardness of Water

It is defined as soap destroying power of water. It is attributed to the presence of carbonates, chlorides and sulphates of calcium and magnesium in the water.

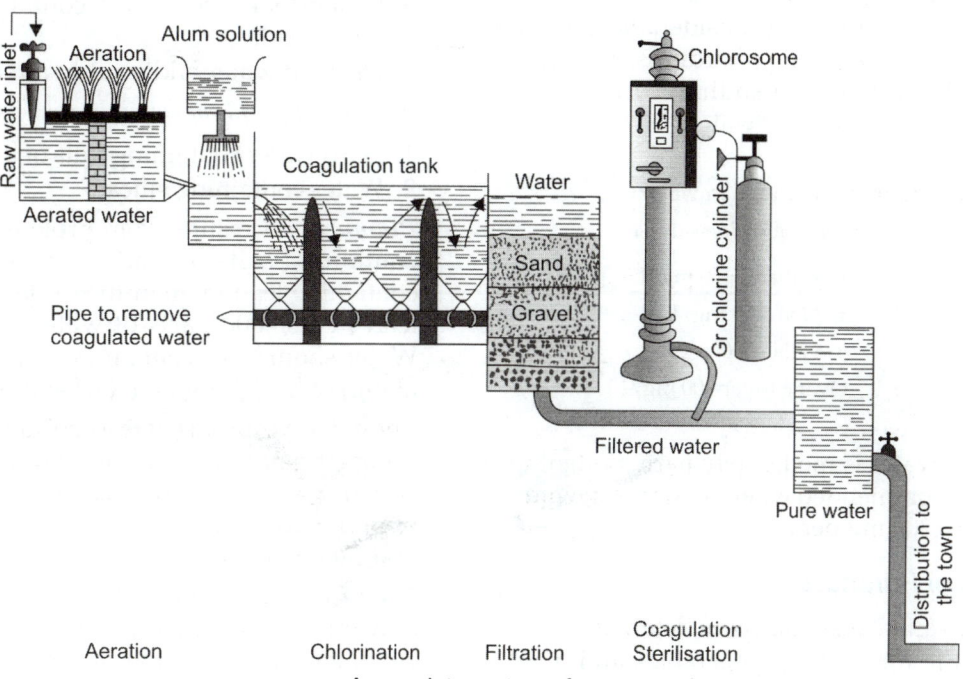

Fig. 1.5: A complete system of water supply

Types of Hardness

It is of two types—temporary and permanent.

Temporary hardness

This can be got rid of by removing coagulated water, aeration, chlorination and boiling the water. It is chiefly due to the presence of calcium carbonates (chalk) or magnesium carbonate in water held in solution by carbon dioxide.

They exist in solution as bicarbonates and as carbonates and are insoluble in water. On boiling, carbon dioxide escapes and insoluble carbonates separate out and sink to the bottom.

$$CaH_2(CO_3)_2 \xrightarrow{\text{on heating}} CaCO_3 + CO_2 + H_2O$$

$$MgH_2(CO_3)_2 \xrightarrow{\text{on heating}} MgCO_3 + CO_2 + H_2O$$

Permanent hardness

It persists even after boiling. It is due to the presence of chlorides and sulphates of calcium and magnesium. It is removed by the addition of lime and soda either in the form of hydrate or carbonate which converts some of the sulphate of calcium and magnesium into sodium sulphate, thus:

$$CaSO_4 + Na_2CO_3 = CaCO_3 + Na_2SO_4$$

The total hardness is estimated by finding the amount of standard soap solution which will neutralise the hardness and produce lather. The water is then boiled, when the temporary hardness is removed and again the amount of soap solution necessary is found.

The temporary hardness can be estimated, by subtracting the second figure from the first.

In the case of water containing considerable amount of permanent as well as temporary hardness, a mixture of both calcium hydroxide and sodium carbonate is often used to remove hardness of water.

Classification of hardness in water	
Classification	*Level of hardness (mEq/L)*
i. Soft water	Less than 1 (50 mg/L)
ii. Moderately hard water	1–3 (50–150 mg/L)
iii. Hard water	3–6 (150–300 mg/L)
iv. Very hard water	Over 6 (over 300 mg/L)

Good drinking water is moderately hard. Softening of water is only recommended when hardness in water exceeds 3 mEq/L (300 mg per litre).

Disadvantages of Hardness

1. It wastes soap and consumes more detergents.
2. It is unsuitable for cooking vegetables and meat and for making of tea, coffee, etc.
3. Temporary hardness in water causes a deposit of calcium carbonate on the inside of boilers and kettles forming a coat, which interferes with the smooth action of the boilers resulting in its loss of efficiency. In extreme cases, it can cause explosion resulting in serious accidents and deaths.
4. Excessive hard waters may cause dyspeptic symptoms leading to diarrhoea and other digestive disorders.
5. It shortens the life of pipes and fixtures in industrial concerns.

Advantages of a hard water supply are that calcium carbonate and magnesium carbonate will neutralise any acid present in it and hence will not dissolve lead or other metals as soft water may.

The soft water on the other hand is good for domestic purposes of cooking, drinking, washing, etc. Besides, it is good for commercial purposes for use in the boilers and laundries, provided no lead pipes or vessels are used. However, use of soft water for drinking purposes has shown to be associated with heart disease due to presence of low sodium in it.

1.5 METALS IN SOLUTION (Table 1.1)

a. **Lead** is most important metal pollutant in water. The following kinds of water act on lead:
   1. Soft water by virtue of its dissolved oxygen forms oxyhydrate of lead, which is dissolved more rapidly by acidulated water. Peaty waters are acidic in character thus have higher plumbo-solvency and so dissolve lead from lead pipes.
   2. Water containing nitrates or nitrites in solution or an excess of carbon dioxide.
   3. Upland surface waters containing humic and ulmic acid.
   4. Distilled water and muddy river water.

   The following kinds of water do not act on lead

   1. Hard water containing salts of lime or magnesia.
   2. Water containing silica.

   Plumbism: It results from prolonged use of water containing salts of lead. Consumption of water containing lead in quantities as less as 0.09 parts of lead in 1,00,000 parts of water has proved fatal. Water should not contain more than 1/20th grain (3 mg) of lead per gallon (4.546 litres).

   The chief symptoms of lead poisoning produced by taking repeated doses of lead are anemia, constipation, colic, wristdrop, and other manifestations of peripheral neuritis as depression, renal disease and finally death.

b. **Iron:** Contained in the strata of earth may find its way into the water supply. It may be derived from rusting of inner coating of pipes when iron pipes are used. It gives rise to gastritis, dyspepsia and

Table 1.1: Substances and parameters in drinking water that may give rise to complaints from consumers

Constituents or characteristics	Levels likely to give rise to consumer complaints	Reasons for consumer complaints
Physical parameters		
Colour	15 TCU	Appearance
Taste and odour:	Should be acceptable	
Temperature	–	Should be acceptable
Turbidity	1 NTU	Appearance; for effective terminal disinfection, median turbidity ≤1 NTU
Inorganic constituents		
Aluminium	0.2 mg/L	Depositions, discolouration
Ammonia	1.5 mg/L	Odour and taste
Chloride	250 mg/L	Taste, corrosion
Copper	1 mg/L	Staining of laundry and sanitary water (health based provisional guideline value 2 mg/L)
Hardness	–	High hardness: Scale deposition, scum formation; low hardness; possible corrosion
Hydrogen sulfide	0.05 mg/L	Odour and taste
Iron	0.3 mg/L	Staining of laundry and sanitary were
Manganese	0.1 mg/L	Staining of laundry and sanitary ware (health-based provisional guideline value 0.4 mg/L)
Dissolved oxygen	–	Indirect effects
pH	–	Low pH: Corrosion; high pH: Taste, soapy feel preferably <8.0 for effective disinfection with chlorine
Sodium	200 mg/L	Taste
Sulphate	250 mg/L	Taste, corrosion
Total dissolved solids	1000 mg/L	Taste
Zinc	4 mg/L	Appearance taste

constipation. The presence of not more than 0.01 part of iron per 100,000 part of water is allowed in drinking water.

c. *Zinc*: May be found in water in small quantities. It gives rise to obstinate constipation. Such water should be condemned. Zinc, however, is rarely present in water in a proportion considered to be dangerous.

d. *Fluorine*: If present in water in concentration of 1.0 to 1.5 mg per litre per day may cause dental fluorosis, whereas high concentration of flourine in water ranging from 50 to 100 mg per litre may give rise to symptoms of skeletal damage and dental fluorosis in children and adults over prolonged period of consumption. However, complete absence of flourine in drinking water has also been found to be associated with dental caries.

e. *Organic impurities* are derived from animal and vegetable kingdom. These are important from the health point of view because they include the impurities derived from contamination of water by excreta and urine which may contain disease germs capable of living and multiplying in water and communicating diseases to the people, who happen to use that water. These are called water-borne diseases, e.g. cholera, dysentery, enteric fever, including typhoid, paratyphoid A and B and epidemic diarrhoea.

Entozoal diseases due to *Distoma hepaticum, Ascaris lumbricoides*, etc. may be contracted by drinking water containing eggs, larvae, etc. of these parasites. Bilharziasis and guinea worm infection occurs due to drinking of infected water.

McCarrison's view is that goitre is due to the presence of micro-organisms in water, which produce toxin in the intestines of a man, that acts on the thyroid glands and enlarges them. But others consider it due to lack of iodine in water or food. It has, therefore, become a common practice nowadays to incorporate minute quantities of iodine in common salt or in the water supply of such an area.

WHO recommend different levels of metals in drinking water (Table 1.2).

1.6 PURIFICATION OF WATER

Purification of water has two steps, filtration and disinfection. Both steps are necessary to remove or kill all bacteria, viruses, and parasites and make the water safe to drink. As filtration only removes soil particles and plant material that can interfere with disinfection,

Table 1.2: Drinking water standards

Sl. no.	Parameters	Prescribed by			
		BIS IS 10500–91		ICMR	
		Desirable limit	Max. permissible limits in the absence of alternate source	Desirable limit	Max. permissible limits
1.	pH	6.5 to 8.5	No relaxation	7.0–8.5	6.5–9.2
2.	Total dissolved solids mg/L	500	2000	500	1500–3000
3.	Total hardness as $CaCO_3$ mg/L	300	600	300	600
4.	Calcium as Ca mg/L	75	200	75	200
5.	Magnesium as Mg mg/L	30	100	50	–
6.	Chloride as Cl mg/L	250	1000	200	1000
7.	Sulphte as SO_2 mg/L	200	400	200	400
8.	Nitrate as NO_2 mg/L	45	100	20	100
9.	Iron as Fe mg/L	0.3	1	0.1	1
10.	Fluoride as F mg/L	1	1.5	1	1.5
11.	Arsenic as As mg/L	0.05	0.05	–	0.05
12.	Manganese as Mn mg/L	0.1	0.3	0.1	0.5
13.	Zinc as Zn mg/L	5	15	0.1	5
14.	Copper as Cu mg/L	0.05	1.5	0.05	1.5
15.	Chromium as Cr mg/L	0.05	0.05	–	–
16.	Lead as Pb mg/L	0.05	0.05	–	0.5
17.	Mercury as Hg mg/L	0.001	0.001	–	0.001
18.	Cadmium as Cd mg/L	0.01	0.01	–	0.01
19.	Cyanide as Cn mg/L	0.05	0.05	–	0.05
20.	Minerals oil mg/L	0.01	0.03	–	
21.	Phenolic compounds mg/L	0.001	0.002	–	
22.	Total coliform MPN/100 ml	1	10	–	–
23.	Residual free chlorine mg/L	0.2	–	–	–
24.	Aluminum as Al mg/L	0.03	0.2		
25.	Boron as B mg/L	1	5		
26.	Selenium as Se mg/L	0.01	–		
27.	Pesticides	Absent 0.001			

Source: http://indiawater portal. org

disinfection is needed to remove bacteria and viruses that can pass through filters. Either or a combination of the following methods may be used for purification of water at small scale/household level or at large scale.

a. Natural
   • Pounding or storage.
   • Oxidation and settlement.
b. Artificial
   i. Physical
      • Distillation.
      • Boiling.
   ii. Chemical
      • Precipitation.
      • Disinfection or sterilisation.
   iii. Filtration

• "Biological" or "slow sand" filtration.
• "Rapid sand" or "mechanical" filtration.
• Domestic filtration.

1.7 DOMESTIC PURIFICATION OF WATER

It is the treatment that happens at the point of water collection or use, rather than at a large, centralised location. It improves water quality and reduces diarrhoeal disease in developing countries. Available treatment options are boiling, chlorination, flocculent/disinfectant powder, solar disinfection, ceramic filtration, and slow sand filtration. Besides purification of water, the emphasis should be on safe storage of treated water and behaviour change communication (BCC) to improve water and food handling, sanitation and hygiene practices at home and in the community.

In those places where water works cannot be constructed, water may be purified on a small scale by the following methods.

a. Distillation

This method is used in chemical laboratories and on board in the ships. Such distilled water being flat and insipid owing to loss of dissolved gases, requires to be aerated before use. It also acts readily on metals such as zinc, copper, lead, etc.

b. Boiling

It removes solid matter such as chalk, obnoxious gases, organic matter and kills all bacteria, cysts, ova and spores. Boiling involves a large expenditure on fuel. Boiled water is flat and tasteless. It should be aerated before use. It is adopted as a precautionary measure during presence of an epidemic of water-borne diseases. Boiling makes temporary hard water soft by the precipitation of calcium salts. It helps in removal of ammonia and sulphuretted hydrogen gases, which renders the water suitable for cooking and washing purposes.

c. Filtration

- *Straining through a muslin cloth:* It cannot prevent passage of bacteria, foul gases and finely divided solid particles. Besides, the cloth itself may serve as a source of potential infection.

- *Other filtering materials* used are charcoal, sand, silicated carbon, porous iron, etc. Charcoal is largely used as a filtering medium. It is, however, not the ideal material, as it absorbs impurities from water or air and becomes a source of infection, if not often cleaned with boiling water.

- *Filtration of water by three pitchers' system:* Three pitchers are placed one above the other on a wooden stand. The top pitcher containing sand, is filled with water which percolates through a hole made at its bottom, along with a piece of cloth or cotton plugged into the hole, into the second pitcher which contains a mixture of sand and vegetable charcoal. Water passing through the layers of sand and charcoal percolates through a hole at its bottom into the third, viz. the lowest pitcher. This last pitcher now contains filtered water. This system of filtration is not recommended as it is very difficult to look after the cleanliness of the contents of these pitchers during the process.

- *Domestic filters:* These are made of porcelain, clay and infusorial earth and moulded into bougies or candles. They keep back all germs. The essential features of a good filter are:

  i. It should be strong, compact and simple; all parts being easily accessible for cleansing.

  ii. It should be efficient to keep back all germs.

  iii. It should be cheap and its purifying power fairly lasting.

  iv. The filtering medium should not require frequent changing.

  v. It should not impart anything injurious to water.

- *Diatomite filters:* These are generally used in industrial concerns, but sometimes they may be used in mobile installations also.

The main types of these filters are

i. *Pasteur Chamberland filter* (Fig. 1.6): It consists of a cylindrical vessel fitted with an unglazed porous porcelain candle. The water gets filtered through the pores of the filter candle and is collected into a separate reservoir. The filter candle should be cleaned by brushing with hot water and then sterilised with boiling water. Muddy water should be first cleared, by passing it through closely packed coarse sand filter.

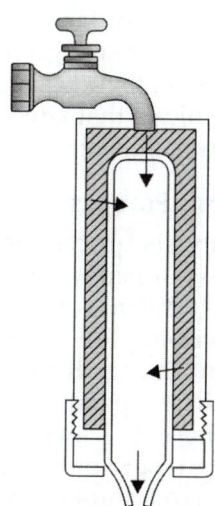

Fig. 1.6: Pasteur Chamberland filter

This filter holds back all kinds of bacteria and suspended impurities present in water but does not affect the chemical composition of the constituents dissolved in water. Its action is merely mechanical.

ii. *The Berkefeld filter* (Fig. 1.7): In this type of filter, the candle is made of infusorial earth known as *kieselguhr*. However, on long-term use and constant cleaning, the candle wears thin and gradually ceases to filter efficiently. It is more rapid in action and does not require an additional pressure. Candle should be cleaned by scrubbing with a brush under running water and boiled at least once a week.

iii. *Combined filters (Aqua Guards/reverse osmosis filters)*

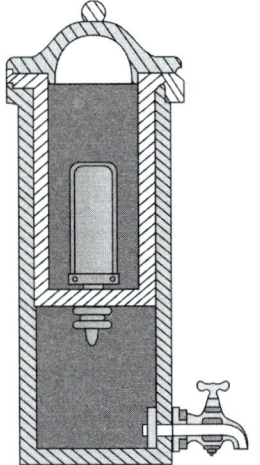

Fig. 1.7: Berkefeld filter

Reverse Osmosis

The reverse osmosis water treatment method has been used extensively to covert brackish or seawater to drinking water, to clean up waste water, and to recover dissolved salts from industrial processes. It is becoming more popular in the home-market as homeowners are increasingly concerned about contaminants that affect their health, as well as about non hazardous chemicals that affect the taste, odour, or colour of their drinking water.

The Reverse Osmosis Process

IN the reverse osmosis process as cellophane-like membrane separates purified water from contaminated water. An understanding of osmosis is needed before further describing RO. Osmosis occurs when two solutions containing different quantities of dissolved chemicals are separated by a semipermeable membrane (allowing only some compounds to pass through). Osmotic pressure of the dissolved chemical causes pure water to pass through the membrane from the dilute to the more concentrated solution (Fig. 1.8). There is a natural tendency for chemicals to reach equal concentrations on both sides of the membrane.

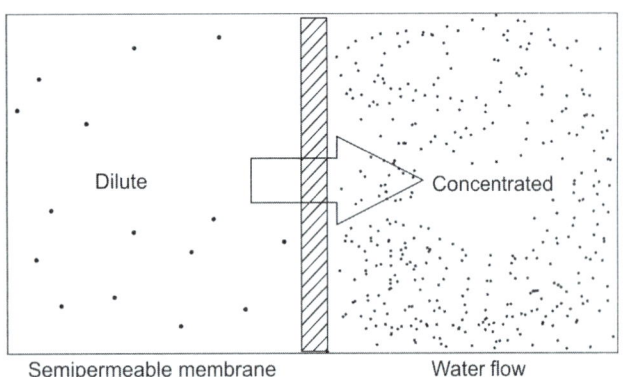

Fig. 1.8: In osmosis, water across the membrane from the dilute to the concentrated solution

In reverse osmosis, water pressure applied to the concentrated side forces the process of osmosis into reverse. Under enough pressure, pure water is "squeezed" through the membrane from the concentrated to the dilute side (Fig. 1.9). Salts dissolved in water as charged ions are repelled by the RO membrane. Treated water is collected in a storage container. The rejected impurities on the concentrated side of the membrane are washed away in a stream of wastewater, not accumulated as on a traditional filter.

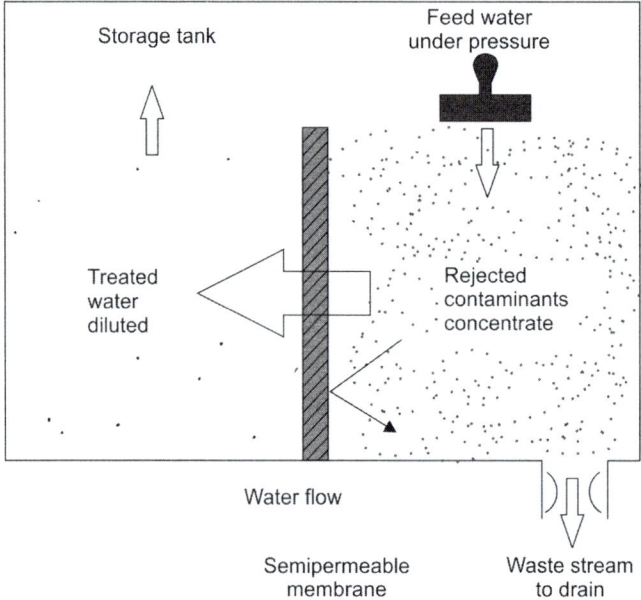

Fig. 1.9: The reverse osmosis, pressure is applied to the concentrated solution reverting the natural direction of flow, forcing water across membrane from the concentrated solutions into the more dilute solution

The RO membrane also functions as an ultra-filtration device, screening out particles, including micro-organisms that are physically too large to pass through the membrane's pores. RO membranes can remove compounds in the 0.0001 to 0.1 micron size range (thousands of times smaller than a human hair).

Figure 1.10 shows the diagrammatic form and the various elements of a typical multistage reverse osmosis process.

d. *Chemicals*: Following chemicals are used for purifying water:

- *Flocculent (alum)*: It is largely used to purify muddy water. Only 1–4 grains (60–240 mg) are sufficient to add to each gallon (4.56 litres) of water. Alum when added to water containing calcium carbonate, which is present in all kinds of water is decomposed and insoluble salts of calcium sulphate and aluminium hydrate are precipitated carrying with them suspended impurities and bacteria thus leaving the water purified and clear.

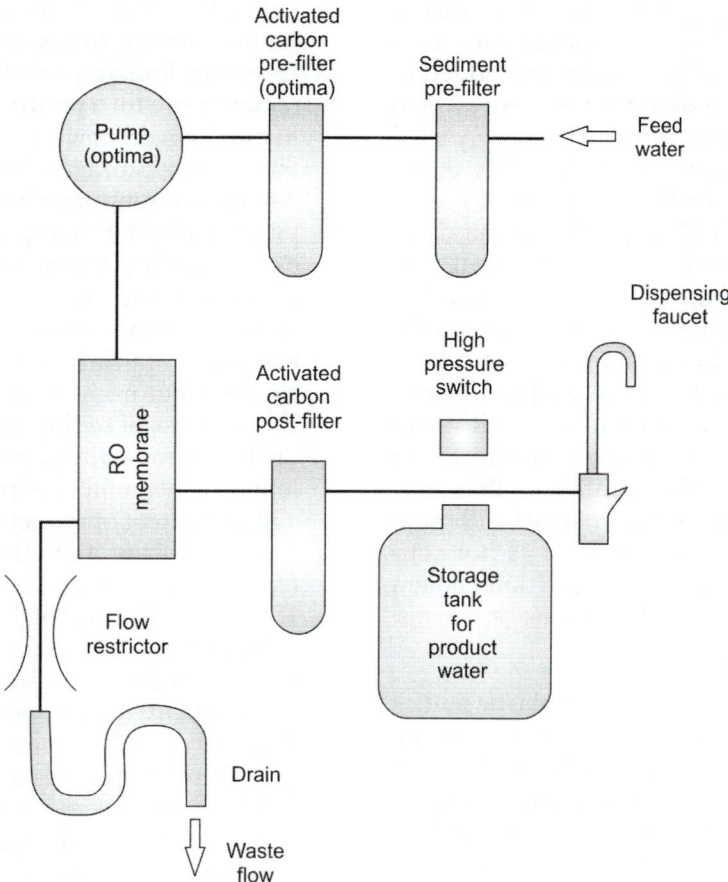

Fig. 1.10: Schematic of a typical RO system

- *Copper sulphate:* It is not a germicide in the true sense, but when used in the proportion of 0.1 to 0.25 parts to 1,000,000 parts of water prevents the vegetative growth including algae that gives rise to odours and unpleasant taste in water. It has, however, no effect on organisms of water-borne diseases, e.g. cholera, typhoid, dysentery, etc. Copper chloride is considered more efficacious to stem them.

- *Calcium oxide (quicklime):* Some people prefer dry slaked lime to ordinary lime. The quantity of slaked lime for sterilising water is proportionately reduced if the period of its contact with water is prolonged. 6 grains (360 mg) of slaked lime will sterilise a gallon (4.546 litres) of soft water. Quick-lime is cheap, easily procurable and is highly recommended for disinfecting the water of a well or a tank at the time of an outbreak of cholera in villages. It hastens the process of precipitation of iron in water. Its disadvantage is that comparatively heavier doses are required for efficient disinfection of water. Its dose is about 20 times to that of bleaching powder.

- *Chlorine:* When added to water in the strength of 1 in 2 million parts, chlorine gas is said to kill disease producing germs. It is a very cheap and convenient method. Instead of chlorine gas, bleaching powder or hypochlorite of lime may be used in proportion of 30 grains (1.8 gm) to 100 gallons (454.60 litres). Chlorination inactivates most bacteria and viruses that cause diarrhoea, however, it may not be effective against protozoa like Cryptosporidium.

- *Bromine:* 0.06 grains (3.6 mg) of bromide when dissolved in potassium bromide and added to a litre of water kills bacteria in five minutes. The offensive smell of bromine may be removed by further treatment of water with sodium sulphate and sodium carbonate solution.

- *Iodine* is used in doses of 2 parts per million to destroy micro-organisms present in water in emergency cases. Sodium hyposulphite should be added after 15 minutes to neutralise the free iodine of sodium which renders water fit for drinking.

- *Nesfield tablets:* A 2 grains (120 mg) tablet of iodine and iodate of sodium and the same quantity of citric acid when added to 4 gallons (18.18 litres) of water will kill cholera and typhoid germs in a few minutes. The free iodine present in water may be removed by the addition of sodium hyposulphite.

- *Potassium permanganate*: It is a strong oxidising agent thus oxidises organic matter and also serves as a deodorant. 0.5 part of this salt added to 100,000 parts of water is sufficient to destroy 98% of micro-organisms in 4 to 6 hours. It is largely used for disinfection of wells. 4–6 oz (113.40–170.10 gm) of it used for a well, so that water will give a proportion of 1/2 oz (14.17 gm) of the chemical per 1000 gallons (4546 litres) of water in the well. It is better to treat water of the well with the chemical in the evening so that it may be ready for use on the following morning, when it should have a faint pink tinge, if the dose has been added in right proportion. If smell reappears in the well water after 2 or 3 days, potassium permanganate treatment should be repeated. Its disadvantage is that taste and odour of the water treated changes, although temporarily. Moreover, the method is not considered very dependable, since it may kill cholera vibrios, but it does not destroy other disease organisms.

Solar Disinfection (SODIS)

This can be done by filling 0.3–2 litres of plastic bottles with low turbidity water, shake them to oxygenate and place the bottles on the roof in a rack for 6 hours, if sunny or 2 days, if cloudy. The process inactivated the disease causing organism by combined effects of UV-induced DNA alteration, thermal inactivation and photo-oxidative destruction. Over 2 million people in 28 developing countries use this method for purification of drinking water.

Slow Sand Filters

Filtration of Water Supply on a Large Scale

Filtration cleans the water by removing suspended matters, ova, cysts, spores and bacteria by the use of filters, which are of the following two types (Table 1.3):
1. "Biological" or "slow sand" filters (Fig. 1.11).
2. "Rapid sand" or "mechanical" filters.

1. *Biological or slow sand filters*: This system was first introduced in England about more than a century back and it is, therefore, often termed as "English System".

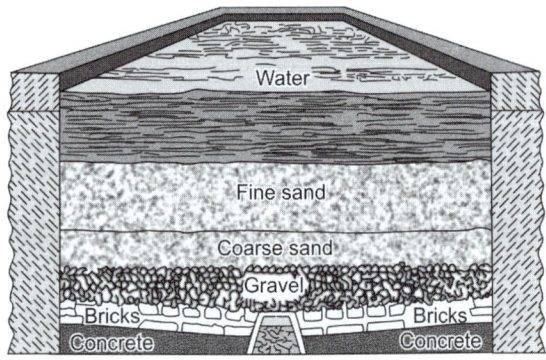

Fig. 1.11: Section of a slow sand filter

The raw water from the source, usually a river, canal or stream is collected and stored in large open reservoirs known as *settling tanks* and is allowed to remain there for a period of 24 to 48 hours. The solid matter present in water as suspension gravitates to the bottom. Storage of water for a period of about 3–4 weeks renders the water supply pretty safe prior to filtration. The process of sedimentation can be hastened by adding a flocculent/coagulant such as alum or sulphate of ammonia, which is specially done in rainy season, when the water becomes turbid, in specially constructed circular mixing troughs, before its entrance to the settling tanks. This process of sedimentation has a great influence on bacterial counts and life thus significantly reducing their numbers, may be as much by 90% with a higher extent of reduction of *coliform bacteria*.

The water is now allowed to circulate slowly from a higher level and then to gravitate from above into the filter beds downwards.

Filter beds are watertight rectangular masonry tanks or reservoirs usually arranged side by side and ordinarily kept open. These are usually about 9–12 feet (2.74–3.96 metres) deep. They are filled up from bottom upwards as follows:
a. There are two layers of bricks placed one above the other on their edges which are arranged in the form of drains and channels for the passage of filtered water. Over the bricks, layers of the following materials are arranged systematically one after the other.
b. 6" (15.24 cm) to 12" (30.48 cm) gravel, broken stones or pebbles (size 1" or 3.81 cm) cubes.
c. Coarse sand 6"–12" (15.24–30.48 cm).
d. Fine sand 36" (91.44 cm).
e. Water from settling tanks 36" (91.44 cm).

Thickness of these materials varies at different places, but an important thing is that the thickness of sand layer is never less than one foot (0.3 metre). To ensure uniform filtration, these filter beds are provided with valves at outlets and inlets. The size of filter depends upon:
a. The size of the community to be supplied with water.
b. The quantity of water to be supplied per head.

The action of slow sand filter is three-fold:
a. *Mechanical obstruction or physical*: The suspended impurities are strained off by upper portion of the filter.
b. *Chemical*: The organic matter in water is oxidised by the presence of air and nitrifying micro-organism in the sand.
c. *Biological action is carried on in the vital layer*: After the filter bed has been working for 2–3 days, a thin green slimy gelatinous layer of low vegetable organisms, thread-like algae and fungi, etc. called *Schmutzdecke vital layer* forms on the surface of the

Table 1.3: Comparative study of slow sand and rapid sand mechanical filtration

Slow sand filter	Rapid sand mechanical filter
1. It is an old and English method. Filtration is slow	1. It is recent and an American method. Filtration is rapid. It is usually 40–50 times more than that of a slow sand filter
2. A large piece of land is required and, therefore, employed only at places where plenty of land is available	2. Very little space is required and, therefore, especially adopted at places, where the cost of land is high
3. Initial cost is high for installation; but running expenses are less	3. Intitial cost is less but running expenses are more
4. Suitable for clear or slightly turbid waters	4. Suitable for turbid waters
5. Provision for settling tanks is a necessity	5. Provision for settling tanks is not a necessity
6. No coagulant is required	6. Coagulant such as aluminium sulphate is required
7. Depreciation of plant is less	7. Depreciation of plant is high
8. The action in the filter is physical, chemical and biological	8. Working process is mainly mechanical
9. Delivery rate is slow, i.e. 2½ to 4 million gallons (11.36 to 18.18 million litres) per acre (0.405 hectare) per day	9. Delivery rate is rapid, i.e. 100–200 million gallons (454.60–909.20 million litres) per acre (0.405 hectare) per hour
10. Cleaned by scraping of superficial layer of sand, washing and replacing it after drying. The renewal and resetting of filter is required after 3 years	10. Cleaned very quickly by mechanical agitation of sand bed by compressed air and filtered water. No renewal or resetting is required
11. There is a danger of contamination from labourers	11. There is no such danger
12. Algae growth hampers the action	12. Algae do not grow
13. Results are good and uniform so chlorination of water is not a necessity	13. Results are not so good and uniform so there is the necessity of sterilising water with chlorine

superficial layer of sand. The formation of this vital layer is known as *ripening* of the filter. It generally takes several days for the vital layer for its complete formation and at this stage it extends for 2–3 cm into top portion of sand bed. This layer retains all the bacteria of water so it should not be disturbed. Denser the film becomes in course of time, slower becomes the rate of filtration and consequently greater becomes the pressure head necessary to ensure delivery of the requisite amount of water. In fact, this vital layer is the "heart" of slow sand filter and until this layer is fully formed, the filtrate from first a few days of operation of the filter is usually allowed to go waste.

Water should be tested for bacteriological examination by drawing out a sample of water every week to see that the filters are working efficiently, i.e. arresting the passage of bacteria efficiently. An adequately filtered water should not contain more than 1–2 coliform bacilli per 100 ml of water.

2. Rapid sand or mechanical filters: These are less expensive, simple, easy to operate and require less space. These are small and thus can be fixed inside a covered shed. They consist of large wooden, iron or concrete cylinders about 7 feet (2.13 metres) deep containing a filtering medium consisting of quartz or sand, 4 to 5 feet (1.22 to 1.52 metres) in thickness, supported on broken pieces of stones or pebbles.

These are capable of filtering water at a very high rate, i.e. 100–130 gallons (454.60 to 590.98 litres) per sq foot (0.092 sq metre) per 24-hour or 150 inches (3.81 metre) or more per hour.

There are many varieties of rapid mechanical filters. These may be either of pressure type, e.g. Candy's filter or gravity type, e.g. Paterson's filter. In pressure filters, the chamber is closed and the coagulated water is driven through sand under its own head of pressure. Whereas in gravity filters, the water is passed through a coagulating basin to open filter through which it gravitates.

In this process of rapid filtration, following steps are involved:
a. Coagulation and formation of *floc*.
b. Filtration.

In this system, the place of vital layer of the slow sand filter is taken by a filtering layer artificially made by producing a flocculent precipitate, which with colloidal silt settles on surface of the sand and fills up the sand interspaces.

The raw water is pumped into settling tanks, where heavier material of silt is deposited and certain amount of natural purification takes place.

There are 4 distinct processes involved in the gravity (Paterson) system of rapid filtration, which are as follows:

a. **Coagulation:** The water from settling tanks is led continuously into the plant, after passing through the measuring gear. Then a chemical coagulant, usually aluminium sulphate in proportion of 1–4 gr (60 to 240 mg) to a gallon (4.546 litres) is added. It flows down the trough, where it gets thoroughly mixed up with the chemical by means of baffle plates and reacts with the calcium bicarbonates. There is a flocculent white gelatinous precipitate of aluminium hydrate is formed.

$$Al_2(SO_4)_3 + 3Ca(HCO_3)_2 =$$
$$Al_2(OH)_6 + 3CaSO_4 + 6CO_2$$

b. **Sedimentation:** Water enters into another tank where most of the suspended and colloidal matters are precipitated. As the flocculent precipitate settles down, it carries with it other suspended matters and bacteria which may be present in water. It also affects decoloration. Here water is allowed to remain for 3–6 hours, which varies depending more or less upon the prevailing season and the quality of water required.

c. **Filtration:** Water is then admitted into a series of rapid filters. The coagulant in the water helps to form a gelatinous layer on the surface of sand through which water is forced.

d. **Chlorination:** From the filters, it passes through an automatic regulating gear into a chlorinating chamber, where chlorine gas is added and water is sterilised. Besides its germicidal effect, chlorine oxidises iron, manganese and hydrogen sulphide. Moreover, it controls algae formation and helps in coagulation also.

Cleansing of the Filters

Owing to high rate of filtration, the filtering medium becomes loaded with micro-salt, organic matter and bacteria, which interfere with the efficiency of filters. So these filters require frequent cleansing where the frequency varies according to the quality of water and season of the year. Cleansing of the filter is done by shutting the inlet valve and passing a reverse current of filtered water from the clean reservoir through the bottom of sand bed and simultaneously stirring up the sand by means of rotatory metal arms, rakes or a blast of compressed air. The wash water flows away to the waste over the top. A thorough cleansing of filter takes places within 15–20 minutes and a satisfactory film is formed in another 20 minutes and filter becomes ready for service again.

The bacterial purification, however, is not so constant and uniformly high as that of the slow sand filter.

Filtration head: The rate of filtration through a slow sand filter is controlled in such a way that the flow is maintained at a steady rate of 4 vertical inches (0.1 metre) per hour. The filtered water from the filter bed is led into a filter well and if the water in the well is allowed to run out, it is found out that half an inch (1.27 cm) of the lower level of water in the well causes sufficient flow of water at the desired rate through the filter. This half an inch (1.27 cm) difference in the level is known as *filtration head* or *working head.*

Loss of head: It is the frictional resistance offered to the passage of water through the filter beds by the vital layer formed on its surface and its interstices, so that

after sometime half an inch (1.27 cm) difference of the working head becomes insufficient to draw water at the standard rate through the sand. The remedy is to increase the working or filtration head by lowering the still until even a difference of about 18″ (45.72 cm) to 24″ (60.96 cm) is reached.

1.8 DISINFECTION OF WATER ON A LARGE SCALE

This is effected on a large scale by the following methods:

Chlorination

It is most efficient, cheap, reliable and easily available method. It destroys pathogenic micro-organisms but does not remove its turbidity. So the raw water is first filtered and then chlorinated. Chlorine is used in the following forms for the sterilisation of water.

a. Bleaching Powder or Chlorinated Lime (CaOCl₂)

It is prepared on a large scale by passing chlorine gas over slaked lime. It is, therefore, also known as chlorinated lime.

$$Ca(OH)_2 + Cl_2 = CaOCl_2 + H_2O$$

It is of the consistency of white amorphous powder of brittle lumps having a faint odour of chlorine and disagreeable saline taste. When fresh, it contains 33% of available chlorine but deteriorates soon, if it is not protected from air. Roughly speaking 2.5 gm of good quality bleaching powder would be required to disinfect 1000 litres of water. It may be added that chlorinated lime will not clarify turbid water. Polluted water should, therefore, first be treated with preliminary filtration and then subjected to chlorination.

A filtered water supply requires not more than 0.25 part of chlorine per million parts of water which is equal to 8 lb (3.63 kg) of bleaching powder. But a higher strength/concentration is required for water containing iron or peaty matter having high oxygen absorbing capacity.

The exact nature in which bleaching powder acts on water is complex. Its germicidal effect is due to the following factors:

1. Some of the hypochlorides in the presence of carbon dioxide and water evolve nascent oxygen chemically; the reaction may be expressed as:
$$Ca(ClO)_2 + CO_2 + H_2O = CaCO_3 + 2HClO$$
$$2HClO = 2HCl + O_2$$

2. Free chlorine is liberated which acts as a germicide.

3. When hypochlorites come into direct contact with ammonia or amino acids of the organic matter, *chloramine* (NHCl) is formed, which is a less powerful germicidal agent than chlorine, but prevents change of taste, odour, etc. which chlorination may give rise to.

When bleaching powder is used for purification of water on a large scale, the requisite quantity of powder is dissolved and mixed with water in a mixing tank. The mixture is allowed to flow into a storage tank, from where it is taken to the main water supply.

In India, bleaching powder is largely used as an effective method for sterilising wells, tanks, canals or rivers especially when cholera is raging in the rural areas.

Phases of Chlorination (Fig. 1.12)

Phase I: Formation of chloramines

Phase II: Destruction of chloramines

Phase III: Appearance of break-point

Phase IV: Accumulation of free residual chlorine.

In the case of a well: Calculate the amount of water available in gallons (1 gallon being equal to 4.546 litres) by the formula:

$D^2 \times W \times 5$ = *Number of gallons of water in a well*

D = Diameter of well in feet.

W = Depth of water in feet.

Roughly speaking 2.5 gm of fresh bleaching powder would be required to disinfect 1000 litres of well water. This will give a dose of about 0.7 mg of applied chlorine to per litre of water.

However, Horrock's apparatus can be used to calculate exact requirement of bleaching powder. The required quantity of bleaching powder is dissolved in a bucket of water and the solution poured in the well; the water is then agitated thoroughly.

As already mentioned, the most effective method of disinfecting wells is by bleaching powder. The use of other chemicals for disinfection of wells should, therefore, be discouraged.

For disinfection of well water, volume of water in a well can also be worked out as under:

a. Depth of the water column is measured ....(h) metres
b. Diameter of the well is measured ..... (d) metres.

Average of several readings of the above measurement is taken.

c. *h* and *d* are substituted in the following equation:

$$\text{Volume (litres)} = \frac{3.14 \times d^2 \times h \times 1000}{4}$$

(One cubic metre = 1000 litres of water)

In the case of a tank: A cubic foot (196.65 cu cm) of water contains 6 gallons (27.27 litres). Calculate the amount of water in the tank in gallons (1 gallon being equal to 4.546 litres) by the following formula:

Length × breadth × depth × 6.25 = gallons of water.

In the case of a big tank: Two ounces (56.70 gm) of bleaching powder is required for sterilising 10 running feet (3.048 running metres) of water. Supposing there is a square tank with each of its sides 120 ft (36.58 metres) long.

The total length of the sides will be 120 × 4 = 480 running feet (146.30 running metres).

So, it will require $\frac{480 \times 2}{10 \times 16}$ = 6 lb (2.72 kg) of bleaching powder.

In the case of a running stream: 66 lb (29.94 kg) of bleaching powder is required per mile (1.6 km) of stream water. The requisite quantity of bleaching powder is taken in a sack and is allowed to dissolve in the stream water at a higher point.

b. Electrolytic Hypochlorites

These are formed by electrolysis of water containing definite proportion of sodium and magnesium salts. Electrolytic chlorogen is recommended for sterilisation of wells and other water supplies.

c. Chlorine Gas

This gas is formed on a large scale by electrolytic decomposition of salt solution. The moist gas is stored in steel cylinders. One part of chlorine in one million parts of water is usually sufficient to sterilise water successfully in about 30 minutes.

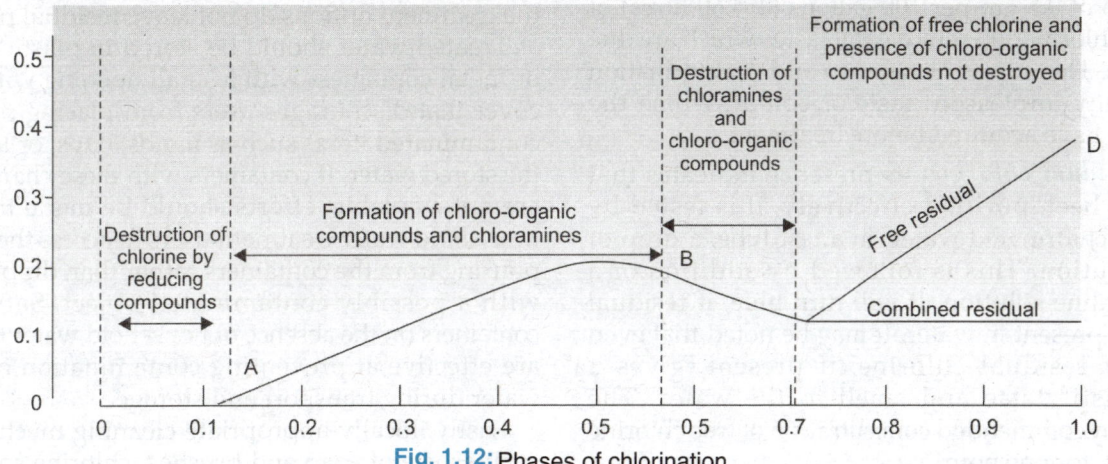

Fig. 1.12: Phases of chlorination

The apparatus used for administering chlorine gas to water supply is known as *Paterson's chloronome*. The gas cylinder is attached to the apparatus, and the gas is conducted through the chloronome to nearly the bottom of the absorption tower. This glazed earthenware tower is filled at the top with a water distributing tray and packed with pumice stone. A small trickle of water is uniformly sprayed over the layer of pumice stone and during its downward flow, it absorbs a measured quantity of chlorine gas. This chlorinated water then flows through a chlorine resisting rubber or earthenware pipe and thus chlorine is uniformly distributed through the main body of the water to be disinfected.

There are several advantages of sterilising water with chlorine gas over hypochlorite solution, especially when a large quantity of water is to be sterilised daily, which are as follows:

1. Chlorine gas is pure and in a concentrated form, it can be stored for a very long period without deterioration, while hypochlorite of lime deteriorates soon.
2. The gas occupies very much less space.
3. A precise dose can be administered without any difficulty.
4. Labour cost is reduced to a minimum.
5. Dry chlorine gas has no effect on metals, but when it comes in contact with moisture it sets up virulent corrosion immediately.
6. It destroys odour producing constituents of water.
7. It controls the formation of algae and slime organisms.

d. Superchlorination and Dechlorination

Here a much larger dose of chlorine is given, *viz.* two parts of free chlorine per million gallon (4.546 million litres) of water with a contact for 15 minutes, in place of 1 part per million gallon with a contact for half an hour. Excess of chlorine is neutralised by the addition of a dechlorinator like anhydrous sodium thiosulphate in the ratio of 0.5 gm per 100 gallons (454.60 litres) of water. Dechlorination removes all tastes which are due to chlorine. This superchlorination and dechlorination destroys any unpleasant taste or colour, which the water may have acquired before treatment.

Free residual chlorine: Its presence indicates that water has been purified effectively, if is tested by adding to chlorinated water, in a test tube, a drop of starch solution. This is followed by addition of a drop of iodine solution. It will turn blue, if residual chlorine is present in water. It may be noted that even a trace of residual chlorine, if present, gives a characteristic taste and smell to the water. The minimum recommended concentration of free chlorine is 0.5 mg/L for one hour.

Horrock's test: This test is carried out for finding out the quantity of bleaching powder required to sterilise a known volume of water. First of all make a standard solution of bleaching powder in the black cup supplied with Horrock's apparatus. The other six white cups are filled with water to be sterilised. The standard solution of bleaching powder is now added, drop by drop, one drop to first cup, two drops to the second, three drops to the third and four drops to the fourth cup and so on. The contents of each cup are thoroughly stirred and allowed to stay for half an hour. Next indicator (cadmium iodide and starch solution) is added to each cup and contents stirred again. Some of the cups out of six white cups will show no colour, while others would show blue colour. Let us suppose cups number 1st and 2nd show no colour. But subsequent cups—3rd, 4th, 5th, and 6th, show blue colour. The number of cups showing definite colour, indicates number of scoopfuls of bleaching powder required to give one part of free chlorine per 100 gallons (454.60 litres) of water, at the end of contact for half an hour with that water. Each scoop has a capacity of 2 gm. In the above case 3 scoopfuls or 6 gm of bleaching powder will be required to sterilise 100 gallons (454.60 litres) of water.

Orthotoluidine test: This test is done after chlorination of water to determine both free and combined chlorine present in water speedily and accurately. The reagent consists of analytical grade orthotoluidine, dissolved in 10% solution of hydrochloric acid. A sample of chlorinated water is taken in a test tube and 2–3 drops of orthotoluidine are added to it. The appearance of yellow colour (flash test) will indicate that sufficient chlorination has been done. Appearance of red colour will indicate presence of chloramine, i.e. excess of chlorination.

Safe Storage of Water

For prevention of water-borne infections, after filtration and disinfection of water, it is important that the water storage and drawing practices are hygienic especially when the treatment options do not leave residual protection.

Treated water should be stored in plastic, ceramic, or metal containers with a small opening with a lid or cover that discourages users from placing potentially contaminated items such as hands, cups, or ladles into the stored water. If containers with these characteristics are not available, efforts should be made to educate household water treatment users to access the water by pouring from the containers rather than dipping into it with a possibly contaminated object. Safe storage containers (in the absence of household water treatment) are effective at preventing contamination of potable water during transport and storage.

Lastly, locally-appropriate cleaning mechanisms— such as use of soap and brushes, chlorine solution, or an abrasive—should be developed and recommended to clean the container on a regular basis.

Standards for Water Quality

1. Microbial Water Quality

Analysis of faecal indicator microorganisms, with the organism of choice being *Escherichia coli* or, alternatively, thermotolerant coliforms. *Escherichia coli* provides conclusive evidence of recent faecal pollution and should not be present in drinking water.

2. Chemical Water Quality

Most chemicals are of concern only following long-term exposure; however, some hazardous chemicals that occur in drinking water are of concern because of effects arising from sequences of exposures over a short period, e.g. concentration of nitrate/nitrite, which is associated with methaemoglobinaemia in bottle-fed infants. Assessment of the adequacy of the chemical quality of drinking water relies on comparison of the results of water quality analysis with guideline values.

1.9 EXAMINATION OF WATER

To ensure safety of drinking water, the examination of water is generally done under the following heads:
  a. Physical examination.
  b. Chemical examination.
  c. Microscopical examination.
  d. Bacteriological examination.

Collection of Sample

For chemical analysis, water should be collected in a Winchester quart bottle of 200–250 ml capacity, provided with a stopper or a perfectly fitted neat and clean cork. The bottle should be cleaned with dilute acid and then washed thoroughly with distilled water. Before it is filled with the sample, it should be rinsed 3–4 times with the water to be collected. When the sample is taken from a tap, the water should be allowed to run for at least 5 minutes, before the actual sample is taken. When the sample of water is taken from a well, river or a lake, the sample should be taken by placing the bottle well under the surface, i.e. about 25 cm below the surface and sufficiently away from the bank.

  a. *Physical examination*: Note the colour, clarity, lustre or brilliance, taste and smell. This should by no means be attributed as final and should not form the basis of opinion.

  b. *Chemical analysis of water*: Analysis is made to determine:
    i. The amount of organic salts which determine the hardness of water and type of hardness.
    ii. The nature and amount of organic pollution.
    iii. The percentage and amount of poisonous metals.

The chemist determines the reaction (by means of a litmus paper or phenolphthalein), the type and degree of hardness, the presence of chlorides, nitrites, nitrates, ammonia (free and albuminoid) and metals such as lead, copper, iron, calcium, etc. before giving his final opinion.

  c. *Microscopical examination of water*: The sample of water is centrifuged whereby all its suspended matters fall at the bottom of the tube and the deposit is seen under a microscope. The presence of spores of mycelia, if found, is due to the contamination of water with sewage and the most suspicious elements are the remnants of vegetables used for food and fibres of cotton, linen, wool, etc. Animal substances, i.e. wool, hair, yellow elastic tissue, etc. generally indicate recent contamination.

  d. *Bacteriological examination of water*: The main objective of bacteriological examination of water is to find out the contamination of water with excreta. The value of single examination is to justify condemnation of water drinking quality. A routine examination consists of plate count and presumptive *Coli*-aerogenes count, as organisms of coliform group have been found to be most useful for this purpose. The sewage bacteria can be divided into three groups, *viz*.
    i. *Colifom organisms*: They include all aerobic and facultative anaerobic, non-sporing, gram-negative, motile and non-motile groups.
    ii. *Faecal streptococci*: They occur in faeces. But they are generally in much smaller numbers than *E. coli*.
    iii. *Cl. perfringens*: They also usually occur in faeces, but are in much smaller number than *E. coli*.

Special Examination of Water

Examination for radiological substances, both toxic and metallic and presence of virus are not carried out as a routine. However, when their presence in water is suspected these tests may be performed in specialised laboratories having facilities for the same.

Water Standard for Filtered Pipe Water

1. Excellent water = No coliform bacteria in 100 ml
2. Satisfactory water 1 to 2 coliform bacteria in 100 ml
3. Suspicious water 3 to 10 coliform bacteria in 100 ml.

Tube wells and deep wells should conform to the above standards. It is very difficult to lay out standards for shallow wells and tanks.

1.10 PUBLIC BATHS/SWIMMING POOLS

Model baths/pools should be architecturally made to allow easy cleansing. The margin of the bath should slope away as to prevent contamination by dirty water.

The surface should be kept free of growths and deposits. There should be a channel around the bath for the bathers to spit into. There should be ample urinal and water closet accommodation, along with shower baths and dressing-rooms. There should also be a foot bath with hypochlorite solution.

Persons entering the bath/pool must shower using soap. Special care must be taken by the users of the pool to avoid spitting or passing urine while swimming. No person having any skin (including fungal and viral infections of feet) or intestinal infection, any other contagious disease like cough, cold, sore eyes, running ears, etc. should be not allowed to use the public bath/pool until completely free from infection.

There should be continuous water supply to ensure fresh flow through the bath or preferably a system where the water in the bath circulates continuously from the bath through a filter and back again to the bath.

The water in the swimming pools/baths should be transparent enough to show up the bottom and the sides of the pool clearly. The water should be dosed for a few days with 1 to 2 parts of copper sulphate per million parts of water avoid any danger of growth of algae. The water should also conform to the standards of drinking water, i.e. no *Bacillus coli* should be present per ml of water.

Continuous chlorination during the entire season of use is the best way to ensure safety of water in the swimming pool/public bath. Proper free chlorine level (1–3 mg/L or parts per million [ppm]) and pH (7.2–7.8) maximizes germ-killing powder, and provides adequate protection against viral and bacterial infection. Filtration through Katadyn filter or treatment by ozone is also useful.

1.11 HYGIENE OF ICE-MAKING

Though most food poisoning organisms do not readily multiply in foods below 8°C, however, scientific research has shown that certain bacteria and viruses can survive freezing for many hours and can also remain viable in very strong alcoholic drinks.

Ice may become contaminated during production in the factory or during delivery by poor quality of water used for making ice, airborne particles, food handlers or from dirty utensils. However, inadequate cleaning of the ice-making machine or equipment and poor hygiene practices when handling ice are the ones that are most commonly responsible reasons for contamination of ice.

The water used for ice manufacturing must qualify minimum standards for drinking water quality. The ice machine should be connected to a "direct" wholesome mains water supply.

The ice should be sampled at the factory for bacteriological examination from time to time. The containers in which water is frozen should be scrubbed out weekly and sterilised by steaming to keep scrupulously clean.

The workmen should wear clean overalls during work and cleanliness as regards to their hands and nails should be observed. The person dispensing ice from the machine should wash and dry their hands thoroughly before starting this task. The ice should always be removed from the machine preferably using a clean utensil such as a scoop and never using hands.

Adequate latrine accommodation should be provided for the staff. No typhoid carrier should be allowed to work in the ice factory. Spitting should be strictly prohibited. Delivery of ice should be effected in closed vans.

There is always a possibility of pollution of ice even in a well-cared establishment. Public should never keep foodstuffs in direct contact with ice or put ice directly into drinks to cool them. Food stuff or drinks should be cooled by keeping them in an ice chest in which there are two separate compartments; one for keeping ice and the other for food drinks.

1.12 AERATED WATER FACTORIES

Aerated waters are prepared by dissolving in ordinary drinking water, salts of lime, soda magnesium, etc. and then charging them with carbon dioxide gas. Three processes are involved in the preparation of aerated waters: (a) Cleansing of bottles, (b) preparation of syrups, and (c) bottling of the products. During any of these processes, nuisance or danger to public health may arise so these factories must be licensed. It is preferable to have separate rooms for each of these processes. The factory should be well lit, adequately ventilated and fly-proof. All workers must wear scrupulously clean clothes and observe cleanliness regarding their hands and nails. The floor should be made up of smooth impermeable material and flushed regularly at the end of day's work. The internal walls should be painted with waterproof paints. Adequate lavatory and washing accommodation with soap and nail brushes should be provided for workers separately from the factory.

Bottle washing: Three tanks should be provided for washing the bottles. The first tank is filled with pure water to which washing soda has been added—1/2 oz (14.17 gm) to a gallon (4.546 litres) of water. All bottles on return to the factory should be immersed in this solution to soak. When the labels have come off, the bottles are transferred after having been well scrubbed with brushes to the second tank, which contains clean water mixed with potassium permanganate. These are scrubbed internally with good bottle brushes, rinsed out and placed in the third tank with plain water. Here these are again rinsed, inverted on a draining rack and allowed to dry.

Syrup room: It must be fly-proof. It should have a table having smooth, clean and washable top. Strainers should be washed daily in clean water, boiled and kept in a dust proof cupboard when not in use. Syrup containers should be kept in an ant and fly-proof cupboard. The water supply of the factory must comply to the drinking water standards and preferably be sourced from the municipal water supply.

Bottling: There are two types of bottles in use. The crown-capped bottles are hygienic because the whole of the top of bottle is covered over by the cap. Capping machines are needed for the insertion of the caps. There are two types, one fed with a supply of caps automatically, which is the best and the other requiring the insertion of each cap by hand, which may get infected by forefingers of the operator. The other type of bottles, made gas-tight by means of a glass ball fitting against a rubber ring, are most insanitary and are extremely difficult to clean.

1.13 WATER-RELATED DISEASES

Water-related diseases can be due to biological agents:

a. Those due to micro-organisms and chemicals in water people drink.
b. Diseases like schistosomiasis which have part of their life cycle in water.
c. Diseases like malaria with water-related vectors.
d. Drowning and some injuries.
e. Others like legionellosis carried by aerosols containing certain micro-organisms.

Water-borne diseases: These may be classified as hereunder:

a. *Caused due to the presence of an infective agent*:
   i. Bacterial: Cholera, typhoid, paratyphoid, diarrhoea, bacillary dysentery.
   ii. Viral: Poliomyelitis, viral hepatitis.
   iii. Leptospiral: Weil's disease.
   iv. Helminthic: Roundworm, threadworm, whipworm, hydatid disease.
   v. Protozoal: Amoebiasis, giardiasis.
b. *Caused due to the presence of an aquatic host*:
   i. Cyclops: Guinea worm, fishworm and tapeworm
   ii. Snails: Schistosomiasis
c. *Due to chemical contaminants in drinking water*:
   i. Dental and skeletal fluorosis: The presence of fluoride at about 1 mg/litre in drinking water has protective effect on dental caries, but consumption of water with higher levels fluoride for long period of time causes dental mottling and skeletal fluorosis.
   ii. Cyanosis in infants: High nitrate content of water is associated with methaemoglobinaemia.
   iii. Cardiovascular diseases: Hardness of water has beneficial effects against cardiovascular diseases.

Water-borne diseases: Occur due to drinking water contamination, transmitted by faeco-oral route.

Example: Typhoid, cholera, dysentery, viral Hep A.

Water washed disease: It includes infection of the outer body surface which occurs due to inadequate use of water or improper hygiene.

Example: Scabies, trachoma, typhus, bacillary dysentery and amoebic dysentery.

Water based disease: Refers to infections transmitted through an aquatic invertebrate animal.

Example: Schistosomiasis, dracunculiasis (Guinea worm disease)

Water-related disease (water breeding diseases): An infection spread by insects that depend on water.

Example: Malaria, filaria, dengue, yellow fever, and onchocerciasis.

Air and Ventilation

2.1 IMPORTANCE OF AIR

Air is absolutely essential for the maintenance of life. Besides supplying the life giving oxygen, atmospheric conditions, air serves several useful functions. The human body is heated or cooled by contact with air and special senses of smell and hearing act through air-transmitted stimuli. The two main functions of air are interchange of gases in the process of respiration and regulation of body temperature.

Air is a mechanical mixture of gases and not a chemical compound. It is enveloping earth as atmosphere. Pure air has approximately the following composition:

Oxygen	20.93%
Nitrogen	78.1 to 78.2%
Carbon dioxide	0.03 to 0.04%
Water vapour and ammonia	Varies with temperature
Argon, neon, krypton, helium, bacteria, spores, etc.	Variable in traces

In the open air, this composition remains more or less remarkably constant, owing to diffusion of air currents and due to the fact that the plants by virtue of their chlorophyll content, take up carbon dioxide from the air and give off oxygen, thus compensating for the consumption of oxygen and formation of carbon dioxide, which is always going on as a result of the existence of animal life, combustion, etc. This process, however, is reversed at night. Moreover, the rain as it falls washes the air free from most of the suspended impurities. The wind also helps in producing a uniformity of composition of air and renders assistance in the removal of impurities by dispersing them. Oxygen is an essential constituent of air necessary for all life, the inert nitrogen simply acts as a diluent of oxygen; the only exception to this rule being certain types of bacteria which thrive only in the absence of oxygen and anaerobic bacteria. Water vapour is always present in the air. Its amount varies widely and depends mainly upon the quantity of water available for evaporation,

i.e. on rainfall. It is present more at sea than at land. At a certain temperature, air can hold only a definite amount of water vapour. The air is said to be saturated when it can hold no more amount of water vapour at a particular temperature and at that point, its humidity is said to be 100%. About 65 to 75% humidity is considered as conducive to health.

2.2 VARIOUS FACTORS

The factors responsible for purification of air are given below:
1. Wind, which dilutes, sweeps away or aspirates the impurities and gets replaced by pure air.
2. Rain, which washes the air and removes gases as well as suspended impurities.
3. Oxygen and ozone, which oxidise the organic matter present in the air.
4. During sunlight, chlorophyll present in green leaves of the plants absorbs carbon from carbon dioxide of the atmosphere and gives off free oxygen, but at night this process gets reversed.

2.3 IMPURITIES OF AIR

The chief impurities in the air are due to:
1. Respiration.
2. Combustion.
3. Decomposition of organic matter.
4. Dust.
5. Bacteria.

Impurities due to Respiration

These are chiefly carbon dioxide, water vapour and organic matters. The proportion of gases in inspired and expired air per 100 parts is given in Table 2.1.

On an average, a man respires about 18 times a minute and at each breathing an adult gives out about 22 cubic inches (360 cc) of air. The expired air contains about 4.4% carbon dioxide. The air in the atmosphere loses about the same percentage of oxygen. On an

Table 2.1: Proportion of gases in inspired and expired air (per 100 parts)

	Inspired air	Expired air
Oxygen	20.93	16.51
Nitrogen	78.1	79.09
Carbon dioxide	0.03 to 0.04	4.41
Water vapour	Varies	Saturated
Temperature	Varies	At body temp.

average about 10 ounces (283.50 gm) of water vapour are given off from the lungs of a man within 24 hours, whereas skin excretes about 20–30 ounces (566.98–850.47 gm) within the said period. Respiration also raises the temperature of air. When the amount of carbon dioxide in the air of a particular room rises from its normal percentage, i.e. 0.03 to 0.06%, air becomes perceptibly stuffy to a person entering from fresh air environment and the occupants of the room begin to suffer from the usual symptoms complained of in over-crowded rooms, e.g. drowsiness, headache, nausea, vomiting, etc. These symptoms are caused by either or in combination of these factors, i.e. increase of carbon dioxide above 0.06% or organic poisons from the expired air or the decrease of oxygen along with stagnation of air in the room.

Impurities due to Combustion

The chief impurity derived from coal in the process of combustion by the oxidation of carbon in the air is carbon dioxide. Under certain conditions, carbon monoxide is formed by combustion. The burning of coke especially in cast iron stoves is a source of carbon monoxide. As carbon dioxide is passed over hot coke, it is reduced to carbon monoxide, which is expressed in the following equation:

$$CO_2 + C = 2CO$$

The other products of combustion are carbon bisulphide, sulphurous and sulphuric acids, sulphuretted hydrogen, ammonium hydrogen sulphide and water.

Air pollution by industrial smoke can be considerably prevented by adopting the following methods:

i. Use of smokeless fuels, e.g. coke in boilers and furnaces.
ii. Use of mechanical stokers or employment of skilled labour, for careful stoking of furnaces.
iii. Provision of efficient furnace plants with accurately maintained draughts.
iv. Enforcement of laws relating to smoke nuisance.
- An ordinary gas burner consumes 6 cubic feet (0.17 cubic metres) of gas and vitiates about 7200 cubic feet (203.875 cubic metres) of air. This vitiation approximates the contamination of air to the breathing of three adults.

- Burning of candles and oils chiefly paraffin oil adds to the impurities of air as they produce soot, carbon dioxide and water.
- By the term "One candle power" is meant the light given out by a sperm candle burning at the rate of 120 grains (7.20 gm) per hour. This gives out 0.4 cubic foot (0.01 cubic metre) of carbonic acid and also about the same quantity of water.

Electricity is the best source of light and heat since it is not dependent on the oxygen of air and, therefore, it is not conducive to vitiating atmosphere, like combustion of coal, etc.

Impurities due to Decomposition

Animal and vegetable matters, when they putrefy, give off offensive poisonous gases such as carbon dioxide, hydrogen sulphide, ammonium hydrogen sulphide, carbon bisulphide, ammonia and marsh gas. These mostly emanate from cesspools, sewers, drains, stables, cowsheds, etc. Bacteria, moulds and fungi grow rapidly in such air. Presence of 0.2% of hydrogen sulphide in the air may sometimes produce unconsciousness.

Impurities due to Dust

These constitute inorganic matter, organic matter and bacteria. More or less poisonous gases and volatile effluvia and suspended matters are given off by certain trades and manufacturing concerns. The inorganic particles of dust to be met with, in the atmosphere, are chiefly composed of silica, aluminium silicate, carbonate or phosphate of calcium, magnesium, sodium chloride, carbon, etc. Those found in the air of houses are due to debris arising from the wear and tear of articles in domestic use, such as dust, soot and ashes. Mineral particles from the neighbouring factories may likewise find access into the houses.

Bacteria

Micro-organisms are found in the normal atmosphere. The great source of aerial bacteria is the soil, which is teeming with micro-organisms. They are emitted by coughing or speaking and after floating in the air at the most about 10 feet (3.04 metres) high, they again fall on the ground. Pathogenic micro-organisms are not present in the atmosphere except in close proximity to patients whose expired air is charged with viruses and bacteria as in cases of persons suffering from common cold, influenza, etc.

2.4 KATA THERMOMETER

The word "Kata" is a Greek word, which means "down". It is essentially an alcohol thermometer, with a glass bulb 4 cm long and 1.8 cm in diameter. It was contrived by Leonard Hill and consists of a large bulbed spirit thermometer graduated from 95°F to

100°F (35°C to 37.8°C) and it is meant for measuring rates of cooling. Two such generally used instruments are (Fig. 2.1):

1. **Dry kata:** In this instrument, the bulb is uncovered and it records the cooling power of air obtained by radiation and convection.

2. **Wet kata:** In this instrument, the bulb is covered with a piece of wet silk cloth or fine cotton. It records cooling power of the air obtained by radiation, convection and evaporation.

Reading: The bulbs are immersed in test water of about 150°F (65.6°C) temperature until the spirit rises into the small bulb at the top of the instrument. The excess of water is then jerked off the wet bulb and the other part of the instrument is subsequently dried with a piece of cloth.

The time required for alcohol to fall from 100°F to 95°F (37.8° to 35°C) is noted in seconds by a stopwatch. At least four such readings are recorded with each thermometer. The first reading is discarded and the average of other three readings is taken. Each thermometer has a factor and is marked with a letter F on the stem. This factor divided by the number of seconds consumed in 5° temperature drop gives the rate of cooling expressed in millicalories per sq cm per second.

A fresh comfortable room has a dry kata cooling power of 6 and above and a wet kata cooling power of 20 and above, whereas in a perceptably cool room, the figures will be 8 and 22. These figures will come down

to 4 and 16 in case the room happens to be warm and stuffy.

Globe thermometer: The globe thermometer was introduced by Vernon in 1930 as a means of assessing the combined effects of radiation, air temperature and air velocity on human comfort. It consists of a hollow copper sphere painted matt back to absorb radiant heat, with a temperature sensor at its centre. When it reaches a steady state (after 15 minutes or so depending on the size of the globe and the environmental conditions), the heat exchanges by convection and radiation will be in equilibrium, and the temperature recorded by the sensor will be somewhere between the air and radiant temperature. This is referred to as the globe temperature (tg) or black globe temperature and resembles the thermal conditions felt by the human body (Fig. 2.2).

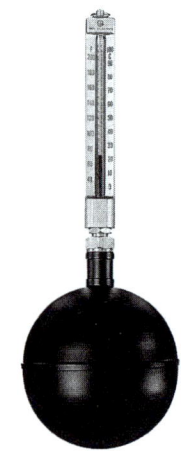

Fig. 2.2: Globe thermometer

2.5 EUPATHEOSCOPE AND EUPATHEOMETER

These are the latest types of "comfort indicators". The former is rather cumbersome so the Eupatheometer is commonly used. It consists of two thermometers filled with spirit, one having a glass bulb and the other a silver metal bulb. Heat the bulb of each thermometer with warm water, till the spirit rises up in the top bulb. Wipe out the bulb, dry it and suspend the black thermometer. Stand at a place as far from the instrument as is convenient and observe the fall of spirit from the upper mark on the scale to the lower mark. Use a special stopwatch to time this and take the reading from the small scale. Now suspend the silvered instrument and time its cooling. Note the reading upon the silver scale of the watch.

The equivalent temperature in degrees Fahrenheit is obtained by adding the two readings together. Thus the stopwatch shows 35 when the black thermometer cools in 30 seconds and 20, if the silvered thermometer cools in 27 seconds. Hence the equivalent temperature is 35°F + 20°F = 55°F. Three or four such readings should be recorded and the average obtained.

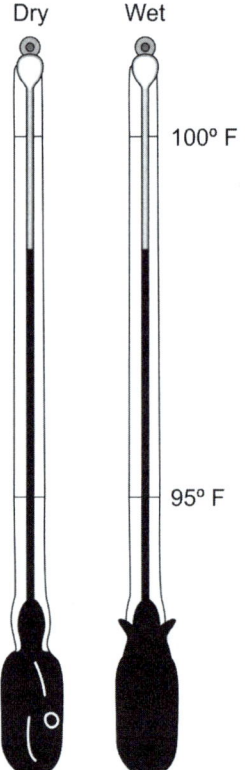

Dry   Wet

100° F

95° F

Fig. 2.1: Kata thermometer—dry and wet

Effective temperature: It is defined as "that temperature of saturated, motionless air which would produce the same sensation of coolness as that produced by the combination of temperature, humidity and air motion under observation." Places or zones with effective temperature from 65° to 70°F (18.3° to 21.1°C) may be safely termed "comfort zones".

Indices of Thermal Comfort

Thermal comfort is defined as: "That condition of mind which expresses satisfaction with the thermal environment. Fanger (1970) defined 3 parameters for a person to be in thermal comfort:

a. The body is in heat balance
b. Sweat rate is within comfort limits
c. Mean skin temperature is within comfort limits.

Thermal stress is an important factor in many industrial situations, athletic events and military scenarios as it can seriously affect the productivity and the health of the individual and diminish tolerance to other environmental hazards. However, the assessment of the thermal stress and the translation of the stress in terms of physiological and psychological strains are complex. Many indies that have been suggested can be categorized into one of three groups: "Rational indices" (based on heat balance equation), "empirical indices" (based on objective and subjective strain), or "direct indices" (based on direct measurements of environmental variables). The first 2 groups are sophisticated indices, which integrate environmental and physiological variables; they are difficult to calculate and are not feasible for daily use. The latter group comprises simple indices, which are based on the measurement of basic environmental variables. In this group 2 indices are in use for over four decades: the "wet-bulb globe temperature" (WBGT) index and the "discomfort index" (DI).

2.6 AIR POLLUTION

Air pollution is a major environment-related health threat to children and a risk factor for both acute and chronic respiratory disease. While second-hand tobacco smoke and certain outdoor pollutants are known risk factors for respiratory infections, indoor air pollution from solid fuels is one of the major contributors to the global burden of disease. In poorly ventilated dwellings, indoor smoke can be 100 times higher than acceptable levels for small particles. Exposure is particularly high among women and young children, who spend the most time near the domestic hearth.

Sources

1. Automobiles
2. Industries
3. Domestic.

Outdoor Air Pollution

Outdoor air pollution is large and increasing a consequence of the inefficient combustion of fuels for transport, power generation and other human activities like home heating and cooking. Combustion processes produce a complex mixture of pollutants that comprises both primary emissions, such as diesel soot particles and lead, and the products of atmospheric transformation, such as ozone and sulphate particles.

About 1.3 million deaths worldwide per year are attributed to urban outdoor air pollution. Children are particularly at risk due to the immaturity of their respiratory organ systems. Those living in middle-income countries disproportionately experience this burden. Exposure to air pollutants is largely beyond the control of individuals and requires action by public authorities at the national, regional and even international levels.

Indoor Air Pollution

Indoor cooking and heating with biomass fuels (agricultural residues, dung, straw, wood) or coal produces high levels of indoor smoke that contains a variety of health-damaging pollutants. There is consistent evidence that exposure to indoor air pollution can lead to acute lower respiratory infections in children under age five, and chronic obstructive pulmonary disease and lung cancer in adults.

Indoor air pollution is responsible for 4.3 million deaths annually. Acute lower respiratory infections, in particular pneumonia, continue to be the biggest killer of young children due to indoor air pollution and this toll almost exclusively falls on children in developing countries.

Common Air Pollutants

The six common air pollutants are particle pollution (particulate matter), ground-level ozone, carbon monoxide, sulphur oxides, nitrogen oxides, and lead. These are called "criteria" air pollutants because the Environmental Protection Agency sets human health-based and environmentally-based criteria for setting limits on the amount of these pollutants that are permissible in the ambient air. These limits are called primary and secondary standards.

In 1997, particle pollution was divided into two divisions: (a) Particulate matter (PM) 10, i.e. particles equal to or smaller than 10 micrometers in diameter, and (b) Particulate matter (PM) 2.5, i.e. particles equal to or smaller than 2.5 micrometers in diameter. Ozone and particle pollution are the most widespread health threats. The smaller or pulverized particles actually have more serious health effects because microscopic particles get deep into the lungs.

Hazardous Air Pollutants

Various international agencies like US EPA and Iowa DNR regulate 187 air pollutants known or suspected to cause cancer or other serious health effects such as reproductive effects or birth defects, or adverse environmental consequences. These pollutants are called hazardous air pollutants (HAP) or air toxics. National Emission Standards for Hazardous Air Pollutants (NESHAP) have also been set up as national standards for regulating sources of HAP.

Air toxics are generally more localized than the criteria pollutants and the highest levels are close to their sources. Most air toxics originate from man-made sources, including cars and trucks, factories, power plants and refineries, as well as some building materials and cleaning solvents.

Prevention and control of air pollution: The Air (Prevention and Control of Pollution) Act, 1981—an Act of the Parliament of India to control and prevent air pollution was amended in 1987. This Act provides for the prevention, control and abatement of air pollution.

Air quality index (AQI): The AQI is an index for reporting daily air quality. It tells about the quality of air and its associated health effects. The AQI focuses on health effects you may experience within a few hours or days after breathing polluted air. AQI is calculated for five major air pollutants: Ground-level ozone, particle pollution (also known as particulate matter), carbon monoxide, sulphur dioxide, and nitrogen dioxide. For each of these pollutants, national air quality standards have been set up to protect public health. Ground-level ozone and airborne particles are the two major pollutants that pose the greatest threat to human health.

2.7 VENTILATION

It is replacing the vitiated air with fresh outdoor air along with control of quality of incoming air with regard to its temperature, humidity and purity to provide a comfortable thermal environment which is free from risk of infection.

Internal ventilation: Means the removal or dilution of the atmosphere which has become stagnant, warm and moist through the vitiating process by air which is comparatively fresh and in motion.

In order to admit fresh air into the houses, it is necessary to take into consideration the ventilation of streets and surroundings of the buildings, also *external ventilation*. This is ensured by making the streets wide and straight, keeping sufficient open spaces and parks especially in the congested part of the towns and by building houses detached or separate from each other. This can be also helped by watering the streets to lay down the dust, prevent nuisance from smoke and also by speedy removal of street and other refuse.

Amount of air required for ventilation: When the amount of carbon dioxide present in air increases above 0.03 to 0.06%, stuffiness begins to become perceptible. Thus 0.06% of carbon dioxide is regarded as a permissible limit of respiratory impurity. It has been assumed that air vitiated to the extent of 0.2 parts per thousand, which is still fresh and does not differ sensibly to smell from the outer atmosphere, can be breathed with impunity.

Satisfactory ventilation means supply fresh air to the rooms, maintenence of proper temperature and humidity and removal of gases, odours, bacteria and other impurities by continuous circulation of air. Accordingly standards of ventilation have been set based on the efficiency of ventilation in removing body odour.

However, ideal ventilation is said to exist when the supply of pure air to a room is sufficient enough to prevent the amount of respiratory carbon dioxide increasing beyond a limit of 0.2 parts per thousand parts since the permissible limit of the impurity in this regard is 0.2 parts per thousand of air which means 0.0002 cubic ft of carbon dioxide per cubic ft of air (1 cubic ft being equal to 0.028 cubic metre).

$$Efficiency\ D = \frac{E}{R}$$

Delivery of the amount of fresh air available in cubic feet per hour per head

$$= \frac{\text{Amount of carbon dioxide exhaled per hour per head}}{\text{Respiratory impurity } (CO_2) \text{ per cubic foot of air}}$$

If $E = 0.6$ and $R = 0.0002$

$$D = \frac{0.6}{0.0002} = 3000 \text{ cubic ft (84.95 cubic metres)}$$

Each individual requires 3000 cubic feet of air per hour so that respiratory impurity may not exceed 0.2 part per 1000 parts.

1. **Fresh air supply per cubic space:** The widely quoted standard is that of De Chaumont who advocated a fresh air supply of 3000 cubic feet (84.95 cubic metres) per person per hour.

2. **Rate of air change:** It is recommended that the per hour air exchanges should be 2–3 times in the living room and 4–6 times in workrooms and assemblies. Excess air change, i.e. more than 6 times per hour, is likely to produce a condition like draught. It should thus be noted that where the available cubic space is large there is a comparatively lesser need of frequently changing the air.

3. **Floor space:** The optimum floor space requirements per person is even more important parameter to analyse the status of ventilation. This is based on the

fact that the need of ventilation depends upon the fact that the warm vitiated air rises up and gets cooled after rising about 12 feet (3.65 metres) and falls down again. So in calculating cubic space, any height above 12 feet (3.65 metres) has to be discarded because products of respiration tend to accumulate at the lower levels of rooms of the buildings. Thus for mechanical methods of ventilation also, height above 12 feet (3.65 metres) is regarded as useful. By keeping 12 feet (3.65 metres) as the limit of height, it will follow that the floor space would be equal to 1/12th of the total cubic space. Ideally it should vary between 50 and 100 sq feet (4.64 to 9.29 sq metres).

Amount of fresh air required for artificial lights: As candles, kerosene oil lamps, coal gas burners, etc. consume oxygen from the air while burning, so these must also be taken into consideration when arranging for provision for the ventilation of rooms. For an ordinary oil lamp and a gas burner, 2000 and 2250 cubic feet (56.63 and 63.70 cubic metres) of air is required per-hour respectively. Electric light is considered best from hygienic point of view as it has practically no effect on air of the room. All other lights are more or less dependent upon the absorption of oxygen from the air and vitiate the atmosphere by certain products, which affect health to a greater or lesser degree.

Amount of fresh air required for the sick: On an average, 3750 cubic feet (106.18 cubic metres) of air per hour is required for a sick person, in a hospital.

2.8 SYSTEMS OF VENTILATION

Natural Ventilation

This is greatly achieved by building houses having sufficient open space and by having a large number of windows opening direct into the open air. It largely depends on the following three natural forces.

1. Diffusion of Gases

Gases diffuse inversely as the square root of their densities, so the air of room diffuses through the cracks and crevices of various doors and windows of a room, even though they are closed. Since under the ordinary circumstances, diffusion is very small and is thus not a dependable source of ventilation. Diffusion causes the gaseous impurities of the respired air to mix up with the fresh air of the room until homogeneity is established with no effect on the suspended matter present in the air which tends to fall back towards the earth in the still atmosphere, due to gravitational force.

2. Effect of Temperature

When air gets heated from the products of respiration or by fire, it expands and becomes lighter. This hot air rises up and the outer cold fresh air rushes in through outer openings until temperature of both outside and inside air becomes same. Therefore, in all methods of ventilation based upon the force, suitable and adequate inlets for fresh air and outlets for the escape of impure air must be provided. This method is more relied upon in cold countries where coal fires are used and the external and internal difference of temperature of the room is relatively high. But in hot countries, where difference in temperature between the external and the internal air is less, ventilation is imperfect.

3. Perflation and Aspiration

Winds are very powerful ventilating agents and they act in two ways, *viz.* (i) perflation, and (ii) aspiration.

  i. *Perflation* means the setting up of masses of air in motion and forcing them through open doors, windows and porous bricks into the room as a result of movement of natural air currents for rapid and continuous flushing with fresh air. Cross ventilation means free perflation between windows and other openings, placed opposite to each other. But natural cross ventilation is not feasible in the case of houses having back to back construction and in countries having warm climates, as in India, where the inside and outside temperature of a room is more or less the same. Thus in such cases, ventilation is promoted by perflation of air through doors and windows facing each other. Similarly pervious walls such as bamboo matting also allow free perflating without any harm whatsoever.

  ii. *Aspiration* means the suction action of the wind, which draws air out of a space, creating therein a partial vacuum and thus fresh air rushes in to take its place and a continuous current in perpendicular direction is thus set up. The aspirating action of wind is utilised to ventilate rooms by means of provision of chimneys. When fire is kept burning in the grates, the aspirating action of chimneys is further increased.

In tropical countries, during hot weather, particularly when the humidity is high and there is air stagnation, ventilation becomes imperfect. Electric fans, therefore, are used for agitating the air of the room which cause evaporation of respiration imparting thereby a feeling of comfort. In addition, these fans help circulation of air of the room and force the vitiated air out through the ventilators, etc. They may be used in the form of ceiling fans or table fans. They are also sometimes called as *agitator fans.*

Inlets and outlets: The openings through which the process of ventilation is carried out are known as inlets and outlets. Inlets are intended for the entrance of fresh air and the outlets for the escape of vitiated air.

Inlets: The area of inlets per head should be about 24 square inches (154.838 sq cm) and the total inlet area should be always greater than the total outlet area in order to reduce the tendency for draught. Inlets should be provided preferably at a height of 5–6 feet (1.52–1.83 metres) above the floor level so that the entering cool air is admitted at about the level of the head of a person sitting in a room. These should be placed in such a positon so that the air supplied is pure and not polluted before admission. The incoming air should be given an upward direction so that it slowly comes down and becomes slightly warm during the process. The objective being to prevent cold draught coming to the feet. Whatever devices may be employed as inlets these should be so arranged that they take in fresh air direct from the outer atmosphere.

Outlets: These are meant for the escape of impure air and should be made of the same size as the inlets. As a general principle, the outlets should be provided opposite to the inlets. These are best provided on the upper part of the room, to serve as outlet openings for the respired air, which has a tendency to go upwards. Rooms with sloping roofs can have outlets in the form of ridge openings along the entire top as in the case of Indian huts.

Artificial Ventilation

Natural sources of ventilation are not practical in case of large buildings, where a number of people are congregated for a considerably long period and where conditions do not permit free use of open doors and windows. Consequently, artificial ventilation is largely resorted to in places such as shopping malls, theatres, cinemas, auditoriums, examination halls and schools. In this system, mechanical means are used to facilitate the renewal of air.

The systems of artificial ventilation are as follows

1. *Plenum or propulsion ventilation:* In this system, the air is forced into a room by mechanical forces like centrifugal fans, blower's steam heated coils forming steam jets and other appliances. Air is forced under pressure and consequently all doors and windows are kept closed. The motor power is installed in a central chamber. The air is washed in a water screen or filtered through a viscous filter, then warmed or cooled, according to the season and finally humified. It is driven along passages to inlets of the rooms. The air in this method is introduced at a low level near the floors, so that the breathing line is completely bathed by the incoming air. This method has many advantages:
   i. The incoming air can be delivered at any level and at any rate.
   ii. It can be warmed in cold weather by passing through heated pipes.
   iii. It can be cooled and humified by passing through cold sprays of water.
   iv. Air can be filtered and made free from dust by passing through the filtering screens of wool.

   Though it is an excellent method, the disadvantage in adopting this mechanism is that the windows have to be kept closed and that the incoming air being treated loses its freshness. This system, however, is used with advantage in public halls, factories and printing presses, etc.

2. *Vacuum or exhaust ventilation:* It consists of the mechanical suction or extraction of vitiated air out of the rooms by means of ducts communicating with the main shaft in which motor power is derived from an electric exhaust fan. This method is generally employed in areas for providing local exhausts to extract dangerous dusts or fumes away from work rooms or benches. Generally, exhaust fans, called propeller fans, are used for extraction as they can be regulated easily and the amount of their draught can be controlled.

   In coal mines, ventilation is done by means of furnaces. The vitiated air is exhausted through a chimney. The hot air being lighter and having been reduced in density goes up through the chimney and fresh air rushes in to take its place.

   Apart from the disadvantages of the artificial methods of ventilation, the other disadvantages to its use are as follows:
   i. The rooms situated near the upcast shaft have the air extracted well, but those situated at some distance may have comparatively a little or no extraction at all. Thus the extraction of air from all the rooms is not uniform.
   ii. It is very difficult to regulate the incoming air, although suitable inlets are provided, yet air tends to be sucked in through all cracks and holes and may result in the creation of an undesirable draught.
   iii. It is not possible to heat or cool the incoming air. Theatres, public halls, hospitals and mines are often provided ventilation on this extraction principle.

3. *Balanced or combined ventilation:* This is probably the best method. It is a combination of the plenum and the vacuum systems. This system is largely used in air-conditioning, where conditioned air under controlled conditions of temperature and humidity is driven into the room by means of ducts. Warmed fresh air is delivered at a height of about 7 feet (2.13 metres) from the floor, by the plenum method (i.e. a fan is used to force the air in) and all the outlets are connected with an upcast shaft, where extraction is done by means of a fan or a furnace. Since electric fans are the motive force in this case, thus their regulation depends on the success of the whole system. For the efficient

working of this system, it is essential that there should be no leakage through windows or doors.

Advantages of Artificial Ventilation

The air can be warmed, cooled, filtered or humified before allowing it to enter the building. It can be supplied at any rate and at any level inside the room. In factories and other trades where dust and other gases must be rapidly removed, natural ventilation cannot be depended upon. In these cases, law provides that each machine should have an air extraction cover. Evidently in some cases, artificial ventilation becomes indispensable, particularly in large establishments, factories, cinema houses and large halls with extensive sitting capacity.

Disadvantages of Artificial Methods of Ventilation

  i. These methods are expensive, thus can be adopted only in large buildings on co-operative basis.
 ii. These should be designed as a part of the building at the time of its construction and can be rarely adopted to the existing buildings.
iii. These require skilled supervision and skilled mechanics.
 iv. None of the artificial methods of ventilation can make the air of a room as fresh and in vigorating as that by the incoming of a good draught by keeping doors and windows of the room opened.

2.9 METHODS OF VENTILATION SUITABLE FOR INDIA

1. *Ventilation of houses*: The natural method of ventilation is efficient, cheap and satisfactory. Any of the various inlet and outlet devices may be employed to achieve effective ventilation in the houses. Under the present conditions, the best that can be done to achieve the object is to introduce the free use of windows and to rely upon ventilators provided near the ceiling of the rooms to serve as outlets.

2. *Ventilation of schools*: The classrooms should be adequately ventilated, as air of rooms may become vitiated on account of respiration of students and teachers, by the putrefaction of animal or vegetable matter and dirt from the shoes, etc. Besides, there is the danger of germs of communicable diseases located in the respiratory tract of students, being added to the exhaled matter. The natural methods of ventilation should be relied upon in the case of school buildings. In planning buildings for the schools, the windows and doors should be placed opposite to each other and kept open to allow a cross-exchange of air. The perflation action of the wind can be effectively utilised by opening windows facing wind. Such a method is of unquestioned utility for rapidly changing the air of an unoccupied classroom and may generally be put in operation. In inhabited rooms during the summer season, when the temperature inside and outside the house approximates, Sheringham's valves or Tobin's tubes may also be employed.

3. *Public buildings*: Natural methods of ventilation are rarely considered satisfactory for public buildings, where people are congregated for considerably long periods, e.g. theatres, lecture rooms, examination halls, etc. In such cases, adoption of artificial methods of ventilation considered as desirable.

2.10 EFFICIENCY OF VENTILATION OF AN INHABITED ROOM

The following points should be kept in view

1. Make the visit at the time of maximum contamination, e.g. in a sleeping room, just before a person rises. Note the *"Sense impression"*.

2. Calculate the cubic space of the room by the following formula:

$$Length \times Breadth \times Height = Cubic\ area$$

   Deduct the cubic space occupied by solid articles in the room such as big trunks, solid furniture, etc.

3. Ascertain the number of occupants of the room. The total amount of cubic feet of air per hour supplied can be calculated thus:
   Number of occupants × allowance of cubic feet of air per hour per head.

4. Floor space per head is ascertained.

5. The rate of velocity of air can be ascertained by means of an anemometer.

6. The inlet provision for fresh air is considered as 24 square inches (154.84 sq. cm) for each person. The direction of air current must be determined which can be conveniently done by examining the situation of inlets and outlets of the room. These can be distinguished by observing the direction of smoke emanating from smouldering brown paper.

7. Efficiency of proper ventilation can be tested by smell test or Pattenkofer's test (e.g. lime or baryta water test) estimate the percentage of CO_2 in air.

8. Find out the number of artificial lights used in the room and the amount of fresh air required for these per hour.

The number of bacteria or dust particles in a room may be estimated by a slit sampler.

Effects of living in stuffy, over-crowded and ill-ventilated rooms: The physical changes noticeable in vitiated air, therefore, are: (1) A rise in temperature, (2) increased humidity, and (3) stillness. These are apt to produce headache, inability to concentrate, drowsiness, lassitude, depression, loss of appetite, higher incidence of viral and bacterial infections like common cold, flu, tuberculosis of lungs and diminished resistance to infectious diseases.

Airborne Diseases

The airborne diseases are grouped as: (1) Airborne infections and (2) airborne other harmful agents.

1. **Airborne infections** are distinguished as: (a) Droplet infections, (b) droplet nuclei and (c) infected dust.

   a. *Droplet infections* are transmitted by coughing, sneezing or talking loudly through droplets containing a large number of organisms. These droplets are projected up to 20 to 30 ft (6.09 to 9.14 metres). Examples of diseases transmitted by droplet infections are TB, diphtheria, smallpox, chickenpox, measles, mumps, whooping cough, viral and pneumococcal pneumonia, etc. Overcrowding and thus inadequate ventilation especially limitation in air exchanges favour droplet infections.

   b. *Droplet nuclei* are constituted by rapid evaporation of droplets leaving behind minute residues or nuclei (less than 0.1 mm) which may be mostly bacteria or virus. Diseases spread by droplets can also be spread by droplet nuclei.

   c. *Infected dust* is constituted by infected moisture droplets or droplet nuclei becoming a part of dust. Diseases transmitted by droplets or droplet nuclei are also transmitted by infected dust, especially if the organisms survive on dust particles under conducive conditions of temperature and moisture. Tuberculosis, pneumonia, streptococcal and staphylococcal infections, etc. are examples of dust-borne infections transmitted through air or dust infected food, milk, etc.

2. **Other airborne harmful agents** are dust, industrial wastes and air pollutants. Inhalation of non-infective dust leads to irritation and hence is very conducive for subsequent lowered resistance to eye infections and respiratory infections. Toxic as well as non-toxic particles of industries and polluted atmosphere of cities with heavy industries and vehicular traffic lead to pneumoconiosis problems like siderosis, silicosis, byssinosis, anthracosis, lead poisoning through inhalation of lead fumes, etc.

2.11 HEATING OF ROOMS

This is commonly done by the combustion of some sort of fuel, and the heat produced, thereby is distributed by the following methods:

1. *Conduction*: As a general principle, solids are good conductors of heat, while liquids and gases are bad ones. Good conductors rapidly transmit heat to the surrounding air and to the articles they come in contact with.

2. *Radiation*: By this process, heat is transmitted from hot bodies like open fire spaces to colder ones through air in straight lines on all sides with equal intensity.

3. *Convection*: In this case, heat is transmitted through gases and liquids.

The common methods of heating houses or buildings are:

1. *Open fire places*: Where wood, charcoal or coal is used. This method is popular in England and hill stations of India.

   The advantage of open fire places is that they are cheerful in appearance and form a useful attraction for the family. The disadvantage is that heating of the room is unequal; most of the heat falls on those objects near the fire. The heat is uneven as the fire burns, alternately bright and dull and needs periodic replenishing of the fuel. And also coal yields a good deal of smoke and is thus a serious cause of atmospheric pollution.

2. *Closed fires or stoves*: These stoves are made of cast iron in which coal, coke, kerosene oil, etc. are used as fuel. They give a more uniform heat because they emit heat by convection. The disadvantages are that they are less cheerful, dry the air and are not as efficient for ventilation as open fires.

3. *Heating by hot air, hot water or steam*: These methods are not commonly used in India. In case of hot air, mechanical methods are used to heat the air, which is used for warming the buildings. When hot water or steam is used, it is circulated from a central source to the various parts of the buildings. This is called central heating.

4. *Electric fires or radiators*: They heat by radiation. They have advantage of being clean, easily regulated and do not give off any impurities; but if used continuously they are more expensive forms of heating than modern solid fuel fires. Their disadvantage is that they dry the air. Oil-fired furnaces and heaters are a popular choice in areas of the country with limited access to natural gas, such as the Northeast. Oil-fired furnaces and boilers present an opportunity to use renewable fuels to heat your home.

5. *Panel heating*: In this system, heating units (*viz.* hot water, pipes or electric coils) are embedded during the construction of buildings in the floors, ceiling and walls. This method is generally used in schools, hospitals, and other public places and is expensive. There is a uniform transmission of heat in this method, which is not possible with open fires or ordinary types of radiators.

However, it is important to maintain proper ventilation to ensure air quality in the indoor environment due to combustion systems.

Combustion air is needed by all electric, oil and gas heating systems to support the combustion process.

This air is provided in some homes by unintentional air leaks, or by air ducts that connect to the outdoors. The combustion process creates several byproducts that are potentially hazardous to human health and can cause deterioration of the indoor air leading to indoor air pollution. To protect yourself from these hazards as well as maintain energy efficiency, the heating system should be adequately ventilated and the chimney system should function properly. Properly functioning chimney systems will carry combustion byproducts like carbon monoxide out of the home. The combustion gases exit the home through the chimney using only their buoyancy combined with the chimney's height. Naturally drafting chimneys often have problems exhausting the combustion gases because of chimney blockage, wind or pressures inside the home that overcome the buoyancy of the gases.

Atmospheric, open-combustion furnaces and boilers, as well as fan-assisted furnaces and boilers, should be vented into masonry chimneys, metal double-wall chimneys, or another type of manufactured chimney. Masonry chimneys should have a fireclay, masonry liner or a retrofitted metal flue liner.

2.12 ARTIFICIAL COOLING

It has been found that artificial cooling not only applies to the need for thermal comfort but also to improve indoor air quality. There are various methods of artificial cooling used in rural and urban areas. A few of them are as follows:

1. Prevention of heating by direct radiation from sun by closing doors and windows or fixing blue cloth over glass panes during daytime.
2. Use of fans and coolers.
3. *Khus-khus tatties or chiks*: These are used as a screen during summer. They are kept continuously saturated with water. The dry air of the atmosphere causes evaporation and the heat of the room is absorbed and thus it keeps the rooms cool. Moreover, they have the additional effect of acting as filters by preventing the suspended impurities of the air from coming in. As this method reduces the temperature but increases the relative humidity, it can be used only in areas where the air is hot and dry, but is not suitable for places where the climate is hot and humid.
4. Refrigeration, condensation and rarefaction.

2.13 AIR-CONDITIONING

Air-conditioning implies to control of both physical and chemical conditions of the atmosphere within any confined space or room. These factors include temperature, humidity, air movement, dust, bacteria, toxic gases, that affect the human health and comfort in greater or lesser degrees.

Comfort zone: It may be defined as the range of effective temperatures over which people feel comfortable. There is no unanimous opinion on a single zone of comfort for all people and it varies from person to person. In tropical countries after adequate air-conditioning, the air of a room should have a temperature of about 70°–72°F (21–22°C) and relative humidity of 60%. This varies due to certain factors, such as the individual, the nature of the clothes he is wearing and his state of health.

The problems of air-cooling in the tropics differ in principle according to the local conditions of weather and climate. In Northern India, the air in hot weather is excessively hot over 100°F, but is dry; thus reduction in temperature alone will give comfort, even if accompanied by a rise in relative humidity. Whereas in hot moist climates at sea ports like Kolkata, Mumbai and Chennai, discomfort is experienced both due to high temperature and humidity. Therefore, here reduction in both temperature and humidity is necessary.

2.14 LIGHTING

The lighting of buildings may be natural or artificial.

Natural lighting should be used where possible both for economy and for its beneficial effect on health. It is obtained by providing windows, which should have an area of at least one-tenth of floor space. The rays of sun include light rays, heat rays and invisible ultraviolet rays.

Artificial lighting should provide adequacy, consistency, and uniformity of illumination without flickering or glare and complete absence of shadows. Light may be produced by the combustion of substances, which burn with a flame or by an electric current. The commonest form of artificial lights are as follows:

1. **Non-electric lighting by flames like candles, paraffin lamps and gas lights:** These are most ancient forms of lighting used in places where there is no electricity. They give a very soft and poor light with a certain amount of flicker. They involve a great deal of labour in cleansing, trimming the wicks and filling the lamps with kerosene oil/gas. They have the disadvantage of blackening the walls and ceiling and emits light smell of petroleum. If there is not enough oxygen for complete combustion of coal gas, carbon monoxide may be formed and this gas is highly dangerous. Moreover, the great danger of coal gas is the risk of its escape, causing explosions or death from carbon monoxide poisoning.

2. **Electric lighting:** It does not involve combustion and, therefore, no oxygen is taken from the air and no waste substances are produced. Two types of lamps/bulbs—filament and fluorescent lamps are used for lighting. In first type, the electric current

heats up the tungsten filament of the electric bulbs and the light emitted depends upon the temperature produced. Fluorescent electric lighting is produced in fluorescent tube consisting of a glass tube filled with mercury vapour and an electrode fitted at each end. The inside of tube is coated with fluorescent chemicals, which absorb ultraviolet radiations. It produces better light with less heat and is advocated for certain purposes where a steady light, with a minimum of shadow is required.

Effects of bad lighting: The most common are: Eye strain, headache, tendency of deformity such as wry neck, round shoulders, poking head and lateral deviation of spine, irritability of temper, great liability to accidents. Poor lighting affects the quality as well as the quantity of work.

School lighting: This must be satisfactory because the continued strain of trying to see in an inadequate light is especially harmful to young children. The light should enter, if possible, over the left shoulder of the student and there should be an absence of glare from the blackboard and schoolbooks.

Artificial lighting of workshops and factories: It has been found in industry that inadequate lighting is uneconomical as the output tends to fall and there is an increased accident rate. If lighting is below certain level, the workers complain of discomfort and eye-strain. Poor lighting in coal mines is an important cause of miner's nystagmus.

Requirements for good lighting: The illumination should be adequate, constant and uniform. There should be no flicker or variation; glare and shadows due to bright light. Shadowless lighting is essential for certain types of fine work. Direct gaze at bright light must be avoided and every effort should be made to see that glaring light does not enter the eye even obliquely. Where possible fluorescent lighting should be provided, as it, besides being economical in the consumption of electric energy, avoids shadows and contrasts and, therefore, is helpful in increasing the efficiency of workers.

Disposal of Refuse: Human and Animal Excreta

In every town, public health largely depends on the efficiency with which all waste products are collected, removed and disposed off.

The waste products which require removal from human habitation are:

1. Excretal refuse, i.e. faeces and urine.[1]
2. Waste water from houses, works and factories.
3. Refuse:
   a. Dry refuse such as ashes, house dust, cinders, pieces of wood, iron, etc.
   b. Solid and liquid refuse from stables, cow sheds, slaughter houses, etc.
   c. Street sweepings such as rages, horse and cow-dung, etc.
   d. Garbage, leaves, vegetables, rotten fruits, kitchen waste, grease, etc.

Scavenging: It means the collection and removal of town and domestic refuse and other waste material, which is not carried away by sewers. This is done by manual labour.

Household and street refuse: This includes dry refuse from houses, streets and roads. It comprises mineral matter from sweepings, ashes, organic matters, waste scrapings of wood, paper and garden refuse, mainly consisting of leaves and other vegetable matter.

Trade refuse: It consists of refuse from any of the manufacturing trades or business concerns.

Consequences of incomplete removal of house and street sweeping are:

1. The contamination of the soil and pollution of subsoil water from which drinking water is derived.
2. Fly breeding.
3. Dissemination of filth diseases.
4. Dogs, birds, cattle, etc. scatter the refuse and increases nuisance.

3.1 COLLECTION AND REMOVAL OF REFUSE

It consists mainly of household, stable, cattle shed and street refuse. The nature of refuse depends upon the habits of the population.

1. **Household refuse collection:** The standard method is to put all domestic refuse into galvanised iron cans or tin tubs provided with handles and well-fitting lids. The lids prevent blowing away of refuse by wind and keep out the rainwater. On account of the organic matter contained therein, the domestic refuse will ferment and putrefy thus producing foul smell, which action is hastened by the presence of moisture. The lid of the tub also prevents flies from getting in and breeding in the refuse. It should be provided with a rim at the base so as to raise the bottom of the bin from the ground just to prevent its rotting due to dampness of the ground. The dustbins or tin tubs should have handles on each side and should be of sizes as can be handled conveniently by the conservancy staff. Moreover, these should be suitably placed at a fair distance from any dwelling house so that they can be reached conveniently by the conservancy staff without causing annoyance to the inhabitants. These should be emptied out daily, once in winter and twice in the hot weather in countries like India, where due to hot climate and rains, refuse decomposes rapidly and flies multiply enormously.

   For better and hygienic disposal of refuse, instead of conventional metallic dustbins, "paper sacks" are used. Domestic refuse is stored in the paper sacks and the sack itself is removed along with its contents by the conservancy staff for disposal/destruction at a far off place and a new storage paper sack is substituted in its place.

   Removal: The refuse should be collected in properly covered wheel barrows (Fig. 3.1) and refuse carts,

---

[1] In the case of adult Europeans, it amounts to about 4 oz of solid and 50 oz of fluid each day. While an Indian, owing to his vegetarian diet, passes 8–16 oz or more, on an average, 12 oz of solid excreta. In India, water is used instead of paper and this ablution water together with liquid excereta is about 80 oz.

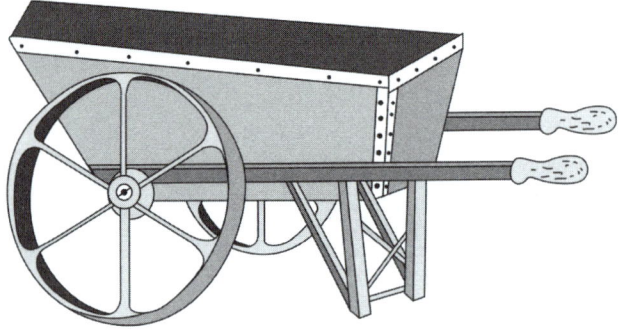

Fig. 3.1: Wheel barrow

provided with closed lids to prevent the refuse from being blown away by air. The wheel barrows are hand driven small carts and are used to collect refuse from narrow lanes and streets where ordinary refuse carts drawn by bullocks cannot go. The refuse collected through the agency of wheel barrows is eventually deposited into dustbins.

2. **Special refuse (i.e. from stables, cattle sheds, etc.):** It consists of grass, straw mixed with dung and moistened with urine. It ferments rapidly giving rise to objectionable smell. The more it is disturbed, the more it emits smell. The method adopted for its removal is that an iron conservancy cart is kept in the proximity, i.e. in the premises and this refuse is at once packed into the cart, which is removed at frequent intervals as and when required and an empty one left in its place.

3. **Street refuse collection:** It consists of droppings of animals, horses, and other cattle together with mineral matter swept along with street sweepings. In India, dustbins made of corrugated steel sheet are placed on raised concrete platforms, away from the dwelling houses. They should be of standard size and provided with handles for lifting. The street sweepings should be collected in these dustbins.

Removal: This is done by municipalities covered carts, tempo trucks and tippers fitted with mechanical means of tilting for quick and speedy removal of the refuse. The refuse should ideally be removed twice daily, both in the morning and evening.

3.2 DISPOSAL OF REFUSE

The refuse after collection should be disposed of in such a way that it does not create any nuisance. There are four methods for its disposal:

1. **Incineration:** It is one of the best methods of disposal of refuse at places, where suitable land for trenches is not available. It is rendered harmless by burning and the refuse reduced to one-fourth of its original weight. The organic matter is transformed into carbon dioxide and nitrogen. The residue left behind after the burning of refuse is a mass of hard material

called 'clinker'. After getting it thoroughly powdered and mixing it with lime, it has a great cementing action and is thus utilised for road making, an incinerator or the destructor furnace consists essentially of the following parts:

i. A furnace or a combustion chamber, built of fire-proof bricks with cement lining.
ii. A suitable arrangement with a platform for tipping the refuse through a series of feeding holes through which the refuse falls into the cells below.
iii. The stokers for raking the refuse forward to the fire.
iv. A baffle plate so placed that all fumes are driven through the hottest part of the incinerator's combusion chamber, before passing up through the chimney.

Various types of incinerators, *viz.* double cell Meldrum and single cell Horsfall destructors are available in the market, though they work on the same principle.

The **advantages** of incineration are that the cost of carting refuse is minimised to a very large extent. It is reduced to one-fourth of its original volume and residual ash or clinker can be used for making roads, mortar, cement or filter beds.

However, the **disadvantages** are that the disposal of refuse by burning deprives the community of the much needed manure. Also during rains or due to high moisture content, the refuse in the incinerators may not burn properly.

The incinerator will give off offensive smoke, which will obviously create nuisance, if the chimney of the incinerator is not sufficiently tall and the draught of the air is inadequate, to support the temperature of 1200°F (648.8°C) in the furnace for effective combustion (Fig. 3.2).

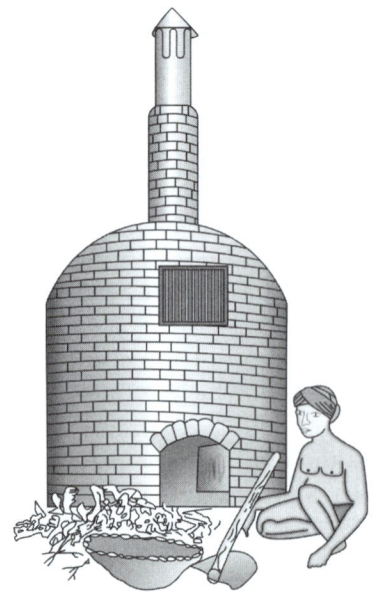

Fig. 3.2: An ordinary incinerator

2. **Dumping tipping:** In this method, the refuse is generally utilised in filling up clay pits or hollows, insanitary tanks or in reclaiming low lying lands. When these are filled by the refuse, the ground is called "made soil". This method creates a great nuisance to the neighbourhood on account of the production of offensive gases, breeding of flies, harbouring of rats and other vermin. The loose and uncovered refuse is often dispersed and scattered by the action of wind. The land selected should be situated outside the limits of the town, i.e. 100–150 feet (30.48–45.72 metres) away from the nearest habitation, to avoid unsightly scenes and nuisance to the nearby localities.

If dumping is done under proper supervision and during dry season, it is called "controlled dumping". In this method, the work of filling up should be started from one end and gradually continued on to the other end. Refuse material should be deposited in layers but not in any case exceeding 6 feet (1.83 metres) in depth and should be covered with about 9 inches (22.86 cm) thick layer of earth. No refuse should be left uncovered for more than 72 hours. Each layer of refuse along with the layer of earth lying over it should be allowed to settle, before the next layer is deposited upon it. Filling should be done 2 feet (0.6 metre) above the level of the surrounding area to allow subsequent settlement. When the work of filling is completed, cultivation should be done for about 10 years before the site is used for construction of residential houses.

Controlled tipping ⟨ Trench method / Ramp method / Area method

The World Health Organisation Expert Committee (1967) has disapproved dumping and characterised it as "a most insanitary method, which creates public health hazards, a nuisance and leads to pollution of environment". The WHO has recommended that dumping should be outlawed and replaced by other sanitary methods of refuse disposal.

3. **Compost formation:** This method is used mainly in towns, where refuse has to be disposed off with nightsoil and its main objective is to convert the waste matter into humus or compost of high manurial value.

Compost formation ⟨ Bangalore method / Mechanical composting

4. **Sorting:** This method consists of sorting the refuse into three parts:
   i. *Breeze:* It consists of cinder and small particles of coal. It is used in brick making.
   ii. *Soft core:* It consists of animal and vegetable organic matter. It is used as a manure.
   iii. *Hard core:* It consists of broken bottles, crockery, tiles, etc. It is utilised for metalling roads.

3.3. COLLECTION, REMOVAL AND DISPOSAL OF HUMAN EXCRETA

For this purpose, the following systems are adopted:

A. **Unsewered areas**
   1. Conservancy system (service type): Its efficiency depends upon the methodical collection, removal and disposal of night-soil.
   2. Non-service type (sanitary latrines):
      i. Borehole latrine
      ii. Dug well or pit latrine
      iii. Water seal type of latrines (PRAI, RCA, Sulabh Shauchalaya)
      iv. Septic tank
      v. Aqua privy
   3. Latrines suitable for camps and temporary use.
      i. Shallow trench latrine
      ii. Deep trench latrine
      iii. Pit latrine
      iv. Borehole latrine

B. **Sewered areas:** Water carriage system (*see* Chapter 4).

Health hazards of unhygienic refuse disposal: Health hazards may be listed as: (a) smell nuisance, (b) un-aesthetic sights, (c) fly breeding, (d) rodents breeding, (e) hogs feeding, (f) water pollution, (g) soil pollution, and (h) contamination of food. Putrefying organic refuse is very conducive for creating above mentioned health hazards.

3.4 CONSERVANCY SYSTEM, COLLECTION OF NIGHT SOIL

In this system, the excreta has to be collected and removed by manual labour. This method is an old system and is employed in underdeveloped towns, however, it is being replaced by water carriage system in the developed towns and cities (Fig. 3.3).

The efficient working of this system is of great importance. The principle aimed at is that filth, refuse and all other putrescible matters should not be exposed to flies or allowed to contaminate the sources of water and should be transported and disposed off safely without causing even the least possible nuisance.

1. **Privy system:** The privy is meant for private use. It is simply a place where excreta is deposited until removed. It should consist of a brick built and cement lined chamber and should be of a small size and provided with a proper seat. The object of cement lining is to make it waterproof, so that the contents should not permeate into the ground and contaminate the underground water. It should be well ventilated having a window of not less than 3 square feet (0.28 sq metre) and have a provision

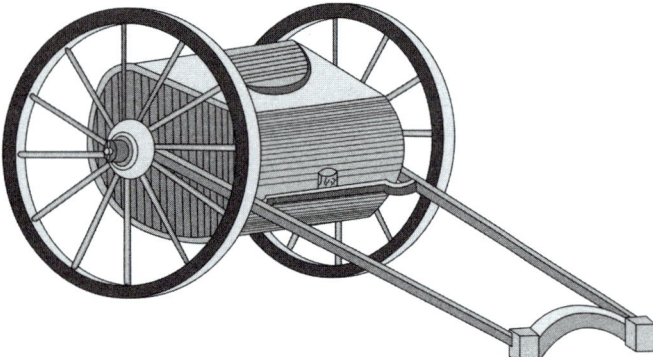

Fig. 3.3: Night soil or crawly cart

for an adequate supply of air and an external wall to permit light ventilation. It should be protected from flies by providing wire-gauze to the windows and doors so that they may not be a source of infection especially disease germs of dysentery, typhoid, cholera, etc.

Privy system is most objectionable as it gives rise to nuisance of smell especially when it is cleaned out. In addition, there is a danger of fly breeding. Although privy system is the simplest, yet at the same time most insanitary out of all systems. Besides, there is a likelihood of leakage and thus it may lead to water and soil pollution.

2. **Pail system:** This is an improvement over privy system. Here a pail or any other removable receptacle is placed underneath the seat which is removed as soon as possible after the use of the privy, and immediately after that emptied out by the sweeper in a storage pail provided with a well-fitting lid, cleaned and kept ready for reuse.

3. **The commode:** Its use is very common at places where there is no adequate water carriage system. It consists essentially of a hinged wooden seat fitted with a self-closing lid to make it fly-proof and is provided with a big circular hole in its centre under which removable enamelled steel, porcelain or steel receptacle is placed. The pail from the commode is removed by the sweeper immediately after use. It is taken off by him in a basket to a place of secondary collection. Here the contents of the pail are emptied out into a large collecting drum. The pail is cleaned and refitted to the wooden seat. In most houses, some suitable disinfectant is also supplied to the sweeper for scrupulous cleansing of the pail.

4. **Earth closet:** This is an improvement over the pail system to the extent that mechanical arrange-ments are provided for disposing of a large quantity of earth into the pail after use. The earth acts as a deodorant; prevents the emittance of foul smell, and is mixed with faeces who ensures complete disintegration in a short time.

5. **Pit latrine:** A pit or a well-like hole 10–20 feet (3.05–6.09 metres) deep is dug in the ground to receive the excreta. At the top of it, a masonary platform having provision of a seat and a superstructure is built. In such a privy, the septic tank action goes on, if there is some water in it and the night-soil is liquified. This system is objectionable from sanitary point of view as not only foul gases are evolved but there is a risk of pollution of water supply of the surrounding area through soakage, especially after a rise in the level of subsoil water during rainy season.

6. **Borehole latrine (Fig. 3.4):** This is a modification of a pit latrine. It was first introduced by the Rockefeller Foundation during 1930 while campaigning for the control of hookworm disease. It consists of a circular hole of 14–16 inches (0.35–0.41 metres) in diameter sunk 18–20 feet (5.49–6.09 metres) deep under the ground by means of a machine called Auger, until the surface of subsoil water is reached.

   The opening of the hole is covered at the top with a concrete slab of about 2 feet 9 inches (0.84 metre) in diameter for squatting. It is provided with a central slot 5.5" (139.7 mm) wide and 12"–15" (0.30–0.38 metre) long and is fitted with footrests on either side. The hole structure is enclosed with mud or a brick wall about 5 or 6 feet (1.52 or 1.83 metres) high for screening purposes.

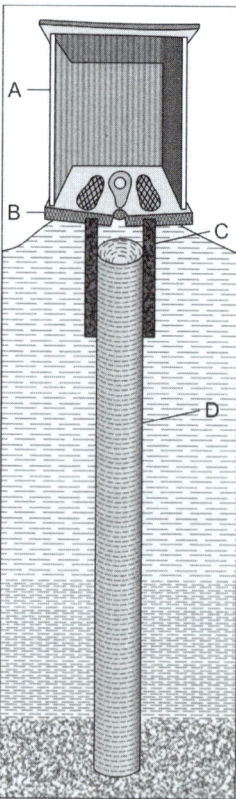

Fig. 3.4: Borehole latrine: A—superstructure, B—squatting plate, C—concrete cylinder, D—bamboo basket

Care should, however, be taken that the hole penetrates about 2–3 feet (0.6–0.9 metre) below the surface left out of subsoil water, which helps to dissolve the excreta and in setting up septic tank action. This dilution of excreta with water is very essential.

A lining of split-up bamboo is put inside the wall of the latrine hole to prevent the earth from collapsing or falling in. That is why it is essential that the latrine should be sunk in a hard soil.

A small quantity of pestrine should be sprinkled or a solution of crude oil 4 parts and kerosene oil one part sprayed into the hole of the latrine once a week to keep away flies, etc. When the hole gets filled up with excreta up to 3 feet (0.9 metre) from the ground level, it should be filled in with dry earth and the squatting plate removed and fitted over another freshly dug borehole latrine.

7. **Dugwell latrine:** It is another form of a well privy commonly advocated in rural areas for preventing the spread of hookworm infection. It consists of a pit 15 feet (4.5 metres) deep with a diameter of 3 feet (0.9 metre). It is provided with 0.5 inch (12.7 mm) water seal and a squatting plate of 3.5 feet (1.07 metres) diameter. It can be flushed with half a gallon (2.273 litres) of water. Septic tank action takes place. One latrine is enough for about 5 years for a family of 5 persons without any attention. A superstructure made of mud bricks and bamboo or palm matting is provided for privacy. It is better than a borehole latrine because:

   i. It is free from nuisance of fly breeding.
   ii. There is no pollution of subsoil water.
   iii. It does not give out offensive gases and smell due to presence of waterseal.
   iv. It can be constructed with an ordinary spade by a mason or a mistry. No special implement is required, as say, an Auger required for a borehole latrine.
   v. It is comparatively cheaper and has a longer life than borehole latrine.

Well, pit, borehole or dug well latrines should not be constructed within 50–100 ft. (15.24–30.48 metres) from any source of water supply (practical aspects previously discussed). When they are filled up to 2.5 ft. (0.76 metre) from the ground level, they should be filled with earth and new ones should be constructed. These latrines are useful for small villages, isolated houses and tea gardens. They are cheap and if properly constructed, last for a long time.

8. **Trench latrines, shallow type:** These consist of rows of parallel trenches. The trenches are 3 feet (0.9 metre) long, one foot (0.3 metre) wide and 1–2 feet (0.3–0.6 metre) deep and are dug at a distance of two feet (0.6 metre) away from each other. These may be provided with privacy screens. The faeces, urine, and ablution water fall directly into the trench. The trench after use should be filled up by excavated earth, and heaped above ground level and suppressed. The trenches are suitable as a temporary measure during fairs, etc. in rural areas.

9. **Trench latrines, deep type:** Each trench should be about 3 ft. (0.9 metre) deep and of a suitable length, usually 13 ft. (3.96 metres). The sides should be rivetted with sand bags, wire-netting or bamboo-matting to prevent their collapse. A fly-proof wooden super-structure with a hinged lid opening is placed in position over the top. The seats are properly screened. The person using the trench latrine should place one foot on each side of the trench. He should squat in such a way that the faeces and urine fall directly into the trench.

10. **Chemical closet:** It consists of a seat resting on the top of a metal tank which is filled with a liquefying solution of caustic soda and phenol and covered with a layer of crude oil. The excreta falls into this solution, which gets disintegrated in soda solution. Phenol kills bacteria and oil acts as a deodorant. Throwing of anything into the chemical closet, except toilet paper should be strictly prohibited. If water is thrown into the closet, the chemical solution will get diluted and consequently the closet will not function properly. When the tanks get filled up, they are emptied and the contents are either taken out and thrown away or discharged into a dump hole. These are mostly used in aeroplanes, trains, buses, etc. and in places where they are not frequently required. Chemical closets are of two types:

   i. *Portable chemical closet:* It occupies comparatively less space, and is, therefore, very suitable for use in motor coaches, small ships, aircrafts, etc. It can also be installed in houses, where there is no water carriage system. It is in the form of a pail closet, where receptacle is placed inside a portable metal container. Chemicals in the form of an emulsion are placed inside the pail, which completely covers the excreta. It subsequently deodorises, liquifies and sterilises, rendering the excreta harmless, which is disposed off into the earth through a simple soakage pit later.

   ii. *Permanent chemical closet:* In the case of permanent camps, sports grounds and country houses, where there is no water carriage system, permanent chemical closets are installed. It differs from the portable type that excreta instead of being collected into a removable pail falls into a tank, which is permanently installed.

11. **Aqua privy:** It is a miniature water tight septic tank consisting of a masonry tank or a water tank reservoir of an approximate size 3 × 2.5 ft. (0.9 × 0.76 metre) provided with a 2.5 ft. (0.76 metre) long tube merged into the tank. A platform and a squatting plate is provided on the top. The effluent is allowed to percolate into the soil or taken out in a receptacle and used for irrigation purposes. This method is suitable for isolated private houses having small gardens. Water is to be added every time during and after its use and the ventilation tube is to be kept open to provide exit, for the foul gases. A capacity of 1 cubic ml is recommended for a small family, allowing a period of 5–6 years for cleans-ing purposes.

12. **Cesspools:** These are built for the reception of waste waters and sewage in those places where sewers have not been installed. These consist of underground pits made of bricks, and lined with cement for water-proofing. When filled up, they are emptied out into sewage carts or trolleys and the contents disposed off in the fields, for use as a manure. However, their drawback is that if they are badly constructed, the waste water may percolate through the soil and thus contaminate the subsoil water.

13. **Soakage pits:** In this system, a pit is dug into the ground approximately 5–6 feet (1.52–1.83 metre) deep and 2.5–3 feet (0.76–0.91 metre) wide and filled to the top with small stones and pebbles. Waste water is carried to the pit by means of a drain, after entangling the fat and oil from kitchen waste by means of a grease trap. The waste water percolates and soaks away into the ground from the pit. Soakage pits should not be constructed near the wells, for fear of contaminating the sub-soil water.

Settling tank and grease chamber: Waste water from the house contains a lot of grease and some solid materials as well, which when allowed as such into the pit, clogs the pores of soaking bricks, and after sometime reduces the soaking capacity and efficiency of the pit to a large extent. To get rid of it, it is recommended that a settling tank and a grease chamber should be provided just before the pit. It means that drain containing waste water first empties itself into the settling tank which screens the solid material and screened water containing grease, finds its way to the grease chamber, where grease is arrested by the projecting wall of the chamber and greaseless water gets into the pit.

Etawah-type soakage pits

i. Here a hole of diameter 16" (0.4 metre) is made at a raised ground with the help of an 'Auger' (a boring equipment), which can be purchased by Gram Panchayats or other local institutions, up to a minimum depth of 16" (the more the depth the more the life of the pit). At about 6", i.e. 15 cm below from the top, an earthen pot is fixed, which serves as a grease chamber and leads the contents of the drain through the mouth, and passes it down to the bored pit through the hole made at the pit-side of the earthen pot.

ii. *Precautions*
   a. The top of the bored hole is to be covered properly to prevent any accident.
   b. It should be at least 25 ft. or 7.6 metres away from the well site as far as possible to prevent any pollution.
   c. Ground should be raised and pit should be disconnected in the rainy season.

iii. *Cost and durability:* It involves no cost except the earthen pot. It does not work for more than 2 years, after which it has to be shifted to another site.

iv. *Advantage:* It requires minimum of space and involves no cost.

14. **Public latrines** (Fig. 3.5): A latrine is a privy meant for public use consisting of a number of seats for several persons. These may be constructed temporary or permanent according to the requirements. The temporary ones are generally used in fairs, *melas,* camps, temporary settlements, etc. more commonly in dry parts of India. The receptacle for night-soil is placed on the ground and the latrines are provided with masonry footrests. These require no plinth or roof. They have corrugated steel sheet partitions. The site should be high and there is no other masonry construction. The permanent latrines should never be located within a distance of 20 feet (6.1 metres) from any dwelling house, public road or within a distance of 50 feet (15.24 metres) from any source of water supply.

Construction: The floor should be cemented or made with any other impervious material such as

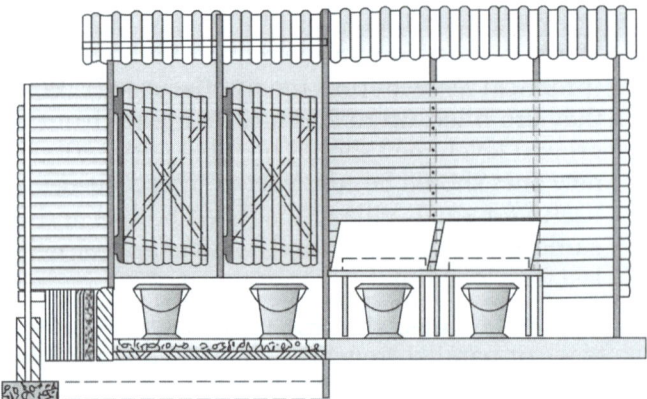

Fig. 3.5: Public latrine—four-seated

stone or slate so as to make it waterproof. It should be properly sloped backward up to an open channel leading to a collection pit dug at one of the corners of the latrine. In the pit, a removeable bucket is placed and connected to a delivery pipe to catch surface drainage of the latrine. It should be roofed over to provide shelter from sun and rain and be provided with privacy screens. These privacy screens should stop short, about 1 ft. (0.3 metre) from the cemented floor all round to allow entrance for sun rays and free ventilation. The roof should be sloped or curved to facilitate draining of rainwater. The walls may be either of brick work or corrugated steel sheet and strict privacy should be maintained. They should preferably be pigeon holed towards the upper half for proper ventilation, or else provided with ventilators. The seats should be arranged in a row. A flap door is provided at the back for removal of the bucket by the sweeper. The entrance doors should be labelled conspicuously for men and women separately with diagrams of respective sexes for easy understanding.

The standard type latrine seat is simply an elevated platform of galvanized iron with footrests, a central hole and under this hole a bucket, a pail or a *kimali* is placed. It must be wider than the size of the hole, so as to obviate possibility of excreta missing the bucket. The seat must be kept clean and occasionally coal tarred to prevent the ammoniacal fermentation due to decomposition of the urine. Footrests must be made in the right position and they should be reasonably wide apart so that the faeces may fall direct into the receptacle below. In order to prevent splashing, the receptacle should be placed directly below the opening at a distance of about 2–3 feet (0.6–0.9 metre) although in some cases this distance may be even more. In order to keep the latrine clean, a sweeper must be constantly present there on duty especially during the time when latrine remains much in use. The duty of the sweeper should be to empty the pail into the collecting drum and after cleaning the pail, to keep it back at its place. There must be dry earth stored near the latrine which

should be sprinkled in the pail in order to avoid the excreta adhering to it. If pails are not kept clean, they will emit foul smell due to decomposition of urine, etc. Similarly, if the surface drainage is not attended to, there will be a constant nuisance from smell and it will provide a breeding place for flies, but if proper lids are provided on the drains, these dangers will get considerably diminished. The storage or collecting drums are either removed in a cart or their contents emptied out into a crawly cart.

RCA Latrine

The RCA latrine comprises a squatting plate, made of an impervious material like cement concrete. This is easy to clean and maintain. Raised footsteps are included in the squatting plate. There is a pan directly underneath the squatting plate. The pan receives the night soil. Pan is connected to the trap, which is a bent pipe. RCA latrine the trap holds water and serves as a water seal. The depth of the water seal is 2 cm. The trap is connected to the pit through a connecting pipe. When the pit fills up another one can be dug up and pipe may be accordingly shifted. The pit can also be made directly underneath the pan. An appropriate superstructure can be made. It is easy to maintain the latrine. Latrine is hand flushed by pouring 1 to 2 litre of water every time the latrine is used. The squatting plate should also be washed clean every day. Water seal prevents access to flies and avoids release of odour (Fig. 3.6).

It is said that for these latrines, at least two sweepers are required to adequately look after each set of latrines to be kept constantly clean. Otherwise, being unclean they will not be much used by the public because of unsightly scenes and nuisance of foul smell, fly breeding, etc.

3.5 DISPOSAL OF NIGHT SOIL

It can be done by any of the following methods in a conservancy system:
a. Trenching
b. Incineration of night soil
c. Compost or manure making.

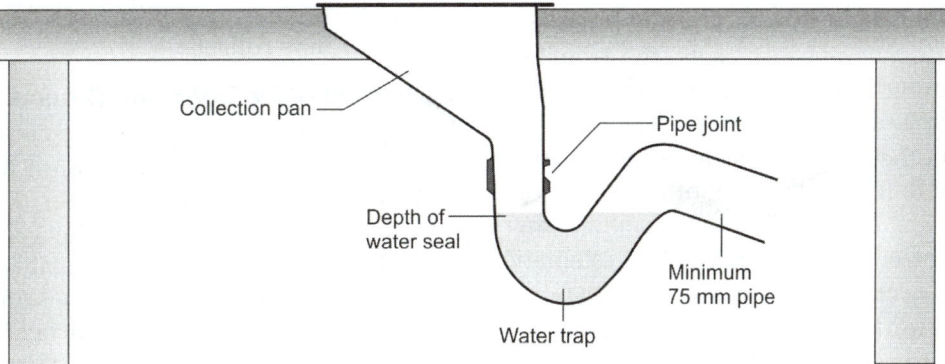

Fig. 3.6: RCA latrine

Trenching

This is a standard method which is compulsorily adopted in all the cantonments and military stations in India, but this system is not very much resorted to by most of the municipalities probably because it does not bring any revenue and a difficulty is experienced by the authorities in procuring land near the towns, for this particular purpose.

Selection of Site for Trenches

The ground for the trenches should be selected at a suitable distance from the town and should not be too close to it. The ground should be at a higher level because the low lying land is liable to be encroached upon by floods during rainy season or may become waterlogged. The soil should be loamy, alluvial and sturdy. Even clay soil is good, provided it is not wet and sticky. It should be situated in the neighbourhood of a source of water supply but should be at least 300 yards (274.32 metres) away from it. Moreover, it should be about 600 yards (548.64 metres) away from all human habitation. The ground should be situated on one side of the town away from the prevailing winds and should be separated from the town by means of some quick growing trees. The approach to the trench ground should be easy and accessible, preferably by a coal tarred road.

Preparation for Trenching Ground

The selected area is levelled and drained and is then divided into 12 parts, thus earmarking one part for each month of the year. It should be intersected with properly planned metalled roads to be used for carts. The plot which is once trenched should not be used again for making trenches for at least 2 years.

Emphasis should be laid on the following points in the management of an ideal trenching ground:

1. There should be an adequate arrangement for the systematic drainage of rainwater.
2. There should be a provision for one or two roads for carts to reach right up to the trenches.
3. Some source of water supply should be made available in the neighbourhood of the trenching ground to facilitate washing of carts and buckets.
4. After filling the excreta into carts, the trenches should be immediately covered with earth to prevent breeding of flies.
5. The carts and other appliances should be cleaned periodically with liquid disinfectant like crude oil, phenyl, etc.
6. The process of trench filling should be systematic and should proceed from one end to the other.
7. Cultivation should not be allowed at least for 3 months after trenching. It is preferable that dhoop grass be cultivated first.

Kinds of Trenches

The following kinds of trenches are generally used:
1. *Shallow:* These are dug 2 feet (0.6 metre) wide and 9 inches (22.86 cm) deep. In these trenches, 2 inches (5.08 cm) thick layer of filth is spread, at the bottom of the trenches having been previously loosened. It is then covered with earth.
2. *Deep:* These are also 2 feet (0.6 metre) wide but are 12 to 18 inches (0.3–0.45 metre) in depth. These should be situated 2 feet (0.6 metre) apart from each other. In these trenches, 8 inches (20.32 cm) thick layer of filth can be spread and then covered with excavated earth.
3. *Allahabad system of trenching:* This is really the shallow trench system and is used in cantonments. Each trench is 16 feet (4.88 metres) long and 5 feet (1.52 metres) broad but is only 3 inches (7.62 cm) deep. The base of the trench is dug up and the soil loosened up to the depth of 9 inches (22.86 cm). The filth is then put into the trench and thoroughly mixed with the loose earth. The trench is finally filled up with earth.

Area of Ground Required

In shallow trenching system 180 square feet (16.72 sq metres) of ground area per day is required for a population of 1000. This area includes the trenches as well as the ground between them used for making roads, etc. 1.5 acres (0.60 hectare) of land is required for making such type of trenches to cope up with the requirements of a population of 1000 for full one year.

In deep trenching system, one-fourth of the above area is required or about one-third area of land per 1000 population. This calculation will permit trenches being left undisturbed for a year.

Filling of Trenches

These are laid out in a line and the night soil is poured down into them from the storage pails or crawly carts by manual labour. These are filled up with an excess of earth, so as to form elevated mounds or domes above the surface of ground. This would allow some amount of sinkage, due to subsequent settling of the earth, without forming any hollows or depressions, where rainwater may collect.

Cultivation of the Trenching Ground

It is very important for the success of trenching ground, as otherwise the ground becomes sewage sick and unfit for retrenching. So, three months after filling up of the trenches, the ground should be ploughed and sown with any suitable crop. Practically any crop will grow but the general rule adopted is that the vegetables usually eaten uncooked should not be grown. In Punjab, crops like tobacco, sugarcane, lucerngrass, etc. are usually sown. The objection to growing vegetables is based upon the assumption that they might pick up infection from the soil. It has been also stated that the eggs of intestinal parasites, i.e. worms may be carried by vegetables grown in the trenching ground. In very dry climate, the trenching ground should be irrigated to prevent soil becoming dry and hard. Moreover, trenches should not be too shallow, otherwise the wind may blow away the surface and expose the trenches to fly-breeding. This is the main objection put to the Allahabad system of trenching. The ordinary housefly quickly lays its eggs on human excreta and if the trenches happen to be superficial, then the hatching larvae will have no difficulty in developing into adults which would be congenitally infected with pathogenic germs, i.e. typhoid, etc. and may retain the germs for some time in their bodies. Shallow trenching is preferable because deep trenching requires very deep ploughing to yield mamirial value of filth.

Objects of Trenching

Soil is a great bacteriological laboratory and the bacteria present in the soil very rapidly break up the organic constituents of the night soil into simple non-putrefiable compounds, which are used up by the plants in the process of metabolism. Various gases are given off in this process but these are absorbed by the pores of the earth and so once the filth has been buried underground, it gets satisfactorily and economically disposed of without causing any nuisance owing to its foul smell. Experiments reveal that the soil bacteria or the nitrifying organisms which are most active in breaking up the filth and converting the organic nitrogen in the excreta into nitrates are contained in the superficial layer of the soil and this is the greatest requirement of shallow trenching system because the process is quick. The deeper the trenches, the slower is the process. In the case of deep pits, the filth may remain unaltered for years together, because the deep layer of earth contains very few bacteria. In addition, the bacteria of soil very quickly kills all pathogenic germs present in faeces and the urine.

Dangers of Trenching

These are:
1. Pollution of groundwater and wells.
2. If trenches are not sufficiently deep, eggs of flies, which have been laid on the faeces may develop.
3. Superficial trenching of human excreta may lead to exposure of the night soil in consequence of earth getting dried and blown away.
4. If not properly supervised, it may give rise to the nuisance of obnoxious smell.

Incineration of Night Soil

If properly carried out in a well-designed furnace, it will be found to be sanitary and the danger of polluting the water supply or the air through its smoke vapours will be reduced to the minimum. The incineration of night soil may or may not be combined with the incineration of street refuse. Where street refuse contains a large proportion of dry grass, straw, rags, paper scrapings, etc. these may serve as fuel. The incinerator should be installed near the latrines or near the pail depot. The sweeper should be present there constantly. The night soil should always be placed on the fire in small quantities at a time. A covered shed for the collection of dry fuel (viz. wood shavings, saw dust, dry grass or straw, etc.) should be constructed near the incinerator. The incinerator is started by placing a small quantity of dry refuse and setting it on fire. When the combustion has proceeded for some time, the contents of latrine pans, etc. are poured over the smouldering material. For efficient working of the incinerator, the chimney should be large and sufficiently high. Moreover, the number of air inlets must be adequate to ensure good draught. It is preferable to render the smoke inodorous either by providing a baffle plate or by placing a horizontal grid below the entry of flue. On the whole, this method requires supervision and is costly.

Compost or Manure Making

Composting is the process of biological fermentation and decomposition by which bulky organic refuse (may be animal or vegetable in origin), is changed into manure by the aid of living organisms such as bacteria, protozoa, actinomycetes, fungi, etc. During the process over a period of several days, the heat produced exceeds 60°C temperature, which is sufficient to destroy pathogenic agents, including eggs and larvae of flies.

The essential requirements of proper composting are:

1. Suitable carbon–nitrogen ratio 30:1. The dry refuse obtained from town and household sweepings is usually deficient in nitrogen while night-soil and cow dung are rich in it. For proper composting, a suitable admixture of the two, viz. the dry refuse and night soil or cow dung is desirable. An admixture of about equal weight, of the refuse and night soil, would give the desirable carbon–nitrogen ratio of 30:1. If the proportion of night soil is less, the decomposition will be slow. But when it is more than the actual requirements, then there is a danger of loss of nitrogen taking place.

2. Presence of a suitable amount of moisture is essential for its proper decomposition. The quantity of water should be as much as can be retained by the material. If the amount of moisture is deficient, the rate of decomposition would be slow, but if there happens to be an excess of moisture, there

would be a danger of water logging with consequent loss of nitrogen.

3. Aeration of the night soil in initial stages is beneficial but excessive aeration promotes rapid decomposition; resulting in unnecessary loss of the material and its nutrients. For proper decomposition, the mass should be neither too compact nor too loose.

Procedure

The following procedure is recommended for the preparation of compost manure in different cases:

a. *Trenching ground:* It should be situated at a distance of about 2–4 furlongs (402.32–804.64 metres) away from the nearest habitation. It should be on a raised ground, so that it is not waterlogged during rainy season. To avoid obnoxious smell coming into the town, it should be located on the windward side.

b. *Trenches:* The size of trenches should be adjusted according to the amount of refuse likely to be available daily so that one or more trenches are completely filled up on each day. The breadth of the trench should be 6–8 feet (1.83–2.44 metres), so that an average-sized cart or a truck could be emptied out into the trench conveniently. The depth of the trenches should be about 3 feet (0.91 metre). Given the breadth and the depth, the length of the trenches should be adjusted to suit the amount of material likely to be available. Trenches are arranged in rows, so that longer sides are parallel and shorter ends are in the same line. There is an intervening space of 4–8 feet (1.22–2.44 metres) "between one trench and the other". A suitable earth bund should be provided on all sides of the trenches to prevent rainwater from flowing in.

c. *Methods of working*
   1. *For places when refuse and night soil are collected in a mixed state:* The material containing proper proportion of refuse and night soil (i.e. equal weight of each) should be dumped directly into the trench. While the cart is being emptied out into the trench, two men should be deputed (one on each side) for raking up and spreading the material evenly in the trench with long-handled rakes. After the material is properly raked and spread over, sufficient amount of water is added to moisten the material. The addition of water should be done before another cart load is emptied into the trench. This procedure is carried on till the trench is filled up to 6–9 inches (15.24 to 22.86 cm) above the ground level, then a thin covering of earth or old manure, varying from 1 to 2 inches (2.54–5.08 cm) thick should be evenly spread over the material.

   2. *For places where night soil and refuse are collected separately:* In this case at first a layer of 9 inches (22.86 cm) thick dry refuse (free from brick-bats and other inert material) is spread over at the bottom of trench. Then a layer of 2–3 inches (5.08–7.62 cm) emulsion of night-soil is spread over it by means of long-handled *phaudas.* This is followed by another layer of dry refuse and alternative layering repeated with night-soil and dry refuse till the trench is filled up to 9–12 inches (22.86–30.48 cm) above the ground level. The top layer in all cases is the dry refuse which is covered with 1–2 inches (2.54–5.08 cm) thick layer of dry earth. This topmost layer of earth will prevent loss of moisture, breeding of flies and smell nuisance. If the earth covering is more than 2 inches (5.08 cm) thick, it is likely to hinder proper aeration of the mass.

   After a period of about 2–4 weeks, the material in the trenches would settle down by 6–8 inches (15.24–20.32 cm). In this case, if need be, some more fresh material can be put on the top and covered with a thin layer of earth.

d. *Aftercare:* During the hot weather, there is a danger of the trenched material getting dry and, therefore, some water should be again evenly sprinkled over the filled trenches from time to time. The compost should be ready for use within four to six months depending upon the type of material used and the prevailing season.

e. *Sanitary and economic aspects of composting:* If the system of composting is adopted as a routine method for disposal of habitation wastes not only a quantity of good quality manure is made available for cultivators but the sanitation of the town also gets improved considerably. The smell and fly nuisance is also greatly reduced.

During the process of composting, considerable heat (60°–70°C) is produced in the mass and it destroys most of the pathogenic organisms, fly larvae, weeds, seeds and other obnoxious constituents and thus renders the resultant material practically innocuous.

In most cases, the income from the sale of refuse after composting is much more than it is from the sale of raw refuse.

3.6 DISADVANTAGES OF THE CONSERVANCY SYSTEM

These are as follows:

1. The night soil remains in privies and latrines for a long time and putrefaction starts from removal. This gives rise to nuisance due to smell, atmospheric and soil pollution.

2. Night soil carts emit foul smell when wheeled on the roads, so in some places they are moved on the road at night.

3. Latrines at different places cause inconvenience.

4. Conversion of unstable inorganic compounds of excreta into stable organic matters requires anaerobic conditions and an open place.

5. Insanitary conditions prevail due to employment of human beings for the removal of excreted matter.

6. It is not economical from financial point of view as it is very slow and involves dependency on labour at various stages as compared to the automatic functioning of water carriage system.

7. The wear and tear of the night soil carts, pails and other appliances is very great.

8. The system is manifested with dangers of contamination of air and water and spread of infection through flies, etc.

9. Rats may breed in open privies wherein addition to excreta, there is generally an abundance of general household refuse.

*Health hazards of unhygienic faecal disposal:*Health hazards are many. In fact hygienic faecal disposal, if possible to implement scrupulously in a community (as has been done by developed communities) can lead to complete control of faecal-borne infections. The health hazards may be listed as (a) enteric infections transmitted through contaminated water and food, e.g. diarrhoea, dysentery, typhoid and paratyphoid group of fevers, food poisoning, cholera, infected hepatitis, poliomyelitis, amoebiasis, ascariasis, and other infections, and (b) soil transmitted infections and infestations, e.g. ankylostomiasis and other enteric infections transmitted through soil to food and water.

Water Carriage System

In a great majority of large towns, human excreta and urine is now removed along with the liquid waste of dwellings by a flush of water by force of gravity through a network of underground pipes called sewers leading to a far off place outside the town. This is the cleanest and the most sanitary method of removing night soil provided there is plenty of water available for the purpose.

Sewage: It comprises excreta, urine, house waste and rainwater, together with solid refuse from cow-sheds, stables, houses and factories, etc. It contains 99% or even more of water. Its offensive nature is due to presence of organic matter, which undergoes put-refaction and emits foul smell.

Sullage: Waste water from houses, etc. unmixed with human excreta is usually known as 'Sullage'.

Conditions essential for the successful working of water carriage system are:

1. Availability of an abundant supply of water for flushing water closets.
2. Provision of good underground drains and sewers with proper ventilation.
3. Sufficient fall to give required velocity to the sewage.
4. Proper means of utilisation of sewage.

A complete layout of water carriage system consists of:

1. A system of house drainage leading to sewers.
2. A system of sewers.

A complete system of house drainage consists of water closet, soil pipe, house drain with manholes or inspection chambers, leading to a public sewer.

4.1 WATER CLOSET

It is a sanitary installation for the reception of the human excreta and is connected with a sewer through the soil pipe. It may be broadly divided into two types, viz. Indian squatting type and Western commode type.

It should fulfil the following conditions:

1. It should be made of hard, smooth and impermeable material as glazed stoneware, fire clay or porcelain.
2. It should be of wash-down pedestal form.
3. The posterior wall should be vertical.
4. It should have 2 inches (5.08 cm) of water-seal.
5. It should have flushing rim all around.
6. Trap and pan should be of one piece.
7. The trap should be of S or P type.
8. It should have a hinged seat.
9. Height of the closet should be more than 18 inches (0.46 metre).
10. Closet should be fixed in a compartment with at least one external wall and a window of the size of 2 feet × 1 foot (0.6 × 0.3 metre) opening to the outer air, half of which must remain open. There should be a provision for cross-ventilation.
11. Flushing should be efficient to wash the basin clean and remove all traces of excreta with the minimum amount of water.

Parts of a water closet: These consist of the following:

1. Closet proper with a basin and a trap.
2. Flushing apparatus.

Bidet: In India, most of the people use water instead of paper for cleansing purposes and this ablution water spoils the seat and footrests. To obviate this, an appliance known as *bidet* has been introduced for washing the anal region and perineum. It is provided with a flushing and circulating rim, an open stream outflow and a plug outlet. It is generally connected to the waste pipe and not directly to soil pipe or the drain.

Situation of water closet: It should be situated near outer wall of the house. The floor should be made up of white tiles which should be carried around the wall also up to a height of 3 feet (0.9 metre). The closet should be mounted bare, without any wooden structure and the supply pipe should be kept free on the wall and painted white. A window opening directly into the open air must be provided. The rest of the wall should be distempered with a waterproof paint. The room should contain nothing else except the water closet. The practice of putting bath tub in the same room is now being stopped. The water closet is connected to the spoilable by an S-shaped bend called the trap.

Flushing apparatus: Since the water closet should be flushed immediately after use, it is essential that a provision should be made for the storage and discharge of water. The water for flushing the water closet is provided by means of a separate flushing cistern of about 12.5 litre capacity with the minimum capacity should be 2 gallons (9.09 litres). The water closet is constructed to work with that amount and the cistern is placed above the closet at a height of not less than 6 ft (1.83 metres). It is connected directly to the closet at the flushing rim. The cistern is connected to the house water supply and is controlled by a ball valve. The cistern delivers its water by siphon action which is set in motion by pulling a chain and letting it go. The flushing rim must go all around the closet and for the satisfactory operation of the flush system it must be distributed evenly over the entire surface of the closet (Fig. 4.1).

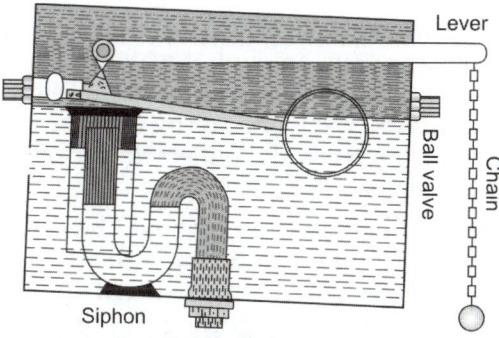

Fig. 4.1: Siphon flushing cistern

4.2 SOIL PIPE

It is a circular pipe carrying the contents of water closet to the house drain. It is made of cast iron or milled lead. It has an internal diameter of about 4 inches (10.16 cm). It is carried clear of the window 6–8 ft (1.83–2.44 metres) above the roof for escape of foul gases. Its end may be covered with a gauze dome. To prevent oxidation or rusting, iron soil pipes are coated either with a paint containing magnetic oxide of iron called *Barffs Process* or may be dipped in Angus Smith Varnish, which is composed of pitch, asphalt and tallow. Lead pipes can be more conveniently and expeditiously fitted. These pipes should be laid as straight as possible and preferably be fixed on the shady side of the house so that the joints may not be damaged in the heat of the sun. The soil pipe should be placed against the outer wall of the house so that it may

be easily inspected and extended beyond the roof. To allow a free circulation of air and escape of foul gases generated, the loose end of the pipe should open over a disconnecting trap outside the house. Moreover, its upper end should be carried on to at least 5 ft (1.52 metres) above the roof of the house. It has been found through experience that the soil pipe should open directly into the house drain without intervention of a trap, as it imposes a useless barrier to the sewage and prevents the soil pipe acting as a drain ventilator.

Anti-siphonage pipe: When the soil pipe happens to be common for the various closets (Fig. 4.2) constructed for different storeys of a multi-storeyed building and are placed one above the other, there is always a risk of the water being sucked in or siphoned from the traps of lower closets at the time when the upper ones are

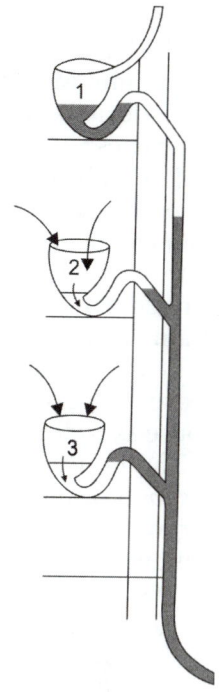

Fig. 4.2: Three closets at different levels explaining siphonic action

flushed. This siphonic action can be prevented by carrying a ventilating pipe, called anti-siphonage pipe from beyond the trap of every closet through the house wall and is connected with a vertical pipe 2 to 2.5 inches (5.08–6.35 cm) in diameter placed along the side of soil pipe, after it has received the anti-siphonage pipe from the highest water closet.

4.3 HOUSE DRAIN

It is an underground pipe, connecting the soil pipe of water closets with the sewer. It also receives waste water from the house or the compound and the rainwater.

The main house drain is made of glazed stoneware or earthenware socketted pipe, 2 ft (0.6 metre) in length or when placed under the road it is made from socketted caste iron pipes coated inside with a paint containing magnetic oxide of iron (*Barffs process*). Stoneware pipes are connected with cement and cast iron pipes are caulked with molten lead. It is laid on a bed of concrete about 15 cm below the ground level in a straight course with the socket end looking towards the house and the spigot end towards the sewer with sufficient gradient towards the main drain. It should be laid without any angle or bends on a smooth inclined surface to facilitate easy transit of its contents. Its interior should be without any projections and perfectly smooth to prevent accumulation of filth. House waste, kitchen and rainwater pipes are connected to the house drain at an acute angle and never at right angles. The joints should be made both air- and watertight. Moreover, these pipe connections should be made in the direction of flow of contents of the pipe. A 4 inches (10.16 cm) drain should have a fall of 1 in 44 and a 6 inches (15.24 cm) drain a fall of 1 in 60. Thus for all practical purposes, the fall should be 10 times the diameter of the house drain. It should also be provided with inspection openings or manhole chambers at convenient intervals. It should be noted that a small drain is more liable to self-cleansing than a large one but care should be taken that it is wide enough to prevent blocking and to carry off all the sewage of the house as well as rainwater.

The house drain should not be allowed to pass through or under a house. There should be a proper arrangement for flushing the house drain. The requirements of a good house drain are:

1. Perfectly fitting joints to eliminate danger of leakage of any sewage or foul gases.
2. The provision of a proper flushing arrangement.
3. A fall to provide velocity to the current.
4. The pipes should have smooth internal surface.
5. The pipes should have Y joints, i.e. they should form an acute angle and not a right angle.
6. It should be easily accessible.
7. It should be laid on a bed of cement concrete to prevent cracking and loosening of pipe joints due to uneven settling of the underneath foundation.

4.4 INSPECTION CHAMBER, DISCONNECTING CHAMBER OR A MANHOLE

These are square-shaped, brick built and cement lined underground chambers. These are provided for inspection and cleansing of sewers, at every point, where two or more drains meet and at distances of 100 metres in the long straight runs. The main house drain is continued along the floor of the chamber in a half channelled glazed pipe, which discharges itself into an intercepting trap. The branch drains and the subsidiary drains are also made of glazed channelled pipes and are connected to the main chamber. The chamber is closed by an iron lid and from its side a ventilating shaft provided with a mica flap, lets the air in, but not out. As a rule, inspection chambers should be laid in open spaces and not actually in the main building.

At the distal end of the chamber, an interception trap is provided which has on it an inspection arm which is closed by a lid. The object is to permit rodding of the short length of pipe leading from the trap to the sewer. This intercepting trap is interposed between house drain and the sewer. It prevents reflux of foul gases from the sewer and the entrance of sewer rats into house drains, but allows a free circulation of

air through the drain and soil pipe. The house drain must be adequately ventilated at intervals by providing an air shaft passing up to gratings at the surface of the ground or these may be carried away to side of the house to prevent nuisance. Arrangement for the provision of inlets and outlets (Fig. 4.3) should be made to ensure free circulation of fresh air.

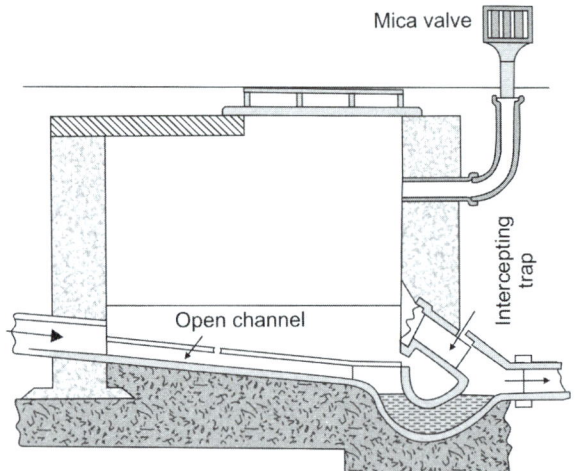

Fig. 4.3: Inspection chamber

4.5 TRAPS

A trap consists of a pipe, bent upon itself in such a way so as to retain certain amount of water in the bend. It prevents the reflux of sewer air or gas into the house and acts as a barrier. It is effected by water seal. A good trap should completely disconnect the air of one pipe from the air of another pipe.

Qualities of a good trap: It should be constructed out of strong, smooth and non-absorbent material. It should be provided with a base, so that it may be firmly fixed, to prevent it from getting out of position. It should not corrode. It should be free from all angles and corners so as not to allow readily the accumulation of filth. It should be self-cleansing. It should have a water seal of at least 2 cm and the body of the trap should be smaller in section than the inlet and outlet. It should not be liable to silt but self-cleansing and should have an opening for cleansing, etc.

A trap is apt to be unsealed and may fail to perform its functions due to the following reasons:

1. **Evaporation of the water seal:** It happens if a trap is little used or the house remains vacant and the use of the trap is discontinued for some time. It may be also due to the bend being too shallow.
2. **By momentum for flushing water:** Being maintained to the vertical line, in different storeys of a multi-storeyed building and if the closet in the upper storey is flushed, then water of the traps in the closet fitted in lower storeys will get aspirated. This is prevented by the provision of anti-siphonage pipes.

3. **By momentum of flushing water:** Being maintained to the very end of flushing, due to sudden and violent discharge of water.

4. **By backward passage of gases:** When the drain is not adequately ventilated.

5. **By capillary action:** Caused by a foreign substance like pieces of cotton, thread, jute, etc. which may be caught in the trap and act as a siphon. The remedy is adequate flushing.

6. **Trap:** May be rendered useless on account of getting blocked with deposit of solid matter due to imperfect setting or insufficient fall in the house drain.

Varieties of Traps

1. **Siphon trap:** It is simply a bent tube, placed under the basin of each water closet. It is of the P or S type trap according to the outward or downward direction of the outlet (Fig. 4.4). It is the best type of trap as it maintains siphonic action and keeps a constant level, of water. In this case water collects at the lower bend of S and the water seal should be 1.5–2 inches (3.81–5.08 cm) deep. Anti-D type of trap is generally condemned as it is not self-cleansing.

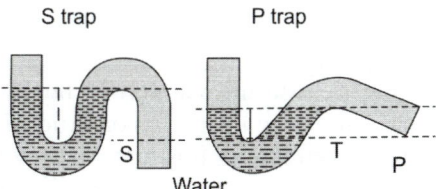

Fig. 4.4: S and P traps

2. **Gully trap or intercepting trap** (Fig. 4.5): It is interposed between the house drain and public drain. It is fitted at a distance of about 18 inches (0.46 metre) from the wall of the house, is intended to arrest the solid suspended matter in its downward passage and allows the rain or muddy water to flow into the drain. It is required to be cleaned periodically by removing the suspended matter which settles down at the bottom.

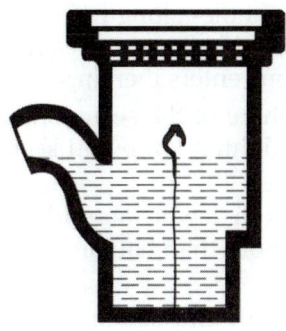

Fig. 4.5: Gully trap

3. **Grease trap:** It is fitted to the kitchen sink to prevent the choking of drains, due to collecting and congealing therein of grease. The trap is made up of earthenware or iron and contains a large volume of water which allows the grease contained in it to float to the surface and solidify. It thus arrests its inward flow, by allowing the dirty water to flow away from its under surface.

4.6 SEWERS

A sewer is an underground trunk channel, in which house drains empty their contents. It carries them to the place of disposal. It is also required to carry household and trade effluents, rain or storm water and the water used for municipal purposes. It is provided with manholes and flushing gates for inspection and cleansing. It is generally built of glazed bricks and given the shape of an egg on cross-section. The idea being that it flushes better by providing that shape.

There are two systems of sewers

a. *The combined system:* In this system, the sewer carries away sewage and all the storm or rainwater from the streets, along with factory drainage, excreta, etc. The sewer in this system should be very large, which creates great difficulty in places, where there is less rainfall.

b. *The separate system:* In this system, all storm or rainwater is taken away by separate drains and disposed off separately from the sewage. It is an expensive method but undoubtedly the best. It is now being adopted largely because in this case no difficulty is experienced with regard to the sewage disposal.

The advantages claimed by the separate system are

1. The sewers required are of smaller dimensions and can, therefore, be easily flushed; consequently there is less deposit.

2. The sewage is uniform in quality and smaller in quantity.

3. Purification and utilisation are affected with less difficulty.

4. In a known population, estimation of total bulk of sewage can be made from allotment of water per head.

5. It is cheaper to run than the combined method.

The disadvantages are

1. Two sets of pipes are required for every house, so wrong connections may be established through an oversight.

2. The rain and storm water may wash away impurities that would contaminate a stream.

3. The flushing effect of rainwater on the sewage is lost.

Under no circumstances, a public sewer should be less than 9 inches (22.86 cm) in diameter. Sewers up to 18 inches (0.46 metre) in diameter are constructed of glazed earthenware or stoneware pipes and are circular in shape. They should be laid on a bed of concrete to prevent subsequent sinking. Large sewers of 2–3 metres in diameter are made of glazed bricks or cement and are oval- or egg-shaped with their narrow end downwards, as they provide a greater depth to sewage and comparatively less contact with inside surface of the walls, which obviously minimises friction.

Sewers are placed underground, usually at a distance of 10 feet (3.05 metres) from the surface of roads. All sewers must be laid with as few bends as possible and the junctions are made at acute angles to allow the sewage to pass in the direction of the flow. Curves, if any, should be gradual. The joints of the sewers should be thoroughly cemented and their inside surface must be perfectly smooth. Sewers should be self-cleansing and provided with sufficient gradient. The size should be proportionate to the volume of sewage they have to carry.

Inspection, Cleansing and Ventilation of Sewers

For periodical examination and cleansing of sewers, manholes or inspection openings are provided. These are side entrances into sewers provided at an interval of 100 yards (91.44 metres) throughout its course through which workers can descend into the sewers for periodical examination, cleansing and removal of deposit, etc. It consists of a masonry chamber down to the sewer through the centre of which the main sewer runs. The branch sewers are made to join the main sewer in the manhole chambers.

Flushing gates: These are contrivances placed at the ends of sewers for purposes of efficient flushing and to prevent stagnation of sewage material at their bottom. For efficient flushing, automatic flush tanks may be constructed or a housepipe be run into a manhole from a hydrant or water carriers be engaged for this purpose. The sewers may also be flushed by pouring large quantity of water into them through manholes.

Self-cleansing: It is considered essential that sewers should be as much self-cleansing as possible. An even flow of sewage should be aimed at, so that it does not "pond" or accumulate at any spot. Ponding or obstructing may cause the sewage to go back into the house drains and may lead to even disturbances of ventilation in the sewer proper with the accumulation of inflammable and poisonous gases. These gases being highly toxic may endanger the lives of workmen in the sewers.

Ventilation of sewers: In a properly constructed sewer, where the sewage is well diluted its flow is rapid and flushing efficient; deposition of deposit does not occur and so the air does not become foul.

In badly constructed and even in other sewers, owing to the constant variation of the flow some deposit forms which putrefies and gives rise to obnoxious gases such as carbon dioxide, marsh gas, hydrogen sulphide, ammonia, carburetted hydrogen, etc. The gases evolved are combustible, so unprotected lights should not be brought in the newly opened sewers. In tropical countries, the temperature of sewer air is lower than that of atmospheric air. Bacteria have a tendency to adhere to the damp surfaces of the internal walls of the sewers. Hence, the provision of ventilation for the sewers is most essential to dilute such gases and to preserve the purity of such air.

The method utilised for the purpose is to fix long iron shafts, at a suitable distance, say 100 yards (91.44 metres), along the entire length of sewers. They are carried sufficiently high above the top of the neighbouring houses for the exit of sewage air or gases into the atmosphere. The other method is to have perforated manhole covers having a tray or a dirt box below it to catch dirt and stones, etc. with the idea that the air which escapes through these would be rapidly diluted by fresh air and rendered inoffensive. They are installed at a distance of 100 yards (91.44 metres). Some of them act as inlets and the others as outlets.

Disadvantages

These are as follows:

1. Sewers might cause effluvia to enter the houses. But, however, if they are properly constructed, flushed, trapped and ventilated, this may be prevented.
2. Any leakage may contaminate water supply. A sewer may begin leaking on account of various reasons, viz. from sinking of foundation, cracked or faulty joints of pipes or by penetration of roots of trees through cracks, etc.
3. Accidents in sewers: Workmen who enter parts of a sewerage system for cleansing them, sometimes die being asphyxiated by poisonous gases from the sewers.

Precautions

The following precautions should be observed before cleansing the sewers:

1. Six of the manholes along with the whole length of the sewer should be uncovered for at least 2 hours before any one enters therein.
2. The atmosphere of the sewer should be tested by letting in a lighted lamp and seeing that it burns brightly.
3. The workers in sewers should not be allowed to remain for more than half an hour at a time in the sewer.
4. If a worker in the sewer gets ill or becomes unconscious, he should be at once taken out and

given artificial respiration and medical aid to restore him.

5. At least two or more workers should enter the sewer at a time. They should be fastened by a stout rope. They should work under the supervision of chief sanitary inspector.

6. The work should be carried out between sunrise and sunset and never during the night.

4.7 PNEUMATIC SYSTEM OF SEWAGE REMOVAL (Fig. 4.6)

In this system, two sets of pipes are used, viz. pipes with smaller diameter for the removal of waste water and the pipes with a larger diameter, i.e. 5 inches (12.7 cm) for the removal of sewage. In low-lying areas where removal of sewage by gravitation scheme cannot be efficiently carried out, for want of proper gradient, some other mechanical means should be adopted. In such cases, periodical pumping to raise the sewage to a higher level should be resorted to. For this purpose, an automatic apparatus such as *Shone's Ejector* is used. This apparatus consists of a closed tank into which sewage gravitates. The motive power is compressed air supplied from a central station. The pressure of the air is sufficient to lift the sewage into a sewer at a higher level.

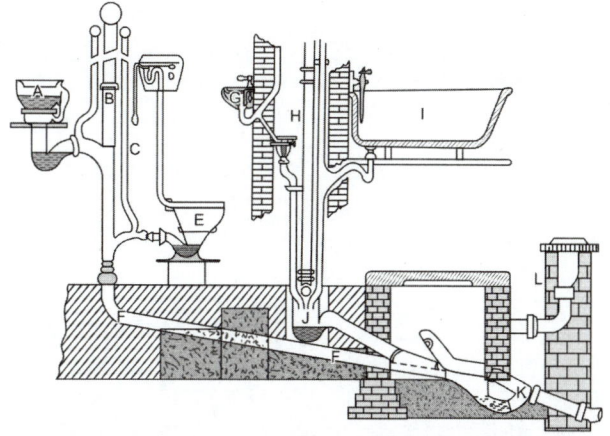

Fig. 4.6: A complete system of house drainage. A and H are two pipes, D. Flushing cistern which opens into closet, E and F. House closets which open into the soil pipe, B and C. Anti-siphonage drain, G. Wash basin, I. Bath tub, J. Gully trap, K. Intercepting trap, L. Inlet opening

In the *Liemur's pneumatic system,* two sets of pipes are used. Pipes with a smaller diameter are used for the removal of waste water, whereas pipes with a larger diameter, say 6 inches (15.24 cm) are used for the removal of sewage proper. The sewage is propelled by means of an air pump installed at a central station.

Disposal of Sewage

The character of sewage depends upon the amount of water consumed, the social habits of the people, admission of rainwater and the character of effluent from different trades and industries. The fresh town sewage has the appearance of dirty odorous water of brownish colour, with solid lumps floating on the surface. The lumps finally disintegrate and fall as the gases of putrefaction are given off. The main object of disposal of sewage consists of changing different organic matters, present in the sewage from unstable into harmless stable chemical compounds.

The chief methods of disposal of sewage are:
1. By dilution.
2. By purification.

5.1 SEWAGE DISPOSAL BY DILUTION

This is done in the following ways

1. **Discharge of sewage into the sea:** This is the readiest, the most economical and the best practical method of disposal of untreated sewage of the towns situated on the sea side. The sewage should be discharged well below the lowest level of the ebb of the tide so that the discharge may not be driven back on the seashore during the incoming tide. Thus great care should be taken to select a position for discharging a large bulk of sewage into the sea. Study of the tide, prevailing wind, weather and float observations should be fully taken into consideration before deciding such a point or else the sewage discharged into the sea is bound to be thrown back to the seashore. A sea outfall should be taken as far as possible from the shore. The liquid of the sewage rapidly becomes diffused in water, but the solid matter may persist for some time, especially as the seawater delays the oxidation of solid organic matter and it is not until some hours after discharge that putrefaction sets in, whereby it gets broken up and dissolved by aerobic bacterial action. The possibility of infecting shellfish layings must always be borne in mind.

2. **Discharge of sewage into rivers:** This was formerly practised in England and the result was most undesirable. In fact, an Act had to be passed in England in 1876 prohibiting the discharge of crude sewage into rivers. This Act is called the *River's Pollution Preventive Act*. The sewage must be partially purified by removing suspended solid matters by screening or by allowing it to settle in sedimentation tanks, or by septic tank action before it is finally discharged into a river, because in England, the rivers are very small and may get readily polluted.

In India, the rivers are much larger, but even here the discharge of crude sewage should be prohibited. Such a discharge is liable to prove still more injurious, if the discharge of the sewage is allowed to take place at a point up the stream so that the people living below are constrained to use the polluted water.

Before discharging sewage into the sea or a river, it should be ascertained whether the dilution will be sufficient or not. Comparatively, less dilution is required in the case of a rapidly flowing river than in the case of a stagnant river. The volume of water should be enough to permit aerobic bacterial action which will effect complete breakdown of the organic matter and at the same time will not kill fish. Thus the oxygen content in the river or the stream should not be allowed to be reduced more than 3 parts per million parts of water and the current must be sufficient to prevent silting up of the stream and there should not be any possibility of the floating materials getting deposited on the shore.

5.2 SEWAGE DISPOSAL BY PURIFICATION

The different methods of sewage purification are described as follows:
a. Direct land treatment.
   1. Intermittent downward filtration.
   2. Broad irrigation of sewage farming.
b. Chemical treatment of sewage.

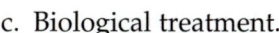

c. Biological treatment.
   1. Septic tank.
   2. Activated sludge process.
   3. Oxidation pond.

Disposal by Direct Land Treatment

It can be done in two ways:

1. **Intermittent downward filtration method:** By this method, sewage is purified by the action of soil which acts as a mechanical filter and for this purpose porous soil should be selected. Sand, clay and peat are unsatisfactory and chalk is dangerous for this purpose. The purification is chiefly effected by the soil bacteria or the nitrifying organisms which exist in large number in the superficial layers of all soils, especially in land rich in organic matter, aided by those contained in the sewage. These bacteria require air and oxygen for their development and on account of feeding of the organic substances of the sewage, cause their oxidation.

   Here the earth is made to act in the same way as a sand filter is used for water purification. The growing of crops, if practised at all, should be a matter of secondary importance.

   For successful filtration, the land should be prepared in a fashion of beds. The bottom of the bed should be properly drained by means of porous earthenware drains laid at a depth of 6 feet (1.83 metres) and about 10 feet (3.04 metres) apart from each other. The surface of the land should be levelled and must have a proper slope to allow an equal distribution of sewage over the whole area. The sewage should be distributed through surface channels. The land should be divided into 4 sections so that each section may receive the sewage for 6 hours and have an interval for aeration for about 18 hours. The surface of each section should be laid out in ridges and furrows and cultivation may be carried on the ridges, while sewage is permitted to flow down the furrows. The effluent, which comes out of the subsoil drain is pure, does not putrefy and can be discharged into any river or a stream. The method is simple and works efficiently, where plenty of suitable porous soil is available. One acre (0.4 hectare) of land is sufficient for treating the sewage of about 3,000 persons.

2. **Broad irrigation or sewage farming:** A considerably large plot of land is required for this system and it is generally adopted where suitable land is available near the neighbourhood of a town. The soil should be porous and the land selected low enough to allow the sewage to flow by gravitation. The untreated sewage is used to irrigate a given area of land on which crops, etc. are grown and the ordinary processes of agriculture are carried out. If proper extent of land is not available and it is overdosed with sewage, then due to lack of sufficient aeration, it stinks, becomes *sewage sick* and it will not be fit for growing any crop at all. So a considerably large area of land is required for efficient manipulation of this system. It becomes difficult to take care of the sewage during heavy rains and to prevent the soil from waterlogging. The growing of crops is the main consideration. The land should be used for growing fodder for horses, cattle and other crops rather than the cultivation of vegetables.

The sewage should be discharged on the land in fresh condition and the coarse portions should be removed by precipitation or sedimentation. Irrigation of sewage should not be continuous but must be intermittent so that the aeration of soil can take place during the period of intermission. The land is laid out in the ridge and the furrow system and the sewage flows down the centre of the ridge towards the furrow. One acre (0.4 hectare) of land is required for about 100–200 persons in temperate climates, if sewage has been previously clarified. Irrigation with crude sewage usually proves to be a failure. Lands irrigated by sewage are termed *sewage farms*.

Chemical Treatment of Sewage

This is effected by the addition of certain chemical agents such as lime, alum, alumino ferric, mixture of lime and alum, etc. These chemicals act as precipitants and carry down suspended matter with some dissolved organic impurities of the sewage.

Crude sewage is first collected in large tanks made of cement called settling tanks. The solid matter gravitates leaving a comparatively clear fluid at the top. This fluid is treated with certain chemical agents which act as precipitants. The *sludge* or the precipitate is then pressed into cakes and sold as manure. The clear, supernatant fluid, at the top is called *effluent*. This may either be discharged into a stream or a river or carried along drains into open land for the purpose of irrigation. The disadvantages of this method are numerous. The sludge which contains organic and mineral matter and about 80–90% of water is very bulky and has very little manuring value. The effluent is not safe as it is not free from pathogenic organisms. Moreover, the method is expensive, requires the provision of tanks and chemicals, besides close supervision. So this method is not much adopted nowadays.

The chemicals commonly used for this purpose are

1. **Lime:** 12–16 grains (720–960 mg) of lime are added to each gallon (4.546 litres) of sewage. It combines with carbonic acid of the sewage forming an insoluble carbonate of calcium and also with some of the sewage. This precipitate falls to the bottom forming sludge. This method is cheap and simple. The disadvantages are that the effluent is rendered more alkaline, more putrescible and the sludge is bulky and decomposable.

2. **Alum or aluminium sulphate:** 5–10 grains (300–600 mg) is used for a gallon (4.546 litres) of sewage. This causes a flocculent precipitate which entangles and carries down most of the suspended organic matter present in the sewage.

3. **Lime and alum:** 5 grains (300 mg) of each of these chemicals are added to a gallon (4.546 litres) of sewage. This method is more efficient than lime or alum when used alone.

4. **Amine process:** Sewage is treated with a mixture of lime and a small quantity of brine. An amine is formed, which acts as a deodorant or an antiseptic and renders the sludge also antiseptic.

5. **ABC process:** The chemicals used are alumino ferric, blood, clay and charcoal. They produce a precipitate which causes sedimentation of the dissolved solids present in the sewage.

6. **Iron sulphate copper:** It forms a precipitate of hydrated protoxide of iron when added to alkaline sewage or to the sewage which has been previously treated with lime. Usually 3–5 grains (180–300 mg) of it are sufficient to treat one gallon (4.546 litres) of sewage.

Biological Treatment

This process does not precipitate suspended matters but reduces the complex organic matter present in excreta into simple substances by the action of bacteria and other microorganisms. Their main action depends upon the two kinds of bacteria present in sewage, i.e. aerobic and anaerobic. The anaerobic bacteria are chiefly concerned in reducing organic substances into simple compounds by breaking down, digesting and liquefying them, which are ammonia and ammonical compounds. The aerobic bacteria convert, by a process of nitrification, the ammonical substances into nitrites and nitrates. The disposal of night soil by trenching, sewage farming, etc. are in fact biological methods, as the ultimate results are obtained through bacteria present in the soil.

There are various methods of biological treatment

1. **Septic tanks** (Fig. 5.1): This system was first devised by Cameron and actually put into practice by Fowler and Clemesha in 1906. By this process, the combined action of two groups of organisms, viz. anaerobic liquefaction and aerobic nitrification is utilised for the purification of sewage. The anaerobic liquidation takes place in a water tight masonry septic tank, whereas aerobic nitrification takes place in the contact beds or the sprinkling filters. The septic tank is covered with a concrete slab of a thickness of about 5 cm and is provided with a manhole. The sewage is at first passed into a *grit or detritus* chamber, where all heavy stones, bricks, etc. fall to the bottom, while hard lumps of faeces float on the surface. The length of the chamber is about

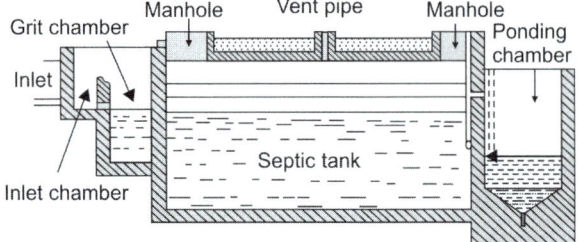

Fig. 5.1: Section of septic tank installation for a house

10 to 20 metres and it is meant to maintain a constant velocity of about 1 ft (0.3 metre) per second with a retention period of 30 seconds to 1 minute.

The digestion chamber is an underground, airtight, rectangular tank made of bricks. It may be kept open or closed but in India it should be closed to suit its climatic conditions. It has an inlet pipe connecting the two chambers at a distance of 1–1.5 feet (0.3–0.45 metre) above the bottom for receiving the sewage, and an outlet pipe for the discharge of effluent. The capacity of the tank should be equivalent to bulk representing 24 hours flow of sewage. In the tank, there should be a provision for plenty of space above the level of fluid to accommodate scum and gases.

In the septic tank proper, some of the solid organic constituents settle at the bottom and the scum about 2" to 6" (5.08–15.24 cm) thick is formed which floats at the surface, which should not be disturbed. Under the scum, anaerobic microorganisms grow and multiply in the tank and these organisms bring about material liquid action of the suspended organic solid matters and split them into soluble and unstable compounds. The black deposit of the sludge accumulates at the bottom of the tank, which is generally small. As soon as it becomes 8 inches to 12 inches (20.32 to 30.48 cm) in thickness, it should be removed and deposited in trenches. The scum further undergoes digestive changes owing to the action of anaerobic bacteria and the organic matter is decomposed into water nitrites, nitrates, and gaseous products, such as carbon dioxide, ammonia, marsh gas, sulphuretted hydrogen, etc. These gases may be employed either for heating or after carburetting for lighting purposes. The flow of sewage in the tank must be slow, and it should be kept in the tank for about 24 hours, so that the bacteria may have sufficient time to act on the sewage.

The effluent from a septic tank is generally dark in colour with faecal smell and contains eggs of intestinal parasites, such as hookworms and as such it should not be discharged into a river or a stream without further purification. It is, therefore, carried on to either contact beds or filter beds where aerobic nitrification takes place; here the aerobic organisms convert the different ammonical compounds into oxidised nitrogenous substances of harmless character, i.e. nitrates. In septic tank installation, no disinfectant should be used.

i. *Contact bed:* It is a water tight masonry tank, rectangular in shape and may be of any depth, but depth of 3–4 feet (0.91–1.22 metres) gives the best results. Its bottom is made up of concrete and slopes from its centre to the sides, which are surrounded by a drain for collecting and carrying away the effluent. Contact bed is filled up with a layer of fine, hard, furnace clinker, quartz or gravel ranging from 1/4 inch to 2 inches (6.35–50.8 mm) in thickness to present a relatively large and rough surface for the growth of bacteria. The material should be removed, washed and replaced periodically.

The effluent from a septic tank which is generally dark in colour, is distributed and allowed to remain for a fixed period generally 2–4 hours. It should not take more than half an hour to get itself filled or emptied out. It should be so arranged that each bed should be allowed rest for 8 hours after functioning for 4 hours so that the bed may be properly aerated, otherwise the organisms may die.

Bacteria, chiefly aerobic, and other suspended solids adhere to the filtering media. The bacteria act on dissolved organic materials, oxidising them to nitrates. It requires some weeks for a contact bed to become efficient, i.e. acquire a suitable bacterial flora. Its useful life is from 5 to 8 years, when it becomes clogged and unfit for further use. This method, however, is costly, as it requires the services of operators to run it.

ii. *Percolating filter, trickling filter or filter bed:* It works on the same principle as contact bed and is used for the same purpose although the method of application of the clarified sewage is different. In the filter, oxidation is assisted by aerobic bacterial action and the effluent is non-putrescible as the micro-organisms (aerobes) develop gradually in the interstices of the filters and these attack the organic matter present in the sewage, since it slowly falls in the form of a thin stream on the filter.

These filters are circular or rectangular in shape usually 6 feet (1.82 metres) deep and consist of a bed of porous material like *jhama,* cinder, etc. graded from above downwards, over which the effluent or clarified sewage is sprinkled through fixed sprinklers, mechanical travelling sprinklers, revolving fans, dripping trays, etc. to ensure uniform distribution. While passing through a filter, the sewage rapidly coats the filtering medium with bacterial growth which is gelatinous in nature. When properly designed and worked out these filters, practically, require no attention except that their surface requires periodic scraping about once a month. It is comparatively cheap and more efficient than a contact bed.

The final effluent is generally discharged into a river or a stream or it may be treated on the land. So when it is discharged into a river or a stream it is necessary to eliminate the danger of transmitting water-borne diseases by proper disinfection. This is done by using bleaching powder or chlorine gas in some form or the other. The fluid should be clear and devoid of smell. It should be non-putrescible, having practically no suspended impurities contained in it.

2. **Activated sludge process or bioaeration process:** This is an aerobic process of disposal of sewage and is claimed to be the most satisfactory method of purifying sewage. It is worked out on the same principle as the contact beds but a higher standard of efficiency is aimed at in this process (Fig. 5.2).

The sewage is first passed through rough screens made of vertical bars fitted at a distance of about 2 inches (5.08 cm) apart from each other to get rid of gross solids, such as stone, bricks, etc. from entering the main aerating tanks. The sewage is treated here with compressed air, in gusts through porous tile diffusers at the bottom of the tank (sheffield) or by means of other devices such as perforated pipes, mechanical agitators or paddles (simplex). The sewage is disintegrated and liquefied with formation of fine emulsion which rises at the

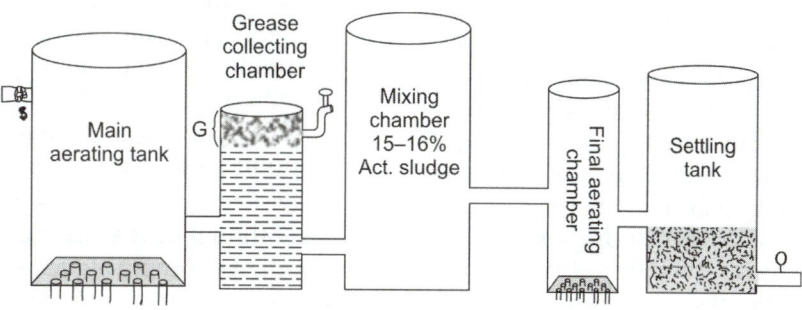

Fig. 5.2: Activated sludge process

top. Subsequently, it is passed through a grease collecting chamber, where any grease collected at the top of the liquid, is trapped.

The treated sewage is drawn off from the bottom and led into a mixing chamber. Here it is mixed intimately with 20–25% activated or ripened sludge, to 75–80% of raw sewage by thoroughly agitating it. Then it is passed into final aeration chamber where the air is forced in by diffusers, at the rate of 1–2 cubic ft (0.028–0.056 cubic metre) per gallon (4.55 litres) so that it rises in the form of minute bubbles in the sewage. Practically an infinite surface of contact is produced. This is done for 6–8 hours till all the ammonia in the sewage is oxidised into nitrates. The aerobic micro-organisms increase in numbers and activity and breakup organic matter of the sewage till all the ammonia is oxidised into nitrates causing formation of sludge, which settles down at the bottom as a precipitate and a clear non-putrescible liquid comes over the top. The sludge which settles down is charged with micro-organisms, which are carried down with it, to the bottom and it is then called *activated or ripened* sludge. A portion of this activated sludge can be used over and over again for the activation of fresh sewage. The sludge obtained from the process is inoffensive and is an anaerobic bacterial culture. It is, therefore, used in the process which takes place in two stages. In the first stage, the organic matter is broken down and carbon is converted into carbon dioxide. The deposit from the screening chamber is used in filling up depressions, pits, etc. as it is inorganic in nature. The sludge from the primary and the secondary settling tank is mixed and is ripened in digesting chamber. These are circular metallic tanks, which are heated by burning gas or petrol and kept at a temperature of 69°F. The sludge is thus rendered innocuous, harmless, and is then dried into cakes and sold as a manure. Here the liquid becomes almost stable but the process is continued till nitrates are formed.

The effluent is drawn off and run into a suitable out fall. There being an enormous amount of sludge, a great difficulty is experienced in its disposal because it contains a very large quantity of water. Since the sludge is rich in nitrogen and phosphates, it is utilised as a valuable manure after getting rid of water. The sludge is, therefore, dewatered by air drying on sand beds or by some other means, made into cakes by composting it with town refuse and is sold for use as a manure. At places barren land may be irrigated through the combined agency of activated sludge effluent and the liquid sludge, which serves as useful manuring agents (e.g. Okhla Sewage Treatment Plant at Delhi).

Maintenance of septic tanks

i. The septic tank must be desludged periodically for its efficient functioning. The bailed out sludge should be disposed off by trenching or by any other suitable method.

ii. The use of soap, antiseptics or disinfectants should be avoided, since they kill the bacterial flora present in the septic tank.

iii. Newly built septic tanks should be first filled with plain water and then seeded with ripe sludge drawn from another working septic tank to provide right type of bacteria to carry out the process of decomposition effectively.

Advantages of activated sludge method: These are:

i. The effluent is fully oxidised and is clear, being free from colloids.

ii. Purification is rapid and perfect.

iii. Putrefaction is quickly stopped and the system is free from the nuisance of flies.

iv. The sludge is inoffensive and forms a valuable manure.

v. A small area of land is required and skilled management with a small staff can easily manage the work. One acre land of activated sludge plant can successfully compete with the working of 10 acre land, required for percolating filter.

An activated sludge plant has been installed at Jamshedpur in India. It is aimed to cover a population of about one and a half lakh and to purify about 5 million gallons (22,729,800 litres) of sewage daily.

Characteristics of a good sewage effluent: These are as follows:

1. It should be clear, bright and free from deposit.

2. It should have no faecal smell. If a small living fish is kept in it, it should not readily die.

3. It must not contain more than 3 parts per 1,00,000 parts of suspended matters as per recommendations made by the British Royal Commission on Sewage Disposal.

4. It must not absorb more than 2 parts of dissolved oxygen per 100,000 parts, kept at a uniform temperature for 5 days.

5. It must not contain more than 0.1 part of organic ammonia per 100,000 parts.

6. When incubated at a temperature of 80°F (26.7°C) in a closed vessel, for a week, it must not undergo any further decomposition or emit foul gases.

3. **Oxidation ponds and oxidation ditches:** Oxidation ponds are being used for purification of sewage of small communities. An oxidation pond is an open shallow pool 3.6 ft (1 to 1.15 m) deep with an inlet

and outlet. For its smooth functioning, it needs sunlight and certain types of bacteria, which feed on decaying organic matter and algae. The sewage organic matter is oxidised by bacteria to carbon dioxide, ammonia and water. The algae utilise carbon dioxide, water and inorganic minerals with the help of sunlight for their growth. Oxygen required for oxidation of organic matter by the bacteria is provided by algae and atmospheric oxygen. The oxidation ponds are mostly aerobic ponds during day and some parts of the night. In the remaining hours of the night, the ponds have anaerobic action especially in the bottom layers. The effluent from the ponds can be discharged into a river or used for growing vegetables. Breeding of mosquitoes in the tanks has to be prevented by removing weeds, etc. An oxidation tank needs about 22 acres (8.9 hectares) of area.

Food and Nutrition

6.1 IMPORTANCE OF FOOD

A food may be defined as any substance, which when taken into the body can be utilised to yield heat or energy, to build up new tissues, repair worn-out tissues, regulate body processes and to aid in the production of important body compounds.

The science of nutrition deals with food values, food processing, its digestion, absorption and metabolism in the body. Nutrients that we obtain from food have vital effects on physical growth and development, maintenance of normal body functions, physical activity and health. Nutritious food is, thus needed to sustain life and activity. Nutrition has been established as one of the most important environmental factors affecting health.

In order to understand this close relationship between food and health, it is necessary to study food facts and their functions. Food as a whole serves three main functions:

1. It provides the material needed for growth and maintenance of the body since the body continues to change throughout life even after growth is stopped. The tissues are continually wearing out and these must be changed or repaired.
2. It provides the body fuels or energy foods, which on oxidation supply heat and energy.
3. It provides the materials which regulate and maintain body functions and processes. They regulate the way, in which various parts of the body act and protect the body from disease.

6.2 DIETARY GOALS: NATIONAL INSTITUTE OF NUTRITION, HYDERABAD

The dietary goals are:

1. Maintenance of a state of positive health and optimal performance in populations at large by maintaining ideal body weight.
2. Ensuring adequate nutritional status for pregnant women and lactating mothers.

3. Improvement of birth weights and promotion of growth of infants, children and adolescents to achieve their full genetic potential.
4. Achievement of adequacy in all nutrients and prevention of deficiency diseases.
5. Prevention of chronic diet-related disorders.
6. Maintenance of the health of the elderly and increasing the life expectancy.

6.3 CONSTITUENTS OF FOOD

Man is omnivorous in diet since the structures and functions of his body are such that it conveniently digests and assimilate both types of food.

Food consists essentially of six constituents, known as nutrients, which are classified according to their functions. These are carbohydrates, fats, proteins, mineral salts, vitamins and water. Carbohydrates, proteins and fats are together termed as proximate principles of food since they form the main bulk of food.

Carbohydrates

Chemically, carbohydrates are composed of carbon, hydrogen and oxygen as the name implies. They form the largest component of diet of most of the people and furnish most of the required energy. Carbohydrates have to be changed into glucose and fructose before they can be absorbed into the body providing 4 kcal of energy per gram. Starches and sugars are, grouped under this head. Wheat, rice, maize, barley, cereals, potatoes, sweet potatoes, turnips, root vegetables, etc. are rich in starches while sugarcane, beetroot and fruits contain the sugars. The original source of all starches and sugars is green plants. When plants have excessive sugar and they need to store it as reserve supply of food, plant body is capable of changing its sugar into starch.

Carbohydrates are classified into simple (mono-saccharides and disaccharides) and complex

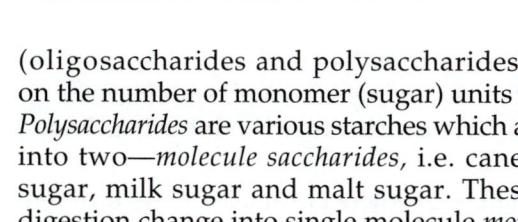
(oligosaccharides and polysaccharides) depending on the number of monomer (sugar) units they contain. *Polysaccharides* are various starches which are converted into two—*molecule saccharides*, i.e. cane sugar, beet sugar, milk sugar and malt sugar. These on further digestion change into single molecule *monosaccharides*, i.e. galactose, glucose and fructose. The Food and Agriculture Organization (FAO) and World Health Organization (WHO) jointly recommend that 55–75% of total energy intake should be from carbohydrates, but only 10% directly from sugars (simple carbohydrates).

The carbohydrates are chief source of energy. Over half the energy requirements of the body are met with by carbohydrates. In the active muscles, the glucose is oxidised for the production of energy and warmth. Glucose which cannot be used immediately is converted into *glycogen* and stored in the liver and muscles or converted into fat and stored under the skin. Carbohydrates and their derivatives play major roles in the working process of the immune system, fertilization, blood clotting, and development. Carbohydrates (dietary fibre) help in digestion and in preventing constipation, mainly by absorbing water, and increasing the bulk of the diet and stool.

Because it facilitates the rapid passage of materials through the intestine, fibre may be a factor in the control of diverticulitis, appendicitis, haemorrhoids. Diets high in dietary fibre are usually associated with lower prevalence of obesity, heart disease, non-insulin-dependent diabetes.

Fats or Lipids

Fats are chemically composed of carbon, hydrogen and oxygen, only in different proportion than they are contained in carbohydrates; the oxygen is less in fats than carbohydrates. Oils are those lipids that are liquid at room temperature such as groundnut or cotton seed oil, while those that are solid are called fats. Chemically, true fats are glycerides of fatty acids. Butter, ghee, vegetable hydrogenated oil, animal fat, etc. are the examples of various fats commonly used by people. Fats are a form of concentrated energy and each gram of fat provides 9 kcal of energy on oxidation. Thus, weight for weight, fats yield more than double the energy as compared to carbohydrates. The process of digestion requires to change the fat into an emulsion form for their absorption into the body as fats are not soluble in water. Liquid fats and those fats which melt at body temperature are somewhat better digested than those which are much harder. A fat-rich diet slows the process of digestion and gives a feeling of heaviness and fullness. In the body, the fat which cannot be immediately used, is partly deposited as adipose tissue under the skin and partly unabsorbed passes out with the faeces. Fat diminishes protein

metabolism and, therefore, is called protein sparing food.

Lipids make an important contribution to adequate nutrition and are thus considered essential for health. Lipids are required for a range of metabolic and physiological processes and to maintain the structural and functional integrity of all cell membranes. The stored lipids in adipose tissue also serve to provide insulation, help to control body temperature, and afford some physical protection to internal organs. They are also required for the absorption of fat soluble vitamins.

For the adults, ICMR recommends that dietary fat should provide at least 15–20% total energy and at least 50% of fat intake should consist of vegetable oils rich in essential fatty acids. Saturated fat intake should be less than 7–10% of total daily calorie intake. The daily diet of an adult should include 25 to 40 gm of fat. However, major health issues concerning intake of fat centred around the role of excessive dietary fat in coronary heart disease (CHD), obesity and certain cancers.

Sterols: Dietary fats also contain minor components such as tocopherols, tocotrienols, sterols, etc. These are the substances which resemble fats only in their physical properties and solubilities. The plant oils also contain certain useful substances such as lignans (sesame oil), sterols, tocopherols (vitamin E), oryzanole (rice bran oil), carotenoids—all of which reduce cholesterol and reduce oxidation damage due to ageing and inflammation which occur in chronic diseases.

Proteins

Proteins are complex organic nitrogenous compounds containing nitrogen and often sulphur in addition to carbon, hydrogen, oxygen. For an adult man who weighs 70 kg, about 16% of body weight is made by protein (i.e. about 11 kg); with 43% in muscles, 16% in blood and 15% in skin. They are thus most essential for the maintenance of animal life and are also known as nitrogenous or flesh forming substances.

The nitrogen in the proteins is needed for the important work of building and repairing protoplasm for body cells, tissues and organs. The body cannot store excess protein consequently the body utilises what it needs, and the excess protein is used as a body fuel. The nitrogenous waste of this protein is excreted by kidneys.

Proteins are complex molecules composed of different amino acids. There are 23 known amino acids in total, each with a specific name. Certain amino acids which are termed "essential", have to be obtained from proteins in the diet since they are not synthesized in the human body. Other nonessential amino acids can be synthesized in the body to build proteins. The essential amino acids are:

1. Tryptophan	6. Leucine
2. Lysine	7. Isoleucine
3. Methionine	8. Valine
4. Threonine	9. Arginine
5. Phenylalanine	10. Histidine

There are broadly two sources of dietary proteins, i.e. animal sources, e.g. milk, eggs, meat, cheese, fish, poultry, butter, and yoghurt and plant sources, e.g. pulses, cereals, beans, nuts, and oil seed.

The presence of these ten essential amino acids in adequate amounts distinguishes the animal proteins as being "biologically complete"/superior *or first class* proteins as compared to the proteins of vegetable origin, which lack in one or more of these essential amino acids. The biological value of protein in egg is highest followed by milk. Thus, a mixed diet containing both animal and vegetable proteins meets with the needs of essential amino acids required by the body. In cases of vegetarian diet, a combination of cereals, millets and pulses provides most of the amino acids, which complement each other to provide better quality proteins.

Proteins perform a wide range of functions like (a) growth and development of the body, (b) maintenance, repair and replacement of damaged tissues, (c) form a part of metabolic and digestive enzymes and hormones, (d) maintenance of osmotic pressure, (e) essential for immunity, and (f) provides energy at the rate of 4 kcal per gram.

Protein requirements vary with age, physiological status and stress. More proteins are required by growing infants and children, pregnant women and individuals during infections and illness or stress. The daily body requirement of protein for an adult is about 1 gm per kg of body weight; and it is desirable that one-fifth of it should be animal protein. Around 10–15% of total calories in a balanced diet must be provided by proteins.

Minerals

Minerals are essential nutrients that are organic and inorganic substances categorized as 'protective foods'. These are required by body in very small amounts, but are essential for growth, repair and regulation of vital body functions. They also maintain the normal osmotic pressure in the fluids and tissues of the body, besides playing an important part in the acid alkali regulation of the body. They are also required to makeup the loss of salts excreted in urine and sweat.

Minerals make up about 4–5% of the body weight. The alkali forming minerals are calcium, potassium, sodium, iron and manganese. The acid forming elements are phosphorus, sulphur and chlorine.

The main functions of minerals in the body are

1. To maintain tone of muscles, nerves and blood.
2. To stimulate digestive secretions.
3. To help general growth of the body.
4. To help in maintaining acid alkali equlibrium.
5. To maintain rigid structure of body such as bones, teeth, etc.

In the human body, there are at least 15–16 different mineral elements and each has its own specific role to play.

There are two kinds of minerals

a. Major or macrominerals are minerals that the body needs in larger amounts. They include calcium, phosphorus, magnesium, sodium, potassium, chloride and sulphur.
b. Trace minerals or elements are required in small amounts. These include iron, manganese, copper, iodine, zinc, cobalt, fluoride and selenium.

The following minerals, however, are most important from nutrition point of view:

1. *Calcium*: It is the chief constituent of bones and teeth. It gives rigidity, and strength to bones and hardness and shine to the teeth. It controls rhythmic activities of the heart and contractile muscles. It is also essential for the coagulation of blood. It is required in much greater amount during the periods of pregnancy and lactation. Calcium metabolism is closely related to phosphorus and vitamin D. Its deficiency leads to poor development of bones and teeth, rickets, osteomalacia, delayed blood coagulation, hyperplasia of parathyroid glands and low calcium tetany. The best sources of calcium are milk, cheese, eggs, dark green leafy vegetables and dried fruits. The calcium in green vegetables, however, is poorly absorbed because of presence of oxalates. Its daily requirement for an average adult is 1 gm and for pregnant and lactating mothers is 1.2 gm. Though recommended dietary allowances for calcium are about 600–800 mg/day, it is desirable to give higher quantities of calcium for adolescents to achieve high peak bone mass.

2. *Phosphorus*: It is contained in every cell of the body and is essential for the multiplication of cells and the growth of body. Its daily requirement in the diet is 1.5 gm but more of it is required during pregnancy.

The roles of phosphorus in the body are

i. Bone structure: 80–85% of phosphorus in the body is located in the bones and teeth.
ii. Energy production: ATP (adenosine triphosphate) and ADP (adenosine diphosphate).
iii. Cell membranes: As phospholipids.
iv. Genetic reactions: In DNA (deoxyribonucleic acid) and RNA (ribonucleic acid).
v. A buffering agent, helping to maintain osmotic pressure.

Deficiency of phosphorus is characterised by softening of bones, arthritis, caries of teeth, muscle

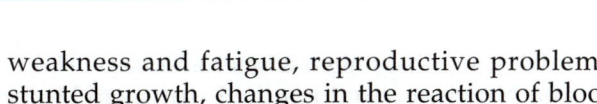

weakness and fatigue, reproductive problems, stunted growth, changes in the reaction of blood and depression of vital processes.

Excess of phosphorus is associated with iron deficiency anaemia, hyperexcitability, arthritis irritability, calcium and magnesium deficiency tremors, diarrhoea and zinc deficiency.

Its chief sources are seafood, meats, cheese, yolk of eggs, grains (oatmeal, millets, rice, wheatbran and germ), nuts and seeds (almonds, pistachio, sesame, peanuts), chocolate, kelp, yeast and vegetables (chickpeas, garlic, lentils, popcorn, soybeans), etc. In cereals, about 50 to 80% of phosphorus is present in the form of phytic acid, inositol hexose phosphoric acid.

3. *Iron:* It is the main constituent of haemoglobin of blood and nuclei of the cells. It is vital for both physical and mental well-being. It acts as an oxygen carrier to the lungs and tissues, maintains a healthy immune system and aids in energy production by playing an important part in the oxidation and catalysis of enzymes.

There are two types of iron in food

1. Haem iron, derived from the haemoglobin and myoglobin found in meat tissue. Haem iron is well absorbed and is influenced to some extent by the body's iron stores. The average absorption of haem iron in meat is about 25%.
2. Non-haem iron, derived mainly from cereals, legumes, fruit and vegetables. Generally, the absorption of non-haem iron is less than 5%.

Recommended dietary allowances for iron in healthy adults varies from 17 to 21 mg per day, however, its requirement is higher in pregnant women and growing children/adolescents. An adult woman needs more of iron to compensate for loss of blood in menstruation and also during pregnancy, lactation, etc. The concentration of iron in an healthy adult is about 30–40 mg/kg body weight, of which about 74–75% is functional iron. About 31 mg/kg iron in men and 26 mg/kg in women exists in the form of haemoglobin and its deficiency causes anaemia. Iron is stored in the form of ferritin and hemosiderin. When the average tissue iron storing content of ferritin approaches about 4000 atoms of iron per ferritin molecules, ferritin is degraded by lysosomal proteases to form hemosiderin. Iron in hemosiderin is less available for mobilization because it is present in the form of amorphous ferric oxide, ferrihydrate; that is chemically less reactive than the iron found in ferritin.

Its chief sources are liver, red meat, eggs, pulses, cereals, onion, green leafy vegetables (Amaranth, Bengal gram, leaves, cauliflower, greens and radish leaves), dry fruits, dates, figs, resins, etc. Human milk is a poor source of iron.

4. *Iodine:* Iodine is an element that is needed for the secretion of thyroxine hormone from thyroid gland. The body does not make iodine, so it is an essential part of diet. It occurs in all the tissues and fluids of the body. The recommended dietary allowance (RDA) for iodine in adult men and women is 150 µg per day. However, this may be increased during puberty, pregnancy, lactation and menopause.

About 167 million population are estimated to be living in iodine deficiency disorder (IDD) endemic areas. In case of insufficient iodine in the body, sufficient thyroid hormone (thyroxine) is not produced, which causes goiter (enlargement of thyroid gland in the neck), neonatal hypothyroidism, cretinism among newborns, mental retardation, delayed motor development, stunting, deaf-mutism and neuromuscular disorders. The most important consequence of iodine deficiency in mothers is cretinism in which the children suffer from mental and growth retardation right from the birth. About 90,000 stillbirths and neonatal deaths occur every year due to maternal iodine deficiency. Around 54 million persons are estimated to have goiter, 2.2 million persons have cretinism and 6.6 million persons suffer from mild psychomotor handicaps.

Iodine is present naturally in soil and seawater. Its chief sources are seafish, cod liver oil, yolk of eggs, onions and fresh vegetables. Iodised table salt is used as a vehicle to supply the iodine in endemic goitre areas. However, excess of iodine in diet can also cause problems especially in individuals that already have thyroid problems, such as nodules, hyperthyroidism and autoimmune thyroid disease.

5. *Sodium:* It is the main salt component of cells, tissues and fluids of human body and is responsible for maintaining osmotic pressure in blood and other tissue fluids. It is essential for the maintenance of pH ion concentration. Sodium independently also has significant role to play in the body in nerve conduction and fluid balance in the body. Sodium is primarily involved in the maintenance of water balance and equilibrium. It also plays an important role in electrophysiological functions of the cell.

Sodium is rapidly absorbed from the gastrointestinal tract and a positive balance is achieved on intakes just above minimal requirements. Requirement of sodium depends on its losses through urine, faeces and sweat. The sweat loss varies according to climatic conditions. High ambient temperatures and vigorous physical exercise increase sodium loss through sweat. Even after 6 hours of hard physical labour, which may generate 3 litres of sweat, the requirement of sodium chloride may not be more than 6 g/day.

Natural diets, in general, provide about 300–400 mg of sodium a day. Cereals, pulses, vegetables, milk, animal and seafoods are the major sources of sodium. Preserved foods such as pickles, sun-dried foods such as papads, sauces/ketchup and canned foods contribute to higher intakes of salt.

Deficiency of salt, chloride of sodium, leads to cramps, marked general weakness, mental lassitude, dyspnoea on exertion and heat exhaustion.

Indian data indicates that per capita consumption of salt ranges from less than 5–30 g/day in different states with almost 40% of population consuming about 10 g/day. Increased salt intake (>8 gm/day) is associated with health risks and may lead to hypertension and heart disease. Since sodium intake needs to be balanced by potassium intake, potassium-rich foods such as fresh vegetables and fruits, decrease blood pressure. Besides increasing blood pressure, excessive salt may also affect stomach mucosa and result in atrophic gastritis and gastric cancer. Higher sodium intake leads to greater calcium excretion which may result in reduction in bone density. Existing evidence reveals a deleterious impact of high salt intake on blood vessels, blood pressure, bones and gastrointestinal tract. Salt is used as a vehicle for food fortification, since it is commonly used in food preparation.

6. *Copper:* Copper is an essential trace mineral presents in all body tissues. It works with iron to help the body form red blood cells. It also helps keep the blood vessels, nerves, immune system, and bones healthy.

Oysters and other **shellfish**, whole grains, beans, nuts, potatoes, and organ meats (kidneys, liver) are good sources of copper. Dark leafy greens, dried fruits such as prunes, cocoa, black pepper, and yeast are also sources of copper in the diet.

Normally, people have enough copper in the foods they eat. Lack of copper may lead to anaemia and osteoporosis.

In large amounts, copper is poisonous. A rare inherited disorder, **Wilson's disease**, causes deposits of copper in the liver, brain, and other organs. The increased copper in these tissues leads to **hepatitis,** kidney problems, brain disorders, and other problems.

Menkes' disease (kinky hair syndrome), another very rare disorder of copper **metabolism,** is a congenital disorder presents in male infants.

The recommendations for requirements depend on age, gender, and other factors (such as pregnancy). Women who are pregnant or producing breast milk (lactating) need higher amounts. The Food and Nutrition Board at the Institute of Medicine recommends the dietary intake of 890–900 µg/day for copper in healthy adolescents and adults whereas it ranges from 200–700 µg/day in children between 0 month and 13 years of age.

7. *Chlorine:* Chlorine is present in food and our body almost entirely in the form of chloride. It is important in maintaining water balance, and is an essential component of gastric juice. Body gets chlorine from food mainly in the form of sodium chloride (salt). Dietary deficiency of chlorine is rare and is only likely to occur in case of excessive losses from the body. This can result from prolonged vomiting, diarrhoea or profuse sweating, or in case of prolonged sodium restricted diet. An estimated safe and adequate amount of chlorine for a healthy adult is in the range of 1700 to 5100 milligrams per day. It is found in common salt, bananas, tomatoes, lettuce and green leafy vegetables.

Vitamins

These are complex organic substances required by the body in small amounts that are very essential for the normal growth and nutrition of animals. Since these cannot be synthesized in the body, they must be present in the diet. However, provitamin like beta-carotene can be converted to vitamin A in the body.

Vitamins are essential for numerous body processes and for maintenance of the structure of skin, bone, nerves, eye, brain, blood and mucous membrane. Vitamins C and E, beta-carotene, riboflavin and selenium act as antioxidants and protect the human body from free radical damage. These do not provide energy but are simply protective foods. The diet devoid of vitamins, if consumed for some time, gives rise to certain diseases known as deficiency diseases and may ultimately even cause death.

Classification of Vitamins

The vitamins may be classified as under:
 i. Fat-soluble
 ii. Water-soluble

i. Fat-soluble vitamins

Vitamins A, D, E and K are fat-soluble and can be stored in the body.

1. *Vitamin A or fat-soluble A (retinol):* Vitamin A helps—form and maintain healthy skin, teeth, skeletal and soft tissue, mucous membranes, and skin. It is known as retinol since it produces the pigments in the **retina** of the eye which promotes good vision especially in low light. It may also be needed for reproduction and breastfeeding. Retinol is an active form of vitamin A. It is found in animal liver, whole milk, and some fortified foods.

Carotenoids are dark-coloured dyes (pigments) found in plant foods that can turn into a form of vitamin A. There are more than 500 known carotenoids. One such carotenoid is beta-carotene which has antioxidant action. Antioxidants protect cells from damage caused by substances called free radicals. Free radicals are believed to contribute to certain chronic diseases and play a role in the ageing processes. Thus, these carotenoids reduce the risk for cancer. Sources of beta-carotene are bright yellow and orange fruits (cantaloupe, pink grapefruit, and apricots), vegetables (carrots, pumpkin, sweet potatoes, winter squash, broccoli, spinach, and most dark green leafy vegetables). The more intense the colour of a fruit or vegetable, the higher the beta-carotene content.

In vitamin A deficiency, the white of the eye (conjunctiva) loses its luster and becomes dry. In severe vitamin A deficiency, the black area of the eye (cornea) gets necrosed, leading to irreversible blindness in young children. Vitamin A also has a role in maintaining resistance of the body to common infections.

Vitamin A is not destroyed by ordinary cooking, although if cooking is prolonged or if the food is exposed to air it gets destroyed. Recommended dietary allowance (RDA) for vitamin A as per Food and Nutrition Board of the Institute of Medicine ranges from 400 to 500 µg per day for infants, 300–600 µg/day for children between 1 and 13 years of age and 700–900 µg in adolescents and adults more than 14 years of age.

For the prevention of vitamin A deficiency under Reproductive, Maternal, Newborn, Child Health plus Adolescent (RMNCHA) programme, vitamin A is given orally to children beginning at the age of 9 months along with measles vaccine and then subsequently at six monthly intervals up to five years of age. The first dose is 1 ml (1 lac IU) and subsequent doses are 2 ml (2 lac IU) each.

2. *Vitamin D (sunshine/anti-rachitic vitamin):* Vitamin D is important for good overall health and strong and healthy bones. Vitamin D is unique compared to other vitamins since it gets turned into a hormone 'calcitriol' referred to as "activated vitamin D".

It can be synthesized by the body from sunlight. However, the vitamin D that is produced in skin from sunlight and as available from supplements, has to be changed by body a number of times before it can be used to manage the amount of calcium in blood, bones, gut and other cells all over the body.

It is thermostable, i.e. withstands high temperature uninjured. It is present in egg yolk, cod liver oil, halibut liver oil, butter fat, ghee, etc. in the form of *cholecalciferol* (vitamin D₃). Cod liver oil is the richest source of vitamin D. In this respect, 5 eggs are equivalent to 1 teaspoonful of cod liver oil.

Vitamin D is essential for absorption of calcium and phosphorus and is thus very important for strong bones. Thus, initially it was believed to prevent a bone condition called rickets in children, however, today it is seen as a vital part of good health. Evidences from recent research show that vitamin D is also important in preventing and treating a number of serious long-term health problems. Its also an important factor in efficient functioning of muscles, heart, lungs, brain and immune system and is also known to have anti-cancer effects.

The condition of inadequate availability of vitamin D is called vitamin D deficiency. Severe vitamin D deficiency is characterised by soft, thin, and brittle bones in adults and children and is known as osteomalacia and rickets respectively. Deficiency of vitamin D has also been linked to some other conditions such as cancer, asthma, type II diabetes, high blood pressure, depression, Alzheimer's and some autoimmune diseases like multiple sclerosis, Crohn's and type I diabetes.

As per Food and Nutrition Board, Institute of Medicine, RDA for vitamin D are 400 IU (10 µg) for infants, 600 IU (15 µg) for ages 1–70 years and 800 IU (20 µg) for ages 70 and above.

3. *Vitamin E:* It was discovered by Dr. Evans of USA. who named it vitamin E. It is also a fat-soluble vitamin. It is stable to heat and light, but is destroyed on oxidation, specially in the presence of alkaline salts.

Vitamin E is an antioxidant that protects body tissue from damage caused by substances called free radicals, that can harm cells, tissues, and organs. They are believed to play a role in certain conditions related to ageing. The body also needs vitamin E to help keep the immune system strong against viruses and bacteria. Vitamin E is also important in the formation of red blood cells and it helps the body use **vitamin K**. It also helps widen blood vessels and keep blood from clotting inside them.

The best way to get the daily requirement of vitamin E is by eating food sources. Vitamin E is found in vegetable oils (e.g. wheat germ, sunflower, safflower, corn, and soybean oils), nuts (e.g. almonds, peanuts, and hazelnuts/filberts), seeds (e.g. sunflower seeds), green leafy vegetables (e.g. spinach and broccoli) and fortified breakfast cereals, fruit juices, margarine, and spreads. *Tocopherol,* an oil extracted from wheat germ, is the most potent known source of vitamin E. In supplement form, however, high doses of vitamin E might increase the risk for bleeding and serious bleeding in the brain. High levels of vitamin E may also increase the risk of birth defects.

Its deficiency in antenatal mothers may lead to prematurity with very low birth weight in newborn babies (<1500 gm). Deficiency symptoms include peripheral neuropathy, ataxia, skeletal myopathy, retinopathy, and impairment of the immune response. Vitamin E deficiency secondary to abetalipoproteinaemia causes such problems as poor transmission of nerve impulses, muscle weakness, and retinal degeneration that leads to blindness. Ataxia and vitamin E deficiency (AVED) is another rare, inherited disorder in which the liver's alpha-tocopherol transfer protein is defective or absent. People with AVED have such severe vitamin E deficiency that they develop nerve damage and lose the ability to walk unless they take large doses of supplemental vitamin E.

Recommended intakes for vitamin E as per the Food and Nutrition Board at the Institute of Medicine are 4–5 mg/day for infants less than 12 months of age, 6–11 mg/day in children up to 13 years of age and 15 mg/day in adolescents and adults. However, in lactation, the requirement is as high as 19 mg/day. The highest safe level of vitamin E supplements for adults is 1,500 IU/day for natural forms of vitamin E, and 1,000 IU/day for the man-made (synthetic) form.

4. *Vitamin K:* Vitamin K, a heat-stable vitamin, is known as the coagulation vitamin, because it is essential for the normal coagulation of the blood. Its main function is the formation of prothrombin. Its deficiency leads to hypoprothrombinemia, occurrence of haemorrhages in the skin and subcutaneous tissues of organs due to prolongation of blood-clotting.

Important sources of vitamin K are green leafy vegetables (kale, spinach, turnip greens, collards, swiss chard, mustard greens, parsley, romaine, and green leaf lettuce), vegetables such as Brussels sprouts, broccoli, cauliflower, and cabbage. Animal sources rich in vitamin K are fish, liver, meat, and eggs. Cereals contain only smaller amounts of vitamin K. It is also synthesized by the bacteria that line the gastrointestinal tract.

The Food and Nutrition Board at the Institute of Medicine recommends adequate intakes (AIs) for vitamin K as 2.0 µg per day in infants less than 6 months of age, 2.5 µg/day in children up to 12 months of age and 30–60 µg/day up to 13 years of age. However, the requirement is 75–90 µg/day in healthy adolescents and adults.

ii. *Water-soluble vitamins*

Vitamin C and B-complex vitamins such as thiamine (B_1), riboflavin (B_2), niacin (B_3), pantothenic acid (B_5), pyridoxine (B_6), biotin (B_7), folic acid and cyanocobalamin (B_{12}), are water-soluble. These cannot be stored in body and get easily excreted in urine. Vitamins B-complex and C are heat labile and are easily destroyed by heat, air or during drying, cooking and food processing.

1. **Vitamin B-complex:** The term vitamin B-complex now refers to all the vitamins split off from the original "vitamin B" and identified chemically or biologically. If all members of this group are absent from the diet, they produce:

   i. Cardiovascular symptoms such as loss of breath on exertion, palpitation and precordial pain.

   ii. Anorexia leading to complex distaste for all food and relieved by aneurin.

   iii. Diminution of nerve excitability leading to peripheral neuritis, hypoaesthesia and pain along the nerve trunks.

From the complex mixture, the following constituents have been isolated:

   i. *Vitamin B_1 (thiamine):* It is sensitive to heat and is considered anti-neurotic and anti-beriberi (dry or wet) vitamin. Deficiency of vitamin B_1 leads to loss of appetite, indigestion, constipation, nausea, weak heart muscles, palpitation, breathlessness and degeneration of nervous system. It is present in brewers yeast, beans, bran, wheat germ oil, sun flower seeds, nuts particularly ground nut, meat, fish, eggs, etc. Milk and highly milled rice are its poor sources. The use of antibiotics and alcohol adversely affects this vitamin. The daily requirement of this vitamin is 1.1–1.4 mg in healthy male and females who are moderate workers.

   ii. *Vitamin B_2 (riboflavin):* It is a water-soluble yellow pigment and is found in yeast, milk, eggs, fish, pork, liver and green leafy vegetables. It is highly heat stable and survives even canning. It has also been artificially synthesised and is essential for the maintenance of normal fat metabolism. Deficiency of Vitamin B_2 leads to ocular manifestations, chelosis, photophobia, burning, itching, angular stomatitis, glossitis and dermatitis of skin, which occurs most commonly in the individuals or communities whose diet mainly consists of milled rice. The estimated daily requirement of this vitamin is about 1.3–1.6 mg in healthy men and women who are moderate workers.

   iii. *Vitamin B_3 (niacin) or nicotinic acid (pellagra-preventing factor):* It is remarkably stable, capable of withstanding heat, oxidation and ultraviolet light. Vitamin B_3 is found in many foods including yeast, meat, liver, kidneys, fish, milk, eggs, whole meal flour, green vegetables, beans, cereal grains, etc. Niacin and niacinamide are also found in many vitamin B complex supplements with other B vitamins.

Niacin is used for treating high cholesterol and diabetes. It is also used along with other treatments for circulation problems, migraine headache, dizziness, and to reduce the diarrhoea associated with cholera. Since it has known to maintain healthy condition of skin and mucous membrane, thus is used for treating skin conditions called bullous pemphigoid, inflammatory acne vulgaris and granuloma annulare.

Its deficiency leads to pellagra which is characterised by 3 Ds—dermatitis, diarrhoea and dementia. The most typical symptom is erythema. Niacin or niacinamide is used for preventing vitamin B_3 deficiency and related conditions such as pellagra.

The daily recommended dietary allowances (RDAs) of niacin are 2–4 mg in infants less than 3 years of age, 6–8 mg in children up to 13 years of age, 12–14 mg in adolescents and adult men and women. However, the requirement is higher in pregnant women (18 mg) and lactating women (17 mg).

iv. *Vitamin B_5 (pantothenic acid)*: Pantothenic acid is widely found in both plants and animals including meat, vegetables, cereal grains, legumes, eggs, and milk. It is important for our bodies to properly use carbohydrates, proteins, and lipids and for healthy skin. Pantothenic acid has a long list of uses, although there is not enough scientific evidence to determine whether it is effective for most of these uses. Usually, pantothenic acid is used for treating dietary deficiencies, acne, alcoholism, allergies, hyperactivity, low blood sugar, insomnia, irritability, low blood pressure, osteoarthritis, rheumatoid arthritis, Parkinson's disease, nerve pain, premenstrual syndrome (PMS), etc.

Recommended daily intake for pantothenic acid (vitamin B_5) is 1.7–1.8 mg in infants, 2–4 mg in children and adults, 5–7 mg in pregnant and lactating mothers.

v. *Vitamin B_6 (pyridoxine or antidermatitis vitamin)*: It is a white crystalline compound, which is soluble in water. It is essential for normal protein metabolism, red blood cells (RBCs) production and haemoglobin synthesis and is required by body for utilization of energy in the food, and proper functioning of nerves. It is also known as an anti-dermatitis factor. It is present in rice polishing, yeast, liver, yolk of eggs, fat, peanuts, wheat germs, whole grain cereals, fish, vegetables, beans, and other organ meat. Pyridoxine deficiency causes blood, skin, and nerve changes. This vitamin is unique in that either deficiency or excess can cause peripheral neuropathy. The RDA for pyridoxine is 2 mg/day.

vi. *Vitamin B_7 (biotin)*: It is also known as vitamin H and metabolises carbohydrates, fats and amino acids. It is also important for normal embryonic growth, making it a critical nutrient during pregnancy. Its deficiency causes symptoms like hair loss, dry scaly skin, cracking in the corners of the mouth (called cheilosis), swollen and painful tongue that is magenta in colour (glossitis), dry eyes, loss of appetite, fatigue, insomnia, and depression. Its chief sources are Brewer's yeast; cooked eggs, especially egg yolk; sardines; nuts (almonds, peanuts, pecans, walnuts) and nut butters; soybeans; other legumes (beans, blackeye peas); whole grains; cauliflower; bananas; and mushrooms. Adequate daily intake of biotin ranges from 5 to 6 µg in infants, 8–12 µg in children up to 8 years of age, 20–25 µg in children and adolescents between 9 and 18 years and 30–35 µg in adults, pregnant and lactating mothers.

vii. *Folic acid, vitamin M*: Folic acid helps tissues grow and cells work. Taking the right amount of folic acid before and during pregnancy helps prevent certain birth defects, including spina bifida. Folate also helps prevent anaemia. Deficiency of folic acid may cause diarrhoea, gray hair, oral and peptic ulcers, poor growth, glossitis and macrocytic and pernicious anaemias. Natural sources of folic acid are dark green leafy vegetables, dried beans and peas (legumes), citrus fruits and juices, liver, kidneys and yeast. Many foods are now fortified with folic acid, including enriched breads, cereals, flours, cornmeals, pastas, rice, and other grain products. Food and Nutrition Board established an acceptable intake (AI) for folate in infants as 65–80 µg/day. However, daily reference intakes (DRIs) for folate in children up to 13 years of age range from 150 to 300 µg, 400 µg in healthy adults and 500–600 µg in pregnant and lactating women.

viii. *Inositol (mouse anti-alopecia factor)*: Inositol is sometimes colloquially known as "vitamin B_8", and is a beneficial nutrient that has been implicated in the treatment of some behavioural or emotional disorders. Inositol can be intrinsically produced by breaking down glucose, however, only dietary inositol can be absorbed and used by the body. It is associated in some way with metabolism or transport of fat thus can be used for treating conditions associated with polycystic ovary syndrome, including failure to ovulate; high blood pressure; high triglycerides; and high levels of testosterone. Its deficiency can lead to loss of hair and is thus important anti-alopecia factor. Inositol is used for diabetic nerve pain, panic disorder, high cholesterol, insomnia, cancer, depression, schizophrenia, Alzheimer's disease, attention deficit-hyperactivity disorder (ADHD), autism, psoriasis, and treating side effects of medical treatment with lithium. Rich sources of inositol are beans (navy and lima), fruits like grapefruit, cantaloupe, citrus fruits and whole grains.

ix. *Vitamin B_{12} (cyanocobalamin):* Vitamin B_{12} is important to maintain metabolism, blood cells, brain and nerves. Deficiency of vitamin B_{12} may result in decrease in red blood cells (pernicious anemia), stomach/intestine problems, and permanent nerve damage. Meat, fish, and dairy products are rich sources of vitamin B_{12} however, vitamin C (ascorbic acid) can decrease the amount of vitamin B_{12}. The RDA of vitamin B_{12} in healthy adults is 1–1.5 mg/day.

x. *Para-aminobenzoic acid (PABA):* It is sometimes called as vitamin Bx, however, it is not a true vitamin. It helps tissue oxidation and is used in sunscreens. It may naturally occur in grains, eggs, Brewer's yeast, liver, molasses, mushrooms, spinach and whole grains.

xi. *Choline:* Choline is similar to the B vitamins. It has variety of roles in human metabolism from cell structure to neurotransmitter synthesis. Choline deficiency is now thought to have an impact on diseases such as liver disease, atherosclerosis, and, possibly, neurological disorders. It can be made in the liver and is also found in foods such as liver, muscle meats, fish, nuts, beans, peas, spinach, wheat germ, and eggs. The average choline intake for humans on an ad libitum diet is about 600 mg/day for men and 450 mg/day for women.

2. **Vitamin C or antiscorbutic vitamin:** Vitamin C is an essential nutrient required for healthy bones and teeth. It also promotes iron absorption, is essential for maintaining capillary integrity and for formation of intercellular substance. It is essential for the maturation of red blood corpuscles. Vitamin C deficiency leads to scurvy, a disease characterised by swelling of gums, anaemia, bad teeth, offensive breath, spongy gums, loss of weight, delayed healing of wounds and haemorrhages.

Vitamin C is abundantly available in fresh amla, citrus fruits, guava, banana and certain vegetables such as tomatoes. Amla is indeed one of the richest natural sources of vitamin C. It has been isolated in pure form from fruit juice, has also been synthetically manufactured and termed as *ascorbic acid or cevitamic acid*. However, it is very susceptible to destruction by prolonged heating, preservation of fruits and by atmospheric oxidation. It is for this reason that when vegetables become dry and stale or cut and exposed to air most of the vitamin C originally present in destroyed.

The RDA for vitamin C is 40 mg per day except in infants (25 mg/day) and pregnant and lactating mothers (60–80 mg/day). Since vitamin C cannot be stored in the body so a daily intake of the recommended dose is necessary for good health.

3. **Flavonoids (vitamin P):** These are not strictly true vitamins, though they possess vitamin-like properties. The body cannot produce this nutrient, and must get it from the diet regularly. These are powerful antioxidants that help neutralize harmful free radicals and prevent oxidative stress which damage cells and DNA, and which can lead to aging and degenerative diseases. Almost all vegetables, fruits, spices and herbs contain bioflavonoids, as do some grains and dried beans. Green tea contains flavonoids called catechins that can reach up to 100 milligrams per cup. Berries, especially black raspberries, have the highest concentrations of the flavonoids anthocyanins. It helps in preventing capillary permeability and its deficiency leads to purpura, spontaneous capillary haemorrhages and infiltration of lungs resembling tuberculosis. Thus, the symptoms of vitamin P deficiency are easy bruising, excessive swelling after injury, frequent nasal bleeds, hemorrhoids/varicose veins, weak immune system.

4. **Water:** Water is the most important nutrient of all and helps in the upkeep of our health. It makes up more than two-thirds of the weight of the human body. It is an important constituent of food and represents the major portion of most food stuffs like fruits, vegetables and milk. But as these sources are insufficient to cope up with body requirements, water must be taken either plain or in the form of other beverages. Water is necessary to make up the loss caused by its excretion in breath, sweat, urine, faeces, and also to renew various fluids and solid organs of the body, into the constitutions of which it largely enters. It serves as a vehicle for the solution and dilution of the solid foods, whereby these are more easily digested and assimilated. It is also essential for elimination of many waste products. Although there is no research to identify the exact amount of water you should drink, experts usually recommend that a normal healthy person needs to drink about 8 glasses (2 litres) of water per day. However, during very hot weather and while undertaking vigorous physical activity, this requirement increases as a considerable amount of water is lost through sweat.

The rise of temperature and humidity of air increases the necessity for intake of water. An insufficient intake of water leads to creation of disturbance in circulation, of heat regulation mechanism and the retention of products of metabolism. It is estimated that about 80 oz (2.27 litres) of water enters the body daily as such or as a part of cooked food, beverages, etc. out of which 48–64 oz. (1.37–1.81 litres) is excreted daily in urine, sweat, etc. Some important uses of water are:

i. As a solvent for transportation of nutrients in the body.
ii. It helps regulating body temperature through evaporation from lungs and skin.
iii. As an aid in removing wastes of metabolism in the urine.
iv. As an aid in functions like osmosis.

Water should be safe and wholesome, i.e. it should be free from disease-causing agents like bacteria, viruses, parasites, etc. and harmful chemical substances like pesticides, industrial wastes, heavy metals, nitrates, arsenic and excess of fluoride. Fluorosis, a disease with bone deformities and dental problems, results from drinking water containing an excess of fluoride over long periods. Generally, a concentration of 0.5 to 0.8 mg of fluoride per litre of drinking water is considered safe.

If a water source is not safe for drinking, boiling it for 10–15 minutes is a satisfactory method of purification of the water. It kills all disease causing organisms and also removes temporary hardness, although it does not remove other chemical impurities. Tablet containing 0.5 g of chlorine can disinfect 20 litres of water. There are many modern gadgets which claim to provide safe and wholesome water (details discussed in chapter on water).

6.4 CLASSIFICATION OF FOODS

These are classified according to their functions under the following heads:

1. **Energy producing foods:** These constitute fats and carbohydrates. They are also called protein sparers. Proteins also produce energy to some extent. Cereals, roots and tubers, dried fruits, sugars and fats belong to this group. They supply heat and energy to the body.
2. **Body building foods:** These are foods rich in proteins, mineral salts and water. Milk, meat, fish, pulses, oilseeds and nuts fall in this category.
3. **Protecting or protective foods:** These constitute inorganic salts, vitamins and minerals. They include proteins and water. Milk, eggs, liver, green leafy vegetables and fruits are included in this group. They build our bones, teeth, muscles, soft tissues, blood and other body fluids. These provide material for repair in the body after wear and tear.

Balanced diet: The rationale of balanced diet is to consume nutritionally adequate diet through a wise choice from a variety of foods. Thus, a balanced diet is one which provides all the nutrients in required amounts and proper proportions. It can easily be achieved through a blend of the four basic food groups. The quantities of foods needed to meet the nutrients requirements vary with age, gender, physiological status and physical activity. A balanced diet should provide around 50–60% of total calories from carbohydrates, preferably from complex carbohydrates, about 10–15% from proteins and 20–30% from both visible and invisible fats. In addition, a balanced diet should provide other non-nutrients such as dietary fibre, antioxidants and phytochemicals which bestow positive health benefits. Antioxidants, such as vitamins C and E, beta-carotene, riboflavin and selenium, protect the human body from free radical damage. Other phytochemicals such as polyphenols, flavones, etc. also afford protection against oxidant damage. Spices like turmeric, ginger, garlic, cumin and cloves are rich in antioxidants.

Recommended dietary allowances (RDAs): The RDAs are estimates of nutrients to be consumed daily to ensure the requirements of all individuals in a given population. The recommended level depends upon the bioavailability of nutrients from a given diet. The term bioavailability indicates what is absorbed and utilized by the body. In addition, RDA also includes a margin of safety, to cover variation between individuals, dietary traditions, practices and physical activity. Thus, our diet must provide adequate calories, proteins and micronutrients to achieve maximum growth potential.

There might be situations where adequate amounts of nutrients are not available through diet alone. In such situations, the foods consumed commonly can be fortified with the limiting nutrient(s). A good example of such fortified foods is the salt fortified with iron and iodine (Table 6.1).

Composition of a balanced diet for adults— sedentary/ moderate/heavy activity males and females is given Table 6.2.

Also, sample menu plans for sedentary adult man and woman are given in Tables 6.3 to 6.5.

Table 6.1: Food consumption (g/day)

	Intake*		RDA#
	CU	Per capita	
Cereals/millets	396	345	400
Pulses	28	24	80
Milk	82	71	300
Vegetables	49	43	300
Oils	14	12	30

* National Nutrition Monitoring Bureau, 2006.
\# RDA (2010) for moderately active person

Table 6.2: Balanced diet for adults—sedentary/moderate/heavy activity (number of portions)

		Type of work					
		Sedentary		*Moderate*		*Heavy*	
	g/portion	*Man*	*Woman*	*Man*	*Woman*	*Man*	*Woman*
Cereals and millets	30	12.5	9	15	11	20	26
Pulses	30	2.5	2	3	2.5	4	3
Milk and milk products	100 ml	3	3	3	3	3	3
Roots and tubers	100	2	2	2	2	2	2
Green leafy vegetables	100	1	1	1	1	1	1
Other vegetables	100	2	2	2	2	2	2
Fruits	100	1	1	1	1	1	1
Sugar	5	4	4	6	6	11	9
Fat	5	5	4	6	5	8	6

To calculate the days requirement of above mentioned food groups for an individual, multiply grams per portion with number of portions.

Table 6.3: Sample meal plan for adult man (sedentary)

Meal time	Food group	Raw	Cooked recipe	Servings amount
Breakfast	Milk	100 ml	Milk	1/2 cup
	Sugar	15 g	Tea or coffee	2 cups / 1 cup
	Cereals	70 g	Breakfast item	
	Pulses	20 g		
Lunch	Cereals	120 g	Rice / Pulkas	2 cups / 2 nos.
	Pulses	20 g	Dhal	1/2 cup
	Vegetables	150 g	Veg. curry	3/4 cup
	Vegetables	50 g	Veg. salad	7–8 slices
	Milk	100 ml	Curd	1/2 cup
Tea	Cereals	50 g	Snack	
	Milk	50 ml	Tea	1 cup
	Sugar			
Dinner	Cereals	120 g	Rice / Pulkas	2 cups / 2 nos.
	Pulses	20 g	Dhal	1/2 cup
	Vegetables	150 g	Veg. curry	3/4 cup
	Milk (curd)	50 ml		
	Vegetables	50 g		
	Fruit	100 g	Seasonal	1 medium

1 cup = 200 ml

Note: For non-vegetarians—substitute one plus portion with one portion of egg/meat/chicken/fish

Use 25 g visible fat and <5 g salt during preparation of meal per day.

Breakfast items: Idli—4 nos./Dosa—3 nos./Upma—1–1/2 cup/Bread—4 slices/Porridge—2 cups/Corn flakes with milk—2 cups.

Snacks: Poha—1 cup/Toast—2 slices

Dhokla—4 nos.

Table 6.4: Sample meal plan for adult woman (sedentary)

Meal time	Food group	Raw	Cooked recipe	Servings amounts
Breakfast	Milk	100 ml	Milk or	1/2 cup
	Sugar	10 g	Tea or Coffee	2 cups / 1 cup
	Cereals	50 g	Breakfast item	
	Pulses	20 g		
Lunch	Cereals	100 g	Rice / Pulkas	1 ups / 2 nos.
	Pulses	20 g	Dhal	1/2 cup
	Vegetables	50 g	Veg. curry	1/2 cup
	Vegetables	50 g	veg. salad	7–8 slices
	Milk	100 ml	Curd	1/2 cup
Tea	Cereals	50 g	Snack	
	Milk	50 ml	Tea	1 cup
	Sugar	10 g		
Dinner	Cereals	100 g	Rice / Pulkas	1 cups / 2 nos.
	Pulses	20 g	Dhal	1/2 cup
	Vegetables	100 g	Veg. curry	1/2 cup
	Milk (curd)	50 ml		
	Vegetables	50 g		
	Fruit	100 g	Seasonal	1 medium

1 cup = 200 ml

Note: For non-vegetarians—substitute one plus portion with one portion of egg/meat/chicken/fish

Use 25 g visible fat and <5 g salt during preparation of meal per day.

Breakfast items: Idli—3 nos./Dosa—2 nos./Upma—1 cup/Bread—3 slices/Porridge—1–1/2 cups/Corn flakes with milk—1–1/2 cups.

Snacks: Poha—1 cup/Toast—2 slices

Dhokla—4 nos.

Table 6.5: Balanced diet for infants, children and adolescents (number of portions)

Food groups	g/portion	Infants 6–12 months	1–3	4–6	7–9	10–12 Girls	10–12 Boys	13–15 Girls	13–15 Boys	16–18 Girls	16–18 Boys
Cereals and millets	30	0.5	2	4	6	8	10	11	14	11	15
Pulses	30	0.25	1	1.0	2	2	2	2	2.5	2.5	3
Milk (ml) and products	100	4*	5	5	5	5	5	5	5	5	5
Roots and tubers	100	0.5	0.5	1	1	1	1	1	1.5	2	2
Green leafy vegetables	100	0.25	0.5	0.5	1	1	1	1	1	1	1
Other vegetables	100	0.25	0.5	1	1	2	2	2	2	2	2
Fruits	100	1	1	1	1	1	1	1	1	1	1
Sugar	5	2	3	4	4	6	6	5	4	5	6
Fats and oils (visible)	5	4	5	5	6	7	7	8	9	7	10

* Quantity indicates top milk. For breastfed infants, 200 ml top milk is required. One portion of pulse may be exchanged with one portion (50 g) of egg/meat/chicken/fish. For infants, introduce egg/meat/chicken/fish around 9 months.

6.5 DIET FOR PREGNANT AND LACTATING MOTHERS

The pregnant woman has increased nutritional demands for the increased growth of her body and to supply the needs of the foetus, thus additional food and extra care are required during this period.

The nutritive requirements of a pregnant woman must be estimated on the basis of her nutritive status, weight, stage of pregnancy and daily activity. It should also afford a reserve for the period of lactation besides compensation of already existing malnutrition in the pre-pregnancy state. Adequate intake of a nutritious diet should ensure an optimal weight gain during pregnancy (10–12 kg) by the expectant woman and the birth weight of the baby as 3 kg.

The daily diet of a woman should contain an additional 350 calories, 0.5 g of protein during first trimester and 6.9 g during second trimester and 22.7 g during third trimester of pregnancy. Some micronutrients are specially required in extra amounts during these physiological periods. Folic acid, taken throughout the pregnancy, reduces the risk of congenital malformations and increases the birth weight. The mother as well as the growing fetus needs iron to meet the high demands of erythropoiesis (RBC formation). Calcium is essential, both during pregnancy and lactation, for proper formation of bones and teeth of the offspring, for secretion of breast milk rich in calcium and to prevent osteoporosis in the mother. Similarly, iodine intake ensures proper mental health of the growing fetus and infant. Though it is possible to meet the requirements for most of the nutrients through a balanced diet, pregnant/lactating women are advised to take daily supplements of iron, folic acid, vitamin B and calcium.

The pregnant/lactating woman should derive maximum amount of energy (about 60%) from rice, wheat and millets. Cooking oil is a concentrated source of both energy and polyunsaturated fatty acids. Good quality protein can be derived from milk, fish, meat, poultry and eggs. Mineral and vitamin requirements are met by consuming a variety of seasonal vegetables particularly green leafy vegetables, milk and fresh fruits. Bioavailability of iron can be improved by using fermented and sprouted grams and foods rich in vitamin C such as citrus fruits. Milk is the best source of biologically available calcium. The diet should be rich in fibre (around 25 g/1000 kcal) like whole grain cereals, pulses and vegetables, to avoid constipation. She should take plenty of fluids including 8–12 glasses of water per day. Salt intake should not be restricted even to prevent pregnancy-induced hypertension (PIH) and pre-eclampsia.

Excess intake of beverages containing caffeine like coffee and tea, smoking and chewing of tobacco should be avoided. Alcohol intake should also be avoided since all these adversely affect fetal growths. Pregnant and lactating women should not indiscriminately take any drugs without medical advice, as some of them could be harmful to the foetus/baby. Wrong food beliefs and taboos should be discouraged.

In addition to satisfying these dietary requisites, a pregnant woman should undergo periodic health check-up for weight gain, blood pressure, anaemia and receive tetanus toxoid immunization. She requires light physical exercise with adequate rest for 2–3 hr during the day.

The most important food safety problem is microbial food-borne illness and their prevention during pregnancy is an important public health measure. Avoiding contaminated foods is important protective measure against food-borne illness.

6.6 BREASTFEEDING

Exclusive breastfeeding ensures safe nutrition and all round development of the infant.

a. Breast milk provides best nutrition, contains all essential nutrients and protects the infant from infections.

b. It is a natural food and is more easily digested and absorbed by the infant as compared to formula milk prepared from other sources.

c. Colostrum, the milk secreted during the first 3–4 days after childbirth, is rich in proteins, minerals, vitamins especially vitamin A and antibodies. In addition, it has a laxative effect as well.

d. Breastfeeding helps in reducing fertility and facilitates spacing of children.

e. Breastfeeding is associated with better cognitive development possibly due to the high content of docosahexaenoic acid (DHA) which plays an important role in brain development.

f. Lactation provides emotional satisfaction to the mother and the infant and improved the bonding between them.

g. Recent evidence suggests that human milk may confer some long-term benefits such as lower risk of certain autoimmune diseases, inflammatory bowel disease, obesity and related disorders and probably some cancers.

Diseases and death among breastfed infants are much lower than those among formula-fed infants. Breastfeeding protects against diarrhoea and upper respiratory tract infections. The bifidus factor in breast milk promotes the natural gut flora. The gut flora and the low pH of breast milk inhibit the growth of pathogens. Breast milk has immunoglobulin A (IgA), lactoferrin, lactoperoxidase and complements which protect the infant from several infections. Antibodies to *E. coli* and some viruses are found in breast milk, which protect the gut mucosa. Breastfeeding also protects infants from vulnerability to allergic reactions.

In addition to providing nutrients, breast milk has several special components such as growth factors, enzymes, hormones and anti-infective factors. The amount of milk secreted increases gradually in the first few days after delivery, reaching the peak during the second month, at which level it is maintained until about 6 months of age. An average Indian woman secretes about 750 ml of milk per day during the first 6 months and 600 ml/day subsequently up to one year.

Early initiation of breastfeeding is very important for successful lactation. The baby should be put to breast immediately after delivery as soon as the mother is comfortable and not later than 30 minutes in a normal delivery and 4 hours in case of a caesarean section. Colostrum should be made available to the infant immediately after birth and no prelacteal feeds, like honey, glucose, ghutti, water or dilute milk, must be given to the baby.

A baby should be exclusively breastfed up to 6 months of age and complementary foods should be introduced thereafter. Breastfed infants do not need additional water. Feeding water reduces the breast milk intake and increases the risk of diarrhoea and should, therefore, be avoided. Additional water is not required for the breastfed infants even in hot climate. Breastfeeding can be continued as long as possible, however, should be preferably continued up to 2 years of age. Breastfeeding should be on demand as 'demand feeding' helps in maintaining lactation for a longer time. Frequent sucking by the baby and complete emptying of breast are important for sustaining adequate breast milk output. If babies are quiet or sleep for about 2 hours after a feed and show adequate weight gain, feeding may be assumed to be adequate.

Even the undernourished mothers can successfully breastfeed, however, composition of breast milk depends to some extent on maternal nutrition. In case of severe maternal malnutrition, both the quality and quantity of breast milk may be affected. Protein content of breast milk appears to be much less affected as compared to fat in malnutrition. Concentration of water-soluble vitamins as well as fat-soluble vitamin A (beta-carotene) is influenced by the quality of the maternal diet. Supplementation of vitamins A and B-complex to lactating mothers increases the levels of these vitamins in breast milk. Zinc and iron from breast milk are better absorbed than from other food sources. Trace element composition of breast milk, however, is not affected by the mother's nutritional status.

It is necessary that the woman is prepared during pregnancy for breastfeeding and is encouraged to eat a well-balanced diet and take adequate rest. Anxiety and emotional stress must be avoided. It is necessary to prepare the breast, particularly the nipple, for breastfeeding. A working mother can express her breast milk and store it hygienically up to 8 hrs. This can be fed hygeinically to her infant by the caretaker. Since, drugs (antibiotics, caffeine, hormones and alcohol) are secreted into the breast milk and could prove harmful to the breastfed infant, caution should be exercised by the lactating mother while taking medicines.

Human immunodeficiency virus (HIV) may be transmitted from mother to infant through breast milk. However, women living in the resource poor settings in developing countries may not have access to safe, hygienic and affordable replacement feeding options. Considering the important role of breast milk in child growth and development, National AIDS Control Organization (NACO) recommends that such mothers should be informed about the risk of transmission of HIV through breast milk vis-à-vis the risks and benefits of each feeding method, with specific guidance in selecting the option most likely to be suitable for their situation. When replacement feeding is not acceptable, feasible, affordable, sustainable and safe (AFASS), exclusive breastfeeding is recommended during the first months of life. Every effort should be made to promote exclusive breastfeeding for up to six months in the case of HIV-positive mothers too followed by weaning, at six months. In any case, mixed feeding, i.e. breastfeeding along with other feeds should be strictly discouraged as it increases the risk of HIV transmission.

6.7 DIET FOR INFANTS AND CHILDREN

Foods that are regularly fed to the infant, in addition to breast milk, providing sufficient nutrients are known as supplementary or complementary foods. These could be liquids like milk or semisolids like *'kheer'* in the case of infants or solid preparations like rice, etc. in the case of children over the age of one year.

For initial six months of life, breastfeed alone is adequate to meet the requirements of growth and development. However, subsequently the requirement of all the nutrients progressively increases with infant's growth with simultaneous reduction of the breast milk secretion. Thus, adequate food needs to be added to promote optimal growth in infants. Easy to cook home-made preparations are hygenic and healthy foods for the growing baby. Low-cost food supplements can be prepared at home from commonly used ingredients such as cereals (wheat, rice, *ragi*, jowar, bajra, etc.); pulses (grams/dals), nuts and oilseeds (groundnut, sesame, etc.), oils (groundnut oil, sesame oil, etc.) and sugar and jaggery. Such supplements are easily digested by all infants, including those with severe malnutrition.

Childhood is the period of continuous growth and development. An infant grows rapidly, doubling its birth weight by 5 months and tripling it by 1 year of age. During the second year, the child increases not only in height by 7–8 cm but also gains 4 times of its birth weight. During the preadolescent period, the child grows, on an average, 6–7 cm in height and 1.5 to 3 kg in weight every year and simultaneously development and maturation of various tissues and organs take place. Thus, an adequate quantity of protein is required for the building of tissues. Besides, iron should also be supplied for the formation of haemoglobin of the blood, and calcium and phosphorus for bone growth and better teeth. Complementary/weaning foods based on cereal-pulse-nut and sugar/jaggery combinations will provide good quality protein, adequate calories and other protective nutrients.

Since infants cannot consume large quantities of foods, they should be given small frequent meals and energy-rich foods like fats and sugars should be included in such preparations.

Green leafy vegetables (GLVs), after thorough cleaning, must form a part of their diet since they are inexpensive but rich sources of vitamins, minerals and dietary fibre. In families that can afford egg yolk and meat soup can be introduced. It is important to ensure that adequate hygienic practices are scrupulously followed at the time of preparation and feeding of the recipes. At about one year of age, the child should share the family diet.

Breastfeeding is the best option to avoid nutritional problems during infancy since improper feeding, under-feeding and frequent infections are the chief causes of malnutrition among artificially fed infants.

6.8 INDIAN FOOD BELIEFS, FADS AND TABOOS

Exaggerated beneficial or harmful claims in respect of some foods, without scientific basis constitute food fads. Food beliefs either encourage or discourage the consumption of particular type of foods. There can be neutral harmless or harmful practices. Most of the food-related prejudices (taboos) are associated with physiological states that make an individual as such vulnerable, i.e. children and women and conditions that need special nutritional care like pregnancy and lactation. The belief of hot and cold foods is widely prevalent. Some nutritious foods like jaggery, dry fruits, groundnuts, fried foods, mango, bajra, jowar, maize, eggs, meat, etc. are considered as heat producing foods and thus are not given to pregnant and lactating mothers and adolescent girls. Papaya is strongly suspected to lead to abortion, though there is no scientific basis and thus is not given to pregnant women thus depriving them of its rich nutritional constituents. Buttermilk, curd, milk, green gram dal, green leafy vegetables, ragi, barley flour and apples are considered as cold-inducing foods which are actually nutritious. Vegetarianism is often practiced in India on religious grounds. Since vitamin B is present only in foods of animal origin, vegetarians remain deprived of B group vitamins unless supplemented. During certain illnesses like measles and diarrhoea, dietary restriction is imposed that can aggravate undernutrition in young children.

6.9 NUTRITIONAL DISORDERS

Nutritional disorders can be caused by an insufficient intake of food or of certain nutrients, by an inability of the body to absorb and use nutrients, or by overconsumption of certain foods. Examples include obesity caused by excess energy intake, anaemia caused by insufficient intake of iron, and impaired sight because of inadequate intake of vitamin A. Diseases include, but are not limited to: Protein energy malnutrition (PEM), scurvy, rickets, beriberi, hypocalcaemia, osteomalacia, vitamin K deficiency, pellagra, cheilosis, Menkes' disease, and xerophthalmia. Some of them are being discussed as follows.

A. Undernutrition

1. **Protein calorie malnutrition (PCM):** It is also sometimes termed as protein energy malnutrition (PEM). The clinical conditions of childhood undernutrition are widely recognised as kwashiorkor, marasmus and the mixed condition of the two, i.e. marasmic kwashiorkor.

    i. *Kwashiorkor*: It results from consumption of very low protein in diets of low biological values, yet providing just enough energy to satisfy the needs of the child. This condition is usually seen in children between the age group of 1 and 4 years. This symptom is characterised by pitting oedema, anaemia, retarded growth, loss of appetite, diarrhoea, scanty hair growth, etc.

    ii. *Marasmus*: It is a clinical condition of protein energy malnutrition, primarily due to total deprivation of the requisite calories required by the body. It usually occurs in the age group of 1/2 to 5 years. This syndrome is characterised by failure to gain weight, wasting of muscles and of subcutaneous fat. The child has good appetite but is irritable.

    iii. *Marasmic kwashiorkor*: Patients suffering from marasmic kwashiorkor show clinical symptoms of both marasmus and kwashiorkor.

2. **Protein deficiency in adults:** Protein stricken deficiency in adults is also quite prevalent in poverty areas. Protein deficiency will result in adults having reduced weight, reduced subcutaneous fat, anaemia, greater susceptibility to infection, frequent loose motions, general lethargy, delay in healing of wounds and oedema.

3. **Mineral deficiencies:** (i) Deficiency of iodine in water leads to goitre, (ii) lack of flourine (<0.5 ppm) in water leads to dental caries, (iii) calcium deficient diets lead to rickets and osteomalacia, (iv) iron deficiency diets lead to anaemia, and (v) there are other important minerals like copper, selenium, etc. Copper deficiency leads to fatigue, anaemia, and a decreased number of white blood cells. Sometimes osteoporosis develops or nerves are damaged. Keshan disease, an abnormality of the heart muscle is caused by a lack of selenium. Kashin-Beck disease, which results in joint and bone disease and myxedematous endemic cretinism, which results in intellectual disability, are also reported to result from selenium deficiency.

4. **Vitamin deficiencies:** (i) Lack of vitamin A results in xerophthalmia, Bitot's spots, night blindness and keratomalacia, (ii) B complex: Deficiency of thiamine leads to beriberi. Niacin deficiency results in pellagra. Riboflavin deficiency symptoms are angular stomatitis, cheilosis, scrotal dermatitis and corneal vascularisation. Other B-complex deficiencies also result in glossitis, cheilosis and angular stomatitis, (iii) vitamin C deficiency leads to scurvy, spongy bleeding gums, haemorrhages in skin and other haemorrhages, (iv) vitamin D deficiency results in rickets and osteomalacia, (v) vitamin K deficiency leads to hypoprothrombinaemia, which further leads to haemorrhages and bleeding tendencies.

B. Overnutrition

Overnutrition problems are especially important for affluent communities, families or individuals:

i. The main features of obesity are overweight and excess fat. It is mostly caused by overeating and intake of abundance of calories. Body mass index (BMI) is a person's weight in kilograms divided by the square of height in meters. A high BMI can be an indicator of high body fat. BMI can be used to screen for weight categories that may lead to health problems but it is not diagnostic of the body fat or health of an individual. BMI is calculated as weight in kilograms divided by height in metres squared (kg/m^2). Cut-off levels for Asians as per World Health Organization (WHO) are given in Table 6.6.

BMI values are age-independent and the same for both sexes. However, BMI may not correspond to the same degree of fatness in different populations due, in part, to different body proportions. The health risks associated with increasing BMI are continuous and the interpretation of BMI gradings in relation to risk may differ for different populations.

Table 6.6: The international classification of adult underweight, overweight and obesity according to BMI

Classification	BMI (kg/m^2) Principal cut-off points	Additional cut-off points
Underweight	<18.50	<18.50
Severe thinness	<16.00	<16.00
Moderate thinness	16.00–16.99	16.00–16.99
Mild thinness	17.00–18.49	17.00–18.49
Normal range	18.50–24.99	18.50–22.99
		23.00–24.99
Overweight	≥25.00	≥25.00
Pre-obese	25.00–29.99	25.00–27.49
	27.50–29.99	
Obese	≥30.00	≥30.00
Obese class I	30.00–34.99	30.00–32.49
		32.50–34.99
Obese class II	35.00–39.99	35.00–37.49
		37.50–39.99
Obese class III	≥40.00	≥40.00

Source: Adapted from WHO, 1995, WHO, 2000 and WHO, 2004.

If the daily food intake is kept at about 500 calories below the energy needs of the body, a loss of one pound (453 gm) of weight per week may be effected, howsoever it is dangerous to reduce weight rapidly than 1/2 pound (226.5 gm) per day.

On the other hand, insufficient intake of food, an unbalanced diet, too little sleep, chronic infections and worry leads to undernutrition and the person looks pale, have poor posture, flabby muscles, dark circles under his eyes, decreased appetite and he often shows irritability.

ii. Hypervitaminosis A is at times caused by excess of therapeutic vitamin A administration. The manifestations are headache, nausea, vomiting, irritability and anorexia. Carotenaemia, a benign condition, is caused by ingestion of excessive amounts of carrots, some yellow and green vegetables, which is characterized by yellow skin with normal conjunctiva.

iii. The toxic manifestations of hypervitaminosis D are anorexia, nausea, vomiting, thirst, polyuria and drowsiness with raised levels of calcium and phosphorus. Calcium may be deposited in many tissues also.

iv. Fluorosis occurs, if fluorine is available more than 1 ppm in water. It is characterised by (a) dental fluorosis: Mottled enamel of teeth and (b) chronic high-level exposure to fluoride can lead to skeletal fluorosis, i.e. dense bone formation, severe spondylitis and even calcifications of ligaments of spine and tendinous inflammation of other muscles in severe cases.

6.10 EFFECTS OF COOKING

Carbohydrates like starch grains in flour, potatoes, rice, cereals, etc. swell up and burst leading to the gelatinisation of starch granules. The protein coagulates (as in the case of white of an egg) and shrinks when heated. Fats, of course, are not affected on moderate heating except that the solid fats liquefy on application of heat and solidify again on cooling. The effect of heat on different vitamins is different as some are destroyed on heating, while others do not.

Thorough cooking kills the cysticerci in measly beef and pork and is a valued defence against pork containing Trichinella worms.

Vitamin D is thermostable and therefore ordinary cooking causes no loss to it, although addition of washing soda or baking powder destroys this vitamin to a considerable extent. Their destructive action can, however, be counteracted to some extents by the addition of tamarind (which is highly acidic) to the vegetables when cooked. Vitamin A is not destroyed in food cooked in the absence of oxygen. Both vitamins A, B_1 and B_2 show remarkable resistance to heat, provided the medium is acidic.

Vitamin C being sensitive to heat is destroyed by moderate heating. The heat stability of vitamin C depends upon the absence of oxygen and the presence of acidity. In whole potatoes, vitamin C withstands boiling for half an hour but in mashed and whipped potatoes it is soon destroyed. In citrus fruits and tomato juice, vitamin C is claimed to be resistant to heat of processing.

6.11 DIFFERENT METHODS OF COOKING

These are

1. **Boiling:** Boiled food might not taste good but is more digestible. A large proportion of mineral salts in vegetable foods are lost as they are soluble in water, thus any surplus water after cooking rice, vegetables, etc., should not be thrown away. It can judiciously be used in cooking pulses and vegetables.

2. **Roasting:** It used to be done formerly by exposing food articles directly to fire but now roasting and baking which are similar methods, are done in *electric tandoors* and oven. As a method of cooking, roasting is popular in many parts of the world for roasted meat and nuts, as it not only enhances taste and digestibility but also retains the nutritional value.

3. **Frying:** This method, in which food is placed in hot melted fat or oil, is the quickest method of cooking because melted fat is brought to a high temperature and food placed in it is quickly fried. But this method is highly destructive, so far retention of vitamins in the vegetables are concerned.

There are two methods of frying; shallow and deep. In the former only sufficient fat or oil is used to cover bottom of the pan. In the latter, the pan contains a large amount of fat or oil and the food is actually boiled in the fat. The food prepared in this way is not so easily digestible as it contains a large amount of oily or fatty matter, although by doing so it becomes tasty. Hot air frying is a new technique to get fried products through direct contact between an external emulsion of oil droplets in hot air and the product into a frying chamber. The product is constantly in motion to promote homogeneous contact between both phases. In this way, the product is dehydrated and the typical crust of fried products gradually appears. The amount of oil used is significantly lower than in deep oil frying giving, as a result, very low fat products. Researches have proved that air frying is more suitable for frying process and produce healthy fried foods than other traditional frying method.

4. **Steaming:** This principle is applied in cookers. It is the best method as it does not involve loss of any of the nutritious ingredients.

6.12 FOOD POISONING

Food poisoning, common name for gastroenteritis, occurs when pathogenic bacteria, parasites, viruses, or pre-formed toxins are ingested via food or water thus encompasses both food-related infection and food-related intoxication. This could be (a) non-infective, and (b) infective.

Non-infective

The non-infective causes of food poisoning are chemicals such as metals from tins, injurious preservatives, insecticides used in agricultural operations, additives and adulterants. Cheap enamel wares may contain antimony and if the enamel comes in contact with fruit, the fruit acids may dissolve the antimony and cause poisoning. The use of commercial acid containing arsenic has resulted in an epidemic of arsenical poisoning amongst beer drinkers.

i. *Neurolathyrism*: It is a disease of nervous system characterised by gradually developing spastic paralysis of lower limbs of an individual. It is generally caused due to consumption of Kesari dal (*Lathyrus sativus*) containing toxin named beta-N-oxalyl-amino-L-alanine acid (BOAA), which is a glutamate analog. The disease is prevalent in landless labourers who consume chickling pea as their staple diet. Deficiencies of zinc, copper, vitamin C and vitamin A are also attributed for neurolathyrism. For prevention of neurolathyrism, possible options are home-based detoxification (soak the pulse in hot water for about 2 hours and then drain off the water completely) or development of new seed lines for genetic improvement of *Lathyrus sativus*. The crop has been banned in India under Prevention of Food Adulteration (PFA) Act.

Infective

The source of infection is food contaminated with wide variety of pathogenic microorganisms like bacteria, viruses, protozoa, fungi, and their toxins. Most cases are caused by common bacteria such as *Staphylococcus*, *E. coli* and *Salmonella*. The infective organism causes acute inflammation of the alimentary tract or an irritant effect occurs on gastrointestinal mucosa due to the toxic substances produced by them. Food infections by bacteria can be divided into two types: (a) Those in which the food does not ordinarily support the growth of pathogens but merely carries them, e.g. Salmonella, Shigella, *Vibrio*, etc. and (b) those in which the food can serve as a culture medium for growth of pathogens to numbers that can infect the person.

Based on the pathogenesis of the infection, the food poisoning by bacteria can be divided into the following categories:

a. Food intoxications resulting from the ingestion of preformed bacterial toxins, e.g. *Staphylococcus aureus, Bacillus cereus, Clostridium botulinum, Clostridium perfringens*.

b. Food intoxications caused by non-invasive bacteria that secrete toxins while adhering to the intestinal wall, e.g. enterotoxigenic *E. coli* (ETEC), *Vibrio cholerae, Campylobacter jejuni*. 'ETEC' is identified to be most common cause for 'traveller's diarrhoea'.

c. Food intoxications that follow an intracellular invasion of the intestinal epithelial cells, e.g. Shigella, Salmonella. These infections usually lead to bloody diarrhoeas.

d. Diseases caused by bacteria that enter the blood-stream via the intestinal tract, e.g. *Salmonella typhi, Listeria monocytogenes*.

The symptoms produced are acute gastrointestinal irritation leading to vomiting, diarrhoea, pain in the abdomen, and collapse. The incubation period varies as it depends on the agent of infection, e.g. salmonellosis usually occurs 8 to 72 hours after exposure to infection, but may at times take up to a few weeks also.

a. **Food intoxications resulting from the ingestion of preformed bacterial toxins:** This is due to the ingestion of toxins formed as a result of the multiplication of bacteria before ingestion. This particularly happens when meat is taken in an uncooked or partially cooked condition, e.g. sausages, pressed beef, etc. However, outbreaks of food poisoning associated with *Staphylococcus aureus* is caused by a heat stable exotoxin that is associated with intake of bakery and dairy products like milk, ice creams, pastries, cakes, etc. The infection could be transmitted by use of infected animals for food, excretion of specific organisms by infected animals to contaminate food, which is kept unprotected or infection transmitted by food handlers like *Salmonella paratyphi* and *Salmonella typhimurium*.

The food concerned is tinned meat or fish. Since ducks may be infected with *Bacillus typhimurium* and *Bacillus enteritidis*—their meat may also be infected and may cause food poisoning.

Incubation period: It is usually short and varies from 12–24 hours.

Botulism: It is severe, neurologic and highly fatal afebrile poisoning caused by ingesting exotoxins produced by the growth of *Clostridium botulinum* in under-processed preserved (tinned) foods, sausages, canned fruits, preserved pickles, etc. The anaerobic environment in the packed food encourages the outgrowth of spores and the toxin is produced in bottled or canned meat, fish and vegetables only. The spores are found in soil also thus contamination of foods by soil may cause botulism. The symptoms of botulism usually appear within 12–36 hours. The incubation period may be as short as 4 hours and as long as 3 days, depending upon the dosage, conditions of eating and severity of contents of botulinum toxin. Common gastrointestinal symptoms include vomiting, thirst, dryness of mouth, constipation and are transitory in nature. The symptoms that cause concern are chiefly nervous in character and consist of distorted vision, diplopia, ptosis, paralysis of accommodation, dysphagia and diminished salivary secretions. Coma or delirium may occur in some cases. Death occurs in 4–7 days due to failure of heart or respiration.

Most people fully recover from common types of food poisoning within 12–48 hours. However, a few like botulism can cause serious complications. With adequate and timely treatment, death is usually uncommon in people who are otherwise healthy. Dehydration is the most common complication. Some serious, less common complications may be arthritis, bleeding problems, damage to nervous system, renal problems and swelling or irritation in the tissue around the heart.

Food poisoning and diarrhoeas can be prevented by hygienic food, water and personal hygiene.

6.13 INVESTIGATION OF AN OUTBREAK OF FOOD POISONING

a. **Preliminary assessment of the situation:** Examine cases to consider whether or not all the cases have the same illness (or different manifestations of the same disease) and determine if there is a real outbreak by assessing the normal background activity of disease. Collect clinical specimens from cases after conducting in-depth interviews with initial cases to identify factors common to all or most cases. Also conduct site investigation at implicated premises to collect food specimens when appropriate. From the available data, formulate preliminary hypotheses to initiate appropriate control measures. If further investigation is required, plan and compose an adequate investigative team comprising of multidisciplinary professionals from clinical medicine, epidemiology, laboratory medicine, food microbiology and chemistry, food safety and food control, and risk communication and management.

b. **Communication:** Effective communication is a crucial aspect of successful outbreak management. Throughout the course of an outbreak, it is important to share relevant information with authorities and other professional groups; local health care providers; media; the people directly affected and general public. Ensure timeliness, accuracy of information and choose best modes for communication with colleagues, patients and the public. Since media is a major interface between the general public and the health authorities and plays an important role in outbreak investigation and control, it should be used constructively.

c. **Descriptive epidemiology:** After establishing case definitions for confirmed and probable cases, identify as many cases as possible. Careful description and characterization of the outbreak should be done to know about the distribution of cases in terms of time, place and person. This is important to develop more specific hypotheses about the source and mode of transmission and frame immediate control measures. To assess the risk of infection in exposed versus non-exposed, the attack rates must be calculated and compared after determining population at risk. The attack rate is commonly used in disease outbreak investigations and is a key factor in the formulation of hypotheses. It is calculated as the number of cases in the population at risk divided by the number of people in the population at risk.

d. **Food and environment investigations:** These are conducted to find out how and why an outbreak occurred and what corrective actions are required to be instituted to avoid similar occurrences in future. The specific objectives of 'sanitary' investigation for a food-borne disease outbreak includes identifying the source, mode and extent of the food contamination and assessing the factors that helped the pathogens survive processes designed to kill them or to reduce their numbers. Each suspect food item that has been implicated in the outbreak should be thoroughly investigated. Laboratory examination of all the samples collected from food must be done for microbiological and chemical contamination.

e. **Analysis and interpretation:** The data from all available sources should be reviewed before developing explanatory hypotheses. Analytical studies should be carried out to test the hypotheses.

f. **Control measures:** Ideally control measures should be guided by the investigation results but this may lead to delay the prevention of further cases. Thus, till the time-specific interventions can be designed, general control measures must be put in place for prevention of further spread of infection. Once investigations have identified an association between a particular food or food premises and transmission of the suspected pathogen, specific strategies should be designed to control the source along with public education programmes to curb the transmission.

g. **Further studies:** Further studies may be conducted after completion of the initial investigations, particularly if new or unusual pathogens were involved or additional information for risk assessment of a particular pathogen is required. Economic evaluations of outbreaks and associated control efforts can be important in assessing the cost-effectiveness of outbreak investigations and food safety measures.

6.14 FOOD HYGIENE

Food being a potential source of infection, food hygiene implies hygiene in its production, processing, handling, distribution and serving. Thus, it involves several aspects—personal hygiene of food handlers and consumers, health control of food handlers, environmental sanitation of food establishment, food preservation, processing, control of adulteration, etc.

1. **Treatment of food and its handling:** Pasteurisation, boiling, cooking and other ways of processing, preservation and handling of food to make it free from pathogens are discussed under their specific headings as well as while discussing individual foodstuffs. Vegetables and foods which are eaten raw pose a problem in food sanitation. Spread of pathogenic organisms, protozoa and helminths is a serious menace to public health, where sewage is used for growing vegetables. Therefore, they should be thoroughly washed if they are to be eaten raw. Cooked ones, if they are eaten just after cooking, are free from such dangers. Harmful and poisonous organisms are killed at temperatures above 50°C. People need education to handle food in hygienic manners including thorough cleansing of utensils, not keeping the food for too long after cooking, storing the food properly covered.

2. **Control of food handlers:** Food handlers are likely to transmit infections like diarrhoea, dysentery, typhoid and paratyphoid fevers, strepto- and staphylococcal infections, diptheria, tuberculosis, enteroviruses, infective hepatitis, protozoal and helminthic diseases. Education of food handlers in basic food hygiene is important. Thus, food handlers should be subjected to thorough medical history taking, examination and laboratory investigations at the time of employment in food and eating establishments, however, routine examination and microbiological assessment is not recommended. Food safety education programmes should aim to improve the knowledge and practice of an entire population (including policy-makers, food producers, food processors, professional food handlers and consumers). However, domestic food handlers who prepare food for the family, particularly expectant mothers and high-risk groups and people preparing food for them, particularly small children, travellers, pregnant women, the immunocompromised and the elderly need to receive greater emphasis in the programme. Professional food handlers should ideally receive

training and education in two aspects of food safety: (a) Principles of good hygienic practice, and (b) application of the hazard analysis and critical control point (HACCP) concept to food preparation.

HACCP is an approach that identifies specific hazards and measures for their control. Its full implementation consists of (a) hazard analysis, (b) determining critical control points, (c) establishing critical limits, (d) establishing monitoring systems, (e) establishing corrective actions, (f) avoiding contact between cooked and raw food, (g) wash hands repeatedly, (h) keep all kitchen surfaces meticulously clean, (i) protect food from insects, rodents and other animals, and (j) use of safe water.

6.15 VEGETABLE FOODS

They contain large proportion of carbohydrates and almost all the vitamins, proteins and fats. They are classified under the following heads:

a. Cereals and millets
b. Pulses
c. Roots and tubers
d. Green vegetables
e. Fruits and nuts
f. Fungi.

a. Cereals and Millets

Cereals, together with oil seeds and legumes, supply a majority of the dietary protein, calories, vitamins, and minerals to the bulk of populations in developing nations. They are in the form of seeds which contain a large quantity of nutritive material condensed in a small bulk and mineral substances like phosphates of calcium, magnesium, etc. with a small amount of iron and silica. The cereals and other plant foods contain significant amounts of toxic or anti-nutritional substances like phytates, enzyme inhibitors, and some cereals like sorghum and millet contain large amounts of polyphenols and tannins. Some of these substances reduce the nutritional value of foods by interfering with mineral bioavailability, and digestibility of proteins and carbohydrates. The seeds are usually ground in a mill which when mixed with water forms a tenaceous mass known as dough, from which breads, etc. are prepared. They have large amount of roughage or the cellulose contents, which promotes peristalsis or the movement of bowels. Smaller grains, which are ground and eaten without having the outer layer removed are called millets. These are mainly maize, bajra and jowar.

1. **Wheat:** It is the most important of all cereals and is extensively used all over the world. It is a staple food in certain parts of India.

It contains 60–70% starch, 8–12% gluten and 15% water. The seeds have an outer envelope called pericarp, which is very hard. It is composed mainly of cellulose and mineral matter and forms about 13% of the grain. A middle layer called endosperm or kernel consists chiefly of starch. It forms 85% of the grain. The germ or embryo forms about 1.5% of the entire grain. It is rich in protein and fat.

Flour is prepared by grinding up wheat. The whole grain is always used; so it is rarely lacking in vitamin B_1. It is customary to reject the outer envelope. It constitutes, what is called bran, which is used for feeding animals such as cattle, horses, etc. Bran contains a very large proportion of nitrogen and fat, viz. 15% and 3.5% respectively. It is rich in mineral matter especially iron and cellulose.

Whole wheat flour is prepared by grinding up whole seed. The only objection to the whole wheat flour is that the bran is indigestible, irritating to gut and may cause diarrhoea. The removal of bran renders the flour fine in texture and white in colour, but deprives it of most of its nutritious and fatty parts.

The flour is divided into 3 portions

i. *Sujee is* the coarse grain derived from the outer coat of wheat. It contains a high proportion of proteins, mineral salts and vitamin B_1.

ii. *Flour* is the next fine layer of grain. It is rich in starch.

iii. *Maida:* It is fine white flour and is produced from the innermost layer of wheat grain. It is deficient in all vitamins and is poorer from nutrition point of view.

2. **Rice:** It is a staple food in some parts of India, particularly Bengal and Chennai. In fact, it forms the staple article of diet for half the population of the world. Rice is a good source of protein, phosphorus and iron. It also contains some amount of calcium. Most of the nutrients and minerals in rice are concentrated in the outer brown layers known as the husk and germ. Therefore, brown rice, which is rice from which only husk has been removed, is the most nutritious type of rice. Unfortunately, many consumers prefer white rice or polished rice, in which the germ and bran has been removed, making it less nutritious.

Rice has about 345 calories per 100 grams. It is very easy to digest rice and hence most of these calories are absorbed by the body. Rice has a large number of health benefits (a) due to its abundance in carbohydrates, it acts as fuel for the body and aids in the normal functioning of the brain, (b) the vitamins, minerals, and various organic components increase the functioning and metabolic activity of all your organ systems, (c) rice is low in sodium, so is considered as good food for those suffering from high blood pressure, (d) whole grain rice like brown rice is rich in insoluble fibre that can protect against many types of cancers like colorectal and intestinal cancers, and (e) rice also has natural antioxidants like vitamin C, vitamin A, phenolic and flavonoid compounds, which also act as or stimulate antioxidants to scourge the body for free radicals.

The outer layer or pericarp contains vitamin B_1 and its complete removal may show the symptoms of its deficiency in rice eating population. When rice is dehusked, shell is removed leaving behind the embryo attached to the rest of the grain. In machine milling, up to 75% of thiamine may be lost in the bran, but in hand pounding the loss is about 25%.

3. **Barley:** It is a staple cereal grain loaded with dietary fibre and proteins, which guarantees an energetic and healthy metabolism. It is rich in manganese, selenium, phosphorus, copper, magnesium, iron, zinc, potassium, vitamin B_6, thiamin, niacin, riboflavin, and folate while calcium, vitamin K and pantothenic acid are only found small quantities. It is available in pearl, flour and malted forms. Pearl barley is used to prepare barley water which is used as a demulcent beverage for the sick and infants. Malt is barley in its incipient stage of germination. Barley has a calorific value of 352.0 calories per 100 grams. Diet rich in barley helps to keep the colon and intestines healthy, while preventing gallstones, diabetes, heart diseases, and osteoporosis. It also supports the immune system and preserves skin elasticity.

4. **Maize or Indian corn:** It is used in some parts of India. It is as nutritious as wheat, and richer in fats than all cereals except oats. The major chemical component of the maize kernel is starch, which provides up to 72 to 73% of the kernel weight. It contains 8–11% proteins, 3–18% fats, 1–2% salts and 14% water. The most abundant mineral found in maize is phosphorus, found as phytate of potassium and magnesium. It contains two fat-soluble vitamins—provitamin A or carotenoids and vitamin E. Maize is poor in lysine and tryptophan. It is deficient in vitamins, the antiscorbutic and anti-pellegra factors being absent and an exclusive maize diet may cause pellagra. It is deficient in gluten so it does not form bread easily. But this difficulty can be overcome by mixing it with milk, eggs, etc. Corn flour is maize flour which has been deprived of its peculiar flavour by a weak solution of soda.

5. **Jowar:** Jowar is the Indian name for sorghum, also known as white millet. Whole jowar kernels can be steamed, boiled, added to soups and stews or ground into a flour that can be used as a substitute for

wheat flour in baked goods. Jowar is a gluten-free, high-protein, cholesterol-free source of a variety of essential nutrients, including dietary fibre, iron, phosphorus and thiamine. It is sometimes eaten as porridge or in the form of thick chappaties or bread. It is midway between wheat and rice so far as its nutritive value is concerned.

6. **Oats or 'Jaow':** These are highly nutritious and are an excellent source of proteins, dietary fibre, mineral salts (manganese, phosphorus, copper, zinc, magnesium, chromium and molybdenum), biotin, vitamins C and B_1. They are deficient in vitamins A and D and gluten. Oats are used as oatmeal porridge and should be eaten with plenty of milk. Oats have proven to be extremely helpful in prevention of adverse cardiovascular events by stabilising blood pressure and reducing levels of blood cholestrol and sugar. However, oats contain naturally-occurring substances called purines, due to which excessive intake of oats may cause some purine- related health problems in some individuals susceptible to purine-related problems. "Gout" and the "renal stone" formation are two examples of purine-related health problems.

b. Pulses

These are mostly legumes and are richer in nitrogenous substances than other vegetable foods. Pulses include peas, beans, and lentils. They are a cheap, low-fat source of protein, fibre, vitamins and minerals. The vegetable protein, which they contain is called legumin or vegetable casein, which is not so easily digestible as milk protein. Compared to meat, pulses are deficient in fat. In their fresh state they contain vitamins A, B, and C, but when dried they lose vitamin C.

Pulses are used in India in the form of *dals*. The common varieties are arhar, moong dal, Bengal gram, green gram, khesari dal, etc. Owing to their richness in proteins, they are called "poor man's meat". Pulses also contain a good deal of carbohydrates but a little fat. Pulses, in dried state, contain no anti-scorbutic properties, but if dried seeds are soaked in water for 24 hours and allowed to germinate for a day or two, they again develop vitamin C. When pulses are sprouted, starch is broken down to dextrin and maltose and proteins are broken to polypeptides and amino acids. Moreover, their concentration of nicotinic acid, riboflavin, folic acid, etc. increase during germination.

Soybeans: Soybeans are very rich in nutritive components. Besides the very high protein content, soybeans contain a lot of fibre and are rich in calcium, and magnesium. The soy protein has a high biological value, contains all the essential amino acids and is easily digestible. It is the richest form of vegetable proteins but with low fat content, a large amount of mineral matter and almost complete absence of starch.

Iron content of soybeans varies from 7 to 30 mg per 100 gm. It contains large quantities of vitamin B_1 but no vitamins C and D. The high fibre content of soy milk helps relieve constipation, while high mineral protein and vitamin (especially B-complex) levels provide "ideal" nutrition. However, American Nutrition Association has reported the presence of several anti-nutrients (phytic acid, anti-trypsin agent, "phytoagglutinins" or "lectins") in raw soybean that inhibit several physiological functions in the body.

c. Roots and Tubers

These are the cheapest sources of dietary energy, in the form of carbohydrates, chiefly in the form of starch which is about 80%. Roots and tubers are deficient in most of the vitamins and minerals but contain significant amounts of dietary fibre. They contain some minerals, that are mainly salts of potash. The common form of tubers are carrots, potatoes, beetroot, radish, onions, arrowroot, sago and tapioca.

d. Green Leafy Vegetables

They consist of leaves, buds, young shoots, leafy stalks and often the entire plants. They have a little nutritive value, but form an important part of diet on account of the presence of vitamins and mineral salts of sodium, calcium and chlorine. In composition, they consist of 90% water, 2% nitrogenous substance or proteins, 4% starch and 0.5% fats. They contain large amount of alkaline salts which act as "buffers" and maintain the alkalinity of the blood. They supply vitamins A, B_{12}, B_2 and C and give relish to the food. Green leafy vegetables are rich in cellulose, so add bulk and are of value in curing chronic constipation. A good rough indication of carotene content of leafy vegetables is their tenderness or say greenness. The greener and fresher are better. Ordinary cooking does not destroy the carotene present in vegetables although it is not stable at high temperatures. Dried vegetables are practically useless as they are not anti-scorbutics. One of the important benefits of dark green leafy vegetables is their low calorie and carbohydrate contents and low glycemic index. These features make them an ideal food to facilitate achieving and maintaining a healthy body weight. Adding more green vegetables to a balanced diet increases the intake of dietary fibre which, in turn, regulates the digestive system and aids in bowel health and weight management. These properties are particularly advantageous for those with type 2 diabetes. Studies have also shown that eating 2 to 3 servings of green leafy vegetables per week may lower the risk of stomach, breast and skin cancer. These same antioxidants have also been proven to decrease the risk of heart disease.

e. Fruits

Fruits contain a large amount of sugar, vegetable acids and salts. These are protective foods. According to their nutritive value, fruits have been divided by Hutchinson into food fruits and flavouring fruits.

Food fruits are those which afford nutrient, and include bananas, dates, figs, grapes, mangoes, etc. Their nutritive value depends on the presence of carbohydrates, which exist in the form of sugar and commonly known as levulose or fruit sugar. Certain fruits such as lemons and oranges are rich in potassium salts, lime and magnesia and contain antiscorbutic vitamins.

The fruits are valuable because

1. These have cooling effect and quench thirst.
2. These contain important mineral salts of potash combined with vegetable salts.
3. These have antiscorbutic properties being the richest sources of vitamin C and for this reason they are included in children's diet, especially in bottle fed infants.
4. These prevent constipation.

f. Nuts

These differ from fruits being rich in proteins, fibre and essential fats. The common nuts are almonds, cocoa nuts, groundnuts, walnuts, etc. These are rich in vitamin B but contain very little vitamin A and no vitamin C.

g. Fungi and Nutrition

Edible fungi: Wild edible fungi are often referred to generically as wild edible "mushrooms". This can be confusing for a number of reasons: Edible species have different forms, some with gills and some with pores, some with stems and some without them. Certain fungi also have medicinal value. Nutritionally, in general, wild mushrooms are rich sources of protein and have low amounts of fat. These have a good amounts of minerals, including trace minerals. On an average, phenylalanine is the limiting amino acid while the highest amount of essential amino acids present in the mushrooms is leucine. One serving of the 250 g fresh weight mushrooms contain an average of 6.12 g of protein, 287 mg of calcium, 9.3 mg of iron and 3.72 mg of zinc. More importantly it had low levels of fat (0.712 g) and sodium (0.077 mg).

Mushrooms are a staple food in the diet of some human cultures (and many vertebrate and invertebrate animals[1]), edible mushrooms are usually considered for their flavor and condiment value. Mushrooms have a fairly high protein content, typically 20–30% crude protein as a percentage of dry matter, However there is extreme variation among species (3.5% in *Cantharellus cibarius*, 44% in *Agaricus bisporus*). High protein content makes them an ideal food because they contain all the amino acids essential to human nutrition. There are about eight essential amino acids, that is, those which cannot be produced by the human body, and so must be consumed in the diet daily. Mushrooms can be an important dietary source of these amino acids.

After moisture, which accounts for 90% of fresh weight, carbohydrates that include glycogen and chitin or "fungus cellulose", a polymer of N-acetylglycosamine, are the main component of mushrooms (average of 4.2% of the fresh weight). Other large carbohydrate polymers are glucans, chitosans and mannans, and including chitin, these polymers are linked together with covalent bonds that cannot be attacked by our digestive enzymes. Therefore, it is suspected that humans cannot utilize a large percentage of the carbohydrate in mushrooms as nutrients and so it functions only as roughage.

Mushrooms contain an average of 85–125 kJ per 100 g whereas an adult male needs about 10,000 kJ per day. This low energy value of mushrooms enables it to be used in low-calorie diets. The low carbohydrate value makes them an ideal food for diabetics.

Mushrooms are characteristically low in fat, comprising 2–8% dry weight. This crude fat includes representatives of all classes of lipid compounds including free fatty acids, glycerides, sterols, and phospholipids. Of existing fatty acids, a high proportion is linoleic acid (the only essential fatty acid required in the human diet), has been found to be 63–74% of total fatty acids. Sphingolipids, important in the brain and nervous system, have also been identified, but appear to represent only a small proportion of total glycolipids. Like vegetable, mushrooms are a cholesterol-free food.

There are many essential vitamins including riboflavin (B_2) niacin, pantothenic acid, thiamine (B_1) biotin, folate and vitamin B_{12}. Besides mushrooms are also reliable natural vitamin D source.

As far as minerals are concerned, in general mushrooms contain significant quantities of phosphorus, potassium, copper, and selenium.

6.16 ANIMAL FOODS

These include meat of any kind, fish, eggs, milk and its preparations, etc.

Meat

It consists of muscle fibres held together by connective tissues. The fibres of meat contain muscle plasma or muscle-juice. It contains salts which are chiefly chlorides and phosphates of potash. The proteins of meat which are present to the tune of about 17 to 20% are myosin, muscle albumen and haemoglobin. Fat is often embedded in the connective tissues of meat.

Meat hygiene: Meat hygiene is expert supervision of all meat products with the object of providing wholesome meat for human consumption and preventing danger to public health. Antemortem inspection of animals should be done, to reject animals if they are apparently unhealthy or to treat them if under any transient illness. It is important to not only inspect the carcase after slaughtering but all procedures from stunning of animal prior to slaughter until the final meat or meat product is offered to the consumer needs to be supervised. Careful examination of the whole and subsequently of all the organs must be done. Mediastinal and bronchial lymphatic glands should be examined for evidence of tuberculosis. If the animal has suffered from jaundice, the flesh will have a yellow tinge.

Meat quality: Meat quality is normally defined by the compositional quality (lean to fat ratio) and the palatability factors such as visual appearance, smell, firmness, juiciness, tenderness, and flavour. The characteristics of good meat are: (a) Muscle fibres are of deep red colour and marbelled with fat, (b) the reaction should be acidic, (c) it should be firm, elastic to touch and there should not be an excess of fluid which indicates oedema, (d) it should have a little or no odour as diseased meat emits odour of putrefaction or sickly smell, (e) the fat should be firm and of whitish or yellowish grey colour, (f) lymphatic glands should be free from all diseases, and (g) any diseased condition, i.e. cysts of tapeworms, etc. should not be present.

Unhealthy meat is the meat which has begun to putrefy. It becomes soft, moist, pale and often has greenish colour. The reaction becomes alkaline and odour of putrefaction may commence in the deeper part of the meat especially near the bones and so the odour may not be apparent from the outer surface. Therefore, in case meat is suspected to be unhealthy, it is advisable to push an iron skewer deep into the meat; pull it out and smell it. The smell should be sweet and agreeable. The juice should be reddish and acidic, since alkalinity is an indication of decomposition. Putrified meat is extremely dangerous, as poisonous substances get developed, which introduce sudden and fatal illnesses due to poisoning due to cadaverine, putrescine and amines. A degenerative substance is called ptomaine is formed as a result of desiccation of cells and tissues, which is a cause of many diseases.

6.17 DISEASED MEAT

The flesh of animals killed by accident, lightning or those who happen to be suffering from diseases like anthrax, rabies, glanders, general tuberculosis, etc. should be condemned. The diseased meat should be condemned and prevented from sending into the market. The chief diseases that can be caused by consuming meat of sick animals are:

1. **Tuberculosis**: It is common in cattle and pigs. It is practically always present in lymphatic glands of the diseased animals. On pleura, it produces shiny deposits like bunch of pearls, while in lymphatic glands it produces lumps of cheesy material. Muscles usually do not get affected and it is extremely doubtful if eating meat, so affected, spreads tuberculosis.

   In tubercular animals when disease is generalised, the whole carcase should be condemned as unfit for human consumption since that meat happens to be poor in quality and unwholesome even though it may not transmit tuberculosis to consumers.

2. **Cysticercus**: This is the name given to the embryos of tapeworms which live in muscles of animals especially oxen and pigs, where they produce a little greyish bladders or vesicles called cysts. In these tiny cysts are contained the heads of tapeworms and when anybody happens to eat such a meat these cysts break into his stomach and let loose the heads, which pass through the intestines, get fixed to the intestinal wall and ultimately grow into full grown tapeworms which may be several metres long. If meat is properly cooked the tiny embryos are killed due to heat and in that case, they may not do much harm. All such infected meats should be condemned.

3. *Trichinella spiralis*: It reaches man on account of eating insufficiently cooked flesh of a pig having worms in encysted form. In pork and ham, these may be seen as white spots, large enough to be visible to the naked eye. The adult worm lives in crypts in mucosa of small intestines. It gives rise to embryos which enter circulation and are carried into the musculature of host, where they encyst. The muscles most often affected are those of the diaphragm, larynx, tongue and abdomen. Encysted larvae remain alive for years. When these cysts are found in the slaughtered animals, the whole carcase should be condemned. Serious illness may result from trichinosis, whose symptoms are pain, nausea, rapid pulse, fever, irregularity of bowels and death occurring due to peritonitis.

4. **Actinomycosis or ray fungus**: In this case, infectious agent is *Actinomyces israelii or Actinomyces bovis*. It is now recognised as a parasite, which occurs in the meat of oxen. It may affect other cattle especially calves, pigs, horses, sheep, etc. It occurs particularly in wet weather. The tongue, jaws and lungs are commonly affected. The postmortem appearances closely resemble tuberculosis. In this, case only the affected parts are condemned.

5. *Distomum haepaticum* or liver flukes: They resemble flat fish, each of them being 2–4 cm long and 1 cm wide. They are brownish in colour and are found

covered with a little bristles. They are very common in sheep and cattle in India. The parasites are found in the liver, bile ducts and give rise to a disease called the *rot*. As cooking always kills the flukes, only a few cases of disease from this parasite are known to occur in man.

6.18 FISH

Fish is much used in certain parts of India. It is easily digested, has a high nutritive value and is less rich in fats and contains more calcium than ordinary meat. It has all the vitamins except vitamin C. Fish liver is a rich source of vitamins A and D. Sea fish is a rich source of iodine.

There are two kinds of fish

1. *Lean fish*: It consists of small fibres and contains fat below 2%. It is easily digested.
2. *Fat fish*: It consists of medium or large fibres with fat content of 2.5% or more. It is somewhat difficult to digest.

A healthy and fresh fish should have bright pink gills, firm glistening scales and prominent lustrous eyes. Its skin should be bright and glistening with a covering of clear slippery mucous. It should be free from any disagreeable odour. When held flat on hand by head, the tail should not droop. It should not feel soft or leave an impression or depressed mark when pressed by a finger. Its skin should be intact and scales should not be easily detachable. If not eviscerated a sound dead fish sinks in water.

A decaying fish has dull grey sunken eyes, grey muddy gills, the scales become detached and have a characteristic putrefying smell. It may cause ptomaine poisoning. It floats in water with belly up. A putrefying fish shows dark blood or dark tarry liquid on cutting and its body becomes flaccid. A large tapeworm called *Dibothriocephalus latus* is conveyed to man by eating insufficiently cooked fish.

Fish poisoning may occur due to toxins produced by *Cl. botulinum.* Its decomposition may give rise to ptomaine poisoning. Some persons may also possess idiosyncracies due to fish consumption especially to muscles, which are said to cause poisoning by mytilotoxin. The chief symptoms produced are dyspepsia, urticaria, swelling of tongue, numbness of limbs, weak irregular pulse, etc.

6.19 TINNED MEAT AND FISH

They are commonly used. It is very essential to see that meat and fish in tins are wholesome, not old and putrefied. The tins should be carefully examined before consumption in the following ways:

1. **On inspection:** There should be no indentations, holes, soldering defects or signs of gross ill-usage. It should not be rusty. It should have concave ends and not be bulging or blowing out indicating putrefaction and formation of hydrogen gas in acidic medium. There should not be more than one soldered hole, since unscrupulous dealers let out the gas from the defective tins by making a hole and solder it again; so if this is done, it can be detected from the presence of two holes. A collapsed tin signifies too much vacuum. All leaking and non-airtight tins should be discarded.

2. **On palpation:** If putrefaction has set in and gas has formed, it gives a springy feel with a sense of resistance. It so happens particularly, when air has entered into the tin through a leaking hole and the vacuum is lost.

3. **On percussion:** If the note is tympanitic, it indicates unsound tin due to formation of gas, while a dull note indicates a sound tin.

4. **On shaking:** A sound tin will produce no sound, but if the contents are putrefied and are partially liquid then a loose sloppy sound will be detected.

6.20 EGGS

A hen's egg weighs approximately 2 oz (56.70 gm) and consists of 10% outer covering or shell, 60% white, and 30% yolk. It is the safest of all animal foods as no infection can be transmissible through it. It is a food containing all the proximate principles of food, except carbohydrates necessary for the growth and development of the body. It is a protective food containing first-class proteins with all the essential amino acids and have the highest nutritive value among dietary proteins. In view of the presence of sulphur in the white of egg, they are considered as acid forming foods and resemble meat in this respect.

It consists of an outer shell with its interior white and yolk. The shell consists of carbonate of lime, the white is made up wholly of proteins, the chief being egg albumen and the yolk contains less proteins and a large amount of fat. Besides, it contains lecithin, vitalin and the organic compounds of phosphorus, lime, and iron. It is rich in calcium salts, antineuritic and antirachitic vitamins. Yolk of egg is a valuable food for anaemic patients, since it contains iron which is very easily digested and assimilated in the body. Since the fat present in the yolk of eggs is in emulsified form, just like milk, it is easily digested and is almost completely absorbed in the intestines; leaving only 3% of residue.

Freshness of eggs can be tested

1. By holding them in the hand in front of a candle in the dark. Fresh ones being more transparent in the centre and stale ones are transparent at their extremities. This process of testing the eggs is known as *candling.*

2. By putting them in 10% salt solution, say 2 oz (56.70 gm) to a pint (283.50 cc) of water; fresh eggs will sink, whereas stale ones will float.

Eggs can be preserved for a long time by drying and preventing the entrance of micro-organisms through their pores, by smearing the shell, when fresh, with wax, gum, fat or aqueous solution of sodium silicate popularly known as waterglass and this process is known as *glazing*. Besides, eggs can be kept fresh for 2–3 months at a temperature of 32°F (0°C) provided the relative humidity of atmosphere surrounding them is controlled to prevent the growth of moulds.

6.21 MILK

Milk is almost complete, an ideal food and contains most of the proximate principles of balanced diet required for human body. It is the best source of calcium in diet both on account of quality and the valuable assimilable form in which it exists. It provides proteins of high biological value to the body.

Milk contains the following proximate principles

1. *Proteins*: 3.5% of total weight, consisting of 3% caseinogen, 0.4% lactalbumen, and 0.1% lacto-globulin.
2. *Carbohydrates*: Lactose or milk-sugar 4 to 5%.
3. *Fats*: 3.5 to 4% in the form of glycerides in emulsified form. When milk is allowed to stand for sometime, fat rises to the surface as cream. Chemically milk fat consists of myristin, olein, palmitin and stearin.
4. *Vitamins*: They contain all the vitamins except vitamins E and K.
5. *Mineral salts*: Phosphates and chlorides of calcium, potassium and sodium. It is poor in iron.
6. *Enzymes*: Amylolytic, proteolytic and lipolytic. These are catalytic in action.

Average composition of milk from various sources is as follows (Table 6.7).

Caseinogen predominates in cow's and buffalo's milk, whereas lactalbumen predominates in human milk.

Table 6.7: Composition of milk

	Buffalo	Cow	Goat	Human
Fat (g)	6.5	4.1	4.5	3.4
Protein (g)	4.3	3.2	3.3	1.1
Lactose (g)	5.1	4.4	4.6	7.4
Calcium (mg)	210	120	170	28
Iron (mg)	0.2	0.2	0.3	–
Vit. C (mg)	1	2	1	3
Minerals (g)	0.8	0.8	0.8	0.1
Water (g)	81	87	86.8	88
Energy (kcal)	117	67	72	65

Average specific gravity of cow's and buffalo's milk is 1.032. Lactometer is used to determine the specific gravity, but it proves to be fallacious, as addition of water lowers the specific gravity, and extraction of fat, before sale, increases the specific gravity. So to a certain extent an addition of water, after extraction of fat, will not show any change whatsoever, so far as lactometer reading is concerned. To arrive at a definite conclusion, a quantitative analysis is necessary which is done by Werner Schmidt's method. By this method, all the fat is extracted from a known quantity of milk, by solvent ether and then ether from this extract is allowed to evaporate. This fat is completely dried and then weighed.

Solids other than fat are estimated by evaporation to complete dryness, a known weight of milk and then weighing total solids and subtracting therefrom the fat previously determined from percentage of solids, which gives percentage of solids other than fat.

6.22 METHODS OF PRESERVATION OF MILK

These are as follows:

Boiling

This method is commonly adopted in Indian homes, as the boiled milk coagulates slowly and the organisms which produce lactic acid, on boiling are reduced in number. The pathogenic organisms (but not spores) are killed. When boiled in an open pan, a thin scum consisting of milk fat, lime salt, partially dried casein and coagulated lactalbumen is formed on this top.

Pasteurization

Pasteurization is the process of heating milk up and then quickly cooling it down to eliminate certain bacteria.

Types of Pasteurization

The original method of pasteurization was vat pasteurization, which heats milk in a large tank for at least 30 minutes. It is now also used in the dairy industry for preparing milk for making starter cultures in the processing of cheese, yoghurt, buttermilk and for pasteurizing some ice cream mixes.

The most common method of pasteurization today is high temperature short time (HTST) pasteurization, which uses metal plates and hot water to raise milk temperatures to at least 161°F for not less than 15 seconds, followed by rapid cooling. Higher heat shorter time (HHST) is process similar to HTST pasteurization, but it uses slightly different equipment and higher temperatures for a shorter time. For a product to be considered ultra-pasteurized (UP), it must be heated to not less than 280° for two seconds. Up-pasteurization results in a product with longer shelf-life but still requiring refrigeration.

Another method, aseptic processing, which is also known as ultra high temperature (UHT), involves heating the milk using commercially sterile equipment and filling it under aseptic conditions into hermetically sealed packaging. The product is termed "shelf stable" and does not need refrigeration until opened. All aseptic operations are required to file their processes with the Food and Drug Administration's "Process Authority." There is no set time or temperature for aseptic processing; the process authority establishes and validates the proper time and temperature based on the equipment used and the products being processed.

6.23 DISEASES TRANSMITTED BY MILK

Milk contains bacillus lactic acid, which sours or ferments milk. The diseases which are commonly transmitted to man by the use of contaminated milk are: Tuberculosis, typhoid, paratyphoid, cholera, dysentery, diphtheria, malta fever, septic sore throat, etc. Bovine tuberculosis in man is generally non-pulmonary. Since the germs find access into the system through alimentary tract the abdomen, joints, bones, nervous system or lymphatic glands get usually affected.

6.24 INFANT FEEDING

World Health Organization (WHO) recommends exclusive breastfeeding for infants up to 6 months of age. The main food of most of the infants is breast milk. It is the most scientific, economic, sterile, nutritious and specific food for infants and it possesses anti-infective properties. The initial breast milk, which is very rich in antibodies and is nutritious called *colostrum* and must be given to the newborns. Human milk yields 20 calories per oz (28.35 gm) so that an average infant in the second month, fed exclusively on the breast milk, would require 20 oz (566.98 gm) of milk a day, 4 oz (113.40 gm) per feed, if it is fed 5 times in 24 hours. The breast milk secreted rarely exceeds 30 oz (850.47 gm) per day. From the age of 6 months, solid food may be supplied to provide the necessary calories (details in 6.5).

6.25 DERIVED MILK

1. **Standardised milk:** It is made by adjusting milk in such a way that it contains 3.7% fat, by adding or subtracting the cream, as the need be.

2. **Reconstituted milk:** Condensed or dried milk is reconstituted to the equivalent composition of fresh milk by the addition of water and vitamin C.

3. **Homogenised milk:** It is so made that the fat does not separate and does not rise to the surface as cream, on standing. The fat globules are reduced in size by passing the milk at a temperature of 150°F (65.6°C) under high pressure through minute apertures and the milk becomes homogeneous in consistency.

4. **Skimmed milk:** It is prepared by skimming of the milk or cream by hand or by centrifugal machines. It usually contains 3% fat. It should contain not less than 8.7% of total milk solids.

5. **Machine skimmed milk or separated milk:** It is milk from which cream has been removed in a centrifugal machine. It contains milk fat less than hand-skimmed milk but contains same amount of total solids.

6.26 MILK PRODUCTS

Cream: It is prepared by allowing the milk to stand for a considerable time in the cold so that butter fat may rise to the top and then removing the top layer. The fat or cream may be separated from milk mechanically through a centrifuge machine known as a *separator* or it may be obtained by churning the curdled milk. Cream may contain about 50% fat as against 3.5 to 5% in milk. Besides milk fat, cream contains proteins and lactose also.

Butter: It is the most nutritious and easily digestible form of all fats. Good butter should neither be rancid nor have an unpleasant odour. Specific gravity of butter fat varies from 0.911 to 0.913. Its melting point is 35.8°C. Its average composition should be:

Water	12–15%
Fat	80–90%
Caseinogen	1–3%
Lactose	1%
Ash	2–3%
Salt and vitamins	q.s.

Common salt is added to preserve and improve the flavour of butter. The use of boric acid or borax as a preservative should be forbidden by law. Annatto, turmuric, saffron or coal tar dyes may be added as colouring agents. Butter is adulterated with other animal fats in Western countries and in India by other vegetable oils. Its chief adulterant is water.

Cheese: It is a very concentrated protein food and methods of making it vary considerably at different places. It is prepared by coagulating caseinogen (chhana) of whole milk or skimmed milk with rennet. The curd is removed from the whey.

The cheese is then rolled and stored under conditions of controlled temperature and humidity and left to mature. The fat contents of cheese depend upon whether it is made from whole milk, skimmed milk or milk to which extra cream has been added. Cheese may contain tubercle bacilli unless prepared from pasteurised milk and typhoid organisms can remain viable for many weeks.

Curd/dahi: It is prepared by boiling milk and adding a little curd to the milk, when it has been cooled down to about 37°C. It is left over night and it ferments at room temperature by the lactic bacilli and bulgaris bacilli.

Margarine: It may be defined as: "Any article of food whether mixed with butter or not, which resembles butter and is not milk blended butter." This is much used in Western countries. It is prepared from animal and vegetable fats. It does not contain fat-soluble vitamins A and D. Margarine is much inferior to butter and contains less fat as compared to butter. It must not contain more than 16% of water or 10% of butter fat.

Ghee: It is clarified butter and is largely used in India in place of butter. It is of special importance in tropical countries where butter cannot be preserved for a long time and it soon becomes rancid and unfit for use. Ghee can be prepared from cow's or buffalo's milk. Buffalo ghee contains more soluble, volatile acids. It is frequently mixed with other animal fats or vanaspati (hydrogenated vegetable oils). The principal adulterants are groundnut oil, animal fat, mohua oil, poppy seed oil, coconut oil, boiled plantains, etc. In the manufacture of ghee from butter by usual methods, some 25% of vitamin A, originally present, may be destroyed. Prolonged heating of ghee in an open pan may cause serious destruction of vitamin A. It is probable that vitamin A value of most samples of pure cow's ghee lies between 1000 and 2500 IU per 100 gm while that of buffalo's ghee, it is usually lower. Vitamin D, however, is more thermostable, is capable of resisting prolonged heating.

6.27 VANASPATI

It is made from edible vegetable oils, which are refined, i.e. deacidified, bleached, deodorized and then partially dehydrogenated in the presence of finally divided nickel, which serves as a catalyst to get a melting range of 31 to 41°C. The product is again filtered, deacidified and washed to remove residual traces of catalyst. Finally vitamin A in the ratio of 25 IU per gm and 5% sesame (*til*) oil are added to it to conform to ISI specifications.

6.28 MUSTARD OIL

It is extensively used in India. It enters into the diet of most of the people, both rich and poor. It is prepared by extraction of seeds of mustard. It is extensively adulterated with some form of mineral oil or argemone oil obtained from the seeds *of Argemone mexicana.* It is a weed which grows wild in jungles and even on bunds of cultivated lands. Certain unsocial elements make it their business to collect argemone seeds and mix them with mustard seeds especially black mustard. Both are black in colour and hence an unwary customer may not easily detect adulteration of the seeds. The practice of adulteration is nefarious and dangerous to public health. It has been shown to give rise to symptoms resembling epidemic dropsy.

6.29 BEVERAGES

These are substances which enable food to be taken with pleasure and relish. They stimulate digestion. Water is considered as the principal beverage throughout the world and all the beverages contain water in varying quantities. They may be divided into three categories:

1. Aerated and mineral waters.
2. Non-fermented drinks as tea, coffee and cocoa.
3. Alcohols and liquors.

1. *Aerated and mineral waters:* Artificial mineral waters are prepared by dissolving mineral salts, and sugar in water and then charging with carbon dioxide gas.

   Natural mineral waters are derived from springs, contain natural ingredients and are impregnated with carbon dioxide gas.

   Mineral aerated waters have sharp pleasant taste. They help digestion and sometimes act as gastric sedatives.

2. *Non-fermented drinks:* The following three items fall under this category:

   1. **Tea:** It is said to be known to the Chinese nearly 1,500 years ago and was later on introduced in England about 300 years ago. It consists of dried leaves 1–2 inches (2.54–5.08 cm) long and 1/2–1 inch (1.27–2.54 cm) broad of a shrub called *Comellia thea* and contains 1 to 6% caffeine, minute trace of theophylline, 0.6% volatile oils and 6 to 12% tannic acid. It is used as a hot infusion. When infusion is prepared, caffeine dissolves out directly and tannic acid dissolves slowly and thus longer the tea is infused, the more tannic acid will be dissolved in it. The addition of milk to the tea infusion precipitates some of the tannic acid. In the case of black tea, the leaves are first fermented for about 20–24 hours before heating, just in order to reduce the astringency due to tannic acid (tannin) which is generally present in the dry leaves in amounts of up to 15% depending upon the type of tea used. Green tea is prepared from the younger leaves which are roasted soon after gathering. It contains more tannic acid, volatile oils and less caffeine than the black tea. In short the flavour of tea depends on its volatile oils content and the stimulating property is due to an alkaloid known as "caffeine", which may be present up to an extent of 5% in its leaves.

      Excessive use of tea leads to bad digestion, as the tannin present is liable to coagulate its albuminous ingredients and thus make the food difficult to digest. It causes gastric irritability, insomnia and dyspepsia. In moderate quantities, it acts as a stimulant and restorative.

Green tea leaves are supposedly richer in anti-oxidants than other types of tea because of the way they are processed. It contains B vitamins, folate (naturally occurring folic acid), manganese, potassium, magnesium, caffeine and other antioxidants (notably catechins).

Green tea is alleged to boost weight loss, reduce cholesterol, combat cardiovascular disease, prevent cancer and Alzheimer's disease.

2. **Coffee:** The roasted coffee contains 1 to 2% of caffeine, a small amount of caffeol and a large amount of tannic acid. It also acts as a stimulant owing to caffeine present in it and reduces fatigue. It contains fat, sugar, etc. It is prepared by roasting seeds of *Coffee Arabica* to chocolate brown colour and then ground into powder. Its chief adulterant, particularly in French coffee, is chicory. Caffeol or the aromatic oil, deteriorates rapidly on heating. It imparts flavour and aroma to coffee. It may be of interest to note that neither tea nor coffee has any calorific value, if only pure infusion is taken. Food value is attached to these beverages only when any sugar and milk are added. Excess use of coffee leads to palpitation, insomnia and nervous disturbances.

3. **Cocoa:** It is a powdery preparation, prepared by roasting and grinding cocoa beans derived from the fruits of the plants *Theobroma cocoa* which contains about 50% of fat and 1.5% alkaloid theobromine which is similar to caffeine. It is nutritive as well as stimulating. It contains much less stimulating properties than tea or coffee; its chief value being as a food and not as a stimulant. It is liked by some persons as it has a palatable taste. Chocolate is a preparation of it, which is made from ripe seeds of cocoa beans after they have been sweetened, dried, roasted and deprived of their shells. It is sweetened with sugar and suitably flavoured with vanilla or any other scent.

Alcohol and liquors. The term alcohol is used to cover a wide group of chemical substances but the one which is referred to under alcoholic beverages is ethyl alcohol (C_2H_5OH). It is produced by fermentation of yeast of monosaccharide sugars, glucose and fructose.

$$C_6H_{12}O_6 = 2C_2H_5OH + 2CO_2$$
Glucose   Ethyl alcohol   Carbon dioxide

Alcohols and liquors contain 2–50% of alcohol.

These are

1. *Beer and malt liquors contain* 3–7% alcohol. These are prepared from fermentation of malt and hops. *Cider and perry* are made by fermentation of the sugar, which is contained in the juice of apples as in the case of cider and pears as in the case of perry.

2. *Spirits:* These are prepared by distillation of alcohol produced by fermentation of various saccharines or starchy materials. Some of the main varieties of spirits are:

   i. *Whisky:* It contains from 45 to 50% by volume of alcohol. It is prepared from malted barley, cereals, rye, etc. It should not be less than two years old and should be free from disagreeable smell.

   ii. *Brandy:* It contains 48 to 54% of alcohol. It is a distilled wine prepared from grapes. It is coloured with burnt sugar and suitably flavoured. It is one of the least injurious forms of spirit.

   iii. *Rum:* It contains 50 to 60% of alcohol. It is prepared by fermentation of molasses or from juice of sugarcane.

   iv. *Gin:* It is obtained by fermentation of rye and malt and is flavoured with juniper berries, cardamoms and other aromatics. It contains 40 to 50% of alcohol.

3. *Wines:* These are the result of yeast fermentation of saccharine fruit juices, e.g. grapes. No yeast is added to liquor as in the making of beer, as yeast spores are always present in the skin of grapes. Lighter wines generally contain 10% of alcohol and the heavier ones up to 20 or even 25%. Since yeast spores present in the skin of grapes cease to bring about further fermentation when the concentration of alcohol reaches up to 15%, higher fermentation is obtained by adding extra alcohol to the wine, i.e. it is fortified. They are *claret, burgundy, sherry, portwine, champagne,* etc.

Alcohol is freely absorbed from stomach and reaches the bloodstream, therefore, it requires no digestion. It is stimulant in small doses. The heart is stimulated and beats more quickly and forcibly for a time. Respiration is also similarly effected. The smaller blood vessels are dilated. However, it is habit forming. It is apt to delay digestion since it gives rise to degeneration of alimentary tract, gastritis, intestinal catarrh, cirrhosis of liver, kidneys, etc. It has an irritant local action and acts as a narcotic. 2% of the alcohol taken is lost by lungs and the remaining quantity is oxidised by the tissues. After taking excessive dose it can be traced in the urine also. Moreover, alcohol if taken in excess, depresses, and paralyses the nervous system and in still larger doses it acts as a narcotic poison like opium and produces insensibility sometimes even causing death. A concentration of 350–400 mg of alcohol per 100 parts of blood may produce unconsciousness and deep anaesthesia.

Alcohol is not a food but is useful in some conditions of exhaustion or wasting diseases. Alcoholic liquors, e.g. beer, etc., have some nutritive value in view of the sugar and yeast they contain. It may give energy and lead to muscular activity, but total output of work is reduced.

6.30 FRUIT DRINKS

When made from fresh fruits such as oranges or lemons, fruit drinks are both palatable and a valuable source of vitamin C. If sugar is added, they provide a source of energy which is quickly absorbed in the bloodstream. The so-called fruit drinks made from chemical powders and some of the liquid fruit drinks sold commercially have no nutritive value other than dissolved sugar, for they contain no vitamin C.

6.31 CONDIMENTS

These are accessory foods such as chillies, mustard, black pepper, etc. Except common salt, they add a little or no food value but they make the food more palatable and are conducive in stimulation of salivary glands. They stimulate the salivary, gastric and pancreatic secretions. They also improve the colour, appearance and taste of food. They expel flatus.

6.32 AROMATICS

These may be classified as spices or plants, roots (used in powdered form), fragrant seeds (used whole, coarsely cracked or powdered), delicate grasses and herbs (fresh and dried), tree bark, etc. These are different from condiments like chillies, black pepper, etc. There are also mixtures or blended aromatics *like garam masalas, curry powders, etc.* Cardamoms, cinnamon, cloves, coriander, anise, etc. constitute some of the most important aromatics which improve colour, flavour and taste of the food.

Since they tend to lose their fragrance, if exposed to air, heat or moisture, it is recommended that only a light dusting should be given to the dish, immediately after it is cooked and is ready for serving.

6.33 NON-CONVENTIONAL FOODS

Population explosion and food shortages have forced man to search newer sources of food. Some of the potential sources are as follows:

1. **Leaves and grasses:** The proteins of green plants in nature are concentrated by passage into seeds or transformation into milk or meat. It has been estimated that protein available from an acre of land per annum is 600 lb as grass or 370 lb as beans or 269 lb as wheat.

2. **Algae:** Algae are capable of building up high concentrations of organic matter from inorganic compounds. Sunlight being the preferred source of energy for the synthesis, algae culture is predominantly suited to the tropical regions of the world. Waste land, not suited for other purposes, can be used for the algae culture which does not, therefore, interfere with the raising of normal agricultural crop.

3. **Phytoplankton:** The large marine algae or sea weeds constitute only 1% of the total marine vegetation. The greater part of oceanic life consists of microscopic phytoplankton.

4. **Yeasts, moulds and bacteria:** Micro-organisms are associated with human nutrition in its several aspects. They are present and they function in the human gut. Such fermentation processes as are involved in the preparation of food are mediated by them.

Yeast is capable of synthesising proteins from simple compounds in the shortest time. Yeast provides an excellent means of producing proteins by utilizing industrial wastes and byproducts such as molasses, skimmed milk, whey, wastes of fruits, groundnuts, potato, starch, paper pulp manufacture and other materials like bananas, wood, straw, seaweeds, putrefied fish and even sewage.

Moulds (fungi) too are capable of synthesising proteins from inorganic salts. They have also been used for obtaining fats from carbohydrates. Many of them are capable of breaking down cellulose for its utilisation to produce proteins from mixtures of fibrous materials and inorganic nitrogenous salts. They thus offer considerable possibilities of use.

6.34 FOOD FORTIFICATION AND ENRICHMENT

Addition of one or more dietary essentials to some foods in amounts which make the total content greater than that found in that particular food in its natural state is known as *fortification*. It also includes addition of one or more dietary essentials which original food does not contain in its natural state. *Enrichment* means addition of dietary essentials to a food to restore the total content of the former. Some of the examples of fortification and enrichment are: (i) Addition of vitamins A and D to milk, (ii) addition of vitamins, minerals and groundnut flour to *atta* (a programme launched in 1970 in Mumbai by the Government of India), (iii) addition of 700 IU of vitamin A per ounce of vanaspati (hydrogenated oil), (iv) addition of potassium iodate to common salt for endemic goitre areas, (v) addition of iron and iodine to common salt, (vi) addition of synthetic amino acids foods, e.g. lysine to wheat flour, etc.

6.35 SUPPLEMENTARY FOODS

A number of cheap supplementary foods is being formulated, which can provide nutrients at low cost, as a supplement to the usual diet. The Indian multipurpose food (MPF), oil seed cakes, 'Balahar' are some of the examples. 'Balahar' contains wheat, groundnuts and dry skimmed milk, fortified with vitamins and minerals supplying about 22% protein.

6.36 FOOD ADDITIVES

Food additives are non-nutritious substances which are added intentionally to food, generally, in small quantities to improve its appearance, flavour, texture or storage properties.

Food additives are generally used as food colours, antimicrobials, antioxidants and as stabilising, bleaching and manuring agents. Their use for a number of technical processes such as the maintenance of the nutritive quality of food, enhancement of storing quality, making food attractive to the consumers and providing essential aids to food processing, is well recognised. However, their abuse is creating serious public health problems, because they are sometimes used to deceive the consumer by disguising the faulty handling and processing techniques. Several food additives are under controversy about their safety, and some are dangerous to health, which are quite often used in spite of not being permitted by law. Some of the examples of food additives: (i) Addition of colours in sweets, (ii) addition of alum to bread to improve its whiteness, (iii) addition of salts of copper and lead to confectionary to give bright colours, (iv) addition of red lead to cheese to increase its attractiveness, (v) addition of ferrous sulphate to beer to strengthen its taste, and (vi) addition of salt, nitre, calcium sulphate to preserve food and so on.

6.37 FOOD ADULTERATION

Food adulteration includes mixing, substituting, abstracting, concealing the quality, selling decomposed foods, misbranding or giving false labels and adding poisonous substances. Motives behind adulteration are mainly economic and its high prevalence today reflects the degree of moral degradation, food shortage and technological advancements in more subtle methods of deception.

Some of the common practices in our country include:

i. *Cereals, pulses and flours:* Stone chips and gravel are used to increase the bulk of grains. Chemical substances such as metanil yellow are added to improve the colour and appearance of old stocks of pulses. Soap stone powders (used for making talcum powders) and cheap flours (e.g. singhara, kesari dal flours) are mixed with flours of wheat or Bengal gram.

ii. *Milk:* Removal of fat and addition of water, starch and skimmed milk, powder, etc. are the common types of milk adulteration.

iii. *Edible oils and fats:* Admixture of cheaper oil, e.g. groundnut oil to sesame oil (or sunflower oil) is widely practiced. Addition of argemone oil to improve the bulk and pungent taste of mustard oil, mineral oils and even lubricating motor oil to increase the bulk and sometimes dyes such as allyl isothiocyanate to improve the appearance are common practices. Ghee is generally adulterated with 'Vanaspati' and cheap animal fats, e.g. pig's fat while tributyrin is added to improve the flavour of adulterated ghee.

iv. *Miscellaneous:* Tea leaves are adulterated with old tea leaves, busker and saw-dust. Coffee is adulterated with chicory. Honey is adulterated with sugar or jaggery and boiled with empty beehives. Papaya seeds are mixed with pepper. Powdered condiments and spices often contain an assortment of innumerable substances including horse dung and brick powder. Lead chromate is added to substances that are passed off as turmeric and so on.

Some forms of adulteration may not be very dangerous, e.g. addition of water to milk, cheap edible oils to expensive ones, cheap flours to expensive ones, etc. However, they may considerably reduce the nutritive value, contaminate the food (e.g. water to milk) and add toxins to the food (e.g. kesari dal flour to other flour and adulteration of edible oils with argemone oil and white mineral oil, use of non-permitted colours in sweets and cordials, and that of lead chromate for spices, etc.

The Prevention of Food Adulteration Act, 1954 (with some amendments in 1963) aims to prevent adulteration and sale of substandard foods. This Act has been revised in 2011 and are now known as Food Safety and Standards Rules, 2011. The rules prescribe standards to which various articles of food must conform, and also lay down what preservatives, colouring agents, antioxidants, emulsifying agents, etc. are to be permitted. The Indian Standards Institution, the Central Committee for Food Standards in the Ministry of Health, and the Directorate of Marketing and Inspection work in coordination for maintaining food quality in India. Although it is a Central Act, its implementation is a responsibility of the state governments and local bodies. "Food inspectors" (in many states, sanitary inspectors work as food inspectors) are appointed, who take samples of food or seize the unwholesome food in certain conditions. If the sample examined by the public analyst of the state government does not conform with the standards prescribed in the rules, the vendor is prosecuted.

Soil and Building Sites

Soils are natural expressions of the environment in which they were formed. They are derived from an infinite variety of materials that have been subjected to a wide spectrum of climatic conditions. Soil development is influenced by the topography on which soils occur, the plant and animal life which they support and the amount of time which they have been exposed to these conditions.

Soil is formed by the disintegration of the underlying rocks, which get mixed up in due course of time with decayed animals and vegetable matters. Often the more superficial soil, consisting of decayed animals and vegetable matter, is called *mould* or *humus.* The depth of this layer varies at different places. Soil scientists recognize five major factors that influence soil formation: (i) Parent material, (ii) climate, (iii) living organisms (especially native vegetation), (iv) topography, and (v) time. The combined influence of these soil-forming factors determines the properties of a soil and their degree of expression.

The subsoil has been derived from disintegration of rocks in the course of millions of years by action of water, gases, etc. The depth of this layer varies from a few feet to hundreds of feet. Soil, in general, is loose and friable and is above the level of groundwater. It contains much air in its interstices. It is like a sponge, the particles being separated from each other by channels and interstices, through which air can pass. Ordinarily these channels are full of air. When rainfalls, it penetrates down into the soil. At varying depths, it forms a continuous sheet of water known as groundwater. When rainfalls and percolates into the soil the air is driven out. Similarly, when the atmospheric temperature is raised, due to sun or by the warmth of the house, air is sucked out of the soil.

7.1 CLASSIFICATION OF SOILS

Soils are classified as follows:

1. **Sandy soils:** These types of soils are of considerable depth and are free from organic matter. With dry ground air, these are considered as healthy soils. If the level of subsoil water is high or the soils are shallow and lie over clay, they are considered as unhealthy soils.

2. **Clayey soils or alluvial soils:** Owing to the retention of water in these soils, they are cold and damp and, therefore, they require adequate drainage. They are rich in humus and very fertile. They are found in Great Northern plain, lower valleys of Narmada and Tapti and Northern Gujarat. These soils are renewed every year.

3. **Granitic, metamorphic and trap rocks:** These are considered as healthy sites for the houses as they are dry owing to good drainage and slopy nature of the soil. Weathered granite, however, is an exception to this rule as it becomes soft and absorbs water.

4. **Chalk, sandstone, limestone and magnesium limestone soils:** All these types of soils are dry and they are considered as healthy soils.

5. **Gravelly soils:** These are the healthiest of all the soils, unless they are water-logged. Water supply from gravelly soil is generally pure.

6. **Loamy soil:** Such types of soils are a mixture of sand, clay and humus.

7. **Filled or made soils:** When depressions of the ground are filled up with refuse, the resulting soil is called "made soil". The refuse undergoes fermentation and putrefaction with formation of certain gases such as marsh gas, hydrogen sulphide, etc. and gives rise to nuisance of obnoxious smell. Such soils are not considered suitable for the construction of buildings there upon for 20–25 years.

7.2 IMPORTANCE OF SOIL TEXTURE FOR BUILDING SITES

Soil texture is an important physical property and a major factor to consider when evaluating the suitability of a lot as a building site. Knowing the texture helps to determine this and offers an opportunity to make site comparisons. The texture of the subsoil indicates the building site potential. If the subsoil is coarse (sand, loamy sand), water drains through it rapidly (assuming there is no high water table). Coarse-textured soils are easily excavated and quite stable during both dry and wet conditions. The properties that make the coarse-textured soils good building sites are the same ones that make them poor for establishing and maintaining lawns and gardens.

The moderate (loams, silt loams) and fine-textured soils generally have a higher inherent soil fertility which makes them desirable for establishing lawns and gardens. Organic soils (peat and muck) make good garden sites, if adequate drainage can be provided. However, the fact that these soils are easily compacted, resulting in settling if foundations are installed, makes them unsuited for building.

Texture has a significant influence on the ability of a soil to accept and treat septic tank effluent. Percolation rates are largely determined by soil texture. Sandy soils tend to have faster rates, while more fine-textured soils have slower rates.

7.3 GROUNDWATER

Groundwater fills spaces between the soil particles and fractured rock beneath the earth's surface. Its depth varies greatly and is determined by the depth of the first impervious strata. If the level of groundwater, for any reason, gets very high, then that particular area should be regarded as unhealthy. The maximum height fixed for the groundwater is 10–15 feet (3.05–4.57 meters) and if that is exceeded then the area should be considered as unsuitable for building houses. The groundwater affects the health in two ways:

1. It supplies water to all the shallow wells. If it is polluted, it may cause several diseases.
2. If its level rises, it gives rise to dampness in houses resulting in rheumatism, catarrh, neuralgia and lung troubles.

It should, however, be remembered that the presence of moisture in the soil favours the decomposition of putrefiable materials. Therefore, a dry soil is comparatively cleaner and its ground air purer than that in the case of damp soil.

The level of subsoil or groundwater can be lowered by launching proper engineering schemes to a safe level. Drainage may have to be carried out on a very large scale and rivers or water courses may have to be opened up, or porous earthenware pipes may have to be laid on a large scale at a depth of 10 feet (3.05 metres) and through them the groundwater over that level is drained away in the direction of the slope of land.

In hot climates, tree plantation has rendered the places healthy. The vegetation abstracts large quantity of water from the soil, which gets evaporated from the green leaves. Eucalyptus trees absorb water 11 times the amount of rainfall over the area which they cover. These have been grown in many malarious districts for purpose of rendering them more healthy and the results have been very satisfactory. The groundwater level rises due to canal irrigation and some time may give rise to waterlogging.

7.4 GROUND AIR

It is present in the interstices of all varieties of soil. It differs from the atmospheric air. It is generally moist and the amount of moisture depends upon the proximity of groundwater to the surface of the soil. If this is a few feet deep from the surface of the ground, the air gets saturated with moisture. But the ground near the surface of the earth in most parts of the world, is moist even after a draught, owing to the capillary action of soil and evaporation taking place from the surface of the groundwater.

The impurities of the ground air are due to the decomposition of various organic matters which are washed into the soil by the rain or which are naturally present in some marshy soils. The gaseous products of decomposition are ammonia, ammonium sulphide, methane and sulphuretted hydrogen. In the neighbourhood of houses, the foulness of ground air is due to the animal contamination and this may be very dangerous.

Leaking cesspools, sewers, drains, animal filth and possibly infected excretions pollute water and air present in the soil. Graveyards permit decomposing dead bodies to exercise a similar pollution, whilst the organic effluvia arising from "made soils" seriously imperil the health of inmates of the houses built on them. It is important that such ground air be prevented from oozing out of the earth by rendering the basement of houses impermeable by cementing or asphalting them.

7.5 DISEASES ATTRIBUTABLE TO SOIL

The pathogens responsible for causing such diseases can be divided into two groups: Euedaphic pathogenic organisms (EPOs), being potential pathogens which are true soil organisms, i.e. their usual habitat is the soil. These include most of the bacterial pathogens and all of the fungal pathogens. The other group consists of soil transmitted pathogens (STPs) (Table 7.1).

Most commonly soil has been held responsible for the spread of infectious diseases such as enteric fever, cholera and amoebic dysentery. Some pathogenic germs are present in the soil which cause anthrax, tetanus, malignant oedema, etc. Soil-transmitted helminth infections are among the most common infections worldwide and affect the poorest and most deprived

Table 7.1: Soil-borne infectious diseases (bold) and their causative agents (italics) split into two groups, "Euedaphic pathogenic organisms (EPOs)" and "soil transmitted pathogens (STPs)", depending on the closeness of their relationship with soil

Euedaphic pathogenic organisms	Soil transmitted pathogens
Actinomycetoma: *Actinomyces israelii*	**Poliovirus:** Poliomyelitis
Anthrax: *Bacillus anthracis*	**Hantavirus**
Botulism: *Clostridium botulinum*	**Q fever:** *Coxiella burnetii*
Campylobacteriosis: *Campylobacter jejuni*	**Lyme disease:** *Borrelia* spp.
Leptospirosis: *Leptospira interrogans*	**Ascariasis:** *Ascaris lumbricoides*
Listeriosis: *Listeria monocytogenes*	**Hookworm:** *Ancylostoma duodenale*
Tetanus: *Clostridium tetani*	**Enterobiasis (pinworm):** *Enterobius vermicularis*
Tularemia: *Francisella tularensis*	**Strongyloidiasis:** *Strongyloides stercoralis*
Gas gangrene: *Clostridium perfringens*	**Trichuriasis (whipworm):** *Trichuris trichiura*
Yersiniosis: *Yersinia enterocolitica*	**Echinococcosis:** *Echinococcus multicularis*
Aspergillosis: *Aspergillus* spp.	**Trichinellosis:** *Trichinella spiralis*
Blastomycosis: *Blastomyces dermatitidis*	**Amoebiasis:** *Entamoeba histolytica*
Coccidioidomycosis: *Coccidioides immitis*	**Balantidiasis:** *Balantidium coli*
Histoplasmosis: *Histoplasma capsulatum*	**Cryptosporidiosis:** *Cryptosporidium parvum*
Sporotrichosis: *Sporothrix schenckii*	**Cyclosporiasis:** *Cyclospora cayetanensis*
Mucormycosis: *Rhizopus* spp.	**Giardiasis:** *Giardia lambila*
Mycetoma: *Nocardia* spp.	**Isosporiasis:** *Isospora belli*
Strongyloidiasis: *Strongyloides stercoralis*	**Toxoplasmosis:** *Toxoplasma gondii*
	Shigellosis: *Shigella dysenteriae, Pseudomonas aeruginosa, Escherichia coli*
	Salmonellosis: *Salmonella enterica*

communities. They are transmitted by eggs present in human faeces which in turn contaminate soil in areas where sanitation is poor. The main species that infect people are the roundworm (*Ascaris lumbricoides*), the whipworm (*Trichuris trichiura*) and the hookworms (*Necator americanus* and *Ancylostoma duodenale*).

Diarrhoea is associated with low-lying alluvial soil, whereas incidence of rheumatism, catarrh and pulmonary diseases including tuberculosis are associated with dampness of soil.

Other non-infectious diseases which can be obtained from the soil or are associated with the soil include silicosis and geophagia which is associated with pica (defined as being a persistent ingestion of eating non-food materials).

7.6 HOUSES AND BUILDINGS

Before constructing a new house or a building, it is most essential that a suitable and healthy site be selected for its construction. The site should be sufficiently elevated from its surroundings, so that it is not subjected to the fury of flood waters during heavy rains. In its selection, consideration should be dryness, warmth, light and air. The height of the groundwater should be determined. If it is higher than 10 feet (3.05 metres) from the surface, the site should be condemned, unless the level of groundwater can be lowered by drainage. Clay and alluvial soils should be avoided as they are

damp and cold. The best soils are rock and well-drained gravel. Filled up soil is unsuitable as it is polluted by sewage or refuse. Places where refuse is thrown or which are situated near the trenching grounds or factories should be avoided. The site should be high with a sufficient slope to allow the rainwater to pass off rapidly and should not be near the marshes, paddy fields, stables, cowsheds, etc.

The buildings should be open on the East and South to allow free passage of light and air and should be exposed to the sun.

Since trees cause evaporation and drying of the ground, there should be vegetation growing near the house, but it should not be so close as to damp the house by obstructing light and air.

Construction of back to back houses should be discouraged, as crossventilation is impossible in such houses and the rooms are naturally dark and ill-ventilated.

Construction of Houses or Buildings

National Building Code, first published in 1970, revised in 2005; is a document containing standardized requirements for design and construction of buildings in the country. These exist to protect public's health, ensure safety and welfare.

General requirements: The following points should be borne in mind, at the time of construction:

Foundation: It must be always solid and substantial, so as to sustain the combined deadload of the building and the superimposed load. It should be dug and a bed of good cement concrete be laid to cover the whole site of the house and should extend 6 inches (15.32 cm) beyond the footings of the walls on every side. The depth of the concrete should depend upon the weight of the wall; which has to be supported and in no case should be less than 18 inches (0.46 metre). This is essential to eliminate the possibility of any subsequent subsidence, which may occur in buildings constructed on a loose soil or with bad concrete structure.

Plinth height is also recommended for 2–3 feet (60–91 cm).

All material and workmanship should be of good quality conforming to the acceptable standards of Bureau of Indian Standards (BIS).

Dampness of houses: It is caused due to three major causes:

1. Rising damp.
2. Percolating damp.
3. Roof leaks.

Damp-proof course (Fig. 7.1): A layer of impervious material should be laid horizontally along the entire thickness of each wall above the point, where the wall leaves the earth but below the level of floor. It imposes a barrier to the upward progress of moisture. By the capillary action, the bricks absorb moisture from the soil even as far as the upper rooms and consequently make the house damp and unhealthy. An effective damp proofing material should be impervious, dimensionally stable, strong and durable, and should be capable of withstanding both dead as well as live loads without damage. Besides it should be free from deliquescent salts like sulphates, chlorides and nitrates.

The materials commonly used to check dampness can be divided into the following three categories:

1. *Flexible materials:* Materials like bitumen felts (which may be hessian-based or fibre/glass fibre-based), plastic sheeting (polythene sheets), etc.
2. *Semirigid materials:* Materials like mastic, asphalt, or combination of materials or layers.
3. *Rigid materials:* Materials like first class bricks, stones, slate, cement, concrete, etc.

In very damp marshy districts, it is advisable to raise the house above the ground on arches open to air.

Walls: These should be constructed of bricks, stones, concrete or wood and should be reasonably strong. The brick walls of the houses should be dry and full of air. The bricks should be properly bounded. Ordinary bricks are porous and very absorbent. The stock size brick of 9 × 4–1/2 × 3 inches (22.86 × 11.43 × 7.62 cm) is capable of absorbing as much as 16 oz (0.453 kg) of water. Stone is non-absorbent and is least affected by

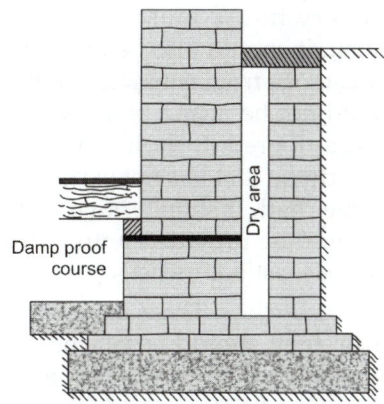

Fig. 7.1: Damp-proof course and dry area

changes in temperature. Timber is not so durable although it is warm but danger to fire, is its greatest disadvantage. Concrete reinforced with steel bars is a most common material used these days. The walls of the houses should be plastered from outside and inside. They should not absorb heat and transmit the same to the rooms. The walls in the rooms are lime-washed or they may be oil-painted to render their face impervious and enable them to be easily washed.

Floors: The base of the floor must have an impermeable layer of concrete or cement to prevent dampness rising from the soil below and as a valuable protection against dry rot, which is caused by the agency of a fungus; which has the effect of reducing timber to powder. They are generally made of bricks with cement, concrete, glazed tiles, asphalt, marble slabs, etc. The floors of upper storeys may, however, be made of wood, cement or tiles. The floor area should be at least 100 sq ft (9.29 sq metres) per person in a living room.

Roofs: These should be sufficiently high and rain-proof and may be flat or sloping depending on the area and climatic conditions. Sloping roofs should be encouraged at hilly places and flat roofs in the plains, which afford sleeping place during hot weather. They should be provided with proper gutters with a suitable fall and sprouts for rapid removal of rainwater.

Doors and windows: Every room must have sufficient number of doors and windows to allow free ventilation of air. Cross-ventilation should be encouraged. Door area as well as window area combined should be equal to two-fifths of the floor area of a room. These should be provided with wire gauze.

Living rooms and bedrooms: These should be of adequate size to permit the assembly of family with comfort. These should be arranged so as to secure the maximum sunlight and outlook should be pleasant as the circumstances may permit. Ventilation is of great importance. A fireplace should be provided which affords a permanent means of ventilation.

Kitchen: Every house must be provided with a separate kitchen. It should also be built on a detached side to prevent smoke from entering into the residential rooms. It should not be near a privy. It should be fly-proof and pucca-floored. It should not open towards the busy road side, so that it is not exposed to dust and impurities of the road. It should have adequate water supply and should be provided with a porcelain sink and water tap for washing utensils.

Food stores or larders: These are essential features of every house; they should be placed on the North wherever possible, or at any rate be protected from full heat of the sun. Good lighting and proper ventilation are indispensable and in rural areas more space for food storage is required than in towns.

Fuel store: It should be sufficient to hold adequate quantity of fuel and it should be in the same block as the outside water closet or kitchen.

Water closets or sanitary privies: These should be built in a detached portion of the building and should be at a sufficient distance from the living rooms and the kitchen. There should be proper arrangement for the disposal of dry refuse, waste water and excreta.

Water supply: There should be a proper arrangement for water supply either from taps or covered deep wells and it should be available for use at all times.

Open space: There should be sufficient open space around each building. A back space of at least 10 feet (3.04 metres) should be kept open.

7.7 HOUSING AND HEALTH

The diseases associated with housing are classified in two groups:

a. **Diseases of overcrowded, ill-ventilated and ill-lighted house,** e.g. poor health, rickets (due to paucity of sunlight), common cold, influenza, tuberculosis, bronchitis, measles, diphtheria, chickenpox, etc. (all airborne infections), and skin infections, e.g. scabies, ringworm, leprosy, impetigo, etc. (diseases of contact owing to overcrowding).

b. **Diseases of houses with poor basic facilities,** e.g. irritation of mucous membranes of ear, nose, throat and lungs owing to smoke nuisance in living rooms, diseases where rodents and arthropods act as vectors in houses with poor refuse disposal, other insanitary facilities, etc.

Climatology and Meteorology

8.1 CLIMATE

It may be defined as the average condition of the weather at any particular place over a considerably long period of time (say 20–30 years) taking into consideration absolute extremes, means how often these are deviated, in the case of temperature, rainfall, atmospheric pressure, sunshine, humidity, fog, mist, etc. Thus if a particular area has a heavy rainfall, it will be spoken of as having a moist climate or if it remains usually hot, it would be termed as an area having a hot climate. In short, it is the sum total of all the meteorological aspects of each individual component. It depends upon the following factors:

1. The altitude or distance from equator.
2. Distance from sea.
3. The altitude, or height, above sea-level.
4. Prevailing winds. East and northeast winds are comparatively cold, whereas southwest winds are rain-bearing.
5. Amount of humidity present in the air.
6. Nature of the soil.
7. Proximity of mountains and hills.
8. Rainfall.

The human body possesses marvellous power of adaptability to various external conditions occasioned by changes of climate and season, and transition from cold to heat, dryness to humidity, and *vice versa*. In all cases, normal temperature is maintained and bodily functions are properly performed. Climates may be roughly classified as cold, temperate, hot, mountainous and oceanic.

8.2 EFFECTS OF CLIMATE ON HEALTH OF THE PEOPLE

Climate change poses a threat to public health. Extreme weather events, heat waves, expanded habitats for disease transmitters, and climate-induced air and water quality degradation can impact human health. Warmer average temperatures will likely lead to hotter days and more frequent and longer heat waves. This could increase the number of heat-related illnesses and deaths. Warmer temperatures could increase the concentrations of unhealthy air and water pollutants. Changes in temperature, precipitation patterns, and extreme events could enhance the spread of some diseases. The climate is an important factor in determining the characteristics of races of mankind. It also affects in the variation of pigmentation of the skin. The impact of climate change on health will depend on the effectiveness of a community's public health and safety systems to address or prepare for the risk and the behaviour, age, gender, and economic status of individuals affected. Impact will also vary by region, the sensitivity of populations, the extent and length of exposure to climate change impacts, and society's ability to adapt to change.

Acclimatisation is affected by slow process of changes taking place either in the individual or in the race by constitutional modifications brought about by the successive generations.

Adaptation should begin now, starting with public health infrastructure. Individuals, communities, and government agencies can take steps to moderate the impacts of climate change on human health. Specific health adaptation approaches include:

1. Monitoring emerging health risks.
2. Planning urban adaptation strategies, such as planting trees to minimize heat buildup in cities and manage storm water, or promoting the use of cool roofs to reduce energy needs and improve air quality.
3. Preparing emergency response plans, which include providing cooling centers for extreme heat events.
4. Improving public communication during specific health risks such as extreme heat events or low air quality days.

Various meteorological conditions bear an important influence on climate and health.

Effects of hot climate on the body: A warmer climate is expected to both increase the risk of heat-related illnesses and death and worsen conditions for air quality.

High temperature will cause diminution of metabolism, so less amount of food is taken and there is an evidence of loss of weight. It diminishes the rate of respiration, retards elimination of carbon dioxide from the lungs and decreases the amount of urea in the urine. It causes reduction in the oxygenation of blood and diminution of digestive power. Moreover, due to hot climate, nerves are enervated, the skin becomes active and excretes profuse secretion. Continued residence in tropical countries may bring about a languor both mental and physical, premature senility and general lowering of the expectation of life. Heat waves can lead to heat stroke and dehydration, and are the most common cause of weather-related deaths.

High temperature in cities would increase the demand for electricity in the summer to run air conditioning, which in turn would increase air pollution and greenhouse gas emissions from power plants. Heat waves are also often accompanied by periods of stagnant air, leading to increases in air pollution and the associated health effects.

Effects of cold climate on the body: It causes increased metabolism, thus the requirement of food is increased to cope up with the change in metabolism. Oxygenation of blood, elimination of carbon dioxide and excretion of urine are increased, the amount of sweat is reduced and the digestive power is sharpened. There is an increase in both bodily and mental activity. Cold season, however, is pleasant invigorating and it tones up the muscles of the body. The expectation of life also increases in cold climate.

Effects of humidity on health: Both very low or high relative humidities may cause some physical discomfort, as the relative humidity of the air directly affects temperature perception. Extremely low (below 20%) relative humidities may also cause eye irritation due to dryness and moderate to high levels of humidity have been shown to reduce the severity of asthma. A large amount of humidity present in the air offers a check to the evaporation from the lungs and skin due to less drying power, thus hindering the process of perspiration and impairing normal functioning of the skin. Moist climate is less healthy than dry one, as it favours the growth and development of micro-organisms and hastens putrefactive changes. About 75% humidity is considered as best for human body.

Effects of warm moist air on the body: These are worse than the dry warm air. Evaporation cannot take place easily and so perspiration does not dry. It lowers the health and working efficiency to a great extent and renders one susceptible to sunstroke. There is a loss of appetite and disinclination to mental and physical work.

Effects of cold and damp air on health: There is a rapid loss of heat and chilling of the body. The research has shown the association of dampness with upper respiratory tract symptoms, cough, wheeze, and asthma symptoms in sensitized persons, i.e. asthma exacerbation. Cold and damp air also affects blood circulation, kidneys, and joints leading to rheumatism.

Effects of warm dry air on body: A relative dry air feels better than moist air at most temperatures. When the air is dry and warm, the rate of evaporation from the body is greatly increased.

Effect of cold and dry air on the body: All the body functions are more active. Breathing is deeper and more frequent, the circulation of blood is increased; processes of digestion, assimilation and metabolism are stimulated. The skin becomes dry and chapped. (This climate is more bracing and invigorating.)

Effects of high altitude on climate: There is diminished atmospheric pressure, rarefaction and purity of air; humidity of the air is lessened. There is a considerable increase of sunlight, on account of brisk blowing of the air. Moreover, there is a large amount of ozone present in the air and it is also free from germs and dirt. There is extreme cold and the temperature is low. As a general rule, temperature falls about 1°F for every 300 feet (91.44 metres) of altitude or 1 degree latitude, and pressure falls, about 1 lb (0.453 kg) for every 1800 feet (548.64 metres) ascent.

A condition known as "mountain sickness" is considered to be due to the rarity of the atmosphere and diminution of oxygen at great heights. Its symptoms are deep breathing, quick pulse, mental fatigue, cyanosis, nausea, headache, intestinal disturbances and fainting. Bleeding from the nose, ringing in the ears and palpitation of heart are also not infrequent symptoms.

Effects of residence at high altitude on health: To compensate for the change in barometric pressure which leads to decrease in the amount of oxygen leading to hypobaric hypoxia, the capacity of chest is increased in all measurements with increased power of expansion and contraction. People living at high altitudes have robust health due to the process of adaptation. It is also good for persons suffering from anaemia, spasmodic asthma without emphysema and chronic pleurisy. High altitude, however, is bad for persons suffering from chronic bronchitis, emphysema, bronchiectasis, diseases of heart and great vessels, infections of kidneys, liver and those of the brain and spinal cord.

Effects of increased atmospheric pressure on health: This is seen in places like mines, submarine works and bridges. There is an increased absorption of oxygen by blood. The effects known as *Caisson's disease* are found in the workers working in the compressed air chambers. The symptoms are pain in the ears, accompanied with disturbance in hearing, excruciating pain in joints and muscles, vertigo, epigastric pain, changed sense of smell, taste and vomiting. There may be appearance of headache, giddiness, epistaxis, paralysis, etc. Sometimes death may occur from internal haemorrhages. These symptoms do not appear, when the men are working inside but appear rapidly when they come outside.

Effects of rainfall on climate: It washes down impurities and microbes contained in the air thus rendering the atmosphere cool, fresh and invigorating. It reduces the atmospheric pressure.

Effects of vegetation on climate: Vegetation, in moderation, improves the climate by keeping the air cool and equitable and counteracts the effects of radiation from earth.

Where there is no vegetation, as in deserts, it leads to a great variation. The deserts are very hot during the daytime but temperature falls during the night considerably owing to rapid radiation.

In cold climates, the trees and shrubs obstruct the passage of rays of sun falling direct on the soil, which, therefore, is liable to be cold and moist but they may prove to be of great help in protecting the place against the cold winds.

In hot climates, the evaporation of water from the leaves of trees tends to dry the soils and lower the temperature. The ground is sheltered from the direct rays of the sun by the leaves of trees which thus keep the place cool. Hence, the heat of summer is reduced, and the cold of winter is tempered with by the presence of trees. Places grown with trees have comparatively lower temperature than other dry places having no vegetation growth at all.

However, the air is generally stagnant in very dense forests.

8.3 METEOROLOGY

It is a branch of science which deals with the atmospheric phenomena in relation to weather. The three basic aspects of meteorology are observation, understanding and prediction of weather, i.e. atmospheric temperature, humidity, wind, rainfall, etc. Weather denotes general condition of the air at any stated period of time, or more scientifically, it may be defined as the state of atmosphere at any particular time in relation to its temperature, visibility, humidity, precipitation or any other meteorological phenomena.

8.4 ATMOSPHERIC PRESSURE

Also called **barometric pressure** is the force exerted by an atmospheric column (i.e. the entire body of air above the specified area) per unit area. It is measured by means of a **barometer** (mercury and aneroid). Meteorologists use barometer to forecast short-term changes in the weather.

The most commonly used is Fortin's standard barometer: It should be fixed and hung vertically in a room, well protected from rain, sun or wind. First, the reading of the attached thermometer is noted. In this type of barometer, the cistern is made of a pliable base of leather, which can be raised or lowered by means of a screw. Before taking a reading, the level of mercury in the cistern is adjusted by means of the rack and pinion at the side of the barometer. The barometer must be fixed in a properly lighted room protected from sun and rain (Fig. 8.1).

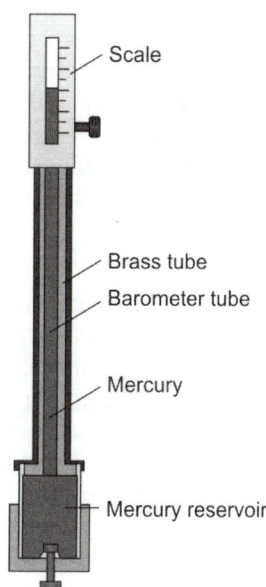

Fig. 8.1: Fortin's barometer

Another type of barometer used is *aneroid barometer* (Fig. 8.2). It contains no mercury or any other fluid. It consists of a small box, which is exhausted of air and

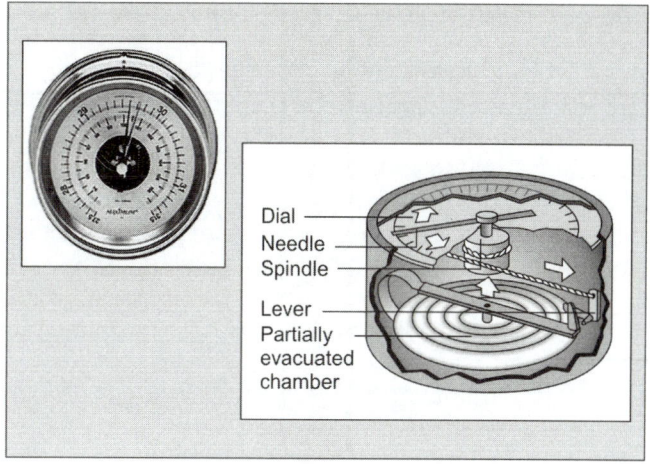

Fig. 8.2: The aneroid barometer

contains a series of springs. The pressure is communicated by these springs on the dial, which has been graduated by comparison with a standard mercurial barometer. When the atmospheric pressure increases, the spring is pulled down, whereas if the pressure diminishes, the spring rises up. This instrument is easy for transport and is used for recording altitudes. But its disadvantage is that it is liable to go out of order and requires periodic maintenance. Moreover, it is not so accurate.

8.5 ISOBARS

In this case, a large number of barometrical readings are taken at the same time over an extended area and the same are telegraphically communicated to a central station, where they are represented on a map. Subsequently on this map, also called *synoptic or weather map*, lines are drawn, connecting the places showing equal barometric pressure and these lines are termed *isobars*. Weather experts use these to interpret the direction of winds, rain, frost, fog and temperature.

8.6 TEMPERATURE

This is ascertained by an instrument called thermometer. It is an instrument used to measure temperature by means of a liquid or a gas contained in a graduated tube. Most commonly used liquids in the thermometers are either mercury or alcohol (ethanol). Mercury is used in thermometers meant for recording high temperatures on account of its uniformity in expansion at different temperatures, easy visibility, high boiling point and low vapour pressure. Alcohol is used in thermometers for recording low temperatures, because it does not freeze even at low temperatures (Fig. 8.3).

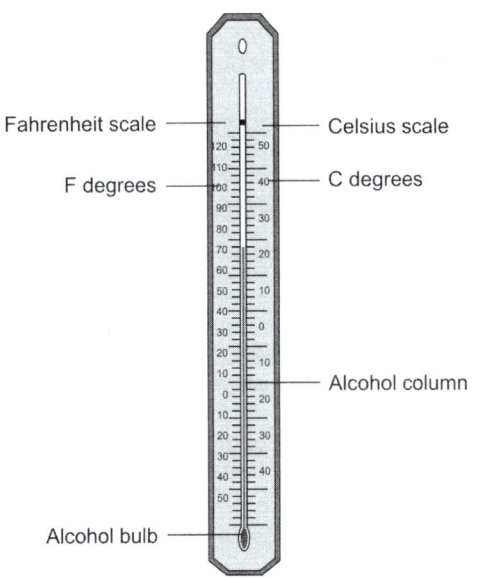

Fig. 8.3: Alcohol thermometer

Various scales, commonly used to measure temperature, are as follows:

Name of thermometer	Freezing point	Boiling point
1. Fahrenheit	32	212
2. Centigrade (Celsius)	0	100
3. Reaumur	0	80

Several kinds of thermometers are used in India. These are:

1. **Standard or dry bulb thermometer:** It is an ordinary thermometer (Fig. 8.4).

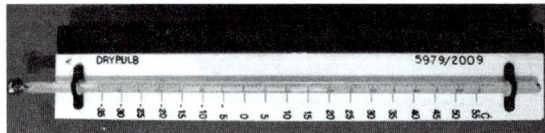

Fig. 8.4: Dry bulb thermometer

2. **Maximum thermometer:** It is used for registering the highest temperature attained in the day or any other period. The thermometer is laid in a horizontal position. In the stem of the thermometer, part of the mercury column is separated by air. When the temperature rises, the mercury expands and pushes this broken column forward. But this column does not recede when the temperature falls and the main mercury column contracts. The reading taken indicates the maximum temperature attained during the day.

3. **The minimum thermometer:** It is used for recording the lowest temperature during the night or during the early hours of morning. A small glass index is enclosed in the spirit, which fills the bulb and a part of the stem. When setting the instrument, the index is first brought to the top of the column of the spirit and the instrument is placed in a horizontal position.

   When the temperature rises, the spirit expands and flows past the index, but when the temperature falls, the spirit contracts and carries the index along with it. The lowest temperature is thus registered. The instrument can be readjusted by tilting.

4. **Six's maximum and minimum thermometer:** It is a combination of maximum and minimum thermometers and gives a double reading (Fig. 8.5). It is, however, not very accurate instrument and, therefore, no more being used now in Indian Meteorological observatories.

5. **Solar radiation or vacuum thermometer** (Fig. 8.6): It is used for measuring the intensity of heat given off or radiated by the sun. It is a maximum, mercurial, self-registering thermometer having a bulb coated with lamp-black to absorb the rays of the sun. The bulb is placed in a glass case in order to prevent the

coating from being washed away by rain. The instrument is placed horizontally about 4 ft (1.22 metres) above the ground, away from the walls, and the trees, and exposed to the direct rays of the sun. The difference between the maximum temperature in the sun and in the shade is the amount of "solar radiation" indicated during the day or of the power of rays of the sun.

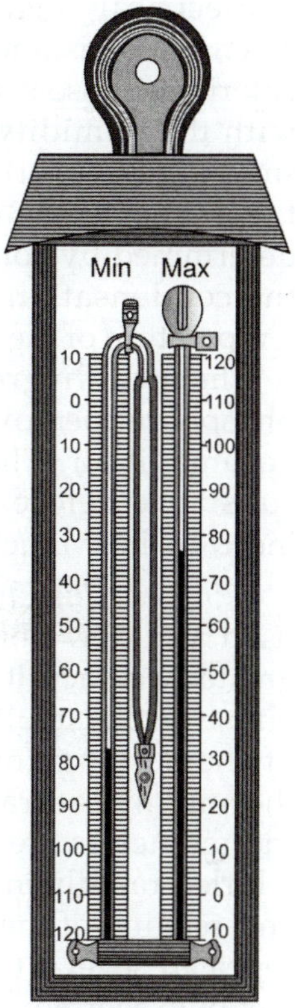

6. **Terrestrial thermometer** (Fig. 8.7): It is a minimum shade thermometer placed close to the ground, with the bulb resting on the grass about 4 inches (10.16 cm) above the ground. The difference between this minimum temperature and the air minimum in the shade is the amount of terrestrial radiation.

7. **Globe thermometer:** It is used to record, the temperature of the atmosphere plus the temperature due to radiant heat. It consists of a yellow metal globe of 6 inches (15.24 cm) diameter. Its outer surface is coated with a dull black paint. The globe has an opening through which a mercury thermometer is inserted. The bulb of the thermometer is suspended in the middle of the

Fig. 8.5: Six's thermometer

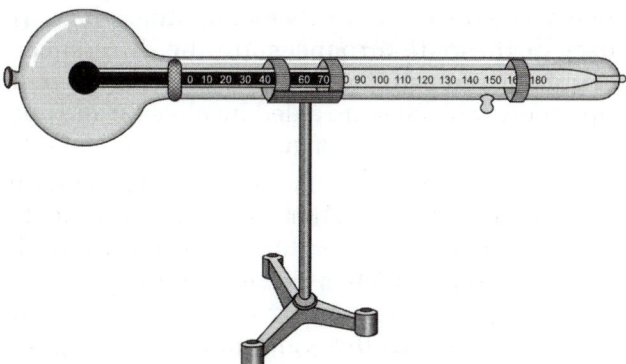

Fig. 8.6: Solar radiation or vacuum thermometer

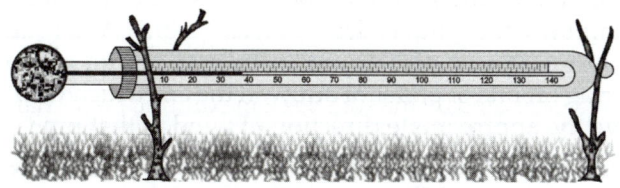

Fig. 8.7: Terrestrial thermometer

globe. This instrument is used indoors, in factories and other places, where there is a source of radiant heat.

8.7 HUMIDITY

It denotes the amount of moisture present in the air. The air absorbs moisture by evaporation of water from the surface of the ocean and other surface collections of water. The amount of water vapour absorbed by air depends on its temperature. The higher the temperature, the greater is the amount of water vapour it can hold. When air at any given temperature can hold no more water vapour, it is called *saturated*.

Absolute humidity: It is the weight of water vapour present in a unit volume of air. It is expressed in kg, or gm per cubic metre of air, i.e. the weight of moisture contained in a known volume of moist air.

Relative humidity: It also measures water vapour but relative to the temperature of the air. It is the ratio expressed as percentage of water vapour actually present in the air at any given temperature, to the amount that would be present, when the air of same volume is saturated at the same temperature. Thus, if the maximum amount is taken as 100 and the atmosphere contains only half that amount of water vapour, we say that relative humidity is 50%. The greater the relative humidity, the nearer the air would be to saturation point.

Dew point: When warm, moist air is cooled to a point at which further cooling will cause condensation, the temperature is known as the dew point. It is the temperature at which air becomes saturated with moisture.

Hygrometers

The amount of moisture present in the air is measured by means of hygrometers and the branch of science that deals with the humidity of atmosphere, is known as hygrometry. These are of two types, i.e. direct and indirect hygrometers. The examples are as follows:

1. Direct:
   a. Daniell's hygrometer.
   b. Regnault's hygrometer.
   c. Dine's hygrometer.
2. Indirect:
   a. Dry and wet bulb hygrometer.

Dry and wet bulb hygrometer (psychrometer) (Fig. 8.8): In this type of hygrometer, two thermometers are mounted side by side on a stand. It is used to measure the pressure of aqueous vapour in the air. The dry bulb thermometer measures the temperature of the air. The bulb of the other thermometer is covered with a sleeve of muslin or candle-wick. The cloth is wetted and the water is then made to evaporate by blowing air over the cloth with a fan or by whirling the psychrometer in

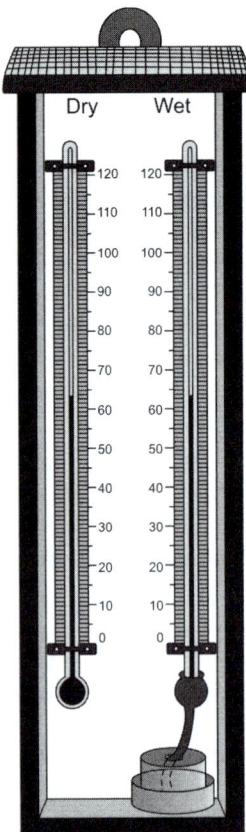

Fig. 8.8: Dry and wet bulb psychrometer

the air. This water, on evaporation, absorbs heat from the thermometer, with the result that the bulb is cooled and temperature indicated by this thermometer is much lower than that indicated by the dry one. In general, the drier the air, the greater is the drop in temperature. The relative humidity is determined by comparing the readings of the two thermometers with published psychrometric tables or charts. The difference in the two, however, depends on the rapidity with which the evaporation proceeds. Since the rate of evaporation depends upon the prevailing temperature and the amount of humidity present in the air; the evaporation will be rapid in case of dry air and the temperature of the wet bulb will be much below that of the dry one. This difference enables one, by means of tables, to obtain the percentage of humidity, the dew point and the vapour pressure of the air. The difference between the dry and wet bulb readings is known as depression of the wet bulb. The instrument should be kept in the shade and protected from air currents and direct sunshine. The dew point is roughly as much below the wet bulb reading as the wet bulb reading is below the dry bulb reading.

Example

Dry bulb reading = 82
Wet bulb reading = 75
Dew point = 75 – (82–75) = 68

Electrical hygrometers typically measure the electrical resistance of a substance, such as lithium chloride, whose resistance to an electric current varies with the humidity. In the dew point hygrometer, a smooth, shiny surface is cooled until water vapour in the air begins to condense on it. The humidity is determined by comparing the temperature at which the condensation occurs (the dew point) with the temperature of the air.

Chemical hygrometers use a substance such as phosphorus pentoxide to absorb moisture from a given volume of air. The difference in the weight of the substance before and after its exposure to the air indicates how much moisture is present.

Sling or whirling psychrometer: This instrument is used as a dew point measuring apparatus. Being of greater accuracy, it is used in preference to dry and wet bulb hygrometer. It consists of two thermometers, one of them being covered. Thermometers should be thoroughly saturated with distilled water. Both the thermometers are fixed in a metallic plate, which is whirled rapidly in the air for 15–20 seconds, stopped and reading of the wet bulb thermometer taken. It is repeated several times till two successive readings of wet bulb thermometer are almost the same. From the difference between the dry and wet bulb thermometer readings, one can calculate the dew point, percentage of humidity, vapour pressure of air, etc. by means of tables.

Kata thermometer: It is used to measure the cooling power of air at a given time and place.

8.8 WINDS

These are produced by the disturbance of equilibrium of two masses of air in a freely mobile atmosphere. The causes of these disturbances are the difference in atmospheric pressure brought about by changes in the temperature and moisture aided by physical and other factors of the two masses of air.

Weather cock or wind vane: It is an instrument by means of which the direction of wind is indicated. It consists of a balanced lever, turning on a vertical axis, the broad end of which is exposed to the prevailing current of wind while the narrower end points to the direction from which the wind may be blowing. It is fixed on the highest point of the building.

The wind vane is provided with an arrow, which turns freely about a vertical axis with the movement of air. If the arrow remains motionless continuously for 3 minutes, the wind is described as "calm". As a rough measure, wind direction can be also found out by letting off bits of paper or straw in the air, which would give the approximate direction of wind at that time.

Anemometer: The velocity of wind is recorded by this instrument. These are of several varieties. One

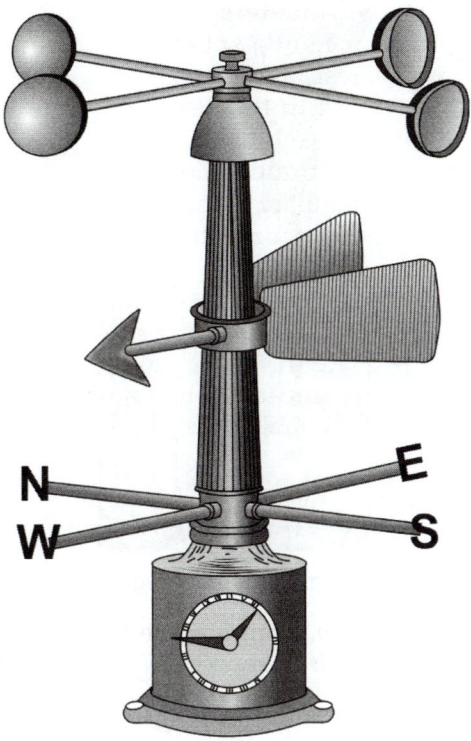

Fig. 8.9: Robinson's anemometer and wind vane

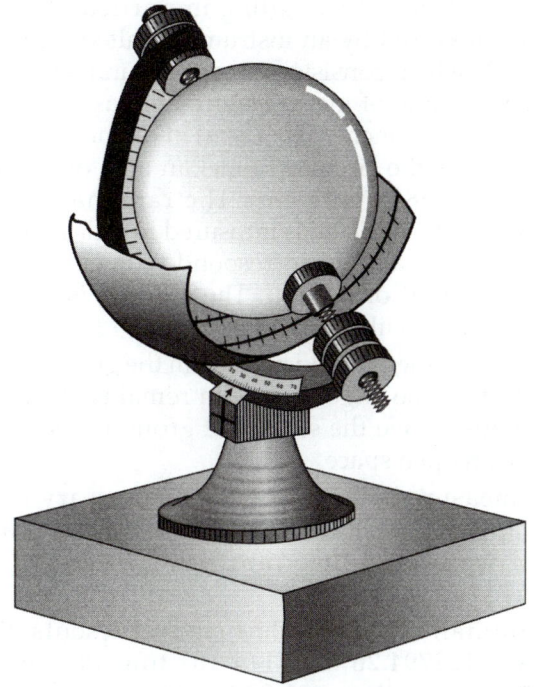

Fig. 8.10: Sunshine recorder

commonly used variety of anemometer is Robinson's wind anemometer (Fig. 8.9). It consists of four hollow hemispheric cups fixed at their ends and moving horizontally on a vertical axis, which by arragement of screws, records the movements on a dial. 500 of its revolutions make up a mile. The velocity can be deduced therefrom. This instrument should be kept clean and properly oiled. It should be fixed at least 20 ft. (6.09 metres) high from the ground. The average velocity of wind is from 6 to 8 miles (9.6 to 12.8 km) per hour.

Some other types of anemometers are

1. Non-mechanical anemometers
   a. Hot wire anemometers
   b. Ultrasonic anemometers
   c. Laser/Doppler anemometers
2. Propeller type anemometers
3. Turbulence measuring anemometers

Sunshine recorder (Fig. 8.10): The hours of bright sunshine are recorded by this instrument. Various types of sunshine recorders, *viz.* Campbell-Stoke, McLeod, Jordon, Isohel, etc. are available in the market. The standard type of sunshine recorder consists of a glass sphere on which the rays fall and the image is received (on a strip or a mill board) at the proper focal distance and makes a burnt track when the sun shines. The sunshine should be measured in hours and tenths of an hour and not in minutes.

8.9 CLOUDS

These consist of masses of vapours condensed into minute water particles which float in the air in the higher regions of atmosphere usually from 1–4 miles (1.6–6.43 km) above the surface of the earth.

A cloud line is the level below which the formation of clouds rarely takes place.

8.10 MIST

It signifies suspended liquid droplets generated by condensation from gaseous state or by breaking up a liquid into a dispersed state. Generally, it is spoken of as a cloud near the earth.

8.11 DEW

In this case, atmospheric moisture gets precipitated or condensed on the solid substances on the surface of the ground. The dew point denotes the temperature at which water vapour, already present in the air, is the maximum quantity the air can hold, or in other words, it is the temperature at which air becomes saturated with moisture.

8.12 FOG

It is a cloud resting on the earth and it is formed where surface of the ground is warmer than the air which is in contact with it. The hot air rises to be condensed into fog.

8.13 RAINFALL

Rain is the result of moisture condensing and coalescing to form drops of water and the rainfall includes all moisture falling in particulate drops. This is measured by an instrument called rain gauge (Fig. 8.11) which consists of a copper funnel leading to a receiver made of glass. The funnel has a sharp rim and is usually 8 inches (20.32 cm) in diameter.

This gives the circular funnel an area of 50 square inches (322.58 square cm). The rain, having been collected in the receiver, is measured in a glass cylinder, which is graduated to correspond with 1/100th of an inch (0.25 mm) of rainfall. The reading is generally taken at 9 AM daily.

The rain gauge should be fixed in the ground to such a depth that the edge of the rim remains at least 1 ft. (0.3 metre) above the surface of ground. It should be fixed in an open space.

To measure hail or snow, it is necessary to melt it by applying heat or by adding a known quantity of hot water and then measuring in an ordinary way.

A rainfall of 1 inch (2.54 cm) represents 22,617 gallons (102794.26 litres) or 101 tons of water per acre or 4.67 gallons (21.22 litres) per square yard

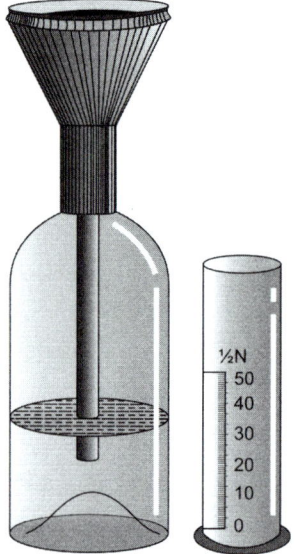

Fig. 8.11: Rain gauge

(0.84 square metre). Roughly one foot (0.3 metre) of snow may be taken to represent 1 inch (2.54 cm) of rainfall.

School Health

Schools lay a country's foundation for the future as what is learnt in this impressionable stage of life has a lasting impact on the entire lifespan of an individual. School is the first experience of group life, where the child meets children coming from different social strata of community, home environment and having different health and immunity status. Children are constantly undergoing changes—physical, mental, emotional and social. Not only ensuring that children stay healthy, school health services also focus on inculcation of healthy habits in children for preventive and promotive health in the future generations.

Historically, the objectives of school health service were:

1. To build schools on modern sanitary lines.
2. To appoint suitable medical inspectors or school medical officers.
3. To make provision of an adequate system of medical inspection of all children at least thrice during the school life or oftener to ascertain the health conditions of students and to detect the presence of contagious diseases and physical defects among them and suggest their remedies.
4. To establish school clinics.
5. To segregate cases of infectious diseases and establish centres for the prevention of spread of these diseases.
6. To provide nutrition, e.g. through mid-day meals.
7. To teach the practice of hygiene and healthy living to students both in school and at home.
8. Provision of special methods of education for children who happen to be disabled in body or in mind.

ASPECTS OF SCHOOL HEALTH SERVICE

9.1 HEALTHY ENVIRONMENT

For healthy schooling, it is important that the site, building, furniture, lighting and privy facilities in the schools are planned adequately.

i. **Site:** The school should be centrally situated, easily accessible to students and should be situated at a distance of at least 60 feet (18.28 meters) from the main street or road so as to eliminate the nuisance of noise, which distracts the attention of students and teachers. The site should be elevated, well drained and should not be overshadowed by tall buildings or trees. If possible, a field or a public park should adjoin it. As per the recommendations of School Health Committee (1961), land area of 10 acres for higher elementary school and 5 acres for primary schools must be provided with a provision of an extra acre per 100 students. A playground of 20 square ft (1.86 sq metres) per child should also be provided.

ii. **Building:** The nursery and secondary school buildings should be single storied as far as possible. The building should be of a pavilion type where the classrooms open into the verandah and the hall is separate so that it provides adequate ventilation, i.e. air and light to all the rooms of the building. The school premises should have a proper boundary wall and should be kept free from all hazards. Corridors should be 6–8 feet (1.83–2.44 metres) wide and the width of the staircase should be about 4 feet (1.22 metres) with a doorway opening outside, provided at the bottom of the staircase as it facilitates the escape of children in case of an outbreak of fire. There should be a separate staircase for each block and it should be protected on the open side by provision of a railing. As far as possible, winding staircase should be avoided. Moreover, fire drills should be installed at prominent places. All parts of the school building should be constructed fireproof, as far as possible. Moreover, it should be provided with a necessary pucca drain surrounding the plinth.

iii. **Space:** A minimum of 150 cubic feet (4.247 cubic metres) space per student is recommended. The floor space should be from 10–15 square feet (0.93–1.39 sq metres) per pupil so that 1500–1800 cubic feet (42.47–50.17 cubic metres) of fresh air per head is aimed at. The height of classrooms should not be less than 12 feet (3.65 metres). Classrooms should be on the sides, away from roads and should preferably face south or southeast for sunlight. Each room should be able to accommodate 25–40 children. Rooms should preferably be rectangular, the width being two-thirds of the length.

A clear space of not less than 7.5 feet extending the full width of the room should be left for the teacher. About one feet of open space should be left between the last row of desks and the wall and a gangway.

iv. **Floors:** Should be made of impermeable material with smooth surface to facilitate easy cleansing. The interior walls should be of white colour and should be whitewashed as and when required.

v. **Ventilation:** Proper ventilation diminishes the chances of infection, lessens fatigue and eyestrain. To ensure adequate ventilation, the windows should be broad with the bottom sill at 2.5 feet from the floor level. The combined area of the door and windows should be at least 25% and ventilators should be at least 2% of floor area Windows should be placed on the opposite sides of the room and possibly open to the external side.

vi. **Lighting:** Natural lighting should be provided to the classrooms preferably coming from the left side or from above.

The colour of the walls of the classroom must be white to brighten the classrooms. Extremely bright light should be avoided as it causes discomfort to eyes.

vii. **Temperature:** The classrooms must neither be too cold nor too hot.

viii. **Water supply:** There should be a provision for the continuous supply of safe and potable water through taps. A small reservoir with one tap for 100 students must be provided. The use of a common glass or a tumbler should be discouraged unless it can be properly cleaned, each time after use.

ix. **Sanitary facilities:** Provision should be made for privies and urinals. Urinals should be constructed of glazed porcelain and should be provided with automatic flushing arrangements. There should be provision for a separate washroom adjoining the bathroom so that the children may use it for cleansing their hands after a visit to the closet.

There should be a provision of at least 5 closets and an equal number of urinals for every 100 students. Arrangement should be seperately made for boys and girls.

x. **Canteen services:** Only licensed vendors who keep food articles clean and covered should be allowed in the school premises.

Mid-day meal scheme: Provision of school meals is important because of several reasons: (i) school age population is a vulnerable group; forms a considerable proportion of the total population and being a controlled community can easily be reached. (ii) The schoolchild often gets hungry in school because the child leaves home after a hurried meal and returns late in the afternoon. In rural areas, the child may have to walk several miles. Thus, school meal will not only correct the malnutrition due to poor diet at home, but would also combat his hunger in the school. (iii) Educational performance of the child would improve by improving nutrition, and (v) school meals provide opportunities for nutrition, education and food hygiene.

With a view to enhance enrollment, retention and attendance and simultaneously improving nutritional levels among children, the National Programme of Nutritional Support to Primary Education **(NP-NSPE)** was launched as a centrally sponsored scheme on **15th August 1995,** initially in 2408 blocks in the country which was later expanded to all blocks of the country. Initially, it was further extended in 2002 to cover not only children in classes I–V of government, government aided and local body schools, but also children studying in EGS and AIE centres. Central Assistance under the scheme consisted of free supply of food grains @ 100 grams per child per school day, and subsidy for transportation of food grains up to a maximum of ₹50 per quintal.

Later in September 2004, the scheme was revised to provide cooked mid-day meal with 300 calories and 8–12 grams of protein to all children studying in classes I–V in government and aided schools and EGS/AIE centres. In addition to free supply of food grains, the revised scheme provided Central Assistance for (a) cooking cost @ ₹1 per child per school day, (b) transport subsidy was raised from the earlier maximum of ₹50 per quintal to ₹100 per quintal for special category states, and ₹75 per quintal for other states, (c) management, monitoring and evaluation costs @ 2% of the cost of food grains, transport subsidy and cooking assistance, and (d) provision of mid-day meal during summer vacation in drought affected areas.

In 2006–07, the scheme was revised to cover children in upper primary classes (VI to VIII) provide assistance for cooking cost at the rate of (a) ₹1.80 per child/school day for states in the northeastern region, provided the NER states contribute Rs 0.20 per child/school day, (b) ₹1.50 per child/school day for other states and UTs, provided that these states and UTs contribute ₹0.50 per child/school day. The calorific value of a mid-day meal at upper primary stage has been fixed at a minimum of 700 calories and 20 grams of protein by providing 150 grams of food grains (rice/wheat) per child/school day. **From the year 2009 onwards,** food norms have been revised to ensure balanced and nutritious diet to children of upper primary group by increasing the quantity of pulses from 25 to 30 grams, vegetables from 65 to 75 grams and by decreasing the quantity of oil and fat from 10 grams to 7.5 grams. Cooking cost (excluding the labour and administrative charges) has been revised from ₹1.68 to Rs. 2.50 for primary and from ₹2.20 to ₹3.75 for upper primary children from 1.12.2009 to facilitate serving meal to eligible children in prescribed quantity and of good quality. The cooking cost for primary is ₹2.69 per child per day and ₹4.03 for upper primary children from 1.4.2010. The cooking cost will be revised prior approval of competent authority by 7.5% every financial year from 1.4.2011, and (c) the honorarium for cooks and helpers was paid from the labour and other administrative charges of ₹0.40 per child per day provided under the cooking cost. In many cases, the honorarium was so little that it became very difficult to engage manpower for cooking the meal. A separate component for payment of honorarium @ ₹1.68 per month per cook-cum-helper was introduced from 1.12.2009. Honorarium at the above prescribed rate is being paid to cook-cum-helper. However, in some of the states, the honorarium to cook-cum-helpers are being paid more than ₹1000/– through their state fund.

xi. **Furniture:** Adequate type of furniture should be provided to prevent the students from developing health problems like myopia due to excess stooping during their school life.

The most important items of furniture of the classroom are seats and desks. Ideally single seats are considered to be the best followed by the dual ones. In the former case, each child can be accommodated with the size that is more suitable for him. The Sheffield type of continuous desk with six separate seats is preferable to a long common seat and a desk.

Desks are classified into three varieties depending upon their relationship to the seats (Fig. 9.1):
1. *Zero desk:* When edge of the desk is vertically in line with the edge of seat.
2. *Minus desk:* When it overhangs it.
3. *Plus desk:* When there is a gap between the two.

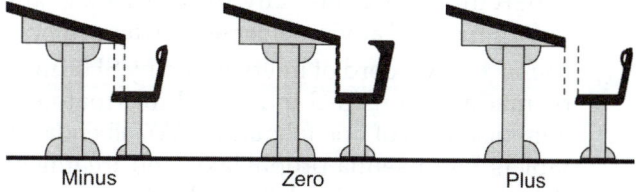

Minus   Zero   Plus
Fig. 9.1: Desks

Zero and minus desks are suitable for reading and writing.

The adjustment of seats and desks is important for prevention of eyestrain, fatigue and to eliminate the risk of developing any orthopaedic defects.

Blackboard and maps: Blackboards should have dull surface. The maps should not be glazed.

xii. **Cleaning of school:** All the school rooms should be cleaned and swept everyday after the day's work. The room and the floors scrupulously scrubbed and swept at least once a week after vacating the room. Every effort should be made to prevent a dusty atmosphere in the classrooms and toilets in the schools.

SCHOOL HEALTH

9.2 SCHOOL HEALTH SERVICE

School health service was started in India in 1909 and is regarded as one of the most important branches of preventive medicine. It provides an opportunity not only for early detection of the health problems in the child but also for health promotion, attitude building and interventions as early as possible. The role of school health services is thus to:

A. Carry out periodic health examinations/inspections of the schoolchildren with adequate intervention. Children detected with health problems require to be followed up.

i. *Health records:* All the findings are recorded on an index card and the records should be maintained. The index card should make a record of personal details (name, age, sex, class, address) of the student, nutritional status and anthropometric data (height, weight), personal habits and hygiene (cleanliness, clothing,) and history of any previous illness/treatment/vaccination.

ii. *Special examinations:* To detect health problems related to teeth, nose, throat (tonsils, adenoids, etc.) eyes, vision, ears, hearing, speech, mental and nervous conditions.

iii. *Screening for diseases or deformities:* All children must be routinely screened for health conditions of heart, lungs, spleen, liver, skin, anaemia, tuberculosis, rickets, any other disease and deformities and advised intervention accordingly.

iv. *Follow-up:* A record of intervention by SHC must be made with regard to referral for treatment, administration of iron folic acid (IFA)/albendazole tablets for anaemia prophylaxis and treatment; directions to parents in relation to diet, treatment, etc.

B. Ensure complete immunization of children for age. As per UIP:

i. *Diphtheria, pertussis and tetanus (DPT):* A booster dose of DPT is required at the age of 5 years, i.e. at the time of school entry if a child is previously covered by DPT along with oral polio vaccine (OPV).

ii. *Tetanus toxoid (TT):* Two doses of tetanus toxoid should be given at 10 and 16 years of age.

C. Health education and awareness: Children should be periodically educated about the importance of personal hygiene, menstrual hygiene, prevention of vector-borne and communicable infections, technique of handwashing, food hygiene and nutrition to build attitude and competencies for their future life.

D. Curative care in case of minor ailments and injuries that occur in school. Arrangement must also made for the follow up of all deviations detected.

School health services are delivered through the school health clinics (SHCs) by the medical officer with or without the help of a trained nurse or teacher from the school. The equipment required for SHCs include a weighing machine, height standards, a tape measure, Snellen's chart for vision testing; a tongue depressor and Holmgren's wool. SHCs also serve as a centre for the control of communicable diseases at the time of an outbreak.

The medical officer (MO) in SHCs should be able to perform following additional duties:

1. Inspect all school premises for healthful school environment with respect to lighting, ventilation, furniture and other sanitary installations and make recommendations accordingly.

2. Arrange a planned immunisation session against infectious diseases common in children and against other anticipated epidemic outbreaks in the area.

3. Investigate into the cases of outbreaks of infectious diseases in schools and take all necessary steps to control and prevent their spread.

4. Ensure periodic disinfection of all school buildings.

5. Train teachers regarding common ailments, defects of scholars through lectures and demonstrations, first aid and observation of hygiene among schoolchildren.

6. Vigilant check on the cleanliness/hygiene in the school canteen and mess and sanitary conditions of the attached hostels.

9.3 SCHOOL HEALTH PROGRAMME

School Health Programme has been launched by Government of India under the ambit of National Health Mission (NHM) and Reproductive, Maternal, Newborn, Child, and Adolescent Health (RMNCH + A) Programme with an aim to universalize the concept of preventive and promotive health, immunization, management of common childhood ailments, micro-nutrient supplementation with improved health awareness and health seeking behaviour. It focuses on effective integration of health concerns through decentralized management at district with determinant of health like sanitation, hygiene, nutrition, safe drinking water, gender and social concern.

This is in response to an increased need to ensure good current and future health, better educational outcomes and social equity. The programme addresses the physical and mental health needs of children along with nutrition interventions, yoga facilities and counselling.

At the national level, the programme provides uniformity/guidance to states that are already implementing or planning to implement their own versions of programme for a coherent strategy through a decentralized framework for implementation. Management structure for effective convergence has been provided for in the guidelines at national, state and district levels. The effective implementation requires an optimum convergence between the Ministry of Health and Family Welfare (MoHFW), Ministry of Human Resources Development (MHRD) and Ministry of Rural Development (MRD). MHRD takes care of capacity building, IEC, monitoring and evaluation. MRD takes care of water, safety education, sanitation education and garbage disposal waste management. The MoHFW is responsible for screening, health care services, immunization, referral, micronutrient management, health education, capacity building, monitoring, evaluation, etc.

Components of School Health Programme

1. Health service provision:

a. *Screening, health care and referral:* Screening general health, assessment of anaemia/nutritional status, visual acuity, hearing problems, dental check up, common skin conditions, heart defects, physical disabilities, learning disorders, behaviour problems, etc.

b. Basic medicine kit has been provided to take care of common ailments prevalent among young school going children.

c. Referral cards for priority services at district/subdistrict hospitals.

d. Immunisation as per national schedule using fixed day activity coupled with health education.

e. *Micronutrient (vitamin A and IFA) management*: Weekly supervised distribution of iron-folic acid tablets coupled with nutritional education. Deworming has to be done biannually under supervision after prior IEC (WIFS under RMNCH + A).

2. Health promotion: Through counselling services, regular practice of yoga, physical education, health education and training of peer leaders as health educators.

3. Adolescent health education: Educating the adolescents for personal hygiene, nutrition, health seeking, life skills along with counselling for their health problems.

4. Nutrition supplementation (mid-day meal scheme).

For implementation, it is proposed that ANM may be spared once a week for school health only if she has either MPW (male) or second ANM to support her at the health subcentre. The multi-purpose worker (male) will be more appropriate for exclusive boys' senior basic schools. If the ANM is not available, the teachers are being trained for screening and counselling the children, and then area ANMs/MPWs will visit one school every week on an average for detailed screening and treatment of minor ailment and required referral. In addition, a medical officer will also visit one school per week for additional screening, treatment and referral.

Further to ensure the effective implementation of the programme, functionaries from various related departments/organisations, such as education, rural development, WCD, NACO, etc. have also been involved. School health coordinator has been hired on contract basis at the state and district level for coordination and monitoring and evaluation.

9.4 SPECIAL SCHOOLS

Special schools for differently abled children (mentally challanged, blind, the deaf and the dumb).

9.5 CHILD GUIDANCE CLINICS

These have been established in many of the large towns, for dealing with children suffering from lesser degree of mental defects, which often comes to the notice on account of behaviour difficulties rather than mental dullness, such as aggressiveness, cruelty, delinquency or nervous manifestations of some kind. The typical child guidance clinic is run on a team basis with:

1. The child psychiatrist

2. The educational psychologist

3. Psychiatric social worker

4. Psychotherapist.

In many cases, a little advice to the parents suffices, in others simple therapeutic measures with some play therapy may be necessary. In the more severe cases, however, the child may be required to leave his home and is then sent to a boarding school or a hostel to attend a different school, where more emphasis is laid on play therapy, easing of mental tension, fear psychosis and re-construction of self-confidence, etc.

10

Maternity and Child Welfare

The National Health Policy (NHP) 2002 aims to provide prophylactic and curative health care services towards building a healthy nation by achieving an acceptable standard of good health amongst the general population of the country. The efforts are directed towards increasing access to the decentralized public health system by upgrading existing infrastructure and establishing new infrastructure in deficient areas.

Despite substantial progress made on many fronts, maternal and infant mortality still remain unacceptably high in several parts of the country. Thus promotion of maternal and child health has been one of the most important objectives of the National Health Mission in India.

10.1 MATERNAL HEALTH

10.1.1 Maternal Mortality Ratio (MMR)

MMR is defined as the number of maternal deaths per 100,000 live births due to causes related to pregnancy or within 42 days of termination of pregnancy, regardless of the site or duration of pregnancy.

10.1.2 MMR Current Status (India)

The national average of MMR is 178 per 100,000 live births (SRS-2013) with highest in Assam (328) and lowest in Kerala (66). Even in the best performing states, the ratio is very high compared to other countries like Sweden (5), USA (24), Brazil (58), Sri Lanka (39) and Thailand (48).

10.1.3 Causes of Maternal Mortality

The major causes of maternal mortality have been identified as haemorrhage (both ante- and post-partum), toxemia (hypertension during pregnancy), anaemia, obstructed labour, puerperal sepsis (infections after delivery) and unsafe abortion. Haemorrhage accounts for more than one-third of all deaths followed by puerperal sepsis and abortion. Anaemia which has

been included in "other conditions" is a major contributory factor. Most of these deaths are preventable with good antenatal care, timely identification and referral of pregnant women with complications of pregnancy and timely provision of emergency obstetric care. Moreover, social factors like illiteracy, low socioeconomic conditions and poor access to health facilities are also contributing factors leading to higher maternal mortality.

10.1.4 Maternal Health Indicators

MMR can only be used as a rough indicator of the maternal health situation in any given country. Hence, other indicators of maternal health status are:

i. Antenatal check-up
ii. Institutional delivery
iii. Delivery by trained personnel, etc.

These indicators also reflect the status of the ongoing programme interventions as well as give a reflection on the situation of maternal health.

10.1.5 Strategies and Interventions to Reduce Maternal Mortality

Government is taking several initiatives under National Health Mission to achieve the goal of reduction in maternal mortality. Some of them are as follows:

a. **Essential obstetric care:** Includes quality antenatal care including prevention and treatment of anaemia, institutional/safe delivery services and postnatal care. To provide essential obstetric care services Government of India is operationalizing the PHCs for 24 × 7 services and also training the staff nurses (SNs)/lady health visitors (LHVs)/auxiliary nurse midwives (ANMs) in skilled attendance at birth.

b. **Quality antenatal care:** A minimum of at least 4 ANCs including early registration and 1st ANC in first trimester along with physical and abdominal examinations, haemoglobin estimation and urine investigation, 2 doses of tetanus toxoid, immunization and ANC in 2nd trimester include consumption of iron folic acid (IFA) and calcium tablets.

c. **Prophylaxis and treatment of nutritional anaemia:** About 55% of women aged 15–49 years are anaemic in the country, 59% during pregnancy and 63.2% lactating. Under the NHM, the current policy is to give one tablet of iron folic acid (IFA) with 100 mg of elemental iron and 0.5 mg of folic acid after first trimester of pregnancy uptil 6 months after the delivery. The dose is doubled, if the women is already anaemic.

d. **Provision of 24 hrs delivery services at PHC:** Under RMNCH + A, all the CHCs and 50% of the PHCs are being operationalized for providing round the clock delivery services by placing at least 3–5 staff nurses and 1 medical officer in these facilities.

e. **Skilled attendance at birth:** Staff nurses/ANMs/LHVs are trained in skilled attendance at birth for a period of 3 weeks.

f. **Provision of emergency obstetric and neonatal care at first referral units (FRUs):** Provision of emergency obstetric and neonatal care at FRUs at the subdistrict, CHC level is being done by operationalizing the critical components such as manpower, blood storage units and referral linkages, etc. MBBS doctors are being trained in life-saving anaesthetic skills, obstetric management and skills including cesarean section for emergency obstetric care. Since emergencies during the process of birth cannot be predicted, it is essential to place effective referral linkages for easy access by pregnant women.

g. **Postnatal care for mother and newborn:** Ensuring postnatal care within first 24 hours of delivery and subsequent home visits on 3rd, 7th and 42nd day by trained ANMs, LHVs and staff nurses for identification and management of emergencies occurring during postnatal period.

h. **Other important interventions:** These are safe abortion services/medical termination of pregnancy, RTI/STI services and setting up of blood storage units at FRUs. Village health and nutrition day (VHND) is organized at the anganwadi centre at least once every month to provide antenatal/postpartum care for pregnant women. Promotion of institutional delivery, immunization, family planning and nutrition are the other various services being provided during VHNDs.

i. **Janani Suraksha Yojana (JSY):** It is a safe motherhood intervention under National Health Mission (NHM) being implemented with the objective of promoting institutional delivery among the poor pregnant women. In low performing states, i.e. states with high maternal mortality and low rate of institutional delivery, all women delivering in government health institutions or accredited private institutions are eligible to receive the cash assistance of 1400 in rural areas and 1000 in urban areas. In high performing states, only BPL pregnant women, aged 19 years and above and the SC and ST pregnant women are eligible to receive the cash assistance of 700 and 600 in the rural and urban areas respectively under the Yojana. The Yojana subsidizes the cost of caesarean section or for the management of obstetric complications up to ₹1500/– per delivery to the government institutions, where government specialists are not in position.

In low performing states (LPS), Accredited Social Health Activist (ASHA) gets ₹600 and 200 in rural and urban areas respectively. Whereas in HPS, cash assistance for ASHA in tribal areas and NE states is ₹600/– in the rural areas and 200 in the urban areas.

Cash assistance for referral transport is over and above the mother's package. The amount is to be decided by individual states keeping in view the terrain and distances to be travelled, subject to a minimum of ₹250. ASHA will get the cash benefit only if she accompanies the pregnant woman to the health centre.

10.2 CHILD HEALTH

Child health comprises morbidity and mortality in children less than 5 years of age. Nearly 27 million infants are born every year, of whom 0.9 million die before completing the first 4 weeks of life. About two-thirds of infant deaths occur in the first month of life. Of these who die in the first month, about two-thirds die in the first week of life and of these two-thirds die in the first 24 hours of life.

The common causes of ill health and deaths among children in India are malnutrition, diarrhoea, diphtheria, whooping cough, etc. On analysis, it has been established that out of 10 deaths among children under 10 years of age, at least 8 are attributable to preventable diseases.

10.2.1 Infant Mortality Rate (IMR)

It is the number of infant deaths in a year under one year of age per 1,000 live births. As per the Sample Registration Survey (SRS) data, September 2014, the IMR is 40 per 1000 live births; with 44 in rural areas and 27 in urban areas. Neonatal mortality rate (NNMR) refers to the number of deaths of children during the period of 0–28 days per thousand live births. NMR stands 29 per 1000 live births in India in 2012. Neonatal mortality thus contributes 56% of all deaths in childhood (up to age 5 years).

10.2.2 Causes of Infant Mortality

a. The primary causes of neonatal deaths are sepsis, low birth weight and asphyxia, whereas for the child deaths are pneumonia, diarrhoea and malaria, meningitis and measles in some states. The maternal causes of infant mortality are toxemia of pregnancy, eclampsia, etc.

b. *Social causes:* Poverty, defective sanitation, bad housing, atmospheric pollution, overcrowding, improper feeding, untrained midwives, ignorance of mothers, etc.

10.2.3 Initiatives for Newborn and Child Health

The reproductive, maternal, newborn, child and adolescent health (RMNCH + A) programme under the National Health Mission (NHM) comprehensively integrates interventions that improve child health and addresses factors contributing to infant and under-five mortality. Reduction of infant and child mortality has been an important tenet of the health policy of the Government of India and it has tried to address the issue right from the early stages of planned development. The National Population Policy (NPP) 2000, the National Health Policy 2002 and the Eleventh Five Year Plan (2007–12) and National Rural Health Mission (NRHM 2005–2012) have laid down the goals for child health.

Key Strategies under RMNCH + A for Newborn and Child Health

1. Increase coverage of skilled care at birth for newborns in conjunction with maternal care.

2. Implement a newborn and child health package of preventive, promotive and curative interventions using a comprehensive IMNCI approach.

3. Strengthen and augment existing services (care at birth/essential newborn care, ARI and diarrhoea control) in areas where IMNCI is yet to be implemented.

4. Implement the multiyear strategic plan for the UIP (Universal Immunization Programme).

5. **Navjaat Shishu Suraksha Karyakram/Basic newborn care and resuscitation:** Basic newborn care and resuscitation, has been launched to address care at birth, i.e. prevention of hypothermia, prevention of infection, early initiation of breast-feeding and basic newborn resuscitation. The objective of this new initiative is to have one person trained in basic newborn care and resuscitation at every delivery.

6. **IMNCI and pre-service IMNCI—facility-based integrated management of neonatal and childhood illnesses (F-IMNCI):** F-IMNCI is the integration of the facility based care package with the IMNCI package, to empower the health personnel with the skills to manage newborn and childhood illness at the community level as well as at the facility. Facility-based IMNCI focuses on providing appropriate skills for inpatient management of major causes of neonatal and childhood mortality such as asphyxia, sepsis, low birth weight and pneumonia, diarrhoea, malaria, meningitis, severe malnutrition in children. This training is being imparted to medical officers, staff nurses and ANMs at CHC/FRUs and 24 × 7 PHCs where deliveries are taking place.

Pre-service IMNCI has been included in the curriculum of medical and nursing colleges of the country. This will help in providing the much required trained (IMNCI) manpower in the public and the private sector.

7. **Early detection and appropriate management of acute respiratory infections, diarrhoea and other infections:** The Government of India in order to control diarrhoeal diseases has introduced the low osmolarity oral rehydration solution (ORS). Addition of zinc has been approved as an adjunct to ORS to reduce the number, severity of episodes and duration of diarrhoea.

Acute respiratory infections (ARI) form 19% of all under-five mortalities in India. Early diagnosis and appropriate case management by rational use of antibiotics remains one of the most effective interventions to prevent deaths due to pneumonia.

8. **Home-based care of newborns and infant and young child feeding (IYCF):** Provision of home-based newborn care has presented valuable opportunity for community health workers to reach out to mothers and newborns at home during the first 6 weeks of life. Village Health and Nutrition Day (VHND), outreach sessions for routine immunisation, management of newborn and childhood illnesses at community level are all entry points for IYCF information and counselling.

9. **Vitamin A and iron and folic acid supplementation:** With the objective of decreasing the prevalence of vitamin A deficiency to levels below 0.5%, 1,00,000 IU dose of vitamin A is being given at nine months followed by 2,00,000 IU (after 9 months) at six monthly intervals up to the age of five years. All cases of severe malnutrition to be given one additional dose of vitamin A.

To manage the widespread prevalence of anaemia in the country, infants from the age of 6 months onwards up to the age of five years shall receive iron supplements in liquid formulation in doses of 20 mg elemental iron and 100 μg folic acid per day per child for 100 days in a year. Children 6–10 years of age shall receive iron in the dosage of 30 mg elemental iron and 250 μg folic acid for 100 days in a year and children more than 10 years will receive the adult doses.

11. **Management of children with malnutrition:** Severe acute malnutrition is an important contributing factor for most deaths amongst children suffering from common childhood illness, such as diarrhoea and pneumonia. Nutritional Rehabilitation Centres (NRCs) are being set up in the health facilities for inpatient management of severely malnourished children, with counselling of mothers for proper feeding and once they are on the road to recovery, they are sent back home with regular follow-up.

12. School Health Programme (discussed in detail in Chapter 9).

13. Implement the multiyear strategic plan for the Universal Immunization Programme (UIP). Under the Universal Immunization Programme, Government of India is providing vaccination to prevent seven vaccine preventable diseases, i.e. diphtheria, pertussis, tetanus, polio, measles, severe form of childhood tuberculosis and hepatitis B. In addition, vaccination to prevent Hib infection is provided in selected states and vaccination to Japanese encephalitis provided in selected districts (Table 10.1).

Government of India declared 2012 as *Year of Intensification of Routine Immunization (IRI)*.

JE Vaccination

- 113 JE endemic districts have completed the JE mass vaccination and are implementing JE under routine vaccination. 2nd dose of JE is also introduced in RI in JE endemic states since April, 2013.
- National Vector-borne Disease Control Programme (NVDCP) division has identified 62 new JE endemic districts. JE campaign in these new districts targeting children between 1 and 15 years of age is planned in a phased manner.
- A total of 101.16 lakh children have been vaccinated during the campaigns in 2012–13 for 17 districts.
- JE mass vaccination planned for year 2013–14 in following states:
  - 14 districts in Bihar
  - 2 districts in Karnataka
  - 2 districts in Tamil Nadu
  - 1 district in West Bengal

JE vaccination is provided as part of routine immunization programme in 113 districts in 15 states.

Measles Supplementary Immunization Activity (SIA)

- Based on National Technical Advisory Group on Immunization (NTAGI) recommendation, Govt. of India introduced 2nd dose of measles under the Universal Immunization Programme (UIP) in 2010 through a two-pronged strategy.

- 21 states with measles 1st dose coverage of >80% introduced 2nd dose directly in their routine immunization.

- 14 states with <80% measles 1st dose coverage have targeted all children between 9 months–10 years age for measles vaccination followed by introduction of 2nd dose under routine immunization after an interval of 6 months.

- Measles vaccination campaigns conducted in all districts of 14 states in a phased manner (Phase I: 2010–11, phase II: 2011–12 and phase III: 2012–13).

- All states have completed measles SIA in all districts (urban areas of Indore and Bhopal are undergoing measles SIA).

Year	Target district	Districts completed	Total target children (lakh)	Achieve-ment (lakh)	% Achieve-ment
2010–11	45	45	138.46	120.77	87.2
2011–12	152	152	401.67	361.02	89.9
2012–13	169	169	854.86	700.10	82
Total	366	1394.99	1181.89	84.7	

- The 66th SEAR regional committee has passed a resolution on 13th sept 2013 to eliminate measles in the 11 SEAR countries including India, by 2020.
- Laboratory supported measles surveillance is enhanced to 15 states.

Polio Eradication Programme in India

- There is a remarkable achievement, particularly considering the fact that in 2009, India accounted for nearly half of the total number of polio cases globally and there were an estimated 2 lakh cases of polio every year in the country in the year 1978.
- *On 25 February 2012, World Health Organization (WHO) removed India from the global list of polio endemic countries.* As on date no wild polio virus cases has been reported in the country after January 2011.

This success can be attributed to the concerted efforts made toward improving both quality and coverage of pulse polio rounds as under:

- **Political commitment** of the highest order Hon'ble President of India inaugurates the national pulse polio round every year and the Union Health Minister provides continuous leadership. 24 lakh volunteers participate in the campaign and 1.5 lakh supervisors monitor activity. More than 17.2 crore children are targeted for vaccination in the national pulse polio round in one go.

- **Assured financial resources** Strong commitment to eradicate polio translated into assured allocation of financial resources. Government of India has not allowed the programme to suffer for want of financial resources.

- **Continuous innovation** India took a lead in introducing bivalent polio vaccine in January 2010. Earlier, it had similarly introduced monovalent oral polio vaccine-1 (mOPV-1) in 2005.

- **Quality of pulse polio rounds** has dramatically improved and the coverage of children has been 99%. This level of coverage is unprecedented and is not witnessed elsewhere in the world.

- **A highly innovative communication strategy** to dispel fears, overcome resistance and refusal and elicit community participation with active involvement of religious leaders, opinion makers and civil society implemented vigorously.

- **Effective partnership** between Government of India, WHO, UNICEF and State Governments, progressively strengthened have been a hallmark of Pulse Polio Programme.

- Mobile and migrant populations were specifically targeted to reach every child.

- India is mindful of the risks that persist, both on account of indigenous transmission and importation. An emergency preparedness and response plan (EPRP) has been put in place under which rapid response teams (RRT) are being setup in very state to identify high risk pockets for timely action.

- **International border vaccination** is being provided round the clock. These are provided through special booths set up at the international borders that India shares with Pakistan, Bangladesh, Nepal and Myanmar.

Current Risks and Challenges to Polio Eradication in India

- **Importation:** Risk of importation of virus from the neighboring countries.

- **Surveillance gaps:** If not maintained and sustained.

- **Population immunity:** The population immunity needs to be maintained in order to mitigate the risk of importation. To maintain the population immunity, high quality of polio campaigns are carried out.

10.3 NEWER INITIATIVES

a. **Introduction of second dose of measles:** States/UTs with >80% measles coverage have introduced 2nd dose of measles in their routine immunization programme. States/UTs with <80% coverage (14 states) are first covering all children between 9 months and 10 years of age through a measles supplementary immunization activity (SIA) in a phase-wise manner followed by introduction of 2nd dose under their routine immunization programme.

Table 10.1: Immunization schedule

S. no.		Vaccine of doses	Protection number	Vaccination schedule
1.	BCG (bacille Calmette-Guérin)	Tuberculosis	1	At birth (up to 1 year, if not given earlier)
2.	OPV (oral polio vaccine)	Polio	5	Birth dose of institutional deliveries within 15 days, primary three doses at 6, 10 and 14 weeks and one booster dose at 16–24 months of age given orally
3.	Hepatitis B	Hepatitis	4	Birth dose for institutional deliveries within 24 hours, primary three doses at 6, 10, 14 weeks
4.	DPT (diphtheria, pertussis and tetanus toxoids)	Diphtheria, pertussis and tetanus	5	Primary three doses at 6, 10, 14 weeks, one booster dose at 16–24 months of age and 2nd booster dose at 5 years of age
5.	Measles	Measles	2	9–12 months of age and 2nd dose at 16–24 months
6.	TT (tetanus toxoid)	Tetanus	2	**Children:** 10 years and 16 years of age
			2	**Pregnant woman:** Two doses given (one dose, if previously vaccinated within 3 years)
7.	JE vaccination (in selected 113 JE endemic districts in 15 states)	Japanese encephalitis (brain disease)	2	1st dose at 9–12 months of age and 2nd dose 16–24 months of age in JE endemic districts after 6 months of campaign
8.	Hib containing pentavalent vaccine (Hib + DPT + Hep B)	Diphtheria, pertussis, tetanus, hepatitis B and *Haemophilus influenzae* type B associated pneumonia meningitis		3 doses at 6, 10 and 14 weeks of age

b. Mother and child tracking system (MCTS): A name-based mother and child tracking system has been put in place which is web-based to ensure registration and tracking of all pregnant women and newborn babies so that provision of regular and complete services to them can be ensured.

c. Janani Shishu Suraksha Karyakram (JSSK): It has been launched with an aim to promote institutional delivery, eliminate out of pocket expenses which act as a barrier to seeking institutional care for mothers and sick newborns and facilitate prompt referral through free transport.

10.4 MILLENNIUM DEVELOPMENT GOALS

A meeting of representatives of 189 countries took place at the Millennium Summit in September 2000, committing their nations to a new global partnership to reduce extreme poverty and setting out a series of time-bound targets, with a deadline of 2015 that have become known as the Millennium Development Goals (MDGs).

There are eight goals under MDGs, where Goal 4 is dedicated to reduce child mortality and Goal 5 is to improve maternal health.

Goal 4: Reduce Child Mortality

Target 4: Reduce by two-thirds the mortality rate among children under-five between 1990 and 2015.

Under the MDG Goal 4, following indicators have been fixed for improving child health:

a. Under-five mortality rate
b. Infant mortality rate
c. Proportion of 1-year-old children immunised against measles.

Other than U5MR, it is important to monitor other key child health indicators like **breastfeeding, exclusive breastfeeding, complementary feeding, anaemia, diarrhoea, underweight, etc.**

10.5 INTEGRATED CHILD DEVELOPMENT SERVICES SCHEME

In persuance of the National Policy for Children, the Government of India in 1975 launched a scheme called Integrated Child Development Services (ICDS) Scheme which aimed at the delivery of a package of services, viz. immunization, periodic health check-ups, supplementary nutrition, health and nutrition education, referral services, etc. in an integrated manner to pre-school children, expectant and nursing mothers and women in the age group of 15–45 years.

The principal worker in the project is the *Anganwadi worker*. In one ICDS project, there are about 100 Anganwadi workers, who provide various basic health services to the mothers and children. They work under the charge of a Child Development Project Officer (CDPO).

Chapter 11

Demography and Family Planning

Demography is the science of composition and distribution of human population and changes in its size and composition over different time periods. Population dynamics can be examined by investigating three main demographic processes: Birth, migration, and ageing (including death) since these three processes contribute to changes in populations, including how people inhabit the earth, form nations and societies, and develop culture.

Demography identifies changes within the population such as, growth of population, mortality and morbidity rates, migration and also marriage. These analyses of these changes can help governments in planning, state and local policy evaluations and to address potential property tax revenue impacts.

11.1 SITUATION IN INDIA

With only 2.4% of world's land mass, India has 17.5% of the world's population. As per census 2011, India's population is **1.21 billion.** India is the second most populous country in the world, being next to China only. The trend in India's growth rate during the present century is given below:

Census year	Total population (in millions)	Average annual growth rate after 1901 (in %)
1901	238.1	–
1911	252.1	0.56
1921	251.4	(–)0.03
1931	279.0	1.04
1941	317.0	1.30
1951	361.1	1.20
1961	439.2	2.00
1971	548.0	2.2
1981	685.0*	2.23*
1991	843.4**	2.11**
2001	1027	1.95

*It does not include the population of Assam, since it could not be recorded due to prevailing disturbed conditions.
**It does not include the population of Jammu and Kashmir due to similar reason.

It is expected that population of India would reach up to 950 million by the turn of this century. It is estimated that 55,000 babies are born in India every day. There are 21 million births and about 8 million deaths in India every year, i.e. about 13 million increase in population every year. The birth rate as per 2011 census is 20.97 and death rate is 7.48 per thousand population. Growth rate in the country is 1.35%. The population of women in reproductive age period (15 to 44 years) is nearly 20–22%.

As per census 2011, the total population of India at 0.00 hours of 1st March 2011 was counted to be 1210.6 million, with 833.5 million (68.8%) rural and 377.1 million (31.2%) urban population. The growth rate in last decade was recorded to be 17.7% with a population density of 382 persons per square km. Number of females per 1000 males (sex ratio) in the country which was 933 in 2001 has increased by 10 points to 943 in 2011. In rural areas, the sex ratio has increased from 946 to 949. The corresponding increase in urban areas has been of 29 points from 900 to 929.

- Child sex ratio under 6 years for females in 919 per 1000 males.
- Literacy rate of India has gone up to 73% from previous figure of 64.83%

The population of India is expected to increase from 1029 to 1400 million during the period 2001–2026—an increase of 36% in 25 years at the rate of 1.2% annually. As a consequence, the density of population will increase from 313 to 426 persons per square kilometer.

The major causes of high population growth are

i. Large size of population in the reproductive age group (estimated contribution 58%).
ii. Higher fertility due to unmet needs of contraception (estimated contribution 20%).
iii. High desire for fertility due to high infant mortality rate (estimated contribution 20%).

116

iv. Approximately 50% of the girls marry below the age of 18 years, resulting in a typical reproductive pattern of "too early, too frequent, too many".

v. Preference for male child.

vi. More children are preferred by poor parents as more workforce.

11.2 NATIONAL POPULATION POLICY 2000

Before the National Population Policy 2000, the *crude birth rate and crude death rates were 26.4 and 9, respectively in 1998 as per SRS data*. The *infant mortality rate* was 72 per 1000 live births (1998, SRS) with a life expectancy to 62 years. Total fertility rate as per 1997 SRS data was reported to be 3.3 with approximately couple protection rate (CPR) as 40% with nearly *universal awareness* of the need for and methods of family planning.

National Population Policy came into being in 2000 with immediate objectives to address the unmet needs for contraception, health care infrastructure and health personnel and to provide integrated service delivery for basic reproductive and child health care.

The medium term objective of NPP 2000 was to bring the TFR to replacement level by 2010 through vigorous implementation of intersectoral operational strategies and on long-term to achieve a stable population by 2045 at a level consistent with requirement of sustainable economic growth, social development and environmental protection.

National sociodemographic goals proposed to be achieved by 2010 were:

i. Address the unmet needs for basic RCH services, supplies and infrastructure.

ii. Make school education up to age 14 years free and compulsory, and reduce drop out rate from primary and secondary school levels to below 20% for both boys and girls.

iii. Reduce infant mortality rate (IMR) to 30/1000 live births and maternal mortality ratio (MMR) to less than 100 per 1000 live births.

iv. Achieve universal immunization of children against all vaccine preventable diseases (VPDs).

v. Promote delayed marriage for girls, at age not less than 18, and preferable after 20 years.

vi. Achieve 80% institutional delivery and 100% by trained personnels.

vii. Achieve universal access to information/counseling services for fertility regulation and contraceptive with wide basket of choices.

viii. Achieve 100% registration of births, deaths, marriage, and pregnancy.

ix. Promote small family norm to achieve replacement level of total fertility rate 2.1.

x. Bring about convergence in implementation of related social sector programmes so that family welfare becomes people-centered programme.

Targets set by NPP 2000 and current status targets under various plans.

The methodwise mode of action, advantages, disadvantages, effectiveness, reasons for failure, side effects and extent of use of various contraceptives are tabulated in Table 11.1.

11.3 SOURCES OF DATA COLLECTION

The important sources of vital statistics in India are:

1. **Population census:** A population census is a total process of collecting, compiling, evaluating, analyzing and publishing or otherwise disseminating social, economic and demographic data pertaining to all persons in a country at a specified time. It is done every 10 years following a defacto canvasser method. It provides valuable information for planning and formulation of policies by the government.

2. **Civil registration system:** The continuous permanent and compulsory recording of the occurrence of vital events, like live births, deaths, foetal deaths, marriages, divorces as well as annulments, judicial separation, adoptions, legitimations and recognitions. Registration of Births and Deaths Act (1969) was enacted by Parliament to enforce uniform civil registration throughout the country under which all births and deaths have to be registered within 21 days of the event.

3. **Demographic sample surveys such as those conducted by the National Sample Surveys Organization (NSSO):** Data on fertility and mortality from the census are not very reliable and they are also available only once in 10 years.

4. **Sample registration system (SRS):** In the late 1960s, sample registration system was initiated based on a dual recording system. Under this, there is a continuous enumeration of births and deaths in a sample of villages/urban blocks by a resident part-time enumerator and then, an independent six monthly retrospective survey by a full time supervisor. The data obtained through these two sources are matched. The unmatched and partially matched events are re-verified in the field to get the correct number of events. At present, the sample registration system (SRS) provides reliable annual data on fertility and mortality at the state and national levels for rural and urban areas separately. In this survey, the sample units, villages in rural areas and urban blocks in urban areas are replaced once in 10 years.

5. **Health surveys:** Such as National Family Health Surveys (NFHS) and District Level Household Surveys (DLHS-RCH) conducted for assessing progress under the Reproductive and Child Health Programme. Three rounds of DLHS and four rounds of NFHS have been conducted.

Table 11.1: Currently available contraceptive methods

S. no.	Method	Mode of action	Advantages	Disadvantages	Effectiveness	Reasons for failure	Side effects	Extent of use
1.	Coitus interruptus or withdrawal method	Prevents in the deposition of semen inside the female genital tract	i. No supplies ii. No particular preparation iii. No cost	i. Makes great demand on the self-control of the male. Some men are physically or emotionally unable to use it ii. The female partner may not reach orgasm prior to withdrawal	Failure rate is high. It may vary from 10–20%. More effective if combined with another method	i. Escape of semen prior to ejaculation ii. Delayed withdrawal iii. Deposition of semen on the women's external sexual organs may result in pregnancy	A wide variety of gynaecological, urological, neurological and psychiatric ills have been attributed to it but the cause and effect of relationship has never been demonstrated	Generally its use is inversely associated with socioeconomic status. It is quite a popular method
2.	Rhythm method or the safe period method	It is based on the avoidance of coitus on the days it could result in pregnancy by the simultaneous presence of a fertilisable ovum and motile spermatozoa	i. No supplies ii. No particular preparation iii. No cost iv. Only method sanctioned by the Roman Catholic Church	i. Unsuitable for women with grossly irregular menstrual cycles ii. Opportunities for coitus greatly reduced especially if cycle is not regular iii. This method is not applicable during post-natal period	Self-taught rhythm haphazardly practised, is very ineffective. If correctly practised it may be quite effective. More effective when combined with another method. Failure rate may be as high as up to 20%	i. Errors in recording menstrual history and recording temperature ii. Errors in computation of the period of ovulation iii. Taking a chance on an unsafe day iv. Exceptionally long survival of the sperms in the female genital tracts	None	Commonly used by Roman Catholics
3.	Condom (Nirodh)	Serves as a cover for the penis during intercourse and prevents deposition of semen in the vagina	i. Protects against venereal diseases (VD) ii. Presence of intact condom after intercourse adds assurance iii. No medical check up required iv. No side effects	i. Some men and women feel it as an obstacle to sexual sensations and pleasure	It is effective (effectiveness depends on the quality of the rubber sheath and use) failure rate 2–14%	i. It may tear or slip off during coitus ii. Escape of semen at open end of the condom if withdrawal is delayed until after detumescene	Extremely rare; an occasional individual may be sensitive to the rubber or to the lubricant used in the condom	Widely used
4.	Vaginal diaphragm	Acts as a mechanical barrier to the entry of jelly	i. Reliable ii. Virtually without side effects	i. Must be fitted and so requires pelvic examination by a physician	Offers a high level of protection if used consistently	i. Incorrect insertion so that it fails to cover the cervix ii. Displacement during the contractions of the upper half of the vaginal vault during orgasm	Rare reactions to rubber or jelly	Usage is more among the middle class women
5.	Spermicidal jelly	Immobilises sperms on contact	i. Simple to use ii. Does not require any pelvic examination	Some users complain of leakage causing messiness and excessive lubrication	Less effective when used alone. More effective with the vaginal diaphragm	Inadequate quantity or quality	Irritation and/or inflammation of the mucous membrane in rare cases	Quite popular

(Contd...)

Table 11.1: Currently available contraceptive methods *(Contd...)*

S. no.	Method	Mode of action	Advantages	Disadvantages	Effectiveness	Reasons for failure	Side effects	Extent of use
6.	Foam tablets	i. Prevents entry of sperms into the cervical canal by mechanical action of foam ii. Immobilises sperms on contact (spermicidal action)	They are clear, harmless and safe	i. Requires waiting time for a few minutes ii. Local irritation	Failure rate up to 20%	i. Failure to observe waiting time ii. Spoilage due to hygrosopic character of the foam tablets iii. Tablets may not dissolve properly if vagina is dry	Local irritation or burning sensation	Quite popular
7.	Intrauterine contraceptive devices (IUCDs)	Interference with movement of sperms through uterus and fallopian tubes or with the fertilisation of the ovum or with its passage through the tubes or with its implantation in the uterus due to local inflammatory action of copper	i. Single action and only one decision is required ii. Sample and highly effective method iii. Its use is disassociated from the sexual act iv. Economical for programme v. Reversible method	i. Not advisable in women with pelvic inflammation ii. Has certain side effects iii. Not suitable in pregnancy or suspected pregnancy	Highly effective Failure rate <1%	Spontaneous expulsion. It can be avoided, if checked periodically for its presence	i. Bleeding or spotting ii. Pain including cramps, backache or discomfort. Bleeding and pain most often tends soon after insertion and occurs to disappear within a few months but may be sufficient to require removal of device in some cases iii. Pelvic inflammation usually due to reactivation of pre-existing conditions iv. Asymptomatic uterine perforation	In India, the initial acceptance rate was high but continuation rate was low on account of the side effects. CuT 380 A with an *in situ* efficacy of 10 years is available under the national programme Post-partum IUCD (PPIUCD) is also a new intervention under the national programme

(Contd...)

Table 11.1: Currently available contraceptive methods (Contd...)

S. no.	Method	Mode of action	Advantages	Disadvantages	Effectiveness	Reasons for failure	Side effects	Extent of use
8.	Oral contraceptives	Suppresses ovulation	i. Highly effective immediately related to sexual activity ii. Application not	i. Require medical examination by physician ii. Have certain side effects	Highly effective, even up to 100% if taken according to prescribed regimen	Omission of one or more tablets during the prescribed cycle of medication	i. Early use is frequently associated with symptoms similar to those occurring in early pregancy, e.g. nausea and vomiting or breast fullness and engorgement, which are primarily related to the oestrogen content of the tablets ii. Break-through bleeding iii. Weight gain iv. Headache, migraine v. Thromboem-bolic disease	Widely used. Available in various combinations Also available free of cost under National Programme (Mala N)
9.	Surgical sterilisations. Tubectomy in females, vasectomy in males	Cutting, ligation and removal of a portion of the fallopian tube in the females or of the spermatic duct in the males	The operation provides maximum protection. No further action is needed at any time throughout in later life	While it has been possible, in some cases, to restore fertility by a second operation, this cannot be counted on and the decision to undergo sterilisation should, in each case be considered carefully	It is virtually 100% effective	Indequate surgery and rare anatomical aberrations	i. The risk of operation and complications are very small especially in the male ii. Adverse emotional reactions occur if individual is not psy-chologically prepared	50% of the total sterilisation in the world have been done in India. The rural areas are covered by sterilisation camps. This method is also being popularised by providing incentives to acceptors

11.4 CURRENT DEMOGRAPHIC SCENARIO IN THE COUNTRY (Table 11.2)

a. Crude birth rate—40.8 per 1000 in 1951 to 21.4 in 2014.
b. Infant mortality rate—from 146 in 1951 to 40 in 2014.
c. Total fertility rate—from 6.0 in 1951 to 2.4 in 2011. TFR declined from 2.9 in 2005 to 2.4 in 2012, with decline more significant in high focus states. 23 states and union territories have a TFR of 2.1 or less. 10 states—Haryana—2.3, Gujarat—2.3, Arunachal Pradesh—2.3, Assam—2.4, Chhattisgarh—2.7, Jharkhand—2.8, Rajasthan—2.9, Madhya Pradesh—2.9, Meghalaya—2.9 and Dadra and Nagar Haveli—2.9 have TFR 2.1–3.0. Bihar—3.5 and Uttar Pradesh—3.3 have TFR above 3.0.
d. Steepest decline in growth rate between 2001 and 2011 from 21.54 to 17.64%.
e. Decline in 0–6 population by 3.08% compared to 2001.

Population added 18.14 crores added during 2001–2011 compared to 18.23 crores during 1991–2011.

Significant decline of 4.1 percentage fall from 24.99% in 2001 to 20.92% in 2011 in the growth rate of population in the EAG states (UP, Bihar, Jharkhand, MP, Chhattisgarh, Rajasthan, Odisha and Uttaranchal) after decades of stagnation.

11.5 DEMOGRAPHIC TRANSITION

There are four stages to the classical demographic cycle:

Stage 1: High stationary: Characterised by high birth rates, and high fluctuating death rates. Population growth was kept low by Malthusian "preventive" (late age at marriage) and "positive" (famine, war, pestilence) checks.

Stage 2: Early expanding: During the early stages of the transition, the death rate begins to fall. As birth rates remain high, the population starts to grow rapidly.

Stage 3: Late expanding: Birth rates start to decline and the rate of population growth decelerates. India is in this stage of demographic cycle.

Stage 4: Declining: Post-transitional societies are characterised by low birth and low death rates. Population growth is negligible, or even enters a decline.

11.6 POPULATION EXPLOSION

Annual growth rate for an area is when we subtract crude death rate from crude birth rate, if no migration has taken place. The world growth rate was 1% in the year 1930–1945 and now it is 1.7%, i.e. 1.7% population is added to the world every year.

11.6.1 Current Scenario of Population and Family Planning in India

a. Expected increase of population of 15.7% from 1210 million in 2011 to 1400 million in 2026.
b. Decline in TFR.
c. Greater investments in family planning which helps to mitigate the impact of high population growth by helping women achieve desired family size and avoid unintended and mistimed pregnancies. The focus is to reduce maternal mortality by 35% and reduce infant mortality and abortions significantly.

Table 11.2: Indicators (current status and targets)

Indicators	Target by 2010	Current status
Population	1107 million	1103 million (2005) 1252 million (2013)
Reduce dropouts at primary and secondary school levels	<20% for both boys and girls	School attendance: 6–10 years—83% 11–14 years—75% 15–17 years—41% (NFHS-3)
Infant mortality rate	<30 per 1000 live births	40 per 1000 live births 40 (SRS 2014)
Maternal mortality rate	<100 per 100,000 live births	170 per 100,000 live births (2013)
Marriage for girls not earlier than age 18	Promote delayed marriage	Marriage: Girls (before 18 yrs)—46% Boys (before 21 yrs)—27% (NFHS-3)
Achieve universal immunization of children		54% of children fully vaccinated (DLHS-3)
Deliveries by trained persons	100%	48%
Crude birth rate	21	19.89 (India demographic profile, 2014)
Total fertility rate	2.1	2.51 (India demographic profile, 2014)

The government of India commits to bring maternal mortality rate (MMR) to <100/100,000, infant mortality rate (IMR) to 25/1000 live births and total fertility rate (TFR) to 2.1 by 2017.

11.6.2 Factors that Influence Population Growth

a. Unmet need for family planning; 21.3% as per DLHS-III (2007–08) and 13.8 as per NFH-III.

b. Age at marriage and first childbirth; 22.1% of the girls get married below the age of 18 years.

c. Out of the total deliveries, 5.6% are among teenagers, i.e. 15–19 years.

d. Marriage below legal age is more alarming in a few states like Bihar (46.2%), Rajasthan (41%), Jharkhand (36%), UP (33%), and MP (29.2%).

e. Spacing between two childbirths is less than the recommended period of 3 years in 57.4% of births (SRS, 2012). However, 46% of women have spacing less than 30 months.

f. 52.5% of women aged 15–24 yrs contribute, to total fertility whereas 46% contribute to maternal mortality.

11.7 POPULATION STABILIZATION

An expert committee of WHO in 1971 defined family planning as, "a way of life that is adopted voluntarily by individuals and couples to promote health and welfare of the family to contribute effectively to the social development of nation and country as a whole". Its main objectives are:

i. To avoid unwanted births and to bring about only desired births.

ii. To limit number of children in a family.

iii. To regulate intervals between pregnancies as per one's own desire.

During 1977–78, major events regarding family planning took place in India. They were (a) change of family planning to family welfare (statement of government policy June 29, 1977), (b) implementation of integrated rural health programme through community health workers (inaugurated on 2nd Oct., 1977) and (c) passing of Child Marriages Restraint (Amendment) Act, 1978 which raised the minimum age of marriage from 15 to 18 years for girls and 18 to 21 years for boys and made its infringement, a cognizable offence.

As per NFHS and DLHS-3 surveys, the small family norm is widely accepted nationwide (the wanted fertility rate for India as a whole is 1.9 (NFHS-3) and the general awareness of contraception is almost universal (98% among women and 98.6% among men: NFHS-3). The data also show that contraceptive use is generally rising. Contraceptive use among married women (aged 15–49 years) has risen by 8.1 percentage points to 56.3% in NFHS-3 vis à vis NFHS-2.

11.7.1 Scope of Family Planning and Contraceptive Methods

With its historic initiation in 1952, the family planning programme has undergone transformation in terms of policy and actual programme implementation. There occurred a gradual shift from clinical approach to the reproductive child health approach and this holistic and target-free approach helped in reduction of fertility.

The objectives, strategies and activities of the family planning division are designed and operated towards achieving the family welfare goals and objectives stated in various policy documents (National Population Policy in 2000, National Health Policy in 2002, National Health Mission) and to honour the commitments of the Government of India (including ICPD: International Conference on Population and Development, Millennium Development Goals (MDG), Family Planning (FP) 2020 Summit and others).

Acc to NFHS-IV, all Ist place station/UTs except Bihar, MP and Meghalaya have achieved/maintained replacement lend of fertility. Government of India has categorised states as per the TFR level as very high focus (more than or equal to 3.0), high focus (more than 2.1 and less than 3.0) and non-high focus (less than or equal to 2.1).

National Family Welfare Programme was launched by Government of India in 1952. Subsequently with the introduction of Copper T/Lippe Loop in 1965 as a more common approach for the implementation of family planning programme, a separate Department of Family Planning was created by the Ministry of Health, Government of India in 1966. The Ministry of Family Planning, however, was renamed as Family Welfare Health in 1977.

However, family planning is not limited to birth control only but has emerged as an intervention for reducing the maternal and infant mortality and overall reproductive. The contraceptive services available under the **National Family Welfare Programme** in India may be broadly divided into two categories, spacing methods and permanent methods. There is another method (emergency contraceptive pill) to be used only in cases of emergency.

11.7.1a Spacing Methods

These are the reversible methods of contraception to be used by couples who wish to have children in future. These include:

i. **Oral contraceptive pills:** These are hormonal pills which have to be taken by a woman, preferably at a fixed time, daily. The strip also contains additional placebo/iron pills to be consumed during the hormonal pill-free days. The method may be used by majority of women after screening by a trained provider. ASHAs are entrusted with a responsibility to provide "Mala N" at doorstep with minimal charge, whereas these are available free of cost at all public healthcare facilities.

ii. **Condoms:** These are the barrier methods of contraception which offer the dual protection of preventing unwanted pregnancies as well as transmission of RTI/STI including HIV. The brand "Nirodh" is available free of cost at government health facilities and supplied at doorstep by ASHAs at a minimal cost.

iii. **Intrauterine contraceptive devices (IUCDs)** are copper containing devices. IUCDs are a highly effective method for long-term birth spacing. Two types of IUCDs are available under the programme—380A for an *in situ* life of 10 yrs and 375B for an *in situ* life of 5 years.

Postpartum IUCD insertion within 48 hours of delivery is a new initiative by specially trained providers to tap the opportunities offered by institutional deliveries. Service providers and ASHAs accompanying clients are being provided with incentive of ₹150/–.

11.7.1b Permanent Methods

These methods may be adopted by any member of the couple and are generally considered irreversible.

A. **Female sterilisation:** Two techniques have been adopted under the programme:

   i. *Minilap:* Minilaparotomy involves making a small incision in the abdomen. The fallopian tubes are brought to the incision to be cut or blocked. Can be performed by a trained MBBS doctor.

   ii. *Laparoscopic:* Laparoscopy involves inserting a long thin tube with a lens in it into the abdomen through a small incision to see and block or cut the fallopian tubes in the abdomen. The procedure can be done only by trained and certified gynaecologist/surgeon.

B. **Male sterilisation:** Two techniques are being used in India under the programme:

   i. Conventional

   ii. Non-scalpel vasectomy (NSV)—no incision, only puncture and hence no stitches.

This can be performed by MBBS doctors trained in the procedure where through a puncture or small incision in the scrotum, two ends of the vas deferens, that carries sperm to the seminal vesicle are cut and tied. However, the couple needs to use an alternative method of contraception for first three months after sterilization till no sperms are detected in semen.

11.7.1c Emergency Contraceptive Pills

Emergency contraceptive pills are available at the rate of ₹3 per packet only to be consumed in cases of emergency arising out of unplanned/unprotected intercourse. The pill should be consumed within 72 hours of the unprotected sexual act.

11.7.1d Other Commodities

Pregnancy testing kits to detect pregnancy as early as one week after the missed period, thus providing an early opportunity for medical termination of pregnancy. These are available at the subcentre level and also carried by ASHA.

All the spacing methods, viz. IUCDs, OCPs and condoms, are available at the subcentre level. However, OCPs, condoms, and emergency contraceptive pills are also distributed at the village level through ASHAs.

Permanent methods are generally available at primary health centre level or above. They are provided by MBBS doctors who have been trained to provide these services. Laparoscopic sterilization is being offered at CHCs and above.

Personal Hygiene

Lifestyle is an aggregation of decisions by individuals which affect their health, and over which they more or less have control. A healthy lifestyle leads to healthy living towards quality of life. The actual definition of 'healthy living' is the steps, actions and strategies one puts in place to achieve optimum health. 'Healthy living' is about taking responsibility for your decisions and making smart health choices for today and for the future. So healthy living would consist of various choices and factors that influence health and causation of disease in one or the other way.

The World Health Organization (WHO) defines health as a state of complete physical, mental, and social well-being, not simply just the absence of disease. Health is the state in which the mental and physical activities of the body are adjusted satisfactorily to the environment. Maintaining personal hygiene is necessary for personal, social, health, psychological or simply as a way of life since poor personal hygiene can result in a risk of infection and illnesses and also cause many social issues to arise as a result of odours and appearance.

Personal hygiene is described as the principle of maintaining cleanliness and grooming of the external body. It comprises washing, oral care, hair care, nail care, wound care, cleansing of personal utensils and prevention of infection. Thus, this concerns with the adjustments, which an individual must make to preserve and improve the health of his body and mind.

Keeping a good standard of hygiene helps to prevent the development and spread of infections, illnesses and bad odours. Personal hygiene is not only concerned with matters pertaining to health of a person but also includes certain personal factors conducive to good health. These are habits, constitution, heredity, idiosyncrasy, temperament, cleanliness, sleep, clothing, exercise, sex, etc. The main objective of personal hygiene is to maintain a high standard of health and prevent infections.

There are many factors that can affect the personal hygiene:

1. **Physical conditions:** Certain disabilities can prevent the person from maintaining an acceptable level of hygiene that is appropriate for them, e.g. amputation, paralysis, patients postoperative, arthritis, back problems restricted physical abilities by plaster casts, surgical incisions, etc.

2. **Psychological conditions:** Depression, anxiety, schizophrenia, Alzheimer's or any other mental conditions are known to have the potential to affect a person's ability to care for oneself. Loss of memory, motivation, social isolation and a lack of self-worth are all contributory factors.

3. **Social factors:** The lack of resources can result in individuals becoming unkept and socially isolated. Poor education and a lack of knowledge are other reasons of poor personal hygiene.

4. **Hospitalisation:** Critically ill patients who are hospitalised or unconscious become dependent on staff and visitors to care for their hygiene needs. Patients often need extra help with bathing and washing, hair care, nail care, pressure area care, toileting needs and oral care.

5. **Personal factors**

   a. *Constitution:* Individual variations in constitution exist in different persons, thus power of resistance to disease also varies over individuals. An individual with strong and robust constitution does not fall prey to an attack of a disease as does a person having a poor constitution. The constitution of a person is partly acquired and partly inherited. A strong constitution may get enfeebled under unhygienic conditions, while a delicate constitution may improve under hygienic conditions.

   b. *Habits:* Play an important part in the preservation of health. Habit is called second nature, because it is readily formed, grows by practice and eventually becomes part and parcel of nature and character. Habits are largely responsible for determining one's quality of life.

1. Personal Habits

a. Eating and drinking: Regular meals should be taken at fixed hours spread out over the course of day as per the calorific requirements of the body. Food should be properly masticated and eaten slowly. Reading should be avoided while talking meals. Heavy fatty meals must be avoided just before mental and intellectual work. Excess intake of food can lead to obesity, apart from digestive and other disorders.

Consumption of water is important as it helps in digestion of food and cellular processes of the body. Water should be sparingly taken along with meals, but should be taken freely between principal meals. At least 6–12 glasses of water must be consumed everyday for healthy metabolism and weight management.

b. Alcohol: The role of alcohol is controversial since some researches have proved that consumption of alcohol in moderate quantities (30 ml a day) is beneficial for heart, aids in digestion and has a calming effect by inducing sleep. However, there are a lot many negative social and health effects of excessive alcohol consumption like gastrointestinal catarrh, fatty degeneration of heart and liver, arteriosclerosis, peripheral neuritis, etc. and has a devitalising action upon the tissues, the symptoms of which range from some impairment of functions to gross degenerative lesions. The excessive consumption of alcohol leads to a condition known as "delirium tremens" which is an alcoholic psychosis with symptoms of delirium, trembling, and mental distress.

Besides alcohol, tea and coffee are also habit forming. In addition to being pleasant beverages, they are useful as stimulants, but excessive use either leads to great mental stimulation and loss of sleep. Thus, are used commonly, in moderation as relaxaing and refreshing drinks.

c. Smoking: Smoking is commonly known to cause lung cancer but has multisystem adverse effects on the body.

It harms digestion, causes sore throat, coughing and wheezing. Chronic smoking leads to bronchitis, an inflammatory condition of bronchus. Many cases of the so-called *"smokers cough"* may be the beginning of bronchitis. The alkaloid nicotine present in tobacco may cause premature hardening of arteries leading to arteriosclerosis and rise of blood pressure, heart beat, palpitation, etc. Pyridine, ammonia, aldehyde and furfurol present in the smoke of tobacco have irritant properties. Pyridine causes darkened teeth; ammonia irritates the throat and carbon monoxide destroys red blood cells.

The *hooka* or hubble-bubble is comparatively a less harmful way of smoking tobacco as smoke in passing through water, loses some of its nicotine and other harmful ingredients.

The tobacco chewing is most condemnable as a great portion of the juice is absorbed directly even if the saliva is not swallowed and thus it must be avoided. Its excessive use may even cause cancer of the mouth, impaired vision (toxic amblyopia), nervous tremor increase in blood pressure and cancer of oral cavity.

d. Sleep: Adequate sleep is important to overcome exhaustion, give rest and rejuvenate body and brain. During sleep, rate of metabolism is lowered, heart rate slows down and the activity of brain is minimized.

The requirement of sleep varies with age. As a thumb rule, the requirement of sleep varies inversely with age. The longer hours of sleep is important for proper growth of infants and children.

Lack of sound sleep may be a sign of poor health in infants and adults. Inadequate sleep decreases the work efficiency and mental alertness in an individual and leaves him irritable.

Ambience has an important role in induction and maintenance of a healthy and sound sleep. The bedroom should be well ventilated and calm. The bed and the mattresses should be firm and elastic to provide comfort to the body with a neat and clean bedding.

Poor physical or mental health is often associated with sleeplessness or insomnia: Other factors like improper food and drinks at bedtime, insufficient amount of exercise, anxiety, constipation or worrying over real or prospective troubles may keep one awake.

Insomnia in many cases can be prevented by having a regular bedtime and calm ambience along with peaceful mental and emotional attitude on retiring. Sometimes, taking physical exercise before bed time for thorough relaxation of the body muscles may also help in induction of sleep. Practising relaxation techniques, like meditation, helps in managing anxiety and helps to induce sleep.

e. Anger: It is a personality trait but is often influenced by the nutritional and mental state of an individual. Exercise, stress management techniques like meditation or even a walk can help to control anger. Anger also leads to physiological changes in the form of increase in blood pressure, and pulse rate along with autonomic stimulation leading to excessive secretion of sweat.

f. Posture: By posture is meant the characteristic form in which the body is maintained during its various activities. Goodness of a posture consists in alignment of parts for relaxation. Correct mechanical use of body permits the internal organs to function efficiently. Good posture is a desirable social asset not only because of its aesthetic value but also for maintenance of vital body functions, i.e. respiration, circulation, excretion, digestion and coordination of body activities can be carried on unimpeded, when the body is in perfect physiological balance. Inherited structural irregularities, malnutrition and insufficient muscular power are some of the factors that can lead to faulty posture. Incorrect posture may interfere with the normal functioning of the diaphragm, thus seriously limiting the amplitude of movements. *"Lordosis" or "sway back"* is a typical postural defect accompanied by a forward and downward tilt of pelvic organs and protrusion of the abdomen. In this position, the last lumbar vertebra rests at too sharp an angle on the sacrum, producing a weak joint at this place. This results in a general strain on the muscles and ligaments of the lumbar region, which may be a frequent cause of low back pain.

2. Body Hygiene

a. Bath: Bath has a beneficient action on the skin and internal organs.

Cold bath: It is invigorating, more refreshing and very stimulating to the nervous system, blood circulation and the metabolism. It tends to improve the texture, tone, firmness and colour of the skin and stimulates the circulation of the blood throughout the body. It stimulates the skin and increases the power of the body to react to variations in temperature.

Warm bath: It helps chiefly to clean the skin, particularly when soap is used. It soothes the nervous system and may be used to induce sleep, if taken just before retiring. When the temperature of water is above that of the body, it is called as hot bath.

Hot bath: It raises the temperature of the surface of the body and causes the blood vessels of the skin to dilate.

Vigorous rubbing of the body with a rough and dry towel, after taking a bath, not only absorbs moisture but also gives massage to the skin and improves circulation of the blood in the skin.

b. Oral hygiene: Since mouth has many types of bacteria, regular brushing of teeth after every meal is indicated for a good oral hygiene. Mouth should be rinsed after every meal to prevent lodgement of food particles and thereby caries of teeth. The movement of the brush should not be from side to side but from above downwards and also on the inside of the teeth. All the inner, outer and biting surfaces should be brushed alike at least for five times. Upper and lower teeth should be brushed downwards and upwards, respectively. The chewing and biting surfaces should, however, be brushed sideways. The gum tissues may be benefited by massaging them with a finger tip smeared with toothpaste. Soft toothbrush should be used and changed regularly. The tongue should be cleaned by a tongue-cleaner every morning.

c. Hands and nails: Hands and nails should be kept clean and should be cut short to prevent infections. The nails should be cut horizontally, because if curved, the skin around them will be pressed over the nails and the pressure of the nails on this enfolding skin will cause symptoms usually attributed to "ingrowing toe nails". Regular scrupulous cleansing of hands with soap and water at least before cooking and everytime before meals and after ablution is essential to prevent spread of infectious diseases like cholera, typhoid, dysentery, etc. They should invariably be washed before taking meals and during handling or preparing food. Hands should be kept free from cracks and roughness.

d. Eyes: Eyes should be cleaned with cold clean water only two to three times a day. Eyes of the school children should be periodically examined and defects corrected and treated.

Unclean environmental conditions, personal hygiene and contact with an infected individual can cause infection of eye commonly known as '*sore eye*'. The infection presents as mucopurulent discharge of the eyes and is transmitted from sick to healthy individuals through fomites like handkerchiefs, soiled towels, door handles, tap heads of washbasin, etc. Indirectly, the infection is spread through flies.

For prevention of transmission of infection, one should avoid contact with open cases of sore eye as the disease is highly infectious. Use of common handkerchiefs and towels should be strongly discouraged.

e. Head and hair: They should be kept thoroughly clean. The scalp needs a good blood supply and massaging for a few minutes daily is of great benefit.

f. Ears: Require proper care and attention. Wax in ears, sometimes gives rise to partial deafness, so it should be removed by a earbud after using wax solving drugs or through syringing. If dirt is allowed to collect for some time, it may develop into a large hard plug causing earache, boils and even deafness. A child with running ears is in constant danger of deafness or mastoiditis.

g. Genital hygiene: The sexual organs require cleaning even more than the other parts of the body. In the case of uncircumcised male organ, the foreskin should be retracted during bath and the secretion washed away. If this is not regularly done, smegma collects and undergoes bacterial decomposition, with consequent irritation, which may lead to infection.

In the case of females, the genitals should be washed with mild soap and water during bath. Girls in their childhood should be taught to wipe the anus from front backwards so as to avoid introducing faecal organisms into vulva or the genital passage. Extra caution on hygiene must be exercised during menstruation. Regular bathing, use of clean undergarments, clean sanitary towels or washed sundried cloth and use of mild soap and water is important for *menstrual hygiene.*

Sex education: Suitable education in elementary biology should be given to every child at an appropriate age to enable him/her to understand the significance of reproduction, family planning and contraception, child rearing and mother craft, evolution to empower them to take responsible decisions as adults. Life skills education should be given to adolescent boys and girls to enable them to make right decisions in life.

Before the onset of puberty, adolescent children must be given adequate knowledge about the forthcoming physical changes. Adolescent girls and boys must be informed about menarchae (first menstruation in a girl) or the first noctural emission in a boy respectively so that they are able to accept the changes normally. The parents and teachers have a role in providing health education to the young growing children regarding genital hygiene, sex and sex- related queries, prevention of sexually transmitted infections, pregnancy and childbirth so that they acquire right knowledge and are able to lead a healthy and productive life.

h. Feet: These must be kept scrupulously clean by daily washing and carefully drying between the toes.

The feet contain many sweat glands, and excessive sweating or *hyperhidrosis* necessitates frequent washing and change of socks or stockings. *Bromhidrosis* is excessive sweating with offensive odour due to decomposition of sweat and soreness of feet. For this condition, the feet should be washed several times a day in boric acid solution, dried, dabbed with methylated spirit mixed with starch and boric powder. Stockings and shoes must be changed each time after use; used stockings washed and shoes should be aired.

Corns: These are caused by pressure of tight fitting shoes. The epidermis thickens and becomes horny and grows inward to a point. If they occur between the toes, they are kept moist and are called "softcorns".

Callosities: These are formed as a result of pointed shoes. The great toe becomes bent in producing an angle at the junction of metatarsophalangeal joint. The head of the metatarsal is thus projecting point on the inner border of the foot and is exposed to pressure, where the callosity is formed.

i. Clothing: Besides aesthetics, clothing serves as a protective covering. To afford protection to the body against effect of heat and cold and to protect the body from external injuries. To a certain extent, clothing influences metabolic change.

The materials used for clothing are derived from animal and plants. Those derived from animal sources are wool, feathers, fur, leather, silk; whereas cotton, linen, artificial silk or rayon, jute, gutta-percha and rubber are derived from products of plants.

Wool: It is a bad conductor of heat and a good absorbent of moisture for which reasons it is regarded as superior to other materials for making garments for the winter. It holds certain amount of air between its interstices thus preventing rapid loss of heat through it, thus forms a valuable garment during winter.

Leather: It is prepared from skins of large animals, e.g. sheep, goats, oxen, etc., a process of tanning renders the skin flexible. This is used as a clothing in very cold countries to protect the body against cold, wind, and rain.

j. Constipation: Factors like sedentary habits, lack of regular exercise and inadequate intake of water and fibre often lead to constipation. Prolonged constipation may cause haemorrhoids. Constant constipation leads to distress that compels the person to use medicines to relieve constipation, which is harmful. Habitual use of purgatives upsets the entire intestinal rhythm.

To prevent constipation, it is important to ensure presence of vitamin B complex in adequate amounts. Movement of bowels is largely a reflex action and training from an early age should aim at establishing this reflux. The habit of evacuating the bowels at the same time each day can also be of great help.

k. Exercise: Exercise not only helps to prevent excess weight gain or maintain weight loss but also boosts high density lipoprotein (HDL), or "good," cholesterol and decreases unhealthy triglycerides. It is also important to improve the demand for oxygen for utilisation of food and to promote the repair of worn out tissues.

Thus, exercise is very essential for the normal growth and development of the body and perfect maintenance of health. Lack of exercises increases susceptibility to diabetes, hypertension, kidney diseases, heart failure, diseases of arteries, liver and gallbladder, cerebral haemorrhage, coronary heart disease and osteoarthritis of spine, hips, knees, etc. Excessive weight of 10% above normal increases the mortality rate by about 20% which lowers life expectancy.

Exercise has effects on various organs and systems of the body

1. *Respiratory system:* During exercise, the number of respirations is increased and breathing becomes deeper. The pulmonary circulation is quickened and brings into use all the air sacs of the lungs. There is a considerable increase in the amount of oxygen inhaled and carbon dioxide and water vapours exhaled.

2. *Circulatory system:* Active exercise increases the force and frequency of the heart. There is improvement in circulation of blood and lymph.

3. *Muscular system:* The blood circulation and oxygenation of the muscles is improved, which contributes to their growth and energy.

4. *Cutaneous system:* There is improved blood supply to the skin with perspiration which improves upon the texture and glow of the skin.

5. *Alimentary system:* Exercise brings about an improved assimilation of food and thus creates a demand for food. The appetite is improved and the action of bowels is stimulated. It plays an important role in the prevention of constipation.

6. *Nervous system:* The mind is refreshed and the powers of observation, precision and tolerance are developed.

A daily moderate exercise like brisk walking of about 35–40 minutes at least 5 days a week may be adequate towards maintaining the healthy body functions. Excessive *exercise* causes either nervous or muscular fatigue or even both. It causes breathlessness, palpitation and hypertrophy of left ventricle and renders pulse small, frequent and irregular. The voluntary muscles become exhausted due to overexert ion, suffer in nutrition and gradually begin to wither away.

1. **Fatigue:** The blood supplies fuel and oxygen to the active muscles and carries off the waste materials formed by the activity of the muscles. If the activity continues for too long or happens to be too strenuous, the blood cannot carry away waste matter sufficiently fast. Therefore, waste materials accumulate in the muscles and make them tired. The feeling of weariness is known as fatigue. Fatigue lowers the resistance of an individual to disease and reduces both the quantity and quality of work which one can normally do.

Balanced vitamin and mineral-rich diet, and relaxation can prevent fatigue. A hot shower or a tub bath is also helpful in removing fatigue. Light massage (rubbing) of body from extremities towards the body will help in removing the waste products from the tissues of broken down muscles and relieves fatigue.

3. Environment

In general, the environment embodies physical, social and the biological components. The physical environment constitutes varying range of natural factors like climate, soils, plains, forests, mountains, lakes, rivers, rainfall, etc. The social aspect of environment is represented by the people and their actions. This is formed by traditions, customs, superstitions, taboos, mores, folklores, etc. Plants and animals including bacteria and parasites that cause diseases comprises biological environment.

Environment has a significant bearing on the health of an individual. The genetic predisposition of an individual for a disease may remain masked for years in a non-conducive environment. The diseases and health seeking behaviour of an individual is largely influenced by the physical, social and biological environment.

4. Cleanliness

There is a famous proverb, "Cleanliness is next to godliness". Special emphasis should be laid on cleanliness with regard to the food we eat, the air we breathe and the water we drink since it is very essential for the up-keep of health and prevention of infections.

Cleanliness is an attitude that involves not only personal hygiene but also environmental cleanliness that should be taught from a very young age to the school children.

5. Genetics

It has great influence upon the health of an individual. The predisposition of an individual to certain diseases is through genes. Multifactorial diseases like hypertension, diabetes and certain types of cancers have their genetic predilection. Similarly, certain diseases like gout, insanity, syphilis, haemophilias, colour blindness, epilepsy, myopia, etc. are transmitted to the offsprings in this way. Mental peculiarities and similarity of features are often inherited.

6. Idiosyncrasy

Means susceptibility to certain medicinal preparations, food items, drugs and morbid agents, e.g. appearance of Nettle rash on the bodies of some members of a particular family as a result of taking shell fish. Food idiosyncrasy is hereditary.

Diseases Caused by Poor Personal Hygiene and Unhealthy Lifestyle

a. Dirty head and hair causes many health problems like seborrhoea capitis and pthisis capitis/head lice.

Head lice are highly contagious and may cause scalp bleeding due to intense itching and anaemia.

b. Poor oral hygiene can lead to tooth decay, if left untreated this can spread and infect your gums. Bad breath (halitosis) can be the sign of a gum infection. The teeth and mouth have to be cleaned because they emit bad odours, cause mouth and dental diseases such as cavities, gingivitis, etc. and stomach disorders due to indigestion.

c. Unpleasant smells and fungal infections are most commonly experienced in areas of the body that are warm and not often exposed to fresh air: The feet; the genitals and some of our sweat glands. Athlete's foot is a fungal infection of feet that causes itching, flaky skin and sometimes a sore, red rash.

d. Skin diseases such as ringworm, scabies, sweat fungi, etc. can also occur.

e. Unclean hands and finger nail germs in between the fingers and finger nails cause contagious diseases such as diarrhoea, worms, etc. and epidermophytosis.

f. Under conditions of sepsis such as carious teeth, septic tonsils, unhealthy mucous membrane or infected sinuses, tongue becomes coated and sordes collect around teeth and lips, which might give rise to parotitis, otitis media, infected sinuses, pyorrhoea.

g. Most of the non-communicable diseases like diabetes mellitus, hypertension, obesity, depression and cardiovascular illnesses are affected by lifestyle of an individual.

Chapter
13

Occupational Health and Offensive Trades

As per ILO/WHO definition, "Occupational health is the promotion and maintenance of the highest degree of physical, mental and social well-being of workers in all occupation". Thus, occupational health is a diverse science applied by occupational health professionals—engineers, environmental health practitioners, chemists, toxicologists, doctors, nurses, safety professionals and others who have an interest in the protection of the health of workers in the workplace. Occupational health is a broad term which emphasises the diagnostic and management approaches for the problems associated with any occupation, e.g. agriculture, industry, varied transport systems, etc. It aims at the maintenance and promotion of physical, mental and social well-being of all workers engaged in different occupations. The discipline covers the following key components:

1. The availability of occupational health and safety regulations at workplace.
2. The availability of active and functional occupational health and safety committee at workplace.
3. Monitoring and control of factory hazards to health.
4. Supervision and monitoring of hygiene and sanitary facilities for health and welfare of the workers.
5. Inspection of health safety of protective devices.
6. Pre-employment, periodical and special health examination.
7. Performance of adaptation of work to man.
8. Provision of first aid.
9. Health education and safety training to the worker.
10. Advice to employers on the above-mentioned items.
11. Reporting of occupational deaths, diseases, injuries, disabilities, hazards and their related preventive measures at working place.

13.1 PROBLEM STATEMENT

According to International Labour Organization (ILO), 1.2 million working people die of work-related accident and diseases every year and more than 160 million workers fall ill each year due to workplace hazards in many developing nations, death rates due to occupational accident among workers are five to six times higher than those in industrialized countries.

13.2 COMMON OCCUPATIONAL HEALTH ISSUES

The most common work-related health problems as per compilation by **National Institute for Occupational Safety and Health** (NIOSH). These are given below.

13.2.1 Occupational Lung Disease (Pneumoconiosis)

Asbestosis, byssinosis, silicosis, coal worker 130s' pneumoconiosis, lung cancer, and occupational asthma.

a. **Pneumoconiosis:** It is a chronic lung disease produced as a result of inhalation of injurious dust particles over prolonged period of time causing lung fibrosis and reducing the working capacity of the individual. Different dusts cause different diseases, e.g. anthracosis by coal dust, silicosis by free silica or silicon dioxide (SiO_2), asbestosis and lung cancer caused by asbestos, siderosis by iron dust, byssinosis by cotton fibre dust and tobaccosis caused by tobacco dust.

Inhalation of these dusts also increases the predisposition of lungs for other diseases like silicosis for tuberculosis and asbestosis for lung carcinomas.

Industrial dust may be mineral, vegetable or animal in origin. The dusty trades and occupations are jute, flax, textile industries, lead, copper, iron, cement and lime works, handling of leather, silk, wool, cotton, paper and drilling of stones, bones, horns, flour mills, etc. The most dusty processes are cording and spinning. Workers in jute, cotton and flour industries suffer from breathlessness, develop, symptoms of asthma and weakness of chest. Millstone cutters, stone masons, pearl cutters, sand paper makers, knife grinders, hair dressers and fur dyers generally suffer from lung diseases. Workers in gold mines inhale rockdust and suffer from silicosis.

Precautions: Inhalation of dust particles may be lessened by the use of mask, oil, water or steam. The nuisance caused by the escape of dust particles should be prevented by providing special boxes for machinery. The dust should be removed by special means, e.g. suction by fans or by special ventilating arrangements. Extraction tubes or magnetic shields may be used. In addition to these, the worker should use respirators.

13.2.2 Occupational Diseases

These are as follows

Wool-sorter's disease occurs in persons who are employed in those industries which deal with wool, cattle hair, hides and skins.

For protection, bales of wool or hair must be opened after immersing in water. Rooms should be provided with exhaust fans. Refuse from wool sorting should be collected in covered receptacles and burnt away. Persons having cuts or wounds on their bodies should not be allowed to work there. Wool should be disinfected first by formalin before handling. Food should not be taken in the workrooms where wool, hair or fibres are handled. There should be a provision of proper washing in that room.

1. **Lead poisoning:** It is one of the most common industrial diseases. Lead is a cumulative poison. When absorbed it is stored in the bones in the form of triple phosphate. Lead is dissolved out of bones by acidosis, especially if food taken by the workers is deficient in calcium, i.e. if it does not contain enough milk and milk products, eggs, green vegetables, etc. It finds entrance into the system in three ways:

   i. *Ingestion:* By swallowing minute particles of lead through drinking water from lead pipes, which are converted by the hydrochloric acid of the stomach into a soluble chloride of lead.

   ii. *Inhalation:* By inhaling dust and fumes of molten lead.

   iii. *By absorption:* Skin absorbs lead particularly when it is mixed with oil, as in paint manufacturing concerns.

   The chief industrial occupations, in which lead poisoning is liable to occur are mining, refining and smelting of lead, white and red lead works, pottery manufacture, electric accumulator works, enamelling and paint manufacturing industries, smelting of metals, glass and file cutting, manufacture of lead pipes, lead rubber compounds and plumbing supplies such as solders, gun shots manufacture, foundries, etc.

   Chronic form of lead poisoning is more common than acute one. The chief symptoms are obstinate constipation, colic, appearance of a blue line on gums, anaemia, rheumatic pains in muscles and joints, paralysis especially of extensors (dropped wrist and dropped foot are common). There may be insomnia, headache, interstitial nephritis, lead insanity, etc.

   Precautions: Hands and fingernails should be thoroughly cleaned and the mouth rinsed before eating. Workers should not take their food in the workrooms, particularly where there is suspicion of lead particles in the air. Workers should use separate clothing while at work. Handling of poisonous materials should be reduced to the minimum by substitution of mechanical methods. Women and children being particularly susceptible to lead poisoning should not be employed in lead factories. Pregnant women are liable to abortion and stillbirths. Workmen should take drinks containing minute doses of sulphuric acid and they should take nutritious food with plenty of green leafy vegetables, eggs, milk and milk products (owing to their high calcium content) and avoid taking alcoholic liquors. Workers should undergo medical examination after short periods to detect absorption and appearance of incipient symptoms of lead poisoning. Factories should be provided with a separate cloakroom and a mess-room having adequate washing facilities.

2. **Mercury poisoning:** It occurs in those who manufacture glass mirrors and workers in lead concerns and plumbers exposed to lead poisoning. Mercury or its compounds are also used in the manufacture of barometers, thermometers, vermillion and in trades like bronzing, guilding, in manufacture of electric metres and lamps, felt hats and fur dressings. It may find access into the body by similar channels as lead.

   Symptoms of mercury poisoning: Stomatitis, salivation, foetid breath, sponginess of gums, falling out teeth, anaemia, muscular tremors, and paralysis.

   Precautions to be observed against mercury poisoning are the same as in the case of lead poisoning. Workmen, while working, should wear overalls and respirators. Carious teeth of workers should be extracted. The floor should be made of asphalt and should be designed and sloped in such a way that the spilt mercury is collected easily and effectively. Since metallic mercury vaporises even at ordinary temperature and produces toxic effects, the work should be conducted in rooms at a temperature below 15.6°C. As far as possible mercury should be kept covered so that the volatilisation of mercury may be minimum. Rooms, where dust and fumes are evolved, should be provided with exhaust ventilation. Any vapours may be neutralised by spraying floors with ammonium hydrate solution, if required.

3. **Phosphorus poisoning:** Phosphorus is used in the manufacture of match sticks and affects those workers who expose themselves to its fumes. *Phossy jaw* or phosphorus necrosis of jaw occurs in workers in match-making industry due to inhalation of fumes of phosphorus.

The dangers of phosphorus poisoning now are much more from its organic compounds, which are used as insecticides or rodenticides.

Symptoms of chronic poisoning: These are headache, loss of appetite, anaemia, dyspepsia, hepatitis, necrosis of the jaw, albuminuria, bronchitis and insomnia. The long bones become brittle and get liable to fracture; a condition known as *fragilitas ossium*. The poison is absorbed through the skin by absorption or inhalation.

Precautions: Special attention should be paid to the teeth. Mouth should be washed frequently with an alkaline solution. Turpentine is recommended as an antidote for phosphorus. Work should be done in well-ventilated rooms and if possible in open air. Workrooms should be provided with exhaust fans or flues to drive away all fumes of phosphorus.

4. **Arsenic poisoning:** It occurs in those persons, who either handle arsenical pigments, viz. lead arsenate, Paris green, inhale arsenical dust from wallpapers or those who mount or cure skins of animals. Arseniuretted and phosphuretted hydrogen is given off from damp ferrosilicon; an impure alloy of iron and silicon, which is used in certain metallurgical processes. Arsenic may enter into the system from the dust of its salts by inhalation, direct contact and from arseniuretted hydrogen gas.

Symptoms: Painful eruptions on the mucous membranes of air and eye passages causing conjunctivitis and oedema of eyelids, vomiting, colic with marked diarrhoea, painful neuritis and anaemia. There may be severe irritation accompanied by acneform or eczematous eruptions on the skin. The salts of metal act as local irritants, particularly around the mouth, nose and armpits.

Precautions: Dyed wallpaper should not be used. The use of arsenic-based dyes should be discouraged. The workroom should have suitable condensing chambers. Workers should not take their meals in the workrooms. Automatic packing machinery should be used instead of personal handling of arsenical pigments.

5. **Brass founders' ague (metal fume fever):** It is the term applied to a condition resembling malarious ague, but usually apyrexial, which affects persons who are exposed to the fumes from molten brass or even brass dust. Brass founders suffer from bronchitis, and asthma, and a disease called "Brass founders' ague" characterised by rigors, fever, and sweating owing to inhalation of fine metal particles of zinc, magnesium or copper oxides.

The workroom should be well-ventilated and should be provided with exhaust fans. Females should not be allowed to work in brass works. Protective clothing should be provided to workers.

6. **Chromate poisoning:** Persons engaged in chromium plating and in the manufacture of chromate and bichromate of potassium and sodium suffer from chronic ulcers on knuckles or at the root of nails. Chromate poisoning particularly affects nasal septum of the workers suffering from it.

The preventive measures are frequent cleansing of the premises, provision of local exhaust fans to draw off the mist, careful dressing of abrasions, use of ointments or rubber gloves and wearing of masks. Workers should be provided with facilities for bath and ablution.

7. **Tobacco poisoning:** Persons working in the manufacture of tobacco suffer from nausea, giddiness and irritation of eyes.

8. **Carbon dioxide (CO_2) poisoning:** It is given during the process of fermentation in breweries, aerated water works, lime kilns, sewers and certain chemical plants. It occurs in mines, lime and brick kilns, in deep wells, cells, etc. Distressing symptoms arise, if the percentage of carbon dioxide increases more than 7–8%.

Its symptoms are headache, chilliness, and symptoms of dyspnea, leading to unconsciousness and death. Oxygen inhalation should be resorted to as a remedial measure.

9. **Carbon monoxide (CO) poisoning:** It is a colourless, odourless and tasteless gas produced by the combustion of carbonaceous materials. It causes distressing symptoms if present to the extent of 0.1%, whereas exposure to the gas if present in the strength of 0.4% or more may cause death due to its combination with the haemoglobin of the red blood cells to form a stable compound called carboxyhaemoglobin. It is also found in "after damp" of mines. This gas is usually found in gas works, blast furnaces, coke ovens, cement and brick kilns, soda water manufacture, in motor exhausts and in manufacture of wood charcoal.

This gas is most poisonous and acts on the tissues of the body by preventing oxygen from reaching up to them.

Symptoms: In acute cases, loss of motor power and loss of consciousness occurs. There may be attacks of pneumonia accompanied with haemorrhage in the central nervous system. Early symptoms of chronic poisoning are loss of power on exertion, headache and fainting.

In less acute cases, dizziness, weakness of knees, roaring in the ears, nausea, vomiting and palpitation of heart are seen. Sequelae are paralysis, loss of memory and in a few cases dementia. The blood assumes cherry red colour. In order to eliminate the dangers of carbon monoxide poisoning, provision of free ventilation and prevention of leaks is essential. Workers engaged in dangerous places, e.g. where leaks are occurring, should invariably wear oxygen helmets. Those affected should be treated with artificial respiration (Shafer's method) and oxygen inhalation, if possible.

10. **Carbon bisulphide (CS_2):** It is used in the manufacture of waterproofs, as a solvent of fats, India-rubber, phosphorus, sulphur and in the preparation of cellulose for artificial silks. It is very poisonous even in minute doses as air containing one part of gas in one million parts of air (1 ppm) is considered to be toxic.

   Symptoms of poisoning: These include headache, giddiness, tremors, hysteria, atrophy and fatty degeneration of muscles and connective tissues with loss of fat. It also causes haemolysis. In some cases, neuritis or paralysis of muscles occur. There may be mania, or dementia. The patient becomes irritable and there may be frequent attacks of colic accompanied by diarrhoea or acute constipation.

   Precautions: Workers should be examined medically once a month. They should not take their meals in workrooms. Carbon bisulphide should be kept in covered vessels and fumes arising from them should be removed by exhaust fans.

11. **Sulphuretted hydrogen (H_2S):** This gas has a peculiar smell of rotten eggs and is dangerous to health even if present in the ratio of 0.2–0.4%. It is found in chemical works, in cleansing of boilers, in soap factories and in treatment of sulphuric acid to remove traces of arsenic therefrom. It is sometimes also found in sewers, privies, filth and manure heaps. It is called "stink damp" in mines, where it is produced due to the decomposition of pyrites.

   Symptoms: These are headache, gastric disturbances and nausea. When inhaled for longer periods, it causes convulsions, paralysis, coma and death. In case of high concentrations, death is sudden and instantaneous. For remediable cares, the measures are artificial respiration and the administration of oxygen.

12. **Sulphur dioxide poisoning (SO_2):** It may occur in those workers, who are engaged in the manufacture of sulphuric acid, process of ore burning and bleaching of cotton.

   Symptoms: Suffocation, dyspnoea, coryza, cough, opacity of cornea, cyanosis, and convulsions.

13. **Arseniuretted hydrogen or arsine (AsH_3):** This gas is found in chemical and galvanising works. Cases of poisoning have occurred from the action of commercial acids containing arsenic on metals and also during roasting of various metallic ores.

   Symptoms: Toxic jaundice or haemolysis may occur. There may be vomiting, haemoglobinuria, haematuria and suppression of urine.

   Remedial measures are the administration of oxygen and transfusion of blood, together with glucosaline solution and diuretics. Free ventilation should be the rule, in stores containing arseniferous materials.

14. **Chlorine (Cl) and hydrochloric acid (HCl) gas:** These evolve in alkali works, bleaching works, paper mills, etc.

   Symptoms: These are spasm of the glottis, cough, dyspnoea, bronchial catarrh, respiratory distress, pneumonia and immediate death due to pulmonary oedema. The precautionary measures to be adopted are the maintenance of gas-tight plant, the wearing of masks and routine medical inspection of workers.

15. **Ammonia (NH_3):** It is evolved in ammonia works, in the silvering of mirrors, tin plating, in manufacture of ice, refrigeration plants, etc.

   Symptoms: Prolonged inhalation of ammonia causes chronic bronchial catarrh, conjunctivitis, salivation, paroxysmal cough but rarely suffocation and death.

16. **Benzene:** It is a coal tar derivative and used in rubber works, drycleaning works, manufacture of aniline, etc. and explosive industries. The vapours of the gas may be inhaled and substances like nitrobenzol or trinitrol (TNT) may be absorbed through the skin. Since women are more susceptible to the effects of benzene than men, they should not be employed in these trades.

   Symptoms: Flushed face, nausea, vomiting, pain in abdomen, giddiness, headache, cyanosis, stupor, coma and death. In chronic cases, fatty degeneration of heart, liver and kidneys are common. Prevention consists of provision of exhaust ventilation and use of overalls, protective gloves, aprons, etc. Since the fumes of benzene are heavier than air, exhaust ducts should be laid below the work level, preferably near the floor. Moreover, scrupulous personal cleanliness should be observed.

17. **Aniline:** It is used in the manufacture of dyes.

   Symptoms: They are due to cumulative action of the aniline on human system. They are eczematous ulcerations, cough, tachycardia, nervous symptoms, insomnia and blindness. Methemoglobinaemia resulting in cyanosis occurs following autoexposure to high levels of aniline. The preventive measures are local exhaust ventilation, mechanical manipulation, periodical medical examination and alteration of employment. Washing facilities should be made use of and protective clothing worn.

13.2.3 Musculoskeletal Injuries

Disorders of the back, trunk, upper extremity, neck, lower extremity, traumatically induced Raynaud's phenomenon.

13.2.4 Occupational Cancers (other than lung)

Leukaemia, mesothelioma; cancers of the bladder, nose, and liver. Chimney sweeps' carcinoma, also known as soot wart, is a form of skin cancer affecting the scrotum.

13.2.5 Injuries Leading to Amputation, Fractures

Eye loss, lacerations, and traumatic deaths.

13.2.6 Cardiovascular Diseases

Hypertension, coronary artery disease, acute myocardial infarction.

13.2.7 Reproductive Disorders

Infertility, spontaneous abortion, teratogenesis.

13.2.8 Neurotoxic Disorders

Peripheral neuropathy, toxic encephalitis, psychoses, extreme personality changes (exposure-related).

13.2.9 Noise

Induced hearing loss.

13.2.10 Dermatologic Conditions

Dermatoses, burns and scalds, chemical burns, contusions and abrasions.

13.2.11 Psychological Disorders

Neuroses, personality disorders, alcoholism, drug dependency.

13.2.12 Vector-borne Diseases

If cattle are kept in over-crowded, ill-ventilated and poorly-drained localities in villages or towns, owing to the decomposition of food grains, putrefaction, soakage of urine and accumulation of dung, etc. on the ground, these localities might serve as a breeding place for mosquitoes, flies, etc. Thus, the inhabitants and workers working in the cattle shed are prone to mosquito and fly-borne diseases.

Thus, to prevent these diseases, the cattle sheds and stables should be built at a distance of about 100 ft (30.48 metres) away from the nearest inhabited area. In pig sites, the food should be stored in impervious vessels provided with proper covers.

13.3 INDUSTRIAL HAZARDS

Besides the offensive trades, other important chemical hazards are dusty trades, occupational poisons, poisonous gases and fumes. Important physical agents creating occupational hazards are temperature (heat as assessed through effective temperature index and cold), light (inadequate or excessive in terms of ultraviolet or infrared), air pressure (high or low), electricity (shock or burn), radiations (local or general), noise and vibrations. Similarly, important biological hazards are occupational zoonosis such as anthrax brucellosis, Q fever, psittacosis, mycotic infections and some parasitic infections. The mechanical hazards are moving machinery parts. About 10% of accidents in industry are owing to mechanical parts. Finally socio-psychological hazards constitute maximum hazards especially in well-organised, automatic and electronically operated industries. Disturbed state of mind as well as industrial tensions are responsible for many health, welfare, production and safety problems.

13.4 OCCUPATIONAL HEALTH IN AGRICULTURE

While a lot of emphasis is given on occupational health aspects in industries, occupational health aspects of agriculture and associated agroindustries, village, cottage and household industries are often neglected. The occupational health hazards in agriculture may be stated as:

a. Agricultural accidents that may occur:
   i. Farm operations with simple and/or sophisticated tools.
   ii. Village home accidents like snake, scorpion and other insects bite or accidents owing to close maintenance of animals, etc.
   iii. Village terrain accidents owing to underdeveloped roads and rickety means of transport.

b. Heavy exposure risks for problems associated with environmental insanitation, zoonosis and cultural lag, poverty, illiteracy and taboos.

c. Hazards of harsh climate and dependence on nature (e.g. floods and draughts).

d. Hazards of toxic chemicals, e.g.
   i. Acute poisoning from toxic organophosphorus compound (parathion), nitrated and chlorinated phenols or chlorinated hydrocarbons like dieldrin, endrin, etc.
   ii. Delayed or prolonged effects of alkyl mercury compounds used for speed dressing organophosphorus insecticides like malathion, etc.
   iii. Hazards of other pesticides, antibiotics and hormonal preparations used for insects and animals.

13.5 HEALTH HAZARDS WITH OTHER OCCUPATIONS

13.5.1 Blood Boiling (blood drying)

Blood collected from slaughter-houses is utilised for preparing blood manure, refining sugar, making blood albumen and manufacturing turkey red pigment. This is done by boiling blood with an admixture of commercial sulphuric acid to bring it into thick consistency.

Precautions

1. Blood should be collected and stored in clean and airtight vessels to prevent escape of offensive gases.
2. Boiling should be done in a place where suitable arrangement is made for the discharge of gaseous products through a chimney, the height of which should be above the height of inhabitable buildings in the vicinity.
3. The floor, vessels, etc. should be kept scrupulously clean.

13.5.2 Bone Boiling

It is done for preparing phosphatic manure particularly for tea gardens. It is also used for preparing gelatine, glue and fat and manufacture of handles of knives, etc.

Following precautions should be observed:
1. The premises should be cleaned daily and all refuse should be collected and removed therefrom.
2. Raw bones should be stored in a suitable shed.
3. Boiling should be done in steam jacketed pans provided with a very high chimney for emanating offensive gases.
4. Walls and floors of the room where boiling is done should be kept in good order and the walls should be lime-washed twice a year.
5. Fresh and dry bones should be treated with lime before they are stored.

13.5.3 Gut Scraping

It is done for the purpose of making sausage skin, catgut, etc. The small intestines of pigs and sheep are first washed, cleaned, softened by soaking in salt solution for a few days and then scraped with a wedge-shaped piece of wood, until only a little of the muscular coat and the peritoneal covering are left. These are finally washed and dried.

Following precautions should be observed:
1. The floors and walls where gut scraping is done should be made of impervious material.
2. Proper drainage arrangements should be provided.
3. The tables should have marble tops.
4. Prompt removal of the waste materials.
5. Proper washing and cleaning of the premises.
6. Prolonged storage should be avoided.

13.5.4 Fat and Tallow Melting (soap manufacturing)

Fats are derived from beef, mutton, pork, kitchen wastes, etc. They are utilised in the manufacture of candles, soap, leather dressings and grease for lubricating machinery. In the soap manufacturing process, fat is boiled with an alkali. These are melted in pans over open fire or free steam or in steam jacketed pans.

Nuisance of obnoxious smell may arise from:
1. Improper conveyance for storage of material.
2. Storage of residual products.
3. General filthiness and unsuitability of premises due to vapours arising during the process of melting or boiling of fat.

Precautions

1. The process should not be carried out near a densely populated locality.
2. By use of steam jacketed pan, the nuisance of foul smell is considerably lessened.

13.5.5 Fell Mongering, Tanning or Leather Dressing

Fresh skins are first beaten to remove dirt and then soaked in large tanks in water. This softens the hair, which are removed by painting the inner side of skin with a solution of slaked lime and sodium sulphide, which has a depilatory action. The process involves putrefaction and gives rise to offensive odours. The process of tanning consists of soaking the hides in progressively stronger solutions of gallnuts and tannin. Since these processes are very offensive, these trades should not be carried out near a thickly-populated locality. The building where tanning is done should have a compound wall at least 6 ft. (1.83 metres) high. All offensive materials should be conveyed in non-absorbent, covered receptacles and should be kept in a special closed room ventilated through air shafts. There should be a satisfactory method of disposal of dirt, scrapings of flesh and waste water.

13.5.6 Brick and Lime Kilns

Release organic effluvia and gases like carbon dioxide, carbon monoxide, sulphur dioxide and hydrogen sulphide, thus these should be installed far away from an inhabited locality. The brick kilns should be provided with proper flues and should be worked at night only. Availability of sufficient amount of water is necessary in the vicinity of brick kilns.

13.5.7 Smoke Nuisance

Large volume of smoke comes out from the chimneys of factories and dwelling houses. The smoke gives rise to a great nuisance, which can be prevented by locating all factories, away from inhabited areas and by having properly constructed furnaces, boilers and chimneys as well as by substituting gas or electricity for coal for the heating purpose.

13.5.8 Paper Making

Paper is manufactured from such substances as cotton, linen, rags, waste paper, straw, bamboo, esparto grass, etc. Esparto grass when used for the manufacture of paper, is reduced to fine pulp by holding it with caustic alkali. Nuisance is caused chiefly by alkali waste, which should not be allowed to run in any pond or ditch near an inhabited place. The collection and storage of the raw material is also a source of danger to health.

13.5.9 Rice Mills

The effluent in which paddy is soaked is putrid and gives out foul smell. It should not be discharged near an inhabited area and should be chlorinated before allowing it to run into any river or a stream. Steps should be taken to install necessary protective machinery against the dissemination of dust.

13.5.10 Oil Mills

These should be well-lighted and ventilated. Their floors should be made of impermeable material. The oil and crushed seed should be stored in covered vessels. There is a nuisance of smell from the oil seeds, oil cakes and noise is produced from the running of the propellers. Therefore, these mills should be located at a distance sufficiently away from human habitation.

13.5.11 Sugar Factories

The factory washings containing cane sugar ferment, decompose readily and give out foul smell. So the effluent should be chlorinated before it is used for irrigation purposes. It should not be allowed to run into a river as it will pollute the water and may kill fish.

13.5.12 Dusty Trades

Certain industries give rise to considerable amount of dust, which causes various ailments and troubles. Constant inhalation of dust particles ranging in size from 0.1 to 100 microns gives rise to pneumoconiosis.

13.6 MEASURES FOR PREVENTION OF OCCUPATIONAL DISEASES

For prevention of occupational diseases measures on three points are needed, i.e. medical, engineering and legislature.

13.6.1 Medical Measures

Medical measures are in terms of (a) preplacement examinations, i.e. placing the right man for the right job through job analysis and other ergonomic techniques, (b) periodical examinations for assessments especially for hazardous jobs, (c) medical care through Employees' State Insurance, welfare and safety aspects through Factories Act provisions, which include first aid, etc. (d) notification of notifiable and compensable diseases, e.g. aniline poisoning, anthrax, arsenic and lead poisoning, etc. and (e) other measures like records maintenance and health education, etc.

13.6.2 Engineering Measures

a. Good designing of buildings
b. Good housekeeping, ventilation, safety and welfare provisions as per Factories Act.
c. Mechanisation of hazardous processes
d. Substitution for hazardous processes
e. Enclosures or wet processing for dusty processes
f. Protective devices, etc.

13.6.3 Legislative Aspects

a. Employees State Insurance Act, 1948 for medical and cash benefits as well as benefits under Workmen's Compensation Act, 1923, and
b. Factories Act, 1948 for health, safety, welfare, first aid, hours of work, employment of young persons, etc.

Occupational Safety and Health Administration (OSHA), an agency of the US Department of labor, was created to improve worker safety and health protection at work. The aim of this organization is to assure safe and healthful working conditions for working men and women by setting and enforcing standards and by providing training, outreach education and assistance. Its mission is to develop job safety and health standards and enforcing them through worksite inspections and providing training programs to increase knowledge about occupational safety and health.

OSHA also provides technical assistance for effective safety and health programs, state plans, workplace consultations, voluntary protection programs, strategic partnerships, training and education, and more.

The Occupational Safety and Health Act of 1970 (OSH Act) encourages states to develop and operate their own job safety and health plans. OSHA approves and monitors these plans.

a. **ESI Act:** The Employees' State Insurance (ESI) Act, 1948 envisaged an integrated need based social insurance scheme to protect the interest of workers in contingencies such as sickness, maternity, temporary or permanent physical disablement, death due to employment injury resulting in loss of wages or earning capacity. The Act also guarantees reasonably good medical care to workers and their immediate dependents. The Act further absolves the employers of their obligations under the Maternity Benefit Act, 1961 and Workmen's Compensation Act, 1923 (central legislation which provides for payment of compensation for injuries suffered by a workman in the course of and arising out of his employment according to the nature of injuries suffered and disability incurred, where death results from the injury, the amount of compensation is payable to the dependents of the workmen).

Under the scheme, all the employees in the factories or establishments to which the Act applies are insured for six social security benefits:

i. **Medical benefit:** Full medical care is provided to an insured person and his family members from the day he enters insurable employment with no ceiling on expenditure on the treatment of an insured person or his family member. Medical care is also provided to retired and permanently disabled insured persons and their spouses on payment of a token annual premium of ₹120/-.

ii. **Sickness benefit (SB):** Sickness benefit in the form of cash compensation at the rate of 70% of wages is payable to insured workers during the periods of certified sickness for a maximum of 91 days in a year. In order to qualify for sickness benefit, the insured worker is required to contribute for 78 days in a contribution period of 6 months.

Extended sickness benefit (ESB): SB extendable up to two years in the case of 34 malignant and long-term diseases at an enhanced rate of 80% of wages. A full wage is payable to insured persons undergoing sterilisation for 7 days/14 days for male and female workers, respectively.

i. **Maternity benefit (MB):** Maternity benefit for confinement/pregnancy is payable for three months, which is extendable by further one month on medical advice at the rate of full wage subject to contribution for 70 days in the preceding year.

ii. **Disablement benefit:** Temporary disablement benefit (TDB) is admissible from day one of entering insurable employment and irrespective of having paid any contribution in case of employment injury. Temporary disablement benefit at the rate of 90% of wage is payable so long as disability continues. However, permanent disablement benefit (PDB) is paid at the rate of 90% of wage in the form of monthly payment depending upon the extent of loss of earning capacity as certified by a medical board.

iii. **Dependents' benefit (DB):** DB is paid at the rate of 90% of wage in the form of monthly payment to the dependents of a deceased insured person in cases where death occurs due to employment injury or occupational hazards.

iv. **Other benefits**
   a. *Funeral expenses:* An amount of ₹10,000/- is payable to the dependents or to the person who performs last rites from day one of entering insurable employment.

   b. *Confinement expenses:* These are available for an insured woman or in respect of an employee's wife in case confinement occurs at a place where necessary medical facilities under ESI scheme are not available.

In addition, the scheme also provides vocational and physical rehabilitation in cases of permanent disability to insured workers. Old age medical care is available for insured person retiring on attaining the age of superannuation or under VRS/ERS and person having to leave service due to permanent disability insured person and spouse on payment of ₹120/- per annum.

Rajiv Gandhi Shramik Kalyan Yojana is a scheme where unemployment allowance was introduced w.e.f. 01-04-2005. An insured person who become unemployed after being insured three or more years, due to closure of factory/establishment, retrenchment or permanent invalidity are entitled to unemployment allowance equal to 50% of wage for a maximum period of up to one year along with medical care for self and family from ESI hospitals/dispensaries during the period.

The contributions are related to the paying capacity as a fixed percentage of the workers' wages, whereas, they are provided social security benefits according to individual needs without distinction.

The contribution payable to the corporation in respect of an employee comprises employer's contribution of 4.75% and employee's contribution at the rate of 1.75%. Employees in receipt of a daily average wage up to ₹100/- are exempted from payment of contribution.

b. **The Factories Act, 1948:** In India, first Factory Act was passed in 1881 applicable for 100 workers, which was later modified in 1891 and extended to factories employing 50 or more workers. Under its purview, it covers safety and security of workers, and regulated their working hours. It also ensures annual leaves with wages and provides additional protection from hazardous processes and for women workmen and prohibition of employment of children.

13.7 SAFETY AND PERSONAL PROTECTION

Personal protective equipment (PPE) is the equipment worn to minimize exposure to a variety of hazards. It includes protective clothing, helmets, goggles, or other garments or pieces of equipment designed to protect the wearer's body from injury or infection. The hazards addressed by **protective equipment** include physical, electrical, heat, chemicals, biohazards, and airborne particulate matter.

To ensure the greatest possible protection for employees in the workplace, the cooperative efforts of both employers and employees will help in establishing and maintaining a safe and healthful work environment. The employers are responsible for performing a "hazard assessment" of the workplace to identify and control physical and health hazards to identify training and providing appropriate PPE for employees. The employers should also maintain PPE, periodically review, update and evaluate and thereby replace worn or damaged PPE, if needed.

The employees' responsibility is to properly wear PPE as per the training given to them for its use and care. They should also inform the supervisor about the need to repair or replace PPE.

Types of PPE: Appropriate *eye and face protection* is indicated, if the workers are exposed to eye and face hazards from flying particles, molten metal, liquid chemicals, acids or caustic liquids, chemical gases or vapours, potentially infected material or potentially harmful light radiation. Safety spectacles with or without side shields, goggles, welding shields, laser safety goggles and face shields are a few PPEs used for eye and face protection.

Head protection: It is a key element of any safety programme. Safety helmet or hard hat is indicated for use to protect an employee's head from injury, impact and penetration hazards as well as from electrical shock and burn hazards.

Foot or leg injuries: Occur from falling or rolling objects or from crushing or penetrating materials. Protective footwear includes *leggings, metatarsal and toe guards combination foot and shin guard and safety shoes.* These protect the lower legs and feet from heat hazards such as molten metal or welding sparks. *Electrically conductive shoes, electrical hazard, safety-toe shoes and foundry shoes* are specially designed shoes for workers predisposed to electrical burns and injuries.

Protective gloves are indicated for *protection of arms and hands* in workers dealing with chemicals, sparks, heat, etc. Sturdy gloves made from metal mesh, leather or canvas provide protection against cuts and burns. Leather or canvass gloves also protect against sustained heat. Chemical-resistant gloves are made with different kinds of rubber: Natural, butyl, neoprene, nitrile and fluorocarbon (viton); or various kinds of plastic: Polyvinyl chloride (PVC), polyvinyl alcohol and polyethylene.

Employees who are at possible risk of bodily injury must wear appropriate *body protection* while performing their jobs. In addition to cuts and radiation, temperature extremes, hot splashes from molten metals and other hot liquids, potential impacts from tools, machinery and materials and hazardous chemicals can cause bodily injuries. There are many varieties of protective clothing available for specific hazards. Like laboratory coats, coveralls, vests, jackets, aprons, surgical gowns and full body suits.

Appropriate *hearing protections* are indicated for workers working in environment with high levels of exposure to noise. Single-use earplugs made of waxed cotton, foam, silicone rubber or fibreglass wool, preformed or moulded earplugs and earmuffs are the protective devices to be used.

Chapter
14

Infectious Disease Epidemiology

14.1 EPIDEMIOLOGY

Epidemiology means epi (among) and demos (people), i.e. among people or in other words, it is a study of a phenomenon among people. It is the basic science of preventive and social medicine that studies the health and health-related events on populations. The health-related events may be communicable and non-communicable diseases, causes of human morbidities or mortalities like accidents, riots, wars, poverty, etc. Epidemiology is studied in terms of multifactorial etiologies and in terms of multiway interactions among agent, host and environment (called epidemiological triad). The main objective of epidemiology is to study the distribution of health/disease and its causal factors to analyse the strength of association between them. Thus, finally striving for control and prevention of disease and thereby its complete elimination.

The methods used in epidemiology are descriptive, analytical and experimental.

a. **Descriptive epidemiology:** Descriptive epidemiology is a study of health and disease and related factors in terms of time, place or person. Time trends may be in terms of secular (over a long period), cyclical (over a few years), yearly (over a year) and seasonal (in a particular season), etc. Place trends may be in terms of topographical or geographical situations. Personal trends may be in terms of age, sex, socioeconomic profiles, occupations, etc.

    Descriptive epidemiology yields data to work out hypothesis of association for going into casual factors and/or modes of transmission.

b. **Analytical epidemiology:** In analytical epidemiology, analyses of hypotheses are usually made in terms of prospective or retrospective studies. Prospective studies are longitudinal studies, i.e. forward studies which are made with a view to highlight risk factors through a comparison of control and experimental groups. Retrospective studies are backward studies which are usually made out from records.

c. **Experimental epidemiology:** Experimental epidemiology may be studied in laboratory for animals, or for control on human population. Evaluation of BCG vaccine on a group of persons is an experimental prospective study with a view to evaluate the role of BCG through a comparison with a control population group without BCG.

Uses of epidemiology: Epidemiology is used both for spelling out disease/other phenomena patterns in groups of people as well as for evaluation of health services.

14.2 INFECTION

Infection means introduction of pathogenic micro-organisms in the body which are capable of multiplying, at the expense of the host without coming into contact with the patient. Diseases caused by these infections are called infectious or communicable diseases. However, an infection may not always cause illness. There are several levels of infection (gradients of infection)—colonization (*S. aureus* in skin and normal nasopharynx), subclinical or inapparent infection (polio), latent infection (virus of herpes simplex) and manifest or clinical infection.

Infectious agent: A micro-organism, i.e. bacterium, protozoon, helminth, spirochete, fungus, virus or other such agents capable of producing infection under favourable circumstances of host and environment.

Communicable disease: A disease that can be transmitted from one person to other in a community. It is a broad term and includes infectious as well as contagious diseases.

Non-communicable diseases: The diseases that cannot be transmitted from one person to the other, e.g. cardiovascular diseases, cancer, diabetes, etc.

Infectious disease: It means a disease of a man or an animal resulting from an infection. The infection may be transmitted through various modes like insect vectors, animal carriers, etc. Infectious diseases that spread from person to person are said to be **contagious diseases,** e.g. scabies, trachoma, sexually transmitted infections, flu, colds, etc.

Infestation: It means the lodgement, development and reproduction of arthropods on the surface or any part of the human body, e.g. helminths in intestines or head louse.

Contamination: The presence of biological, chemical, physical, or radiological substance (normally absent in the environment), in a concentration sufficient to adversely affect living organisms through air, water, soil, and/or food.

Contagion: The material which carries the infection, e.g. in smallpox, contagion is carried through air.

Contact: A contact is a person who has been exposed to the risk of infection as a result of direct or indirect association with a case of communicable disease. Contacts are characterised as immediate, intimate, remote or casual.

Reservoir: Any person, animal, arthropod, plant, soil, or substance, or a combination of these, in which an infectious agent normally lives and multiplies, on which it depends primarily for survival, and where it reproduces itself in such a manner that it can be transmitted to a susceptible host. It is the natural habitat of the infectious agent.

Vector: An insect or any living carrier that transports an infectious agent from an infected individual or its wastes to a susceptible individual or its food or immediate surroundings. Both biological and mechanical transmissions are encountered. The transmission in which the agent undergoes its partial or complete life cycle within the vector is known as a *biological transmission,* e.g. Plasmodium in malaria. Whereas when the transmission of infection occurs where the agent is just physically carried to the host by the vector without undergoing any morphological or developmental change is known as mechanical transmission of infection, e.g. house fly in transmission of typhoid.

Fomites: These are substances capable of absorbing, retaining, or transferring infection. Usually the inanimate objects, like clothing, bedding, are referred to as fomites.

Host: A man or an animal, including birds and anthropods that can provide subsistence or lodgement to an infectious agent under natural conditions. Host can be obligate, primary, secondary or transport hosts. Some protozoa or helminths pass successive stages in alternate hosts of different species. Hosts in which a parasite attains maturity or passes its sexual stage are primary or definitive hosts; those in which the parasite is in a larval or asexual state are called secondary or intermediate hosts.

Epidemic: When an infectious disease becomes largely prevalent, where it previously did not exist, from a common source, it is called an epidemic. More scientifically, an epidemic may be defined as the occurrence of a group of illness of similar nature, clearly in excess of expected frequency in a community or region, and derived from a common or from a propagated source. The excess frequency may arbitrarily be defined as more than two standard errors (+2 SE) of the usual frequency of occurreance of that disease over a period of last three years. When an epidemic is very widely spread over a large geographic area, from country to country or over the entire world, as influenza of 1957, it is called as *pandemic*.

Endemic: When an infectious disease is prevalent in a locality or a community continuously for some time without importation from outside, it is called endemic. It is local and recurs with varying degree of virulence. *Hyperendemic* is when the disease is constantly present at high incidence and/or prevalence rate and affects all age groups equally. Whereas *holoendemic* means a high level of infection beginning early in life and affecting most of the child population, leading to a state of equilibrium such that the adult population shows evidence of the disease much less commonly than do the children (e.g. malaria).

Sporadic: The cases occur irregularly, haphazardly from time to time, and generally infrequently. The a cases are a few and separated widely in time and place that they show no or a little connection with each other, nor a recognizable common source of infection, e.g. polio, meningococcal meningitis, tetanus. However, a sporadic disease could be the starting point of an epidemic when the conditions are favourable for its spread.

Exotic: When a disease is not usually present in a community, area or country but is introduced from outside, it is called exotic, e.g. yellow fever in India.

Zoonosis: It denotes infection or an infectious disease of animals transmissible under natural conditions to man, e.g. plague, rabies, bovine tuberculosis, etc.

Epizootic: An epidemic outbreak of disease in an animal population, often with the implication that it may extend to humans. For example, rift valley fever (RVF) primarily affects livestock and can cause disease in a large number of domestic animals—an "epizootic"— and the presence of an RVF epizootic can lead to an epidemic among humans who are exposed to diseased animals.

Enzootic: An enzootic is an endemic occurring in animals, e.g. bovine TB.

Agents: May be physical, biological or chemical that may cause a disease.

Viruses: These constitute a group of ultramicro-scopic extremely minute-infecting agents. These are of such a small size, that they can even pass through the pores of a filter paper. They depend on living tissues for their growth, e.g. poliovirus, influenza virus, etc.

Bacteria: These constitute the simplest form of vegetable life. They are minute chlorophyll-free unicellular bodies which multiply by transverse fission. They are conducive in breaking down of organic matter into simpler forms. They cannot pass through the pores of a filter paper and can be easily seen under a microscope.

Protozoa: These are unicellular organisms, e.g. *P. vivax*, *P. falciparum*.

Spirochaetes: These are flexible spiral organisms and resemble morphologically to members of the *Spirillum* group, e.g. *Treponema pallidum*, which are the causative organisms of syphilis.

Rickettsias: These constitute small organisms and are intermediate in size between viruses and bacteria. They can be seen under a powerful microscope. They can be cultured, like viruses, in living tissues, viz. chick embryos.

Nosocomial (hospital-acquired) infection: It is an infection originating in a patient while in a hospital or another health care facility. It has to be a new disorder unrelated to the patient's primary condition. Examples include infection of surgical wounds, hepatitis B and urinary tract infections.

Opportunistic infections: These are infections by organisms that take the opportunity provided by a defect in host defense (e.g. immunity) to infect the host and thus cause disease. For example, herpes simplex, cytomegalovirus, *M. tuberculosis* infections in AIDS patients.

Incidence: Number of new cases in a given time period expressed as percent infected per year (cumulative incidence) or number per person time of observation (incidence density).

Prevalence: Number of cases at a given time expressed as a percent at a given time. Prevalence is a product of incidence and duration of disease, and is of a little interest if an infectious disease is of short duration (i.e. measles), but may be of interest if an infectious disease is of long duration (i.e. chronic hepatitis B).

Incubation period: The time interval between invasion by an infectious agent and appearance of first sign or symptom of the disease is called "incubation period". The duration of incubation period varies in each disease and during this period the patient usually remains apparently healthy. Knowing the incubation period of a disease helps in:

a. Tracing the source of infections and contacts
b. Determining the period of surveillance
c. Immunization

d. Identification of point source or propagated epidemics
e. Predicting the prognosis of a disease. Usually the diseases with short incubation period have poor prognoses.

Period of infectivity: It is the duration of communicability of the disease. The power of imparting infection begins with the appearance of first symptom or even before that and lasts until the patient has recovered absolutely or even later. The length of the period of infectivity depends upon a variety of circumstances which differ in each case, e.g. in typhoid and cholera, bacilli continue to be discharged from the body for a very long period, than it is to be usually thought. Hence, such a person becomes a real source of danger to the community for he may go about spreading the germs of the disease for months after he has apparently regained perfect health.

Attack rate: Proportion of non-immune exposed individuals who become clinically ill.

Primary (index)/secondary cases: The person who comes into and infects a population is the primary case. Those who subsequently contracts the infection are secondary cases. Further spread is described as "waves" or "generations".

Eradication: Termination of all transmission of infection by the extermination of the infectious agent through surveillance and containment. Eradication is an absolute process, an "all-or-none" phenomenon, restricted to termination of infection/agent from the whole world.

Elimination of a disease when it ceases to be a public health problem in a given area. The number of cases decreases to certain predefined levels/targets.

Vaccines: These are amino biological substances required to produce specific protection against a given disease. They stimulate the production of protective antibodies and other immune mechanisms against that disease.

14.3 DYNAMICS OF DISEASE TRANSMISSION (CHAIN OF INFECTION)

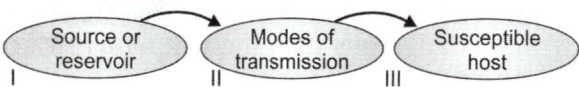

I. Source or Reservoir

The source is defined as "the person, animal, object or substance from which an infectious agent passes or is disseminated to the host (immediate source). The reservoir is "any person, animal, arthropod, plant, soil, or substance, or a combination of these, in which an infectious agent normally lives and multiplies, on which it depends primarily for survival, and where it reproduces itself in such a manner that it can be transmitted to a susceptible host. It is the natural habitat of the infectious agent". Thus, reservoirs may be:

a. Human
b. Animal
c. Non-living

a. **Human reservoirs:** May be either cases or carriers.

Cases: A case is defined as a person in the population or study group identified as having the particular disease, health disorder, or condition under investigation. The cases can be classified as primary, index and secondary depending upon their occurrence. The cases may be clinical, subclinical or latent depending upon the spectrum of disease.

Carriers: A carrier may be defined as "an infected person that harbours a specific infectious agent in the absence of discernible clinical disease and serves as a potential source of infection for others". The carriers, though may not be as infectious as cases, but since these are not recognized, these have a higher significance epidemiologically. The carriers are thus capable of infecting the susceptible individuals, under favourable conditions, for a longer period of time. Depending upon the duration of shedding of the infectious agents, they are divided into temporary and chronic carriers.

1. *Temporary carriers:* Excrete the infective organisms only for a short period. They may be *precocious or incubatory carriers,* or persons during the incubation period of the infectious disease.

    The persons who are in contact with a case of an infectious disease and carry micro-organisms morphologically identical with those causative of the disease are *contact or healthy carriers* and those who continue to shed the disease organism during convalescence are *convalescent carriers.* They are sometimes called acute carriers, e.g. typhoid, cholera, etc.

2. *Chronic carriers:* These are those persons who continue to shed infectious organisms for a long period after recovery from the disease (i.e. more than 3 months). The period of infectivity is often displayed intermittently only. These are far more dangerous than the temporary or acute carriers.

    Depending upon the route of exit of the causative organism, these may be classified as urinary, intestinal, respiratory or others.

b. **Animal reservoirs:** Zoonosis is an infection that is transmissible under natural conditions from vertebrate animals to man, e.g. rabies, plague, bovine tuberculosis.

c. **Reservoir in non-living things:** Soil and inanimate matter can also act as reservoir of infection. For example, soil may harbor agent that causes tetanus, anthrax and coccidioidomycosis.

II. Modes of Transmission of Infection

The infection can be transmitted: (a) Direct or (b) indirectly through vectors, fomites, etc.

a. *Direct transmission:* Occurs without intervention of intermediary host. The infection might occur by *direct contact* when the disease agent is transmitted from an infected individual directly to a susceptible host, through physical contact. The infection may be transmitted from a patient by droplet infection as in tuberculosis, measles, influenza, common cold, whooping cough, etc. Generally infection takes place through an orbit of 2–3 feet (0.6–0.91 metre), but when the discharge from the mouth and nose containing, causative organisms happen to be in the form of very minute particles of fine sprays, the area of infection may exceed even up to 20–30 feet (6.0–9.1 metre). Contaminated hands and fingers spread diseases like cholera, dysentery and typhoid. Another group of diseases are the result of physical contact of moist surfaces of genitalia, the so-called sexually transmitted diseases and includes syphilis, chancroid and granuloma venereum. Tetanus is transmitted from the soil containing spores when it comes in contact with the abraded or lacerated skin. Certain infections, like syphilis and hepatitis B, are transmitted from mother to baby transplacentally.

b. *Indirect transmission:* Infection may be transferred indirectly through the agency of a third person through a vector, vehicle, fomites or airborne. It includes a variety of mechanisms including the traditional **5 Fs**—"**f**lies, **f**ingers, **f**omites, **f**ood and **f**aeces". These may be:

    1. *Inanimate*
        i. Contaminated objects such as dishes, utensils, toys, books, slate-pencils, etc.
        ii. Contaminated foods transmit typhoid, diarrhoea, dysentery, cholera, etc.
    2. *Animate:* Insects which are capable of carrying infection from one host to another as in malaria, plague, etc.

III. Susceptible Host

An infectious agent seeks susceptible host for successful parasitism. There are four stages for successful parasitism: Portal of entry, site of election inside the body, portal of exit and survival in the external environment.

14.4 EPIDEMIOLOGICAL TRIAD

The transmission of an infection from source/reservoir to host depends upon the interaction of agent, host and the environment and their related factors.

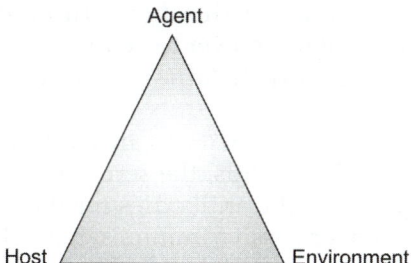

The disease causing agents could be the biological agents (bacteria, virus, protozoa, etc.), physical, chemical, mechanical, nutrient and social.

A. The agent characteristics for the biological agents are:

Virulence: It is the degree of pathogenicity; the disease evoking power of a micro-organism in a given host. This is numerically expressed as the ratio of the number of cases of overt infection to the total number infected, as determined by immunoassay. It denotes the relative infectiousness of a micro-organism or its ability to overcome the defences of the host. *Pathogenicity* means the capacity of micro-organisms to cause disease or morbid symptoms.

When death is the only criterion of severity of infection, attack rate and case fatality rate is important. *Case fatality rate (for infectious disease) is the* proportion of infected individuals who die of the infection. This is a function of the severity of the infection and is heavily influenced by how many mild cases are not diagnosed.

B. The host factors could be biological, socioeconomic and demographic. Susceptibility and immunity to infection are the two major factors that can determine if an individual will catch infections.

Susceptible: It is a person or animal liable to contract a disease if exposed to an infectious agent since he has not acquired immunity to a particular disease by a previous infection or by vaccination.

However, an *immune person* is one who possesses specific protective antibodies or cellular immunity following a previous infection or immunisation, or is so conditioned by such previous specific experience so as to respond adequately with production of antibodies, sufficient to protect from illness following an exposure to the specific infectious agent of the disease.

Immunity: Immunity means non-susceptibility (resistance) of the body to a given disease, or a given organism. Thus, it may not be necessary that all the persons exposed simultaneously to the same infectious agent under similar conditions will develop the disease. These are the ones that are non-susceptible and immune to infection, while in those who develop the disease, the degrees of severity may vary.

The various forms of immunity may be summarised as:

Natural or innate immunity: It is the resistance offered by the body under the normal conditions without any external stimulation of previous infection. It is either possessed from birth or acquired during growth (Fig. 14.1).

Natural protective measures produced in the body against infection: There are three principal means of protection which the body can produce:

1. *Phagocytosis,* which is an action, some of the white blood cells possess, of encircling and ingesting invading organisms.
2. *Antitoxins* are chemical substances produced in the blood serum in the presence of toxins in the body.
3. *Antibodies* are similar to antitoxins but more specific in their action.

Antigen: It is a substance usually protein in nature which when introduced into the tissues stimulates the body to produce specific protective material called

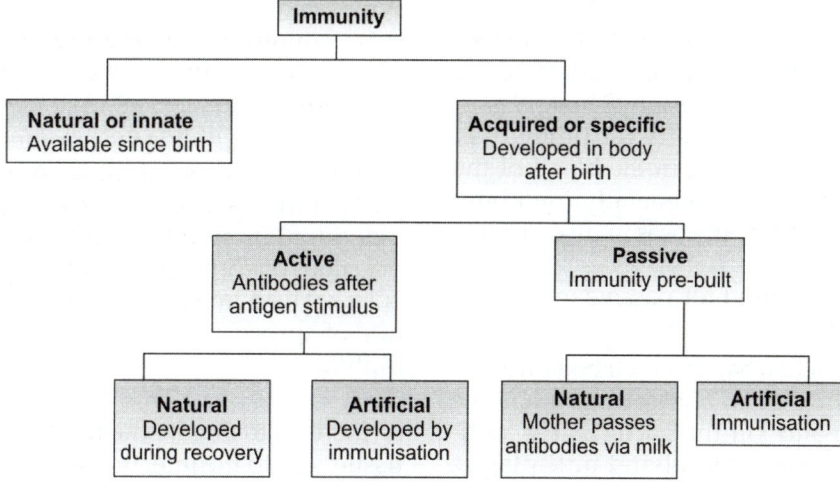

Fig. 14.1 Different types of immunity

antibodies. These are protective entities produced as a result of stimulation of the body's immune system by antigenic substances. Antigens commonly used to produce immunity through vaccines are of three types:

1. Live attenuated organisms, e.g. BCG vaccine
2. Killed organisms against typhoid, cholera, whooping cough, injectable polio, etc.
3. Toxins against diphtheria, tetanus, etc.

Antibodies: An antibody is a substance of the nature of a protein, which appears in the body in consequence of invasion by the antigen.

Acquired immunity: Immunity may be acquired in two ways, i.e. active and passive.

a. *Active immunity*: Antibodies are formed due to reaction of a person's own tissues in acquiring resistance. Body cells are actively stimulated to produce antibodies by natural or artificial means, i.e. antigens from a previous clinical or subclinical infection, or as a result of inoculation with germs or their products. This may be:

   1. *Natural active acquired immunity*: For some diseases, an attack of certain infectious disease confers upon a person, a certain amount of immunity from a second attack, e.g. chickenpox.
   2. *Artificial active acquired immunity*: It is due to inoculation of certain material containing antigen substances derived from bacteria or viruses. It gives an individual, a protection to guard against potential future exposure for a certain period, e.g. toxoids/vaccines.

b. *Passive immunity*: It is acquired by introduction of antibodies produced in some other immune person or an animal of the same or another species. Passive immunity is acquired through:

   i. *Transplacental*: Antibodies transferred to baby from mother through placenta in the intrauterine life.
   ii. Inoculation of sera extracted from immune blood or serum from convalescents or animals.

Passive immunity is effective for immidiate action however, it lasts for a short duration. Thus, it is of particular value in treatment, chiefly for tiding over crisis when antibodies are lacking in the blood of the patient. Passive immunisation is generally used both for curative and prophylactic purposes in diseases like tetanus, diphtheria, etc.

Antisera are commonly used for passive immunity. The anti-serum may be:

Antibacterial serum: When bacterial cell body itself is used in the manufacture of an anti-serum, it has the power to agglutinate and kill the bacteria, e.g. anti-streptococcal, anti-meningococcal and anti-plague serum.

Antitoxic serum: In this type, filtered toxin of bacteria is used. It has power to neutralise toxins of the organisms, e.g. anti-diphtheritic and anti-tetanic serum.

Convalescent or antiviral sera: In viral diseases like measles and poliomyelitis, the serum of convalescent cases contains specific antibodies for the virus. They have been used for passive immunisation. They are not likely to produce any serum reaction, since they have no foreign protein.

Disadvantages of using sera for producing passive immunity is that they may cause allergy or hypersensitivity in the recipient due to the foreign protein introduced into the body by injection. The *hypersensitivity reaction/anaphylaxis* may occur within seconds of injection in humans where the symptoms of a severe shock may set in followed by rashes, joint pains and oedema subsequently. The shock may even terminate fatally. Thus, to avoid anaphylactic shock, the sensitivity is tested by injecting a small dose (2 ml) intradermally before administering the serum in any person who is to be given serum. Sensitivity is indicated by redness and swelling at the site of inoculation which starts appearing within a few minutes and develops into a wheel in less than an hour. In case of no sensitivity, therapeutic dose can be given 4 to 6 hours later or by giving divided doses at hourly intervals until the full amount has been injected. A hypodermic injection of adrenaline administered at the same time will lessen the danger of anaphylactic shock.

Serum rashes and serum sickness: Serum rashes sometimes occur in people with an allergic tendency from 7 to 11 days after the injection has been given. Serum rashes give rise to great irritation, for which calamine lotion has a soothing effect, but they usually fade away within a day or two and there may be no other symptoms. Sometimes the patient has a certain degree of pyrexia accompanied with pains in joints and muscles. This condition, in which the rash is only one symptom, is known as serum sickness and it is much more common than anaphylaxis occurring in about 10% of those patients who have been given injections of serum.

Herd immunity: It is the immunity or the resistance of of a group of people or a community against any particular disease. It has greater importance than individual immunity while studying the spread of an infectious disease. Epidemic occurs when herd immunity is low. Herd immunity is important for lowering the rate of spread of infections in diseases like polio and diphtheria.

Local immunity: This term was formerly employed by Besredka to denote the resistance which is offered by tissue cells to the infecting agents. Its use is being made in creating a local immunity against diseases like poliomyelitis through oral polio vaccine which builds gut immunity and thereby prevent the spread of infection through natural route.

Vaccines: Vaccines are immunobiological substance designed to produce antibodies against specific diseases. These are the antigenic products that are injected in the body to produce desired protective antibody by stimulating the immune mechanism. The vaccines may be prepared from live-attenuated organisms, inactivated or killed organisms, extracted cellular fractions, toxoids or a combination of these.

a. *Live-attenuated vaccines:* *Attenuation* is a process where the capacity of the infectious agent to produce disease (virulence) is reduced whereas the capacity to multiply and stimulate production of antibodies is retained. Live-attenuated vaccines (*BCG against tuberculosis, measles and oral polio*) are produced from live-attenuated organisms. These are more potent as the organism injected multiply and stimulate antibody production without causing the disease in the recipient. The immunity produced from live-attenuated vaccines lasts longer, however, takes some time to come to effect after injection of vaccine. These need to be stored properly to maintain their efficacy. These vaccines should not be given in people with low immunity, e.g. in malnourished individuals, HIV positive patients and other immunodeficiency states.

b. *Inactivated or killed vaccines:* These contain organisms either inactivated or killed by heat or chemicals, e.g. *Pertussis vaccine*. These are usually safer but less efficacious than the live-attenuated vaccines and require a series of doses to bring about the desired effect.

c. *Toxoids:* Organisms, like *Clostridium tetani* and *Clostridium diphtheriae* produce exotoxins that are used for production of vaccine after detoxication. These are safe and highly specific as these produce antibodies against the toxin component and not against the bacteria as a whole.

d. *Vaccines produced from extracts or cellular fractions:* A subunit or component of bacteria is used to produce vaccine as a polysaccharide component of cell wall in case of meningococcus.

e. *Combination vaccines:* More than one type of immunizing agent is used to produce the vaccine, e.g. DPT where diphtheria and tetanus toxoids are used whereas live component of Pertussis is used.

The term '*polyvalent*' is used when two or more strains of same species of bacteria are used in preparing a vaccine.

Immunoglobulin preparations are used for inducing artificial passive immunity. Normal human immunoglobulin (or specific) and antisera are the two types of preparations that can be used for prophylaxis of viral and bacterial infections and in the replacement of antibodies in immunodeficient persons.

a. *Normal human immunoglobulin (HIg) extracted from the serum from convalescent patients of* measles to prevent disease in highly susceptible patients. Live vaccine should not be given for 12 weeks after injection of HIg.

b. *Antisera* are produced from non-human sources like horses as in tetanus, gas gangrene, botulism, diphtheria and anti-snake venom. However, there is a higher possibility of serum sickness and anaphylaxis reactions.

The table regarding the recommended schedule of routine immunization as per the UIP is given subsequently. Table 14.1 summarises immunization schedule as per UIP.

c. Environmental factors include physical, social and biological environment.

Table 14.1: Immunisation schedule

1. For pregnant women, two injections of tetanus toxoid should be given at an interval of one month each, the first one as soon as the pregnancy is detected

2. Interval between two doses should ideally be 4–6 weeks and not less than one month in any case

3. Mild fever and minor cough, colds, etc. should not be considered as contraindications to vaccination

4. Normal gammaglobulins have the value of producing modified measles (when given between 4th and 6th day of the incubation period; and modifying or suppressing attack of infectious hepatitis

5. No vaccine should be ever given intravenously as it can produce death

   a. **Measles** (i) for complete protection, a single dose of gammaglobulin 0.3 ml per kg of body weight within 5 days after exposure, (ii) for attenuation dosage should be 0.05 ml per kg of body weight

   b. **Mumps:** For prevention or attenuation of gamma-globulin in dosage of 0.2 ml/kg of body weight within 3 days of exposure

   c. **Infective hepatitis:** For protection, a single dose of 0.04 ml per kg is recommended

   d. **Serum hepatitis:** Two doses of gammaglobulin 10 ml each at an interval of one month are recommended

In view of costs and short duration of passive immunity, it is recommended only for selective situations.

14.5 STAGES OF AN INFECTIOUS DISEASE

Once a host is infected, all infectious diseases pass through the following stages which vary in duration in different diseases. These stages are:

1. Incubation period.

2. *The onset or prodromal stage:* This commences when the first symptoms appear or are experienced by

the patient and continues until the condition is well developed.

3. *The period of advance or fastigium:* All the symptoms are now increasing in severity, until a climax is reached. In those diseases associated with eruption, the rash becomes fully developed. The term "fastigium" is sometimes reserved for the climax only not for a period as a whole and it lasts as long as high temperature is maintained.

4. *Period of defervescence:* All the symptoms are now decreasing in severity and the patient is feeling quite comfortable.

5. *Period of convalescence:* The patient has completely overcome the invaders and their toxins, but he is suffering from a variable degree of exhaustion and a certain amount of tissue waste. He needs fresh air, nourishing food, tonics and graduated exercise until his health is fully restored.

14.6 PREVENTION AND CONTROL

Thus accordingly, for the prevention and control of transmission of infections, the intervention has to be made at all or either of the three factors.

Levels of Prevention

Leavell's levels of prevention

Stage of disease	Level of prevention	Type of response
Pre-disease	Primary	Health promotion and specific protection
Latent	Secondary	Presymptomatic diagnosis and treatment
Symptomatic	Tertiary	Disability limitation for early symptomatic diseases, rehabilitation for late symptomatic diseases

Primordial prevention consists of actions and measures that inhibit the emergence of risk factors in the form of environmental, economic, social and behavioural conditions and cultural patterns of living, etc. For example, many adult health problems (e.g. obesity, hypertension) have their early origins in childhood, because this is the time when lifestyles are formed (e.g. smoking, eating patterns, physical exercise). The main intervention is through individual and mass education.

Prevention and control of infection: For the prevention and control of infections, the measures to control the reservoir or source of infection, breaking the chain of transmission, and reducing the susceptibility of infection among susceptible by building their immunity.

A. *Control the source of infection or reservoir:* The most important step in prevention and control of communicable disease is its early identification and management.

i. *Early identification and management* of cases is needed for treatment of cases, for epidemiological investigations, to study the time, place and person distribution and thereby institute control measures.

ii. *Notification:* This term means immediate intimation regarding occurrence of every case of an infectious disease to the concerned health authorities. It may be the municipal medical officer of health or district medical officer of health. As per the International Health Regulations (IHRs), certain diseases are notifiable (**notifiable diseases).** Cholera, plaque, yellow fever are notifiable under IHR 1969 whereas louse-borne typhus fever, relapsing fever, paralytic polio, malaria, viral influenza A, SARS, smallpox, etc. are under surveillance by WHO. IHRs have been required in 2005 and now include containment of spread of Public Health Emergencies of International Concern (PHEIC) across the international goods which includes new emerging and reemerging disease conditions.

Any medical practitioner, who examines or diagnoses a case; or guardian or a relation of a case can notify the disease to local health authorities.

Prompt notification not only enables the authorities to find the real source of infection, isolate the patient, treat him and to do necessary disinfection but also helps to control and prevent the spread of infection in the community. Besides it also provides an opportunity for investigating the source of any epidemic disease and investigation of the environmental conditions that lead to the spread of infection.

Surveillance: It is the practice of close supervision of contacts of a communicable disease for the purpose of prompt recognition of its infection or illness but without restricting their movements.

iii. *Isolation:* It is the separation, for the period of communicability of an infected person, from other persons in such places and under such conditions as will prevent the direct or indirect transmission of an infectious agent from infected person to the healthy ones. The period of isolation for a disease should be for the maximum period of communicability of the disease. An infective case may be isolated in an infectious diseases or isolation hospital or at home.

Hospital isolation

- *Barrier nursing:* It is suitable for nursing patients where direct or indirect contact is necessary for the transmission of the infection.

There may be a screen between two patients which should mark "barrier" between the patients. Separate gowns, thermometer, feeding utensils, washing and toilet requisites should be used for each patient under isolation.

- *Cubicle nursing:* It is when the patient beds are separated from each other by partitions. The partitions are usually about 7 feet in height, made almost entirely of glass to provide good light and a common airspace above the partition. When the partition extends to the ceiling so that the patient is quite cut off from others, the system is known as *chamber nursing.* Each cubicle or chamber should contain a washbasin and have a swing door. The nursing technique is the same as in bed isolation.

- *Bed isolation:* It is very similar to barrier nursing except that feeding and toilet requisites are not kept separately for each patient but are sterilised immediately after use and kept with other general equipment of the ward.

- Patients can also be isolated at home in case sufficient space is available for the sick room to be detached, preferably on the upper storey with minimal furniture around.

- *Adequate ventilation must be ensured by keeping* the windows open. Attendants and nurses should be allowed to go in the sick room after optimum asepsis. Attendants selected should be immune to the disease. The soiled clothes of the patient, excreta and remnants of food and utensils should be disinfected properly or buried underground or burnt away. Minimum visitors should be allowed to enter the sick room. Anti-fly and anti-mosquito measures must be taken to exclude flies and mosquitoes from the sick room. After the danger of infection is believed to have ceased, the patient should be well washed and bathed thoroughly with disinfectant. In case of death, the dead body should be completely covered in a sheet soaked in corrosive sublimate or carbolic lotion. Subsequently, it should be buried or cremated as soon as possible. The sick room should be thoroughly disinfected after having been vacated by the patient.

iv. *Treatment:* Treatment of communicable disease in the reservoir aims to reduce the communicability of disease, cut short the duration of illness and prevent the development of secondary cases. However, inadequate or incomplete treatment may induce drug resistance in cases and may interfere with the control efforts.

v. *Quarantine:* It consists of detaining or isolating healthy persons or domestic animals, who have been exposed to communicable disease, for a specified time after their departure from an infected place. The time of quarantine should cover at least the longest incubation period known of a particular disease. The quarantine may be:

a. *Inward quarantine:* When quarantine is imposed on a healthy town for its own protection, or

b. *Outward quarantine:* When it is imposed on an infected town for the protection of the surrounding area.

1. *International quarantine:* It means compulsory isolation at the port, of all persons coming from an infected place or persons who have been in contact with the case of an infectious disease, against which quarantine has been imposed, e.g. 5 days for cholera and 6 days for plague.

2. *Scholastic quarantine:* Children from an infected house during the period of quarantine should not be permitted to attend school until the last case in the house has ceased to be infectious.

3. *Domestic quarantine:* All persons, particularly children, should be strictly prohibited to enter an infected house. All members of such an infected house be kept under observation for a period equal to the incubation period of that disease.

vi. For effective isolation, quarantine and concurrent/terminal disinfection, incubation period and infective communicability period (i.e. the period when infection can be transmitted from one person to another) should be known. This information for some important diseases is given as under:

S. no.	Disease	Incubation period	Infective period
1.	Chicken-pox	2–3 weeks	A week after appearance of the rash, chickenpox is not considered infectious
2.	Cholera	1–5 days	Until stools are negative, usually 7–14 days, long-term carriers have been reported in cholera
3.	Diphtheria	2–5 days	Till 2 cultures taken from nose and throat taken 24 hours apart are negative, usually 14–28 days after onset of the disease
4.	Infectious hepatitis	15–50 days	3 weeks
5.	Influenza	1–3 days	Usually one week from onset

(Contd...)

(Contd...)

6.	Measles	10 days	4–5 days before and after appearance of rash
7.	Mumps	2–3 weeks	Until the swelling subsides
8.	Pertussis	7–14 days	About 4 weeks after appearance of whoop
9.	Poliomye-litis	7–14 days or even more	Probably during later part of the incubation period to 1–2 weeks of the disease
10.	Rubella	2–3 weeks	From onset of catarrhal conditions for 5–7 days
11.	Typhoid	2–3 weeks	Until urine and stools are negative

B. *Interruption in the chain of transmission*: It broadly covers all the mechanisms to re-establish the ecological balance between the agent, host and environment, the disturbance of which has led to the occurrence of the disease. Diseases transmitted by poor personal hygiene like food- and water-borne illnesses can be prevented by improved personal hygiene measures, clean hand washing practices, adequate water treatment ranging from boiling to chlorination. In case of vector-borne diseases, the vector control measures like chemical and biological control of adults and larvae, destruction of breeding places and environmental sanitation measures.

C. *Improving host defenses*: A multitude of factors is important for improving the host defenses that include immunisation (discussed in details previously), adequate nutrition, personal hygiene practices and chemoprophylaxis.

Chemoprophylaxis implies the protection from or prevention of disease. This may be causal prophylaxis (complete prevention of infection by elimination of causal agent) or clinical prophylaxis (prevention of clinical symptoms).

14.7 DISINFECTION

This term means process of application of a disinfectant for a sufficient length of time in adequate quantity and strength, so as to kill the specific organisms of infectious diseases.

Concurrent disinfection: It means immediate destruction of infectious material (*viz.* faeces, urine, sputum, etc.) discharged from the body of an infected person, throughout the course of his illness.

Terminal disinfection: It is the process of rendering the personal clothing and immediate physical environment of the patient free from the possibility of conveying infection to others at the end of illness or soon after his death.

Sterilisation: It is the destruction of all microbial life, i.e. micro-organisms and their spores by physical and chemical means.

Fumigation: It is a process by which destruction of insects and animals, especially anthropods and rodents forms, is accomplished by the employment of gaseous compounds. These compounds paralyse oxygen carrying system of insects and prevent cellular respiration.

Disinfectant: It is a substance which destroys harmful pathogenic microbes, virus, fungi or protozoa (not usually spores) which cause communicable diseases.

Bacteriostatic: It is a substance which inhibits the growth of micro-organisms.

Antiseptic: It is a substance which retards or prevents the growth and activity of micro-organisms, but does not necessarily destroy them. It delays or prevents decomposition and fermentation without destroying the micro-organisms involved in the process, e.g. sugar in jams and salt in fish, etc. Some disinfectants in weaker solutions act as antiseptics, i.e. bichloride of mercury and formalin in the ratio of 1 in 30,000 and 1 in 5,000, respectively.

Asepsis: A state of asepsis is said to exist when an article is absolutely free from pathogenic micro-organisms and their spores. Such an article is said to be sterile.

Deodorant or deodoriser: It is a substance having the power to destroy or to neutralise the unpleasant odour of organic matter undergoing fermentation, or putrefaction, e.g. charcoal. Some deodorants destroy offensive odours simply by substituting an agreeable or a strong smell without destroying the 'organisms giving rise to putrefactive odours. Volatile oils having pungent odours are not deodorants. They simply cover one smell over the other. Formalin is both a disinfectant and a deodorant.

Insecticides: These are chemical substances having specific effects on insects and act as a poison to kill them. They may, however, act as a repellant also.

Residual insecticides: These are poisonous substances, which adhere to the body of insects and they cause a slow progressive paralysis leading to death.

Repellents: They help in keeping the insects away from biting human beings.

14.8 CLASSIFICATION OF DISINFECTANTS

These are divided into three groups:

1. *Natural*	Fresh air and sunlight
2. *Physical*	a. Dry heat, (i) burning, (ii) hot dry air
	b. Moist heat, (i) boiling, (ii) steam
	c. Radiation
3. *Chemical*	a. Solids
	b. Liquids
	c. Gases
	d. Aerosols

1. Natural Disinfectants

Fresh air and sunlight destroy infection and limit the spread of infectious diseases. By drying and desiccation due to the action of air and sunlight, the micro-organisms are attenuated and their multiplication is inhibited. Oxygen of the air plays an important part in killing micro-organisms.

Sunlight is a strong germicide due to actinic rays, especially ultraviolet rays. The action of the actinic rays on the atmosphere is such that they form ozone and hydrogen peroxide, which are powerful oxidising agents. The diphtheria microbes, for example, are destroyed by an hour's exposure to direct sunlight, whereas tubercle microbes are killed even more rapidly. However, the yellow and red rays of the sun possess no disinfecting power.

2. Physical Disinfectants

a. *Dry Heat*

i. *Burning*: This is the best means of disinfection. It should be employed for articles of small value like soiled dressing material, swabs, etc. Burning is done in a small destructor furnace and should be done in open air. Cheap infected dwellings or huts may be burnt away, particularly where a disease like plague has occurred. Cholera and enteric infected excreta should be burnt by mixing it with sawdust and kerosene oil. Sputum and other discharges are best destroyed by burning.

ii. *Hot dry air*: It has very little or no penetrating power to destroy spores. Hence, high temperature has to be maintained for a long time at a stretch, which ruins nearly all fabrics. So it is not employed for this reason. It is, however, useful for the disinfection of surgical instruments, glassware, dressings, etc. which are otherwise spoiled by the action of water or steam. Lice and other insects are, however, effectively killed.

b. *Moist Heat*

i. *Boiling*: It is a very efficient method. Boiling for 5–10 minutes is sufficient for killing ordinary germs, but for spores, boiling should be continued for at least half an hour. Clothes stained with blood or faeces should be first washed with soap and washing soda and then boiled, otherwise a permanent stain will remain behind. Germicidal power of boiling water is enhanced, if 2% of washing soda is added to it. Boiling is not suited for disinfecting woollen material as it shrinks. Linen, hankerchiefs, bed sheets, bed pans, urinals, cooking utensils, etc. are disinfected by this method. This process cannot be depended upon in hills or at high altitudes. The boiling point of water falls at an average rate of 1°C for every 1,000 feet (304.80 metres) ascent. This process is expensive on a large scale but is commonly used on a small scale.

The disadvantage of boiling is that it is a slow process and is not suitable for matresses and thick beddings, etc. Moreover, it fixes albuminous stains.

ii. *Steam*: It is the most efficient method of applying moist heat for disinfection purposes. It is used in three ways:
   a. Current steam
   b. Saturated steam
   c. Superheated steam

   a. **Current steam:** When steam is generated at ordinary atmospheric pressure of 760 mm Hg at a temperature of 100°C and is allowed to escape, it is called *current steam*. This is also called *low pressure steam*. It has got the same disinfecting power as boiling water.

   Current steam disinfector is cheap at the outset but expensive in the long run because it consumes more fuel. Moreover, it has the drawback of delivering articles wet and is therefore not so suitable for rapid work in big disinfecting stations.

   b. **Saturated steam:** When steam is generated by boiling water in a closed vessel, e.g. in a steam boiler or a kettle, steam accumulates under pressure and longer the period for which water is boiled the greater will be the pressure. The steam so generated is called *saturated steam*. It is not only compressed in small volume but is also at a high temperature. There is always a definite relationship between the pressure of the steam, and its temperature, e.g. steam at 20 lb (9.07 kg) pressure, is at 129°C. Steam up to 5 lb (2.27 kg) pressure is low pressure steam and when pressure is increased to 10 lb (4.54 kg) then it is called *high pressure steam*.

   When current steam or saturated steam comes into contact with cooler articles, it immediately gets condensed and in doing so, parts, with its latent heat and shrinks to 1/600th part of its volume. Thus, a partial vacuum is created, which is at once filled up by more steam from behind and so on. It thus raises the temperature in the vicinity to a high degree. This process of condensing will continue until the temperature of the whole bundle of articles to be disinfected is raised to that of the steam. When the disinfection is complete, no further condensation of steam occurs. Saturated steam is better than superheated steam because it is near its condensation point and has got more rapid power of penetration.

c. **Superheated steam:** It can be generated in two ways:

1. If steam is heated without raising the pressure, the temperature of steam is highly raised, it is called *superheated steam.*
2. It may also be generated by boiling saline solution which boils at a higher temperature than ordinary water.

It has got properties similar to those of dry gas and has no value as a disinfectant as it has lost its physical character as vapour. It cannot condense until it has parted with its super heat.

Before using a physical disinfectant, its effects on colour and texture of the articles to be disinfected must be considered. Woollen goods as well as those composed of cotton and linen will not stand high temperature. Woollen materials shrink and acquire a yellow tinge when exposed to steam at about 121°C for half an hour. Most fabrics will stand a temperature of 110°C without undergoing any permanent injury. Cotton and linen will bear 110°C dry heat for four hours but 112°C moist heat only for half an hour. Cotton is scorched at a temperature of 150°C. Scorching occurs comparatively sooner with woollen material. 126°C moist heat applied for 30 minutes turns white woollen blankets yellow, diminishes the tensile strength of hair and causes shrinkage.

Steam disinfecting station: It should be easily accessible and have a van of its own for bringing infected articles for disinfection. Separate sheds should be provided for vans to bring infected articles and for those to return the disinfected articles. The infected articles can be transported in long canvas bags having distinguishing numbers, woven into them or permanently stamped on them. The advantage of putting articles in bags with numbers on them is that the owner on the disinfected side can present his token and receive the articles after disinfection. Infected articles should be put in bags, which are stitched and taken to the disinfecting station in a properly closed tin lined van. The whole bag is put in the disinfector without opening.

Building: The building should be constructed according to improved sanitary principles. The floor should be made of marble slabs, tiles or polished cement; walls should have tiled dado, i.e. 4.5 feet (1.37 metre) of white tiles from the floor and rest of the walls should be distempered with a white waterproof paint. All angles should be rounded and no projections permitted for accumulation of dust. Window space should be ample so as to provide full light and free ventilation.

The actual building is constructed in two halves, completely separated from each other by a dividing wall provided with a fixed observation window. The two halves in no way should directly communicate with each other except through the disinfecting machine since one half is the infected side which is meant for receiving infected clothes articles, etc. The disinfector opens on this side. The workers on this end should wear overalls and the infected clothings, beddings, etc. should be run into the disinfector over a trolley or a sliding cage. The door of the disinfector is closed and steam let in. The time of exposure depends upon the nature and bulk of articles and the pressure of steam employed for disinfection. When the disinfection is complete, the disinfector is opened from the other half of the shed, the disinfected clothes, beddings, etc. are taken out and returned to their owners. A different van, with a separate garage, should be used for this purpose.

There should be some arrangement for ascertaining the efficiency of the disinfector. A raw egg is placed in the centre of the bundle of clothes, and this is inspected after the disinfection. If it is completely boiled, it indicates that thorough disinfection has taken place. If it is not completely boiled, it indicates that the steam has not reached the centre of the bundle of clothes. It can also be tested by placing a culture of suitable mircro-organisms and finding out whether they have been killed or not, by recording thermometers or by the use of a metal thermocouple which makes contact and indicates that a certain temperature has been reached.

Different Varieties of Disinfectors

1. *Washington Lyons (Manlove and Alliott) high pressure disinfector:* In this type, saturated steam under pressure is used at a temperature of 115° to 120°C. It is an elongated cylinder, oval in section, with a door at each end. The disinfecting chamber is surrounded by a jacket and steam is obtained from a separate boiler. The pressure at which it works is 15 to 20 lb per square inch or 1–1.35 kg per sq cm.

   There is an arrangement of producing a vacuum by aspirating air out of the chamber. In working it, steam is first admitted into the jacket to heat the chamber inside so that the steam may not be quickly condensed. Then a vacuum is produced for about 20 minutes. Subsequently steam is admitted inside the chamber for about 20 minutes after which vacuum is again made. A current of hot air is passed in the disinfector to dry the clothes. The disinfecting chamber is sufficiently large to admit beddings, etc. and is built in the partition wall between two rooms.

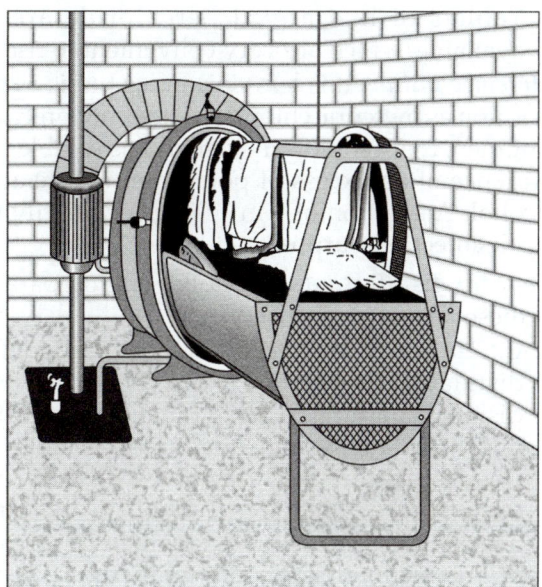

Fig. 14.2: Steam disinfector with cradle

2. *Thresh's current steam disinfector:* It is a low pressure disinfector and does not require the installation of a separate boiler. It consists of a chamber surrounded by a jacket. In this jacket, steam is generated from a saline solution usually calcium chloride solution, which raises the boiling point of water above 100°C without any extra pressure. The boiler is fed with water from a cistern. The time required for exposure of the infected articles is usually 30 minutes. The apparatus is simple, cheap and is best suited for use in small hospitals and municipalities. Although it is a low pressure mechanism, yet the steam is very hot as it is given off from water over 100°C.

3. *Lelean's sack disinfector* (*Fig. 14.3*): It is a current steam disinfector. It is light, simple and is comparatively a cheap apparatus. It consists of a long sack (made up of some material impervious to steam such as canvas), a boiler, a hose pipe and a stove. The sack, which is made up of steam-proof canvas, is suspended like a bell. Its open lower end has a purse string mouth, and the closed end is upward. The infected clothings are suspended by means of hooks fitted at the top of the sack. Steam is admitted at the top through the hose pipe as long as necessary. It is generated in a small boiler heated with a stove. Exposure for 30–60 minutes is sufficient for disinfection. It is easily portable and can be carried on a bicycle, and is used in some municipalities.

4. *Serbian barrel* (*Fig. 14.4*): It was first introduced in Serbia and Bulgaria during the typhus campaign and is the best method of steam disinfection and disinfestation of lice from clothes. It consists of a barrel with perforated bottom which rests on a

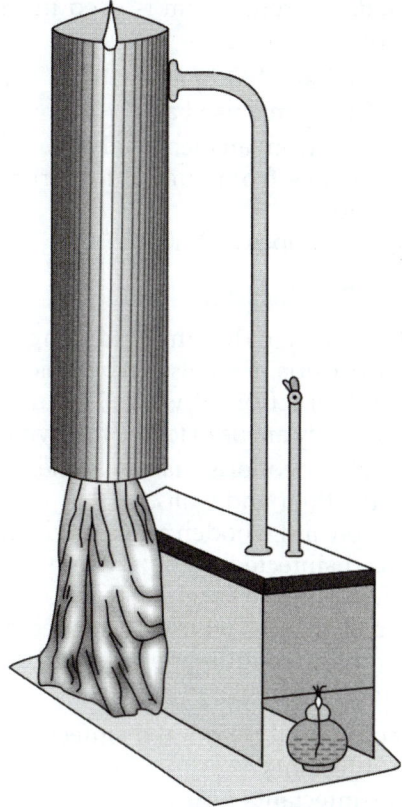

Fig. 14.3: Lelean's sack disinfector

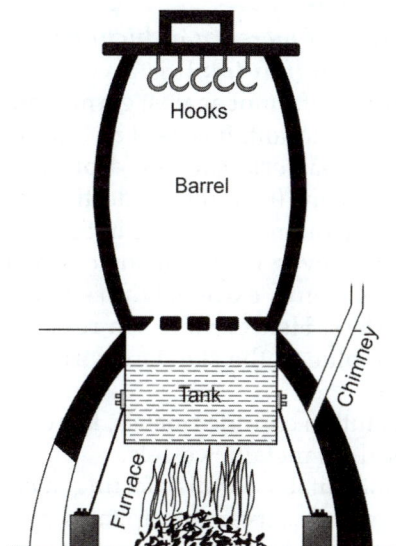

Fig. 14.4: Serbian barrel disinfector

sand bag collar to prevent the escape of steam, which enters the barrel through the perforated holes from a metal tank containing water upon which it rests. The top of the barrel is covered with a removable lid with hooks to hang infected articles, clothes, etc. The barrel with the boiler is placed on a brick-work frame forming the furnace. After about an hour's exposure to steam, the articles will be satisfactorily disinfected and disinfested. Current steam is used in this type of disinfector.

Radiation: It has also been utilised recently for sterilisation. The agents used are:

1. Infra-red rays from an electrically heated element.
2. Ultraviolet rays from sunlight or from mercury vapour lamps.
3. Ionising by isotopes or X-ray.

3. Chemical Disinfectants

They chiefly act by oxidising and coagulating the protoplasm of bacteria. They also act by ionic coagulation, desiccation (abstraction of water) emulsoid action, absorption, etc. They are used for the following purposes:

1. To disinfect or deodorise, faeces, urine, sputum, etc.
2. To wash the floor and walls.
3. To wash iron and wooden articles, which cannot be otherwise disinfected.
4. To disinfect hands in surgical operations and certain cutting instruments, which are spoiled by boiling.
5. Gaseous disinfectants are used for disinfecting houses and buildings.

Most commonly used chemical disinfectants are:

a. Solid disinfectants
b. Liquid disinfectants
c. Gaseous disinfectants

Solid Disinfectants

1. *Perchloride of mercury or bichloride of mercury (corrosive sublimate):* It is a very valuable and powerful disinfectant against germs and spores but it is not a deodorant. It is used as 1 in 1,000 dilution which kills bacteria causing diphtheria, anthrax and typhoid in 10 minutes. It destroys spores, after an exposure of one hour, in 1 in 500 strength. This salt has, however, the following disadvantages:
   i. The solution is extremely poisonous and quite colourless. Hence, there is a reason for adding aniline blue in the standard formula, to impart colour.
   ii. The solution corrodes metals, therefore, it cannot be used for metallic vessels.
   iii. It is not suitable for disinfecting linen.
   iv. All mercuric salts are precipitated by albuminous compounds such as faeces and sputum. This has been overcome in the standard formula by the addition of hydrochloric acid. This solution can be used for disinfecting faeces, sputum, etc. provided they are not kept in metallic vessels. The formula generally used is:

Hydrargyri perchloride	...1/2 oz	(14.17 gm)
Hydrochloric acid	...1 oz	(28.34 gm)
Commercial aniline blue	...3 grs	(0.19 gm)
Water	...3 gallons	(13.62 litres)

Tablets of hydrargyri perchloride are also available, which are very convenient to use.

2. *Mercuric iodide:* It is less poisonous but is as good in action as mercuric chloride. It does not precipitate albumen, is not soluble in water but is soluble in the presence of an excess of potassium iodide and in alcohol. A solution of 1 in 1,000 is ordinarily used for disinfection purposes.

3. *Coal tar disinfectants:* The following preparations of these are generally used:
   i. *Carbolic acid or phenol:* It is obtained from distillation of coal tar. It is a cheap and useful disinfectant. It has a wide range of applications but should not be depended upon to kill spores. Crude carbolic acid dissolves in water with some difficulty therefore it should be thoroughly dissolved before use. It is stable in the presence of organic matter at room temperature. If used in a solution strength of 3.5 to 5%, it will kill ordinary sporeless bacilli within a few minutes to ten hours. It is used for mopping floors, walls and ceilings. Carbolic acid is non-corrosive to metals, so it is used for disinfecting knives, etc. However, it has a caustic effect on hands. It does not harm fabrics or affects their colour nor it coagulates albumin. It is poisonous and caustic.
   ii. *Coal tar derivatives:* These are obtained by the destructive distillation of coal and contain phenol, natural oils, resins, fatty oils and water. They are izal, cyllin, sanitas, iysol, jay's fluid, phenol, etc. They are allied to carbolic acid but are not so poisonous and are used in strength of 1 to 3% in the form of an emulsion. Their activity depends upon the fineness of the emulsion and they are very efficient like carbolic acid.

4. *Potassium permanganate:* Its disinfecting powers are due to oxidation. It is used for disinfection of water especially during the outbreak of cholera. It is generally used for disinfection in 5% solution strength and in less than half per cent strength, it acts only as a deodorant. A weak solution of potassium permanganate is used for disinfecting infected fruits and vegetables during an outbreak of cholera epidemic.

5. *Lime:* It is one of the cheapest and most powerful disinfectants. Freshly burnt quick lime should be used. It is used to disinfect water, stools, floors, stables, etc. 10–20% aqueous suspension of lime called milk of lime kills organisms, other than spores, in a few hours. For stools, equal quantity should be used and thoroughly mixed with a stick and allowed to stand for 2 hours.

6. *Chlorinated lime or bleaching powder:* It is a white hygroscopic powder with a feeble odour of chlorine and bitter saline taste. It readily absorbs

both moisture and carbon dioxide from the air with constant liberation of chlorine and thereby it obviously loses strength. It is prepared by passing chlorine gas over slaked lime. The reaction is represented by the following equation:

$$Ca(OH)_2 + Cl_2 = CaOCl_2 + H_2O$$

It is unstable and deteriorates on keeping. It should be kept in airtight containers. A good quality of bleaching powder should contain about 33% of available chlorine. It is a mixture of calcium chloride and calicum hypochlorite. Owing to its affinity for moisture, which it slowly absorbs from the air, it soon becomes pasty and loses some of its chlorine. Hypochlorites present in lime are then reduced to chlorides and thus it becomes inert. Freshly prepared chlorinated lime should have a very light odour of free chlorine. A strong odour of the gas indicates its deterioration. Chlorinated lime not only bleaches, but is also destructive to fabrics. It may be used as a dry powder or may be dissolved and used in the form of a solution as a surface disinfectant. As a dry powder, it is sprinkled over damp corners of cellars, privies, latrines, drains, etc. where it acts as a deodorant and a desiccant. It is also used in a powder form to disinfect excreta.

Five percent solution of bleaching powder can be used for disinfecting stools. It is mixed with a stick and allowed to act for 1 to 2 hours. 1 in 30 solution of bleaching powder is used for disinfecting rooms.

Liquid Disinfectants

These are very largely used in public health work, in view of the convenience and easy applicability. These consist of solutions or emulsions of certain chemical disinfectants in water.

Requirements of a good disinfectant: These are:
1. It should be homogeneous and should have definite efficiency for a particular type of organisms.
2. It should be a powerful germicide, rapid in action, having a great power of penetration.
3. It should be stable in presence of organic matter. It should not be rendered inert, in the presence of faeces.
4. It should not have any injurious effect on human tissues and material submitted for disinfection.
5. It should easily mix in water and form a uniform emulsion in all proportions.
6. It should be fairly cheap, and should not act on metals, bleach pigments or spoil fabrics. It should be neither toxic nor caustic in action.
7. It should be a high solvent for grease.

Standardisation of disinfectants: Two methods are used for this purpose in judging the germicidal value of liquid disinfectants:

1. *Rideal-Walker or carbolic acid coefficient test*: Through this test, bacteriological property of a disinfectant is compared with that of carbolic acid (phenol) against a standard culture of *Salmonella typhi* in the laboratory for 2½ 5, 7½, 10, 12½ and 15 minutes periods.

Method
   i. Several tubes containing 5 cc of the disinfectant, in different dilutions, are taken.
   ii. To each test tube 5 drops of the culture of bacillus typhosus (*Salmonella typhi*) are added and the tubes are shaken well.
   iii. After every 24 minutes, sub-cultures are prepared from these inoculated tubes into 5 cc broth for 15 minutes, e.g. 2½, 5, 7½, 10, 12½ and 15 minutes, i.e. in all 6 series of sub-cultures are prepared.
   iv. For 48 hours, all subcultures are incubated at 37°C and the presence or absence of the growth is noted.
   v. The same process is carried out within the same time, with same culture, with different dilutions of carbolic acid.
   vi. From the table of result, the two dilutions having the same effects in the same time are seen and thereafter carbolic acid coefficient of the disinfectant is calculated.

2. *The British Admiralty Method for standardisation of disinfectants*: It is the best method and is done as follows:
   i. 10 cc of the disinfectant is diluted to 1000 cc with sterile artificial seawater (32 gm of Tidman's sea salt dissolved in 1 litre of water) and allowed to stand for 24 hours. A portion of this mixture is removed from the middle with a pipette for test purposes. The standard is crystallised phenol, also dissolved in artificial seawater and the test organisms is bacillus typhosus 24 hours' culture in a nutrient broth at 37°C.
   ii. Organisms remain in contact with the disinfectant for 10 minutes. The temperature of the broth and the room being 10°C and 18°C, respectively.
   iii. The germicidal value of the disinfectant is determined in the presence of a definite amount of organic matter consisting of gelatine and finely ground rice starch (0.5% of gelatine and 0.5% of rice starch in suspension in sterile water).
   iv. 0.25 cc of the culture is added to 5 cc of the above solution and 5 cc of the disinfectant. The resultant mixture is shaken thoroughly. After 10 minutes, a sub-culture is made in broth, incubated for 48 hours at 37°C and the presence or absence of the growth is noted.
   v. *Chick-Martin test* is a recent modification in which sterile faeces or yeast is used.

Gaseous Disinfectants

A germicidal gas is an ideal weapon to destroy pathogenic micro-organisms, which are to be dealt with for public health work, especially for the terminal disinfection by reaching all portions of the house. A gas lessens the risk of any surface getting neglected, on which micro-organisms are lodged. The secret of doing successful disinfection with a gas is to obtain a large volume of gas in a short time. Presence of a certain amount of heat and moisture is necessary for carrying out disinfection effectively. The exact amount of moisture which is necessary depends upon the temperature. As a general working rule it may be stated that if the prevailing temperature is below 65°F (18.3°C) or if relative humidity is below 60%, the results become irregular and unreliable, especially if the place is both cold and dry. In cold weather, it may be necessary to artificially warm the room and in dry weather moisture is to be added to the room.

All the openings of the room should be completely closed and all cracks pasted over with thick paper so as to make the room as airtight as possible. The cubic space of the room is calculated, so as to ascertain the amount of the chemical to be used.

The drawbacks in the case of gaseous disinfectants are that most of the gases used are poisonous or irritant. Therefore, when a room is to be disinfected by a gaseous disinfectant, not only that all persons and animals from that room need to be evacuated but very often the surrounding premises are also required to be vacated. This is, therefore, one of the reasons as to why gaseous disinfectants are not much used in residential buildings. They are, however, used for destroying insects and vermin like rats in ships, godowns, etc.

1. *Formaldehyde gas:* It is a powerful disinfectant and is used in the form of vapour. It is generated by pouring liquid formalin over potassium permanganate crystals placed in a deep vessel. It neither tarnishes metal nor bleaches colour. It does not injure textiles even. It is very irritating to eyes and lungs in stronger dilutions. Its smell can easily be removed by sprinkling ammonia in the room. The temperature of the room should be between 60°F and 65°F (15.5°C and 18.3°C) and never less than that. In cold weather, if the room is not warmed and disinfection is performed, its effect will be nullified owing to low temperature. Therefore, in this type of disinfection, the room must be kept fairly warm. Formaldehyde gas is a weak insecticide, so it is useless as an antiplague measure. It, however, kills mosquitoes, house flies, lice and fleas. It has lower density than sulphur dioxide and chlorine gas and so it diffuses better and has greater power of penetration. Formalin vapours are particularly useful for disinfecting blankets, silks, furs, books, leather goods, toys, etc., which will not withstand steam disinfection (Fig. 14.5).

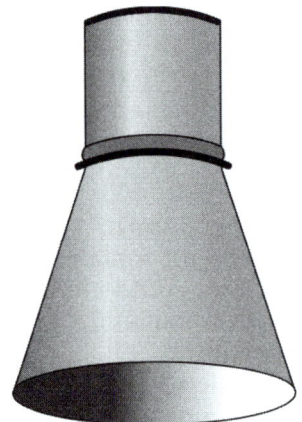

Fig. 14.5: Bucket for generating formaldehyde

It may be used in the following ways/methods

i. *Permanganate method:* Special tin buckets or jars are used for disinfecting 1,000 cubic ft (28.316 cubic metres) of space, 5 oz (141.75 gm) of potassium permanganate is placed in a jar and then on the top of it, 10–15 oz (283.49–425.23 gm) of 40% formalin diluted with an equal volume of water, is poured. There will be a violent effervescence and the formaldehyde gas will be set free in a few minutes. Naked fire should be avoided as it might give rise to explosion owing to inflammable character of the gas. This method is simple and effective and the period of disinfection should be about 6 hours.

ii. *Bleaching powder method:* For disinfecting 1,000 cubic feet (28.316 cubic metres) of space 2 lb (0.907 kg) of bleaching powder and 40 oz (1.13 kg) of formalin are required. The bleaching powder is first made into a paste with water, and formalin is poured into it.

iii. *Paraform method:* For disinfecting 1,000 cubic feet (28.316 cubic metres) of space 25 paraform tablets of one gm each are heated in a special paraform lamp (Alphormant lamp) (Fig. 14.6). By

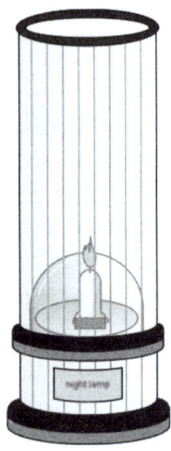

Fig. 14.6: Paraform lamp

heating formalin, the aldehyde changes into solid polymeroid paraform.

iv. *By Trillat's apparatus:* For disinfecting 1,000 cubic feet (28.316 cubic metres) space 0.5 to 1 litre of formochloral is used in this apparatus.

2. *Sulphur dioxide:* It is comparatively less effective than formaldehyde gas and is generally obtained by burning sulphur/except for tuberculous sputum, the results, with sulphur dioxide are as good as when formaldehyde is used. It is highly poisonous to mammalians and insects. Its germicidal action depends upon the presence of moisture, as the dry gas is inert. The moisture changes it into sulphurous acid. It bleaches all vegetable colours as well as aniline dyes. It attacks metals and acts on cotton and linen fabrics. It is especially valuable for disinfecting ships, cars, stables and places infested with vermin. It not only attacks germs, but also the animals concerning their spread. The room should be kept close for six hours after liberation of the gas.

Methods

i. For disinfecting 1,000 cubic feet (28.316 cubic metres) space 2–3 lb (0.907–1.36 kg) of powdered sulphur is put in a pot placed in a tub of water. The sulphur is powdered, then moistened with alcohol and ignited. Sulphur candles may be used in place of powdered sulphur.

ii. The same amount of sulphur powder be sprinkled over ignited charcoal. The walls and floors should be sprinkled with water.

iii. *Clayton's apparatus:* In it, sulphur dioxide and sulphur trioxide are generated. Sulphur is burnt in an iron generator. This gas has a great penetrating power. It is chiefly used for the destruction of vermin, particularly rats, bugs, lice, etc.

3. *Chlorine gas:* It is a disinfectant and a deodoriser as it has an affinity for hydrogen, when it liberates nascent oxygen which has a great affinity for organic matter and bacteria. Since it is a heavy gas, it should be generated as high as possible in a room. A certain amount of moisture is also required for disinfecting a room successfully with chlorine gas. It is more irritant to eyes than sulphur dioxide and bleaches all vegetable and aniline dyes. It is produced by the action of 1 lb (0.453 kg) of sulphuric acid or hydrochloric acid on 2 lb (0.9 kg) of bleaching powder for disinfecting 1,000 cubic feet (28.316 cubic metres) of space. All metal fittings and articles of silk and coloured articles should be removed from the room before chlorination, since it bleaches organic pigments, acts on metals and destroys organic matter.

4. *Cresol fumigation:* For 1,000 cubic feet (28.316 cubic metres) of space, about 6 oz (179.1 gm) of cresol is poured over smouldering cowdung cakes, about 20 in number, placed in a big iron pan in the centre of the room. In the past, this method was used freely for disinfecting plaguestricken houses in Punjab and proved to be of great value in killing rats, fleas. In buildings having high roofs, it is better to fix up a cloth across the room about 10–12 feet (3.04–3.66 metres) from the floor in order to prevent dense fumes of cresol diffusing higher up. The idea being to allow the dense fumes produced to act mainly on the floor. The fumes are absolutely safe for all articles, furniture, etc. It neither tarnishes metal nor bleaches fabrics. It is non-irritating to eyes, easily produced and is inexpensive. It is always preferable to use more than one pan in a big room.

5. *Hydrocyanic acid gas:* This gas has no action on bacteria. It is largely used to destroy rats, fleas, and other vermin on board the ships and pumped into rat holes in combating plague epidemic. It is highly penetrative, is chemically inactive and has no bleaching or tarnishing properties. It has practically replaced sulphur dioxide as a fumigant in the USA. The gas is highly poisonous and should not be used to disinfect any room unless the whole house has been thoroughly evacuated. For efficient disinfection the concentration of gas should be less than 1.5%. It should be used by a trained operator. It is generated by:

i. For disinfecting 1,000 cubic feet (28.316 cubic metres) of space, 5 oz (141.75 gm) of potassium cyanide, 7.5 oz (212.62 gm) of sulphuric acid and 10 oz (283.49 gm) of water are mixed and the gas is generated.

ii. Cyanogen chloride and zyklon B are used.

iii. Cyanogas is largely pumped in rat holes by a cyanogas pump. The gas is slowly evolved and kills rats. 1 lb (0.453 kg) of cyanogas powder is required for disinfecting 1000 cubic feet (28.316 cubic metres) of space.

Disinfection of a first class railway compartment or of an ambulance car

All leather cushions should be mopped thoroughly with 10% formalin solution or washed with 5% izal solution. The water closet and floor of the compartment are to be sprayed with 10% solution of formalin in water. The compartment of the ambulance car is to be hermetically sealed and then fumigated with formaldehyde or sulphur dioxide gas.

14.9 DETERGENTS

These act on the surface of the body and, therefore, are also called "surfactants". The following detergents are generally used:

1. **Soap:** Although much used, its value as a disinfectant is very much limited. Hands, if washed

thoroughly with soap and hot water, the adhering streptococci diphtheria bacilli, if any, will be washed away or destroyed. Soft soaps (potassium soaps) are more effective than hard soaps (sodium soaps) since they lather more profusely.

2. **Cetramide:** It is an ammonia compound and is available in the market under the trade name.

   Cetavlon: It is a very poweful germicide and is used in washing wounds, etc. in 1–2% strength.

3. **Savlon:** It is a combination of a coal tar derivative called hibitane with cetavlon. It is a more powerful disinfectant than cetavlon.

14.10 AEROSOLS

An aerosol is a substance which is capable of being finally sprayed or of being dispersed in the form of a fine mist consisting of very minute particles. High dispersibility, rapid germicidal action and nontoxic action on human beings or animals are properties of a good aerosol. Common examples are sodium hypochlorite, ethylene glycol and propylene glycol. 5 cc of 1 to 2% solution of sodium hypochlorite when dispersed as a fine mist in a room of about 1000 cubic ft. (28.316 cubic metres) capacity kills 90 to 95% suspended streptococci in the atmosphere of a room.

14.11 CONCURRENT DISINFECTION

It is carried out during the course of a patient's illness. Its aim is to prevent transmission of infection to the medical attendants, nurses and the neighbours. Its details are:

1. Attendants' or nurses' hands should be immersed in a phenol solution of 1 in 40 strength, or mercury chloride solution, 1 in 1,000 solution.

2. Clinical thermometer should be kept in a phenol solution of 1 in 20 strength.

3. Feeding equipment, utensils and crockery should be boiled or scalded.

4. Remnants of food should be destroyed by burning.

5. Nasal, facial, ear or any other discharges or secretions should be taken up in gauze swabs and destroyed by burning.

6. Sputum should be received in gauze swabs or paper sputum cups and destroyed by burning. In a tuberculosis hospital, it should be mixed with phenol solution 1 in 20 and allowed to stand for two hours before disposal into a drain or else placed in a sterilising autoclave for 20 minutes.

7. *Faeces*

   i. These are mixed with an equal volume of phenol solution 1 in 20, and bleaching powder, stirred with a wooden stick and allowed to stand for two hours.

   ii. They are sterilised in a steam steriliser.

8. *Urine*: It should be treated with phenol solution 1 in 20 and allowed to stand for half an hour.

9. *Textiles*: If solid with albuminous discharge, they should be cleaned with soap. Except blankets, they should be boiled or disinfected with steam. Blankets may be soaked in 1 in 20 carbolic acid solution for 12 hours or sprayed with formalin or formaldehyde gas.

14.12 TERMINAL DISINFECTION

Its aim is to destroy or disinfect the infected materials after the removal of the patient to the hospital or termination of the case due to his complete recovery or death. Its details are:

1. Books, boots, furs, feathers, etc. are best disinfected by exposure to 3% formaldehyde for 3 hours as they are rendered unserviceable by steam.

2. Dead bodies of persons who have died of an infectious disease should be wrapped in a sheet soaked in a powerful disinfectant. Cremation is very desirable in such cases and should be hastened.

3. Beddings or body linen should be disinfected by steam.

4. Rooms to be disinfected by fumigation.

5. Floors and wall surfaces may be sprayed with coal tar disinfectants 5% solution or with a 2% solution of formalin.

Insects and Parasites of Public Health Importance

15.1 INSECTS

Insects are intimately related to man, and they play an important part in the transmission of disease. They constitute a group of arthropods who have bilaterally symmetrical bodies, jointed appendages, with heart situated dorsally and nervous system ventrally. Their bodies are covered with a tough skin called *exoskeleton* and are divided into 3 parts, namely the head provided with two antennae (viz. feelers); the eyes and the mouth part; the thorax composed of three segments with three pairs of legs and two pairs of wings, and an abdomen composed of 9 to 11 segments, the last two being modified to form the external genitalia. They have distinct sexes and reproduce from eggs. They have visual organs in the form of compound or simple eyes. They are not provided with lungs, but they simply breathe by means of special type of tubular organs called trachea, which communicate with the external air through lateral openings called spiracles.

15.2 CLASSIFICATION OF ARTHROPODS

Sl. no.	Class Insecta	Class Arachnida	Class Crustacea
1.	Mosquitoes Anophelines Culicines Aedes Mansonoideae	Ticks Hard ticks Soft ticks	Cyclops
2.	Flies House flies Sand flies Tsetse flies Black flies	Mites (Chiggers) Leptotrom-bidium mites Trombiculid mites	
3.	Human lice Head lice Body lice Crab lice	Itch mites	
4.	Fleas Rat fleas Sand fleas		

15.3 DISTINCTIVE CHARACTERISTICS OF ARTHROPODS

Sl. no.	Class Insecta	Class Arachnida	Class Crustacea
1. Body division	Head, throax and abdomen	Cephalothorax and abdomen (no distinct division in some cases)	Cephalothorax and abdomen
2. Legs	3 pairs	4 pairs	5 pairs
3. Wings	One or two pairs, some are even wingless	No wings	No wings
4. Antennae	1 pair	None	2 pairs
5. Abode	On land	On land	In water

Wingless Insects

1. Fleas

They belong to the order of *Siphonaptera*. These are small wingless insects 2–3 mm long with laterally compressed hard, chitinous bodies consisting of head, thorax and abdomen. They are of a small size and have bright colour. Both males and females suck the blood. A flea has 3 pairs of legs.

Varieties: There are hundreds of varieties of fleas. But from the point of view of hygiene the following are important.

1.	Rat fleas (oriental)	a. *Xenopsylla cheopis* b. *Xenopsylla astia* c. *Xenopsylla braziliensis*
2.	Rat fleas (temperate zone)	a. *Nosopsyllus fasciatus*
3.	Human fleas	a. *Pulex irritans*
4.	Dog and cat fleas	a. *Ctenocephalides canis* b. *Ctenocephalides felis*
5.	Sand fleas (Jigger fleas)	a. *Tunga penetrans*

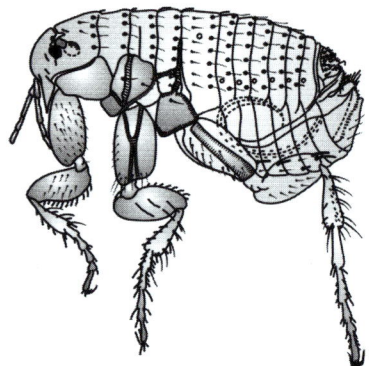

Fig. 15.1: Human rat flea

Life history: There are 4 distinct stages in the life history of fleas, viz. egg, larva, pupa and adult. After a blood meal, a female flea lays about 15–20 eggs per day up to 600 in a lifetime usually in the hair of host, which are small oval, smooth, white and they soon fall to the ground. In summer within 2–4 days and in winter in 1 to 2 weeks time, the eggs hatch up and hairy larvae appear. The larva is very active, thrives on organic matter and develops into a pupa in two weeks' time by spinning a cocoon usually covered with dust and dirt, in which it pupates. It takes another 2 weeks for a pupa to develop into an adult flea.

Habits: They prefer darkness and are very sensitive to light. They freely multiply. In the absence of rats, when starved they bite man. Both the sexes bite and they suck blood. The males carry plague to rats more readily than females. They themselves travel about 20–30 yards (18.29–27.43 metres) but may travel far away, if carried by a host or in the bedding or clothing of men or in grainsacks. They can jump upto 3 inches (7.62 cm) and crawl even up to 8 inches (20.32 cm). They are very active when prevailing temperature is 50°F (10°C) or so. They are most common in dirty, deserted places and in places inhabited by people having unclean habits. Adult fleas cannot survive or lay eggs without a blood meal, but may live from two months to one year without feeding.

Fleas transmit plague: Flea bites cause a persistent, annoying itch. Scratching the area of the bite causes the skin to be irritated. Some fleas, especially the oriental rat fleas, are capable of transmitting diseases such as endemic typhus and bubonic plague.

For prevention from flea bites, lawns and weeds should be trimmed regularly to create a drier environment for flea larvae. Avoid piles of sand and gravel around the home for long periods of time. Fence yards to prevent dogs from roaming freely in heavily infested areas or contacting other infested animals. Discourage nesting or roosting of rodents and birds on or near the premises. Regularly grooming pets and vacuum frequently can remove up to 95% of the flea eggs, some larvae and adults.

2. *Lice*

They are small wingless ectoparasites with hard chitinous covering and have three pairs of legs, each provided with a single claw (Figs 15.2 to 15.4). They live entirely on mammalian blood. They have oval greyish bodies which become brownish, when filled with blood.

Human lice occur throughout the world and thrive under insanitary conditions and standards of personal hygiene are low. Infestation by lice is termed *pediculosis.*

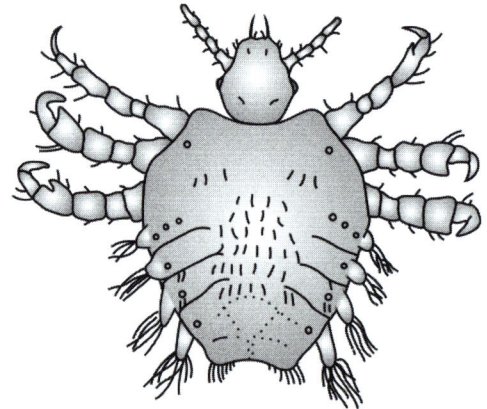

Fig. 15.2: Body louse (female)

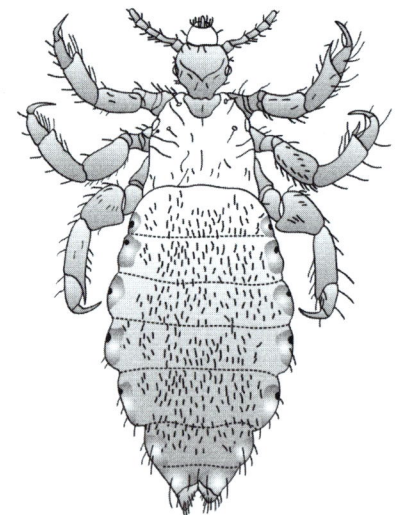

Fig. 15.3: Crab louse (female)

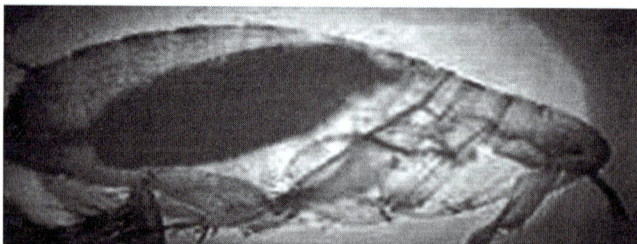

Fig. 15.4: Crab louse (female)

Varieties

a. *Pediculus capitis* (head louse), which infests the hair of the head.

b. *Pediculus humanus corporis* (body louse), or

    Pediculus vestimenti: It prefers to live in the vicinity of the body and is found in the seams of clothes and bedding and hair of the chest and armpits.

c. *Pthirus pubis* (pubic or crab louse), or

    Pthirus inguinalis: It infests the hair of the pubic and perineal regions.

The head and body lice resemble each other and cannot be distinguished so easily whereas crab louse is conspicuous by its small and square body, with blunt and truncated head.

Louse-borne diseases

1. Epidemic typhus.
2. Trench fever.
3. Relapsing fever.

Infestation with head lice may lead to intense itching and secondary bacterial infections of the skin of scalp following minor abrasions that occur after itching the scalp.

Life history: A female louse, within 48 hours of assuming adult form, produces nits or eggs. The body louse lays 300 eggs called 'nits' in her lifetime, whereas the head louse lays 140 and the crab louse 50 in their life-time. In seams of clothing, the eggs may remain alive for 30 days. The male is 3 mm long, whereas length of female body louse is about 3.3 mm. They are attached by a cement-like sticky substance secreted by the female, to the hair. They are oval, greyish white specks and provided with an operculum or granulated cap. The larva emerges in 6 days, begins feeding almost at once. In about 7 days time, during which 3 moults occur, the insects become adults. A louse takes about 15–17 days period to complete its cycle from an egg to the development of adult stage under favourable conditions.

Habits: The average life of a louse is from 35 to 58 days. Both male and female lice are blood suckers. Infection is due to scratching faeces of lice into the skin.

Treatment of pediculosis has 2 aspects—medication and environmental control measures. Environmental control includes improvement in personal hygiene, general cleanliness of the body, hair, clothes and other household articles. Pyrethrins combined with piperonyl butoxide and 1% permethrin are available over-the-counter for treatment of head louse. 5% benzyl alcohol lotion, 0.5% ivermectin solution and 0.5% malathion solution are FDA approved drugs available on prescription. Since lice has become resistant to DDT, dusting the surface of the clothing, socks and the body of persons with 1% malathion powder.

3. Bed Bugs (Fig. 15.5)

They belong to the order *of Hemiptera* and comprise a large number of species. A bed bug measures from 3 to 5 mm in length and 1.5 to 2.5 mm in breadth. It is dark brown, compressed as a thin creature, so it makes its way into narrow cracks. Both male and female bugs bite. Its strong beak inflicts a painful wound. They prefer human blood and in its absence feed on blood of rats and domestic animals. They are nocturnal in their habits retiring during the day in hiding places. No insect is more difficult to eradicate from an infested building than the bed bug. Bed bugs can go without feeding for 20 to 400 days, depending on temperature and humidity. Older stages of nymphs can survive longer without feeding than younger ones, and adults have survived without food for more than 400 days in the laboratory at low temperatures. Adults may live up to one year or more, and there can be up to four successive generations per year.

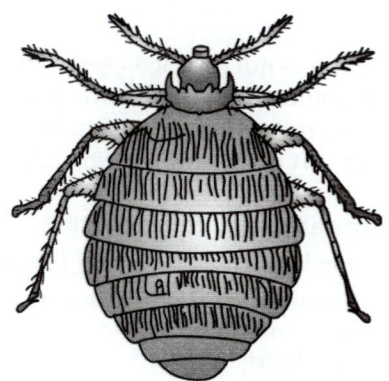

Fig. 15.5: Bed bug (dorsal view)

Management will require employing several non-chemical methods such as vacuuming, washing bedding at a high temperature, using steam or heat treatment, and sealing up hiding places. Insecticides may be required to eliminate serious infestations. Liquid insecticide formulations include products containing the botanical insecticide pyrethrin, which gives quick knock-down but a little long-term control. Various synthetic pyrethroid products (e.g. cyhalothrin, bifenthrin, deltamethrin, and permethrin), mixtures of pyrethroids and neonicotinoids (e.g. temprid and transport), various botanical oils and newer types of products including the pyrrole insecticide chlorfenapyr (phantom) and the insect growth regulator (IGR) hydroprene (gentrol) are more effective in permanent removal. Fumigation using the active ingredient sulfuryl fluoride is highly effective.

Varieties

a. *Cimex lectularius*: In temperate climates (Indian bed bug)
b. *Cimex hemipterus*: In tropics, or
c. *Cimex rotundatus*: (Indian bed bug).

Bed bugs have never been shown to transmit human disease. However, saliva injected during the feeding can later produce allergic dermal reactions such as large itchy swellings on the skin. These may become irritated and infected when scratched.

Life history: Female bed bugs lay 200 to 500 tiny (1/20 inch) white eggs during their lifetimes, usually two to five eggs per day, on rough surfaces such as wood or paper near their hosts' sleeping places, resting places, or both. Glue-like material covers the eggs, which hatch in about 10 to 15 days at room temperature. After hatching occurs, the eggshells frequently remain stuck in place.

There are five progressively larger nymphal stages, each requiring at least one blood meal before molting to the next stage. The entire life cycle from egg to adult requires anywhere from five weeks to four months, depending on temperature and availability of food (blood). Development occurs most rapidly when temperatures are between 70° and 82°F.

4. Ticks

The body of a tick is not distinctly separated into head, thorax and abdomen. Ticks have four pairs of legs and no antennae. There are two types of ticks, i.e. hard ticks (Ixodidae) and soft ticks (Argasidae) (Table 15.1).

Table 15.1: Comparison of hard and soft ticks

S. no.		Hard tick (Ixodidae)	Soft tick (Argasidae)
1.	Scutum (dorsal shield)	Covers entire back in males and only a small portion in front of females	Absent
2.	Head	Seen at anterior end	Not seen from above
3.	Spiracle	Situated behind IV coxa	Situated between III and IV Coxa
4.	Eggs	Several hundreds, or thousands laid at one sitting	Laid in batches of 20–100 over long periods
5.	Nymph stages	One	Five
6.	Feeding habits	Feeds day and night, cannot stand starvation	Feeds during nights. Can stand starvation for many months.
7.	Infestations	Always found on hosts, like dogs and cattle	Can hide in cracks and crevices during day and bite the hosts at night
8.	Important species	*Dermacentor andersoni, Haemophysalis spinigera*	*Ornithodorus moubata*
9.	Diseases transmitted	Viral encephalitis, haemorrhagic fever, tularaemia, tick paralysis, human babesiosis, Indian tick typhus	Relapsing fever

Life history: There are four stages in the life history of a tick:

a. *Eggs:* A female hard tick lays a very large number of eggs at a time. Their number may exceed sometimes 1,000, after which it feels exhausted and dies. The eggs are deposited on the ground and hatch in 1–3 weeks

b. *Larvae:* Larva possesses three pairs of legs. Larvae lie waiting in grass till suitable hosts are found. After a blood meal, they drop off and moult to become nymphs.

c. *Nymph:* A nymph has four pairs of legs like an adult. Nymphs are blood suckers and attach themselves to suitable hosts for blood meals. There are five nymph stages in soft ticks.

d. *Adult:* The duration of life cycle, from eggs to adults, is 2 months in case of hard ticks and 9–10 months in case of soft ticks. Adult ticks may live for a year or longer. Soft ticks live longer than hard ticks. A tick attaches itself to its host by its mouth parts. The rostrum is burrowed in the skin to suck blood. The female tick may remain attached to its host for a long period but the male usually drops off after a few days. Ticks transmit disease by biting blood sucking.

5. Mites (Chiggers)

Mites resemble ticks in having four pairs of legs and its body is not demarcated into head, thorax and abdomen. Two mites are important from public health point of view: (a) trombiculid mite and (b) itch mite (*Acarus scabiei*).

a. *Trombiculid mite:* Its life history consists of four stages:

   i. Eggs are laid singly and hatch in a week's time.

   ii. Larvae have three pairs of legs and attack vertebrate hosts (rodents and man). The larval stage lasts for 1–2 weeks.

   iii. Nymphs: The nymphs have 3 pairs of legs and this stage lasts for 1–3 weeks. Nymphs live on vegetable juices.

   iv. Adults live for six months. Trombiculid mites transmit scrub typhus.

b. *Itch mite (Sarcoptes scabiei or Acarus scabiei):* It is an extremely small, globular arthropod hardly visible to the naked eye. Life history consists of four stages:

   i. *Eggs:* A female burrows its stratum corneum in the skin and lays eggs in the burrows. A female lays up to 30 eggs at the rate of 2–3 eggs per day and then dies at the end of burrows. Eggs hatch into larvae in 3–4 days.

   ii. *Larvae* are three-legged. They leave burrows and come to hair follicles. The larvae mature into nymphs in about 3 days.

iii. *Nymphs* develop into adults in 6–8 days.

iv. *Adults:* The adult mites live for 1–2 months. The life cycle from egg to adult is completed in 1–2 months. The mite causes the disease known as scabies. Scabies is transmitted from person to person through close contact and through contaminated clothes, bed linen, etc. Scabies is prevalent all over India. Rats, mice, bandicoots and shrews play hosts for larval mites. Mite-borne scrub typhus is caused by rickettsial organism.

Control of ticks and mites: Both by personal prophylaxis and chemical treatment of tick infested area with regular spray operations or dusting with insecticide. 50% HCH dispersed in with, 10 litre of water containing 1 kg sprayed over 500 meters or lindane 0.5 kg/hectare can be used. It can be repeated after 8 wks.

Dogs and pets can be treated by wash or spray containing 2% malathion.

HCH suspension should be applied on alternate days on floors and walls surface. Malathion, fenitrothion or carbamate compounds can also be used as 0.5–1% spray or 5–10% dust.

Personal prophylaxis includes wearing of shoes and proper clothing and application of repellants like dibutyl phthalate (DBP), diethyltoluamide (DEET) and benzylbenzoate to clothing and skins.

6. Cyclops

Cyclops or water flea is present in fresh water collections. It is just visible to the trained eye and is not more than 1 mm in length. It has a pear-shaped semitransparent body. It swims on water with characteristic jerky movements. Its average lifespan is 3 months. Cyclops is the intermediate host for dracunculiasis or guineaworm disease. Man gets infestation by drinking water containing contaminated cyclops. The disease has been eradicated in India since 2000.

Control of cyclops

1. Physical separation from drinking water using muslin cloth or domestic nylon stainer.
2. Boiling and superchlorination of drinking water also help to eliminate cyclops from drinking water.
3. Health education and awareness among the affected population has a significant role.

15.4 WINGED INSECTS

1. Mosquitoes

They belong to the order Diptera and are grouped under family *Culicidae* and sub-family *Culicinae*. They are distinguished by the presence of scales on their wings and proboscis. The mouth parts of female mosquito are transformed into a needle-like structure to penetrate the skin for blood meal as females require blood meal for laying the eggs. Males are not blood feeders thus do not act as vectors in transmission of infection. The life cycle has four stages, viz. egg, larva, pupa and adult, of which first three stages are spent in water. The presence of water is, therefore, absolutely essential for their existence.

The body of an adult mosquito is divided into head, thorax and abdomen:

1. *Head* is semiglobular structure and has following structures:
   i. A large pair of compound eyes.
   ii. *Proboscis:* Which is a long needle-like structure with which the mosquito bites.
   iii. *Palpi:* Which is four-jointed structure and may be very short or as long as or even longer than the proboscis, and
   iv. A pair of antennae of feelers. They are plumose in males whereas are pilose in females.

2. *Thorax:* It bears scales and marking which vary according to species. It has three pairs of legs ventrally and a pair of wings dorsally. The arrangement and the colouration of the scales depend upon particular species. Wings are folded when the mosquitoes are at rest.

3. *Abdomen:* It has ten segments, of which two segments at the end are modified to form external genitalia.

The important groups of mosquitoes in India that are related to disease transmission are *Anopheles, Culex, Mansonia* and *Aedes*.

a. *Anopheles:* A lot many species of *Anopheles* mosquitoes are found in India but only a few of them have been identified as vectors for transmission of malaria. Some of them are *A. minimus, A. stephensi, A. culicifacies, A. fluviatilis.* Different species have different habitat. *A. minimus* is a vector in North Bengal, Assam and Southern India.

A. fluviatilis: It is a vector in foot hill areas, from North West Frontier to Assam and other parts of India such as South India, Mysore and Travancore.

A. culicifacies: It is a vector, widely distributed in India except in Bengal, Assam and Jaipur and in hilly tracts. It is found particularly in North West India.

A. stephensi is essentially an Indian species and is widely distributed in India especially in Western and North West India, urban areas of Kolkata, Delhi, Mumbai and Chennai. *A. philippinensis* is a vector in Western and Southern Bengal, Assam and Southern India particularly in rural areas.

A. sundaicus causes malaria in coastal areas of Bengal, Orissa, Andaman and Nicobar, Eastern parts of Kolkata and Bengal.

A. annularis and A. varuua: They are vectors in Assam and Bengal.

b. *Culex mosquitoes:* They are the common disease-carrying nuisance mosquitoes. They frequently breed in cesspools, gully traps, drains, masonry tanks, earthenware vessels and in collections of dirty water around houses and stables. *Culex fatigans* is a highly anthrophilic, strong-winged and feeds at night. Preferable biting site for Culex mosquito is legs below the knees. Culex is a vector for transmission of filariasis.

c. *Aedes aegypti or Stegomyia fasciatus or tiger mosquito (Fig. 15.6):* It is a domestic mosquito and is characteristically marked with white stripes on a black body. Because of the striped character of their bodies, they are called "tiger mosquitoes". It has unhanded proboscis, white marks on the dorsum of thorax called lyre, and the cross band on the abdomen. It is recognised by the broad, flat, imbricated scales completely covering the head and the abdomen which are invariably present on the middle lobe and frequently on the lateral lobe of the scutellum also. The scales impart a satiny appearance, which is characteristic. They are mostly small and have alternate white and black bands on the abdomen. The females are blood suckers and bite both during day and night. Each female lays about 20–25 eggs separately, instead of being cemented together to form rafts, in cisterns or rainwater. They are black. The syphon of the larva is short and dark in colour.

d. *Mansonia:* These are big, black or brown with speckling on their wings and legs. The common Indian species are *M. annulifera, M. longipalpis, M. indiana* and *M. uniformis.*

Life Cycle of Mosquitoes (Fig. 15.7)

The male mosquito feeds on vegetables, whereas the females are blood feeders. During the course of the season, the female mosquito may lay eggs several times and several hundreds at each time. Like other insects, mosquitoes have also 4 stages in their life cycle, viz. egg, larva, pupa and adult.

The male mosquito lives rarely more than 1–3 weeks. The female may live up to 4 months or more. Mosquitoes prefer darkness to light. The Anopheles type of mosquitoes avoid both heat and light and, therefore, during the day, they remain concealed in the corners of rooms, etc. At night, they come out from their hiding places in search of food. In fact, they are most active after sunset and just before sunrise. Only females are blood suckers as they need blood meal for producing a batch of eggs. It takes about a minute for the mosquito to fill her stomach. Anopheles mosquito does not make any noise while flying about. The bite of Anopheles is not very painful. Mosquitoes bite voraciously when the relative humidity of the atmosphere is high. During winter, in cold countries and the hottest months in

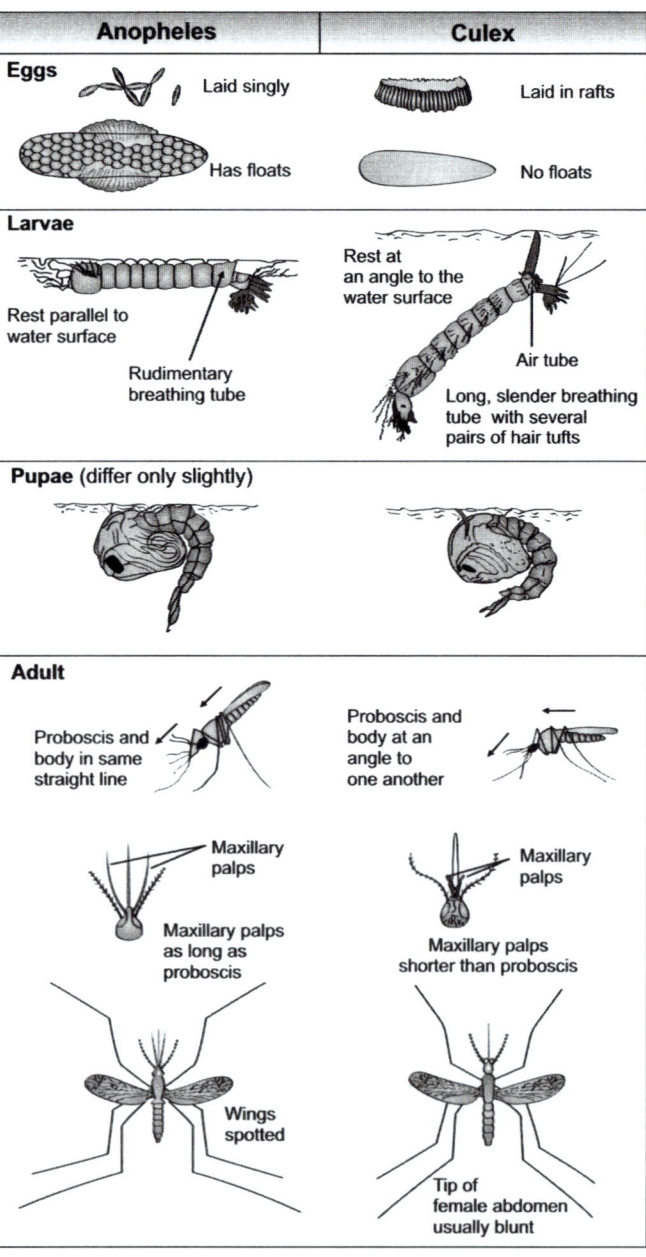

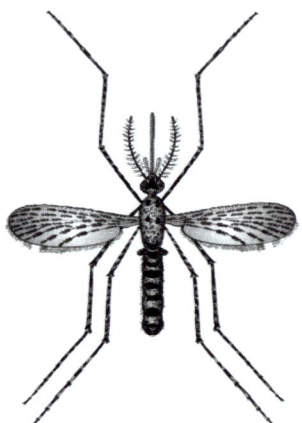

Fig. 15.6: *Aedes aegypti*

Fig. 15.7: Flay of life cycle of mosquitoes

tropics, the female adults hibernate in sheltered places and do not breed. This is known as aestivation.

Life Cycle

The female mosquito, after sucking blood, lays eggs on the surface of water. The Anopheles female lays 100–200 eggs in each batch. They are boat-shaped, with lateral floaters are deposited singly. In the case of female Culex, hundreds of eggs, usually 100–250, are laid at a time and are cemented together in the form of clusters or rafts.

In 2–3 days, the eggs hatch out and a small worm like larva appears from each egg. It consists of a flattened head, with a pair of large eyes, a globular thorax and an abdomen but no legs. They have got respiratory apertures. They are found in stagnant and slow running pools, streams, Anopheles larvae are provided with palmate hair on abdominal segments and they float parallel to the surface of the water. They have no siphon tube. The larva of Culex and Aedes have siphon tubes, so they hang almost vertically with their heads downwards.

The larva casts its skin 2 or 3 times and finally attains its full size in 8–10 days, when it changes into a comma-shaped creature called pupa. It has got a large globular body and a small tail. It is very active and swims rapidly by lashing its hind part. It does not breathe through its tail, like the larva, but does so by means of tubes which project on the dorsal side. It has no mouth and hence it does not eat.

In 2–3 days, it splits up and an adult mosquito or the imago emerges. It has a rounded head with prominent eyes, two antennae, two palpi, a prominent suction or piercing organ—the proboscis, an oval chest, about the size of its head, to which is attached a pair of wings and three pairs of jointed legs. The abdomen is segmented, consisting of 10 segments, of which, however, only 9 can be distinguished. The males are distinguished from the females by the presence of whiskers or plumes on either side (Table 15.2).

Habits of Mosquitoes

A knowledge of habits of mosquitoes is essential for understanding their role in disease transmission and also in control programmes.

a. *Feeding habits:* Only females are blood suckers since they need blood meal once in 2–3 days to lay eggs. Some species prefer human blood (anthropophilic), some animal (zoophilic) whereas some are indiscriminate in their choice and feeds on both animal and human blood.

b. *Time of biting:* Aedes are fearless biters and bite during day time whereas others usually bite in evening or in early part of night.

c. *Breeding habits:* Anophilines prefer clean water for breeding whereas Culex breeds in dirty water. Aedes prefers artificial collections of water as

Table 15.2: Distinguishing features of Anopheles and Culex mosquitoes

Anopheles	*Culex*
Adult	
i. Resting attitude. When at rest inclined at an angle to the surface	i. When at rest the body exhibits a hunch back
ii. Proboscis in straight line with body and head	ii. Not in straight line with the body
iii. Palpi: Long in both sexes	iii. Short in female
iv. Scutellum: Bar-shaped	iv. Trilobed
v. Wings: Spotted	v. Unspotted
vi. Scales: No scales on belly	vi. Scales on belly
• **Breeding:** Breed in clean, fresh water. Some prefer still water, while others prefer running water. Some breed in saltish and brackish water	• In still water, cesspools, gully traps, drains, earthen-ware vessels, around houses and stables, often in collections of dirty and polluted water
• **Eggs:** Boat-shaped, laid singly 100–200 in number, often form patterns on the surface of water, e.g. triangular- and star-shaped. They cannot be detected easily with the naked eye and appear like minute specks of dust particles. They are provided with lateral floats	• Ovate- or cigar-shaped: Laid in batches, 200–500 in number, found cemented together in the form of rafts of hundreds of eggs. They can be easily detected with the naked eye and are about the size of caraway seeds. They are of brown black colour. They are not provided with lateral floats
• **Larva:** Small head has no respiratory syphon or breathing tubes. Rests parallel to surface of water. It has palmate hair (except *A. unbrosus*) on the abdomen	• Large head has a long conspicuous syphon tube suspended with head downwards at an angle to water surface. It has no palamate hair on the abdomen
• **Pupa:** Breathing trumpets are funnel-shaped. Accessory paddle hair grown above the origin of the paddle hair	• Breathing trumpets are long and narrow. Accessory paddle hair grown besides the normal paddle hair or may be even absent

breeding space whereas Mansonia prefers water with certain type of aquatic life for breeding.

d. *Dispersal:* Mosquitoes generally do not fly far from breeding places. The range of flight usually varies up to 11 km in case of Culex mosquitoes. However, these can be transported over various countries, if the breeding sites are present on the aircraft and ships.

e. *Lifespan:* The life of a mosquito ranges from 8 to 34 days and usually males are short-lived. Mosquitoes do not survive extremes of temperatures.

Mosquito Control Measures

The basic strategy to control mosquitoes remains the same as for control of other vectors—environmental sanitation, personal protection against mosquito bites, chemical and biological control of larvae and adult mosquitoes.

A. **Environmental sanitation:** This aims towards reduction in number of mosquitoes by eliminating their breeding places. It comprises minor engineering methods such as filling, levelling of drainage of breeding places for Anopheles mosquitoes. Abolition of domestic and peridomestic breeding spaces for prevention of breeding of Culex, prevention of artificial collection of water for preventing breeding of Aedes mosquitoes and so on.

B. **Personal protection from the mosquito bites**

i. *Mosquito nets:* These offer protection against mosquito bites during sleeping. Rectangular bed nets with the size of net less than 0.0475 inch in any diameter and 150 holes per square inch are effective in protection from mosquito bites. Insecticide treated bed nets (ITNs) are more effective than plain nets.

ii. *Mosquito repellants:* Diethyltoluamide (DEET) has been found to be an all time effective repellent. Indalone, dimethylphthalate and some natural and herbal products are also being used as mosquito repellants.

C. **Chemical and biological control**

i. *Larvae*

- *Biological control: Gambusia affinis* and *Lebister reticulatus* are the small fishes that feed on mosquito larvae and are used for biological control in the potential larvae breeding sites (burrow pits, sewage oxidation ponds, cisterns, etc.).

- *Chemical control:* Fenthion, Chlorpyriphos and Abate are the most effective larvicides. DDT and HCH have long residual effect, potential for contamination of water and chances of developing resistance, thereby are discouraged from use. Paris green or copper acetoarsenite is a stomach poison and has to be ingested to be effective. Thus, it mainly kills Anopheles larva since they are surface feeders. Diesel, kerosene, fuel oil and various fractions of crude oils spreads and forms a thin film on water and kills larvae and pupae within a short time after application.

ii. **Adults:** Anti-adult measures include residual sprays and space sprays.

DDT is the insecticide of choice at the doses of 1–2 gm per square metre, 1–3 times in a year for residual sprays. In DDT resistant areas, malathion, propoxur and lindane are used.

Pyrethrum extracts containing pyrethrin, a nerve poison at the rate of 0.1% per 1,000 cu ft of space is used as space sprays. Malathion and fenitrothion are used for ULV (ultra-low volume) fogging.

2. Houseflies

The commonest variety of housefly is called *Musca domestica*. It belongs to the family Muscidae of the order *Diptera*. It is 1/4 inch (6.35 mm) in length having mouse grey colour and 4 narrow black strips on thorax. It has got a proboscis, which is not capable of piercing but is used for sucking food. When not in use, it is folded upwards into a cavity under the head.

It breeds chiefly on human and animal excreta particularly horse manure, cowdung, decaying and fermenting vegetable and animal matter, carcases and putrefying filth which provides food and home for maggots. Thus, breeding of housefly is indicative of insanitary conditions.

Life Cycle

A female housefly lays 100 to 150 eggs at a time. The favourite site is on the surface of fermenting vegetable matter, on fresh dung of horses, faeces of pigs or men. The progeny of a single housefly will number more than 4,32,000 in seven weeks. The eggs look like tiny grains of polished rice or minute glistening white grains of about 20th of an inch (1.27 mm) in length. Their development depends upon the atmospheric temperature and the characteristics and temperature of food.

Larvae or maggots: Within 3–5 days, the eggs hatch into white legless crawling creatures called maggots. They are 1–2 mm in length at birth. They grow rapidly and burrow into food material on which they feed. The maggots shun light and disappear during the day and come out at night. They eat voraciously.

Pupa or chrysalis: In about 1–3 days, the larva enters into a resting stage. It is passed within a barrel-shaped shell usually 1/4 inch (6.35 mm) in length, which is oval, brown and is quite immovable.

Adult fly: In 5–7 days, depending upon the temperature, it ruptures and a full grown fly comes out, which has a shrunken appearance and is incapable of flying. The wings soon spread out, the outer covering of the body and legs harden and the fly looks quite normal. An adult fly is 1/4 inch (6.35 mm) in length. Its ground colour is mouse grey having black stripes on the thorax and the abdomen. The fly has a short lifespan of 15–25 days depending over weather conditions and in a year 10 to 20 generations are produced. The female is ready to lay eggs in about 4 days after its emergence.

Habits

a. *Breeding places:* The most important breeding places of housefly are fresh horse and other animals manure, human excreta, garbage, decaying fruits and vegetables and rubbish dumps.

b. *Feeding*: A housefly does not bite, its hairy body, sticky feet and wings become covered with filth on which it feeds or crawls. This material which may be infected with pathogenic germs is frequently deposited, subsequently on human food. Furthermore, in the fly's alimentary canal, bacteria live unharmed, until they are discharged in excrement or regurgitated in small drops which are called "vomit spots".

c. *Resting habits*: Flies rest on hanging surface and flies towards light. These are restless and moves back and forth between food and filth. This helps in transmission of infection mechanically.

d. *Dispersal*: Normally, flies remain close to their breeding places and hardly disperse beyond 4 miles from the point of their origin.

Modes of Transmission of Infection

a. The housefly is a mechanical carrier of disease. Its hairy body, sticky feet and wings become covered with filth on which it feeds or crawls. This material, which may be infected with pathogenic germs, is frequently deposited, subsequently on human food.

b. In the fly's alimentary canal, bacteria live unharmed, until they are discharged in excrement or regurgitated in small drops which are called "vomit spots".

c. The flies usually defecates while feeding. Which deposits countless bacteria on the exposed food.

The lifespan of a fly is about 15 days in summer and 25 days in winter. The increase in number of flies is definitely associated with increase in temperature and humidity, prevailing during the summer months of June and July. These climatic conditions favour the rapid multiplication of flies (Fig. 15.8).

Diseases spread by flies: The flies are vector for typhoid and paratyphoid fever, cholera, diarrhoea and dysentery, gastroenteritis, amoebiasis, helminthic infestation, poliomyelitis, conjunctivitis, trachoma, and anthrax.

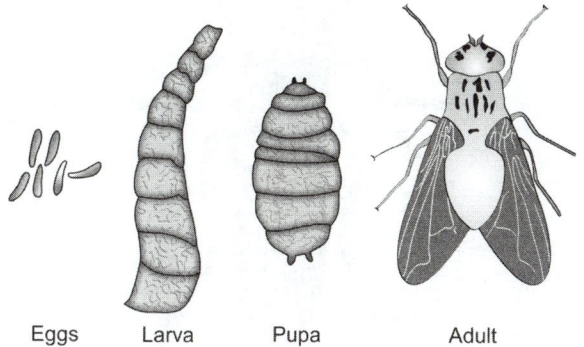

| Eggs | Larva | Pupa | Adult |

Fig. 15.8: Life stages of a housefly

Anti-fly Measures

These are as follows:

1. **Environmental sanitation:** The best way to eliminate housefly is to eliminate the breeding places. This can be done by: (a) Sanitary disposal of human excreta—people should use latrines and stop defecating in the open fields. Flyproof privies and latrines with self-closing seat covers should be used. (b) Storing garbage, kitchen wastes and similar refuse should be placed in garbage receptacles (tins) and not left lying about uncovered or thrown on the ground. (c) Prompt removal and proper disposal of the refuse including horse manure, cow-dung, night soil, etc. The conservancy arrangements should be efficient. (d) Refuse should not be allowed to accumulate in the stables, cowsheds, slaughter houses, fish markets, garbage dumps, etc. They should be regularly cleaned at least once a day and refuse should be removed in covered carts to the closed pits.

2. **Protection of food from flies:** (a) Screens, chiks, wiregauze doors and windows should be provided for all human habitations, restaurants, hotels, confectionary stores, meat markets, etc. to prevent contamination of food by flies. Screens with 14 meshes to an inch would be sufficient to keep out houseflies, but screens of finer mesh; if used, will keep out mosquitoes and other small insects also. (b) The practice of displaying vegetables and other foods meant for eating uncooked, on tables or in stalls, which are open should be discouraged. This can be remedied by placing the food in glass cases or flyproof almirahs or covered with fly-proof covers. (c) Electric fans may be used to force a current of air over the food products on display, to prevent the flies from settling.

3. **Destruction of flies:** (a) For destruction of eggs, larvae and pupae of flies in the manure, an extract of Hellebore say 1/2 lb (226.80 gm) of the powder to every 10 gallons (45.46 litres) of water is best for the purpose. Powdered borax is a more effective larvicide than Hellebore say 1 lb (0.454 kg) for 16 cubic feet (0.452 cubic metre of manure) and it can be applied in solution. Gammexane and chlordane are effective.

Adult flies can be killed in many ways, which are not only expensive but also temporary in value: (a) Sticky fly papers and strings or tangle foot are made by heating together one pint (0.568 litre) of castor oil and 2 lbs (0.906 kg) of resin powder and then spreading in thin layers on glazed papers or strings, while still hot. They are effective as long as they remain sticky. They are placed in rooms. Flies stick to them and die. (b) Flies are killed by wiremesh or leather flaps attached to the handles.

(c) Poisonous baits may be used (2% formalin solution with a little sugar and milk is placed in the rooms to attract flies). Besides, poisonous baits containing 1–2% of malathion, diazinon or dichlorvos have proved quite successful in destroying adult flies. (d) Spraying of DDT, pyrethrum in kerosene, i.e. 5% solution or emulsion will readily kill flies. Two quarts of solution or emulsion are required for 1,000 square ft (92.90 square metres) area to obtain a residual of 200 mg per square ft (0.092 square metres). Since flies soon develop reistance to DDT so dieldrin, chlordane or BHC may be used in place of DDT. Likewise, pesterin is also effective for killing flies. (e) Keating's insect powder is sprinked over table cloths, etc.

4. **Health education:** The lay public should be convinced that the housefly is a carrier of disease, and they must be educated regarding adopting anti-fly measures.

3. Sandflies

Sandflies are extremely small insects, light or dark brown in colour with long proboscis, humped thorax, hairy body and butterfly wings. They possess slender legs and can pass through 18 meshes to an inch (2.54 cm) of mosquito net. In size, they are smaller than mosquitoes and measure 1.5 to 2.5 mm in length (Fig. 15.9).

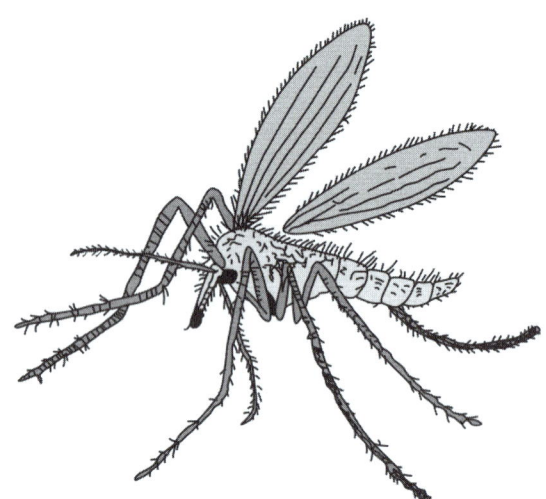

Fig. 15.9: *Phlebotomus papatasi*

They belong to family Psychodidae. They are present in holes and crevices where moisture is present. There are many species of sandflies, however, most common that act as vector for transmission of various infections are *P. argentipes (vector for kala-azar), Phlebotomus papatasi* (vector of sandfly fever and oriental sore) *and P. sergenti (vector for oriental sore).*

Habits: They dislike sun and wind; remain in the dark by day time and bite vigorously at night. The range of flight of the adult is very small and they remain confined to 50 yards of their breeding place. The bite of the female sandfly is irritating and painful, whereas the males are harmless.

Life history: It sucks blood before ovipositing and lays about 40 eggs in moist places like the walls of cellars, latrines, cesspools, embankments and also where food-refuse undergoes decomposition. Eggs hatch into larvae in 7–10 days. The larva lives on organic matter and grows into a pupa in 14 days. Pupa becomes an adult fly in about one week. The whole life cycle takes 6–12 weeks to complete. Since only female sandfly sucks blood, male does not transmit disease.

Diseases transmitted through sandflies: These are sandfly fever, oriental sore and leishmaniasis or kala-azar.

Anti-sandfly measures: The preventive measures consist of:

1. *Sanitation:* Extermination of breeding places, i.e. removal of cattle from dwelling houses or making cattle sheds pucca.
2. *Personal protection:* Sandfly net with 45 meshes to an inch (2.54 cm) may be used to protect from their bites.
3. *Insecticides:* A single application of 1–2 gm/m^2 of DDT or 0.25 gm/m^2 of lindane has been found to be effective for 1 to 2 years and 3 months, respectively.

4. Tsetse Flies (Fig. 15.10)

They are ordinary looking, sombre, brownish flies varying from 3½ to 4 lines in *Glossina morsitans* and to about 5½ lines in that of *Glossina fusca or longipennis* with a prominent proboscis in all species. The wings overlap on the back and cross each other like the blades of a pair of scissors projecting beyond the abdomen, when the fly is in a resting attitude. The commonest ones are *Glossina palpalis,* and *Glossina morsitans.*

Habits: The undergrowth along courses of rivers, ravines and shores of lakes are suitable localities for their breeding. Both the male and female flies are voracious

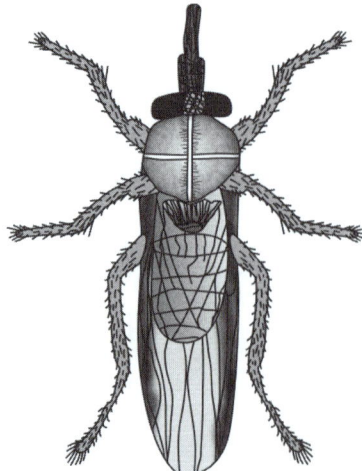

Fig. 15.10: Tsetse flies

blood suckers and attack men as well as animals. They fly low and that is why often bite the ankles and legs. They bite exclusively during the day. The bite is painful. The flies become infective approximately 34 days after feeding, remain infective for 70–80 days and probably even for the rest of their life.

Disease transmitted: Sleeping sickness (trypanosomiasis)

Life history: The female does not lay eggs but gives birth to a living larva one at a time in a carefully selected spot (light soil with some degree of shade). Immediately after birth, the larva buries itself in earth, at a depth of about an inch (2.5 cm) beneath the surface and pupates in 3–4 weeks time.

Control: Use of 25% DDT and 18–20% dieldrin is effective for control of tsetse fly besides clearing of vegetation where tsetse fly lives and breeds.

15.5 NATIONAL VECTOR-BORNE DISEASE CONTROL PROGRAMME (NVBDCP)

The National Vector-borne Disease Control Programme (NVBDCP) is an umbrella programme for prevention and control of vector-borne diseases, viz. malaria, Japanese encephalitis (JE), dengue, chikungunya, kala-azar and lymphatic filariasis. Out of these six diseases, kala-azar and lymphatic filariasis had been targeted for elimination by 2015.

The states are responsible for implementation of programme, whereas the Directorate of NVBDCP, Delhi, provides technical assistance, policies and assistance to the states in the form of cash and commodity.

Malaria, filaria, Japanese encephalitis, dengue and chikungunya are transmitted by mosquitoes whereas kala-azar is transmitted by sandflies. The transmission of vector-borne diseases depends on prevalence of infective vectors and human-vector contact, which is further influenced by various factors such as climate, sleeping habits of human, density and biting of vectors, etc.

The general strategy for prevention and control of vector-borne diseases under NVBDCP is described below:

i. **Integrated vector management:** Including indoor residual spraying (IRS) in selected high-risk areas, long-lasting insecticide treated bed-nets (LLINs), use of larvivorous fish, antilarval measures in urban areas including biolarvicides and minor environmental engineering including source reduction.

ii. **Disease management:** Including early case detection with active, passive and sentinel surveillance and complete effective treatment, strengthening of referral services, epidemic preparedness and rapid response.

iii. **Supportive interventions:** Including behaviour change communication (BCC), intersectoral convergence, human resource development through capacity building.

iv. **Vaccination:** Only against JE.

v. **Annual mass drugs administration:** Against lymphatic filariasis.

15.6 ANIMAL PARASITES

Parasitic animals are those which live within or upon other living organisms, called hosts, for purpose of deriving their nourishment from them. Some parasites nourish themselves on the living material, e.g. the blood or the lymph of their host. Saprophytic parasites derive their nourishment from dead material. Many parasites are pathogenic. Lice, fleas bed bugs, etc. attack external parts of the host and are called *ectozoa*, whereas others live within the body of the host and are called *entozoa*.

There are many ways by which man may get infected; the most common mode being the ingestion of eggs or immature forms of parasites together with water or other fresh food. Infection may occur due to ingestion of immature parasites in an intermediate host. It may be transmitted by the direct agency of the second host as in filaria.

The common animal parasites that affect humans are as follows.

15.7 HELMINTHS

Helminths are triploblastic group of multicellular worms consisting of epiblast, hypoblast and mesoblast. They may be considered under three classes, viz. nematodes, cestodes and trematodes. Ascaris, hookworm, and whipworm are known as soil-transmitted helminths (parasitic worms). Together, they account for a major burden of disease worldwide.

Nematodes or Roundworms

They have slender bodies and have no segments or appendages. They have well developed alimentary canal, with mouth at one end and anus at the other end. They are bisexual. The males are smaller than the females. Following are some of the important parasitic worms found in man.

Ascaris Lumbricoides *(Fig. 15.11)*

It is the large intestinal roundworm, which resembles the common earthworm, being cylindrical and pointed at both ends, with pinkish grey colour, having glistening surface when alive. The adult female measures about 200 to 350 × 5 mm in length and the male about 150 to 300 × 3 mm in length with its posterior extremity curved anteriorly. Adultworms normally do not live

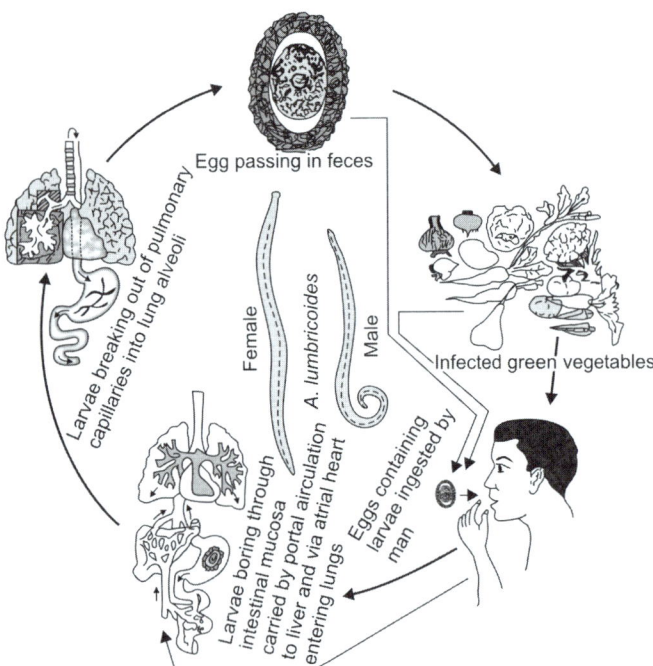

Fig. 15.11: Life cycle of *Ascaris lumbricoides*

cough, asthmatic attacks, etc. are known to occur due to migration of the worms through the body.

Diagnosis: The standard method for diagnosing ascariasis is by identifying *Ascaris* eggs in a stool sample using a microscope.

Prevention and control: The best way to prevent ascariasis is to always:

1. *Sanitary disposal of night soil*: Avoid ingesting soil that may be contaminated with human faeces, including where human faecal matter (night soil) or waste water is used to fertilize crops.
2. Wash your hands with soap and warm water before handling food.
3. Wash, peel, or cook all raw vegetables and fruits before eating, particularly those that have been grown in soil that has been fertilized with manure.
4. Health education for improved personal hygiene and handwashing.
5. Treatment of all infected persons. Antihelminthic drugs like albendazole and mebendazole are treatment of choice for 1–3 days. The drugs are effective with a few side efffects.

Oxyuris vermicularis or Enterobius vermicularis (Threadworms) (Fig. 15.12)

They are tiny, thread-like, whitish worms. The female is 1/3–1/2 inch (8–13 mm) long and the male usually half of its size. They develop from ova in about 3 weeks time.

It most commonly occurs among children, institutionalized persons, and household members of persons

for more than a year. The female lays enormous number of eggs, viz. even up to 2,00,000 eggs a day. They are bile-coloured, oval in shape, having a resistant shell, outside which there is often a clear irregular albuminous sheath. Embryonated eggs remain viable in soil, under favourable conditions, for months and even for years. The egg is noninfective until a larva has developed. The maturation takes a few weeks, while it is lying in the soil.

Mature eggs containing embryos are ingested via contaminated food, vegetables and fingers. When swallowed, these eggs find their way in the duodenum, where the shell dissolves, the embryo emerges, perforates the mucous membrane of the intestine, enters lymphatics and veins and reaches right side of heart from where it passes onto the lungs through bloodstream. It then penetrates the lung alveoli (air sacks), migrates up the trachea, down the oesophagus to reach intestines and becomes an adult to lay eggs. When passing through the lungs they sometimes damage the tissues and cause pneumonia. They may be sometimes found matted in the intestines thus causing intestinal obstruction.

The immediate source of infection is soil containing embryonated eggs, in and about houses and dwelling places, where facilities for sanitary disposal of human excreta are lacking.

Symptoms: There are no well defined signs or symptoms of roundworm infection. General weakness of body, paleness, occasional vomiting and loss of appetite are some of the common symptoms. Some children may get severe stomachache resembling appendicitis. Heavy infections can cause intestinal blockage and impair growth in children other symptoms such as

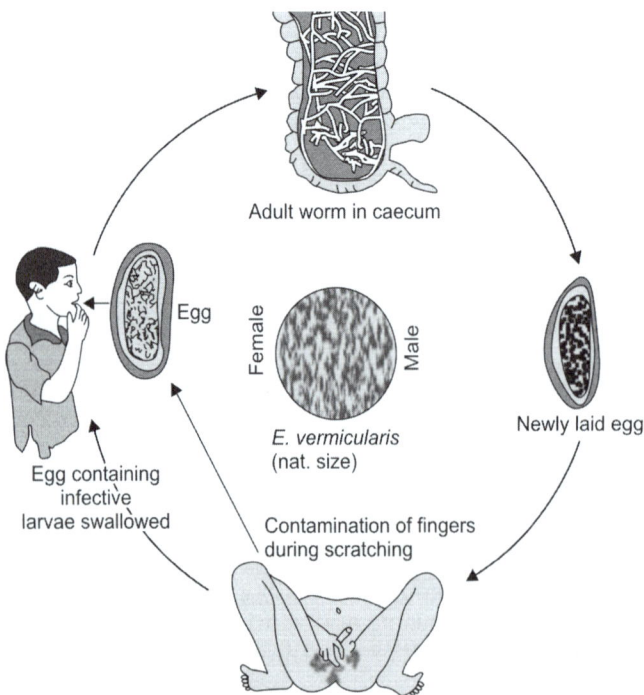

Fig. 15.12: Life history of *Oxyuris vermicularis*

Table 15.3: Insect-wise diseases transmitted and their control measures

Sl. no.	Name of the insect	Disease transmitted	Control measures
1.	Anopheles mosquito	Malaria filaria (not in India)	a. **Environmental control:** Maintain clean tanks by removing the weeds. Drainage of rainwater; installation of dams with automatic flushing devices for big streams. b. Personal protection—prevention of mosquito bites—use of bed nets, repellants like DEET c. Biological measures: *Gambusia affinis* d. Chemical control—*antilarval measures*: Paris green is applied as 2% dust prepared by mixing 2 lbs (0.9 kg) of Paris green, 98 lb (44.452 kg) of diluent, i.e. soap stone powder or slaked lime in a rotatory mixture. Dose—2 lb (0.9 kg) of Paris green dust per acre of water surface **Anti-adult measures:** Residual spray by DDT 100–200 mg per sq ft (0.092 sq m) in the houses. Malathion, propoxur and lindane in DDT resistant areas
2.	Culex mosquito	Filaria (*W. bancrofti*) viral arthritis	a. Environmental measures: Provision for adequate drainage of rain and waste water, removal of artificial collection of water with organic pollution b. Personal protection from mosquito bites c. Chemical measures: *Antilarval measures*: Malarial or crude oil in doses of 10–15 gallons (45.45 to 68.18 litres) per acre (0.4 hectare) of water surface **Anti-adult measures:** DDT 3 to 5% singly or with pyrethrum can be used as a space spray. The effect is very temporary and limited—the mosquito being resistant to chlorinated hydrocarbon
3.	Mansonioides	Filaria (*Brugia malayi*)	Removal of aquatic Pistia plants from the ponds Chemical measures: DDT spray at the rate of 100–200 mg per sq ft (0.092 sq m) is quite effective
4.	Aedes mosquito	Dengue fever, dengue haemorrhagic fever, yellow fever	a. Enviromental control: Clean up or get rid of water holding containers, i.e. old tins, tincans, bottles, etc. b. Personal protection c. Chemical measures: DDT 3–5% with pyrethrum as space spray
5.	Houseflies	Diarrhoea, dysentery, typhoid and paratyphoid fevers, infantile diarrhoea, cholera, gastroenteritis, trachoma	a. Environmental measures: Provision and utilisation of sanitary latrines in every house. Control of open field defecation. Pupa and safe disposal of animal waste, kitchen garbage and refuse b. Chemical measures: Residual spray of 5% DDT in about 4 litres per 100 sq metres of surface. If resistant, use 2.5% diazion in about 4 litres per 100 sq metres of surface. 1–2% of malathion, diazinon or dichlorvos is also effective in DDT-resistant cases
6.	Sandflies	Kala-azar, oriental sore, sandfly fever	a. Environmental measures: Proper construction and regular maintenance of cattle sheds, poultry farms and animal houses Proper disposal of animal waste from their establishments b. Personal protection c. Chemical measures: DDT sprayed at the rate of 100–200 mg per sq ft (0.092 sq m) in human dwellings, cattle sheds and poultry farms is very effective
7.	Lice	Epidemic typhus, relapsing fever, trench fever	a. Environmental measures—personal hygiene: Maintenance of proper personal hygiene by regular soap and water bath, cutting short hairs of axilla, pubic regions and keeping the hair clean and well combed. Use of washed and ironed clothes b. Chemical measures: For body lice, use 10% DDT dusting. Usually 50 gm of DDT will be required. Mass delousing with DDT is done by hand operated dusters. Pyrethrins combined with piperonyl butoxide and 1% permethrin are available over-the-counter for treatment of head louse. 0.2% gama BHC dissolved in coconut oil is a useful application for management of head louse. 5% benzyl alcohol lotion, 0.5% ivermectin solution and 0.5% malathion solution are FDA approved drugs available on prescription. Since lice has become resistant to DDT, dusting the surface of the clothing, socks and the body of persons with 1% malathion powder. Find and treat contacts

(Contd...)

Table 15.3: Insect-wise diseases transmitted and their control measures *(Contd...)*

Sl. no.	Name of the insect	Disease transmitted	Control measures
8.	Fleas	Bubonic plague, endemic typhus	Environmental measures: Do away with rat harbourage, improvement in construction of houses with provision of rat-proof stores
			Chemical measures: Dust the rat runs and burrows with 10% DDT, 15% dieldrin or 2% aldrin solution. In case of resistance, use 5% malathion. Indoor spraying with DDT 10%, dieldrin 1.5%, aldrin 2% floor and walls up to 1 ft (0.304 m)
9.	Ticks—hard ticks, soft ticks	Tick typhus, viral encephalitis haemorrhagic fever, tularemia, tick paralysis, viral fevers relapsing fever, or fever	As insect and tick repellents use diethyl toluamide and benzyl benzoate Environmental measures: Reduce number of animal hosts of ticks such as wild rodents Chemical measures: On dogs, use 5% DDT, 0.5% lindane or 3.5% malathion. In houses, spray cracks and crevices with 0.5% diazinon. For area control, use 5% dusts of DDT at the rate of 20–40 lb per acre and 3% BHC dust at the rate of 16 lb per acre. Use tick repellents Diethyl toluamide, dimethylphthalate by impregnation of the clothings
10.	Cyclops	Dracunculosis (guinea-worms)	Community provision of safe water supply. Use of water after proper staining. Boiling and superchlorination are effective

with pinworm infection. Pinworm infection is transmitted only by humans. They can survive in the indoor environment for 2–3 weeks.

The infection can be transmitted by ingestion through contaminated hands or inhalation. A person can reinfect himself or can be reinfected from others from eggs.

Life cycle: The eggs are colourless and transparent. They are swallowed and larvae hatch out in duodenum. They pass down to caecum where they develop into adultworms and attach themselves to the mucosa of caecum and large gut. The male often dies after fertilising the female, which soon migrates outside the intestinal canal through the anus and deposits her eggs on the perineal skin. The eggs remain attached to the skin, in the grooves, around the anus, in the perineal hair and clothes of the host. These eggs can cause infection to men within 12–36 hours of deposition and contain tadpole-like larvae. The host may be reinfected by contamination of fingers as a result of scratching and other members of the family in many ways. These worms crawl out of anus and give rise to local irritation and often lead to many different types of symptoms, e.g. enuresis, cough, restlessness, convulsions, sleeplessness, disorders of appetite, etc. They may enter the vagina of females and cause vulvovaginitis, pruritus and leucorrhoea.

Prevention: To prevent autoinfection, good personal hygiene should be maintained. Washing hands with soap and warm water after using the toilet, changing diapers, and before handling food is the most successful way to prevent pinworm infection. The nails should be cut short and kept clean If possible, child should wear gloves at night. There should be frequent changing of bed linen, underclothes, pyjamas and towels. The anus should be smeared with dilute ammoniated mercury ointment every night before going to bed.

Treatment: The medications used for the treatment of pinworm are mebendazole, pyrantel pamoate, and albendazole. All three of these drugs are to be given in 1 dose at first and then another single dose 2 weeks later to prevent reinfection by adultworms that hatch from any eggs not killed by the first treatment.

Trichinella Spiralis

It is viviparous and is commonly known as trichina. It causes a disease known as trichinosis or trichinellosis. It passes its entire life cycle in man, rat or a pig. The male is 1.5 mm long, 0.03 mm broad, whereas the female is 3 to 4 mm long and 0.06 mm broad. Their habitat is the small intestine. The parasite differs from others in passing its entire life cycle in each host. The normal common host of *Trichinella spiralis* is the pig, which gets infected by eating rats or directly from infected faeces. The larvae are embedded in its muscles.

Infection is transmitted by consuming raw or undercooked meat of animals infected with Trichinella particularly wild game meat or pork. As the encapsulated larva reaches the stomach, the gastric acid dissolves the capsule, and the larvae are set free in small intestines and in about 2 days time they grow into full mature worms. The adultworms lies in the duodenum and jejunum. The female parasite produces more than 500 young embryos at a time, which pierce the bowels and are carried by circulation to active voluntary muscles. In about 7 to 9 days, the larvae get encysted in the muscles. They may remain in this form for about 8 months, after which they calcify and the larvae finally die.

The first symptoms of trichinellosis are gastrointestinal—nausea, diarrhoea, vomiting and abdominal pain. Classical symptoms of severe muscle pains, fever, swelling of face, weakness or fatigue, headache, rash, diarrhoea, etc. often occur within two weeks after eating contaminated meat and can last up to 8 weeks. If the infection is heavy, persons may have trouble coordinating movements, and have heart and breathing problems. Although rare, death can occur in severe cases.

Prevention and control: Safe food handling and good personal hygiene are two major strategies. The best way to prevent trichinellosis is to cook meat to safe temperatures. A food thermometer should be used to measure the internal temperature of cooked meat. Do not sample meat until it is cooked.

Treatment: Prompt treatment with antiparasitic drugs can help prevent the progression of trichinellosis by killing the adultworms and so preventing further release of larvae. Once the larvae have become established in skeletal muscle cells, usually by 3 to 4 weeks post-infection, treatment may not completely eliminate the infection and associated symptoms. Treatment with either mebendazole or albendazole is recommended.

Wuchereria

The two common species in India are:

i. *Wuchereria (filaria) bancrofti.*

ii. *Brugia malayi.*

They are long thread-like tapeworms with tapering ends and are easily visible to naked eyes. The adult male worms measure about 2.5 cm × 1 mm whereas female worms measure from 8–10 cm × 0.3 mm in length. Both sexes live together, often coiled about each other in lymph channels. The parasite has a fine sheath, in which it moves backward and forward. They complete their life cycle through parasitism in two sets of hosts, i.e. man which is the definite host and mosquito *Culex fatigans,* which is the intermediate host.

The Culex mosquito sucks the blood of an infected person during the night. The embryos exhibit nocturnal periodicity, i.e. during the night; they enter the peripheral circulation; during the day they remain in the lungs and large arteries. If the individual changes his habit and sleeps during the day, the embryos eventually appear in the peripheral vessels only during the day time. So it becomes necessary to examine the blood taken at night, or when the person is asleep, to detect the injection more easily and precisely. The embryos or microfilariae enter the stomach and soon migrate into the thoracic muscles, of the mosquitoes, where they pass through a series of developments lasting for 10–14 days. There is no multiplication of microfilariae. They are so small that they can pass easily even through the walls of capillary tubes. They finally migrate to proboscis of the mosquito. When this mosquito bites a healthy person, the infective larvae find their way into or near the site of the puncture in the skin and eventually reach the large lymphatic trunks, where they slowly grow into maturity (in about a year or so). The embryos are carried via lymphatic trunks into thoracic duct and from there into the general circulation of blood. After entry of infected larvae into the human body, it takes 6–18 months for the appearance of microfilarial in the blood.

Vectors for transmission of filariasis: In Africa, the most common vector is *Anopheles* and in the Americas, it is *Culex quinquefasciatus. Aedes* and *Mansonia* can transmit the infection in the Pacific and in Asia.

Clinical features: Clinical features of filariasis vary according to the stage of development of filarial infections in the human host. There are four stages in the development of filarial infection in man. These are:

i. *Stage of invasion:* This is usually about 1–2 years during which the infective larvae undergo development and reach adult stage. The clinical features during this stage are of allergic nature and comprise early blood eosinophilia, lymphadenopathy and specificity of response of the host to the intradermal reaction. The above parameters compared with history of the host living in the endemic area should suffice to diagnose an early case. Since the microfilariae are absent during this stage, the case does not constitute a public health danger.

ii. *Symptomless or 'carrier' stage:* This period may last for a few months to a few years or even throughout life. No clinical features are manifested by the case during this stage and the disease can be diagnosed only by night blood examination for microfilariae in the blood. While some cases remain in this stage, some proceed to the next stage. This stage is most important from the point of view of transmission of infection.

iii. *Stage of acute manifestations:* During this stage, acute fever with chills and rigor, lymphangitis, lymphadenitis, reversible lymphoedema of various parts of the body and epididymoorchitis and hydrocele in males are noted. These manifestations are considered to be due to reactions to microfilariae or adult worms themselves. In this stage, microfilariae are not always noted in blood although many cases are positive after the acute episode is over. As such, the potential for infection of the case is not very high during the carrier stage. This stage lasts for a few months to a few years and while some cases get over these reactions and become symptomless, others go to the chronic stage of the disease.

iv. *Stage of chronic manifestations:* Due to repeated attacks of acute manifestation, lymphangitis and lymphoedema take place in the dependent parts of the body. This is superimposed often by secondary bacterial infection which leads to elephantiasis of genitals, legs or arms, breasts and hydrocele, chyluria, etc. During this stage, the infection dies out and usually no microfilariae or only a few are noted in the peripheral circulation. Second attacks of infection may, however, take place.

B. malayi infection differs from *W. bancrofti* in that genital lesions like hydrocele, elephantiasis of scrotum or penis or breast are rare and is often less marked. During both the infections, the lower limbs are affected more than the upper limbs and the swelling is mostly unilateral. The frequency and severity of lesions tend to be proportional to the number of worms present in the host.

Filaria survey: A filaria survey consists of four components.

a. **Blood survey:** Peripheral blood (3 drops) is obtained by finger prick between 8 PM to midnight. A thick film is made. The slide is dehaemoglobinised, fixed in 2% acid alcohol solution and stained for microfilaria detection. Three indices are used, i.e. (i) microfilaria rate, i.e. % of persons found positive for microfilaria, (ii) microfilaria density, i.e. number of microfilaria per 20 cu mm of blood, and (iii) average infections rate, i.e. average microfilaria per positive person.

b. **Clinical survey:** When blood is collected, filarial swelling is also recorded. Filarial disease rate is calculated as a percentage of persons giving history of filarial swellings. Filarial endemicity rate is calculated by percentage of persons giving either history of swelling or being microfilaria positives.

c. Skin test for diagnostic purposes by using purified antigen from difilaria immitis is still under experimental phases.

d. **Entomological surveys** are done both for aquatic stages and adults. Indices are in terms of larval stages, adult mosquito densities, percentage of infected mosquitoes and percentage of mosquitoes with infective larvae.

Prevention and control: Since it is a mosquito-borne infection, best way to prevent filariasis is personal protection, prevention of mosquito bites and 'integrated vector control' measures.

Treatment: Diethylcarbamazine (DEC) is the drug of choice. Patients who have already developed lymphoedema should be advised proper hygiene, exercise and treatment of wounds. Conditions like hydrocele may need surgical intervention.

Dracunculus Medinensis or Guineaworm

The male, which is 15–40 mm long × 0.4 mm thick has not been found in man. A fully grown female worm is from 60 to 100 mm long and 1.5 mm in diameter. The worm is round, smooth and has milky white colour. It generally lives in the subcutaneous tissues of man. It is thread-like and nearly the whole of the worm is occupied by uterus stuffed with embryos. Roughly speaking, there are about 3 million embryos per worm. The worm is chiefly found burrowed in the subcutaneous tissues of the leg and sometimes of the back. At the site of entry, the worm secretes an irritant substance, which gives rise to a blister. It breaks the uterus of the worm, prolapses in contact with water and discharges milky looking fluid, containing myriads of embryos. These larvae pass into water and are taken up by minute cyclops, within which they undergo larval development in about five weeks time.

A healthy person (the definitive host) gets infection by drinking water containing the infected cyclops; the gastric juice kills the cyclops and sets free the larvae which burrow and find their way into the subcutaneous tissues. It takes about a year for the worms to mature. Males die after fertilisation and females repeat the cycle.

GWD is the first disease to be eradicated using core public health practices such as surveillance, case containment, and simple interventions, without the use of vaccines or medicines.

Guineaworm disease (GWD) has been eradicated in 198 countries, territories, and areas, representing 186 WHO member states as being free from GWD transmission, with only 8 countries: Angola, Democratic Republic of the Congo, Kenya, Sudan and the four remaining endemic countries of Chad, Ethiopia, Mali, and South Sudan remaining. Only 126 cases have been reported worldwide in 2014. India was declared free of guineaworm disease in 2000 (Fig. 15.13).

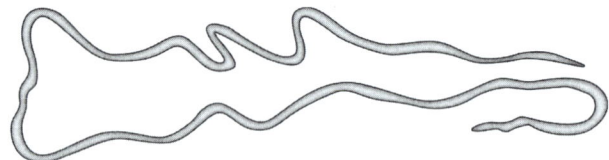

Fig. 15.13: Female guineaworm (half life size)

Ancylostoma Duodenale or Hookworm *(Fig. 15.14)*

Hookworm is a soil-transmitted helminth (STH) and is one of the most common roundworm of humans. Infection is caused by the nematode parasites *Necator americanus* and *Ancylostoma duodenale*. Hookworm infections often occur in areas where human faeces are used as fertilizer or where defaecation onto soil happens. The infection due to this worm is common in Europe, Egypt and India.

Necator americanus is comparatively shorter and more slender, having cutting plates (instead of teeth) whereas *Ancylostoma duodenale* is bigger and has teeth.

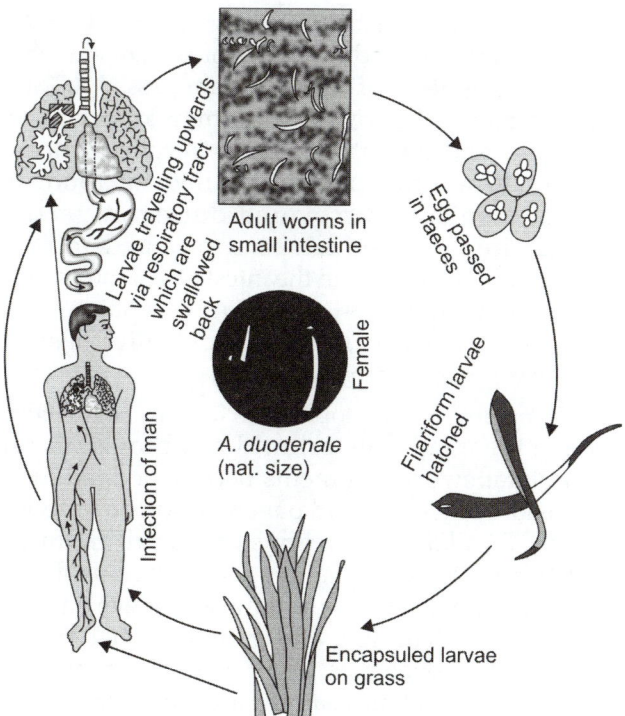

Fig. 15.14: Life history of *Ancylostoma duodenale*

A typical hookworm is almost cylindrical, the male 6 to 10 mm and the female 10 to 15 mm long. Its body is thread-like with a conical-shaped head, a large oval mouth fitted with four claws or hook-like teeth on the ventral side of the buccal cavity and two knob-like teeth on the dorsal side by which the worm fixes itself to mucous membrane of the intestines.

An infected person passes a very large number of ova in the faeces. When they happen to be laid on moist earth, further development takes place and in about 5 days' time, larvae moving about actively in their sheaths are seen crawling up the blades of grass. They can live in this stage for months when moisture and shade are present, but are rapidly killed due to heat and lack of moisture. The larvae pass through two months before becoming infective. So temperature, rainfall, humidity and condition of soil are important factors to influence the spread of infection. This is an infective stage, when the larvae enter human beings through hair follicles, sweat glands or microscopic fault in epidermis. After getting fixed on the skin, it causes dermatitis which is known as ground itch, ground sore or toe itch. After reaching the blood tissues, they enter the lymphatics or veins and thus reach the bloodstream, are carried into the heart and from the heart into lungs and bronchial tubes from where they are swallowed. If swallowed they reach the stomach, lose their protecting sheath, pass into the intestines and develop into an adultworm in about 4 weeks; they then attach themselves to the mucous membrane of the intestines, duodenum and jejunum.

During their journey in the body, they moult twice, which are in addition to two moultings outside. An interval of about 6 weeks is required between the time of initial skin infection and the first appearance of eggs in the faeces. The egg to egg hookworm cycle requires about 6 weeks to complete in the following pattern:

1. Free living in soil	= 5 days
2. Skin to intestines	= 5 days
3. 3rd moulting	= 3 days
4. 4th moulting	= 14 days
5. Maturity	= 15 days
Total	**= 42 days or 6 weeks**

Disease: Haemorrhage which gives rise to anaemia and protein deficiency. It may cause debility, puffiness of face, abdominal pain, flatulance, alternate diarrhoea and constipation, oedema of legs, palpitation, etc.

Prevention and control: The best way to avoid hookworm infection is to avoid walking barefoot and skin contact with soil with fecal contamination where hookworm is suspected. Infection can also be prevented by not defaecating outdoors, installing sanitary latrines and effective sewage disposal systems. Personal, protection using gloves and shoes to prevent infection from soil.

Treatment: Albendazole, mebendazole and pyrantal pamoate (in pregnant females) are the drugs of choice for treatment of hookworm infections. Infections are generally treated for 1–3 days. The recommended medications are effective and appear to have a few side effects. Iron supplements may also be prescribed, if the infected person has anaemia.

Cestodes, Flatworms or Tapeworms

The common forms of tapeworms are:

1. *Taenia solium*
2. *Taenia saginata*
3. *Dibothriocephalus latus* (*Diphyllobothrium latum*)
4. *Hymenolepis nana* or dwarf tapeworm
5. *Taenia echinococcus granulosus*.

They are found in intestines. The worm consists of a minute head, a neck and a row of segments. The worms are devoid of any digestive organs. They are long, flat, tape-like worms and are found in the intestines. They are generally segmented and are white or yellow in colour devoid of any mouth or alimentary canal. The worm consists of a minute head called "*scolex*" the whole body or the "*strobilla*" and the individual segments as "*proglottides*". The proglottides nearing the head are youngest and smaller in size but those on the terminal side are largest and well developed. The length varies. It may be as long as 4 metres or as small as 1/2 centimetre.

They pass through two distinct phases in two different hosts known as definitive and intermediate hosts. Man is a definitive host for the *Taenia saginata* and *Dibothriocephalus latus*; intermediate host for *Taenia echinococcus granulosus* and both definitive and intermediate hosts for *Taenia solium* and *Hymenolepis nana*.

Life History

The proglottides (ripe segments containing uterus) are dislodged from the parent worm, passed out with the faeces when the ova are set free and which retain their vitality for sometime.

The ova at this stage are eaten by some animal which is capable of acting as an intermediary host, i.e. pig, in case of *Taenia solium*, cattle in case of *Taenia saginata*, and fish in case of *Dibothriocephalus latus*, etc. They continue their development till the shell is dissolved in the intestines and the embryo, with six hooklets, is set free. These hooklets enable the embryos to penetrate the intestines to the solid tissue-like muscles of the host, where they develop into cysticercus stage (which is known as *Cysticercus cellulosae* in case of pig) which remains passive in the flesh until it is eaten by man, which acts as a "definitive host". In the stomach of the man, capsule is dissolved by the gastric juice and the scolex or head is set free which finds its way into the intestines. The head, by means of its hook, is fixed into the intestinal wall and develops into a full grown tape worm within eight weeks. It then begins to pass proglottides charged with ova in faeces, which are ready to commence a new cycle.

1. *Taenia solium or pork tapeworm:* The worm is 3 to 4 metres long consisting of 700 or more segments. The head or "scolex" is of the size of a pin and is provided with four suckers. Man is the definitive host and pigs act as intermediate hosts. The egg must be swallowed by the pig. The egg-shell is digested and the embryo is set free, which reaches the muscles (tongue, neck, shoulders and diaphragm), brain, eyes, etc. through lymphatic system where by losing its hooklets develops into a milky white bladder-like larvae (cysticercus). Pig's meat infected in this way is known as "measly pork". Man is infected by taking such insufficiently cooked meat, generally in sausages. The cysticercus is set free by the action of digestive juices and it becomes attached to the intestinal wall and becomes mature within 6 to 12 weeks. Man is also liable to become infected accidentally with the cysticercus stage by swallowing eggs from his own infective feces, or through contaminated water or food.

2. *Taenia saginata, or beef tapeworm:* Its length is 4–8 metres having 1000 to 2000 segments. Head and proglottides are similar to those of *Taenia solium*. The intermediate host is cattle. They become infected by eating grass or drinking water contaminated by faeces of patients in which mature segments of the worm are passed. It forms cysticercus in the bovine flesh, this is known as beef measles and the infected meat is called "measly beef". When the animal is killed for food, the cysts should be discovered during inspection, otherwise if the beef happens to be undercooked, the cysts will develop in the intestines of the persons, who eat it and will thus produce new tapeworms. For *Taenia saginata*, man is the definitive host and cattle serve as intermediate hosts.

Symptoms: Most people with tapeworm infections have no symptoms or mild symptoms. In rare cases, tapeworm segments become lodged in the appendix, or the bile and pancreatic ducts. Infection with *T. solium* tapeworms can result in human **cysticercosis**, which can be a very serious disease that can cause seizures and muscle or eye damage.

Safe food handling and good personal hygiene are the key strategies for prevention of infection. Praziquantel and niclosamide are the drugs effective in teniasis.

3. *Diphyllobothrium latum:* It is the largest ribbon-like tapeworm found in human beings; its length varying from 3 to 10 metres and having about 2500 to 3000 segments. It can grow up to 30 feet long. The cysticercus inhabits some species of fish. The symptoms produced are not always severe. In some cases, the blood produces the symptoms of pernicious anaemia. The eggs when discharged in the faeces of man in water develop into larvae and ingested by a fish. This worm is not found in India.

4. *Hymenolepis nana or dwarf tapeworm:* It is 25–45 mm long and 1 mm broad. It is the smallest tapeworm found in man. It is very slender and because of its very small size, it often escapes notice. Each proglottide contains 80–180 eggs which are set free in the intestines. It undergoes complete development from an egg to the adult stage without any intermediary host. The larval parasite enters the intestinal wall, where it becomes cysticercoid. Later on, it moves into the intestines, where it attaches itself to the mucous membrane and develops. It occurs in hundreds, sometimes even in thousands and may cause symptoms of diarrhoea, epileptiform convulsions, headache, etc. on account of absorption of toxins produced in the system by the parasites. It is most often seen in children in countries in which sanitation and hygiene are inadequate.

Prevention: It consists of adopting the following measures:

i. Cure of the affected person.

ii. Disposal of the human excreta in such a way that cattle, pigs or fish cannot have access to it.

iii. Thorough inspection of meat and pork in the slaughter houses by the veterinary surgeon.

iv. Thorough cooking of meat and fish.

v. Thorough smoking or salting of meat which is eaten raw and avoidance of taking raw meat.

vi. Observance of strict personal hygiene. Hands should be thoroughly cleaned after toilet and before taking food.

Praziquantel and niclosamide are drugs of choice for treatment.

5. *Taenia echinococcus*: It is a minute tapeworm of the dog and is found in its small intestines, which serve as its definitive host. The worm has its cyst stage in man and consists of a scolex, a neck and 3–4 segments only.

The ova are discharged by the dog in its faeces, which are ingested by the intermediary host, i.e. pig, sheep, oxen, horse or man. The shell is dissolved in the stomach of the intermediary host and the embryo is liberated which on piercing the intestinal wall, encysts as a hydatid cyst, chiefly in the liver. This hydatid cyst, attains a great size and forms within itself secondary cysts called daughter cysts. The liquid in the cyst does not coagulate on boiling. Under the microscope, a characteristic head or detached hooklets can be seen.

This disease is common in some countries where men live in close association with dogs and may then be infected directly by them.

Prevention

Following measures should be adopted:

1. A system of licencing of pet dogs should be enforced by the municipalities. Incineration or deep burial of dead animals is recommended.

2. One should avoid the close association between dog and man and contaminating ones hands with the faeces of dogs.

3. Strict personal hygiene should be observed.

4. Rigid control should be enforced on the slaughtering of herbivorous animals so that dogs do not have an easy access to scraps of uncooked meat as dogs are infected only by larval forms of hydatid cysts present in food of mammals.

Trematodes or Flukes

The common ones which infect human beings are:

1. **Distomum or fasciola hepaticum (liver flukes):** It affects sheep causing a disease known as "liver rot". It is 20 to 30 mm long, 8 to 13 mm broad and is heart-shaped. It is of pale-grey colour.

The fertilised egg, when expelled from the bile duct into the sheep's intestines, is passed out with faeces and becomes miracidium, which if it encounters a fresh snail, enters its body where it is transformed into a tadpole-like "Cercaria". It passes out of the snail, sheds its tail and after leaving the water moves up to a grass blade, where it encysts. When this grass is eaten by a sheep, the young fluke is set free in its intestines. It then finds its way to the bile duct, attaches itself to the duct wall and attains maturity. Man gets rarely infected by it. The areas with the highest known rates of human infection are in the Andean highlands of Bolivia and Peru.

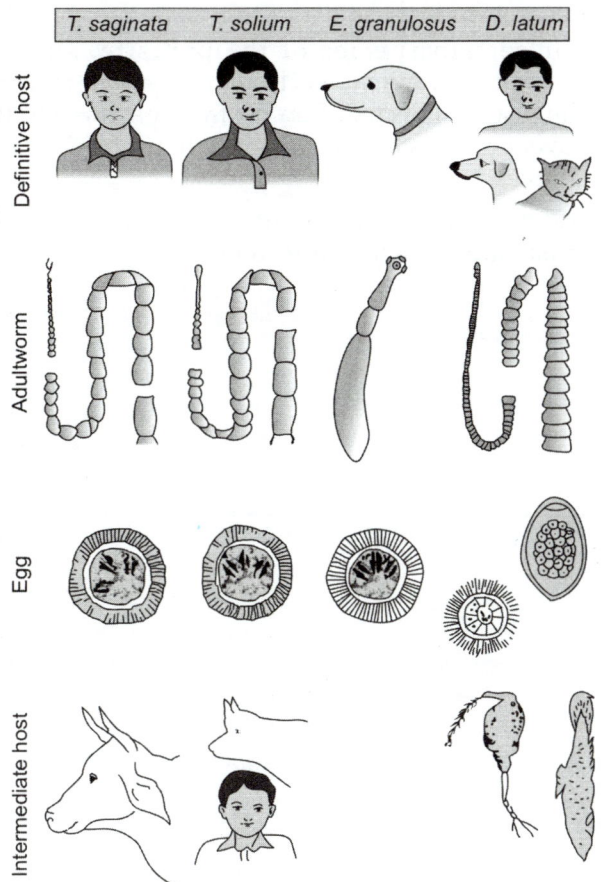

Fig. 15.15: Various types of tapeworms

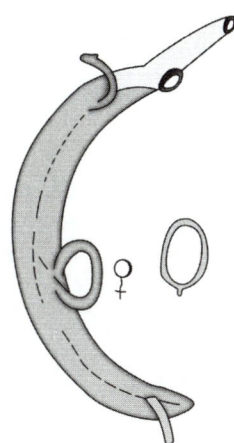

Fig. 15.16: *Schistosoma haematobium* (male and female)

2. **Schistosoma or blood flukes:** Three distinct species of those worms are known to occur in man, but their life cycle is more or less identical. They are:
   a. *Schistosoma* or *Bilharzia haematobium* (urinary bladder).
   b. *Schistosoma mansoni*: The symptoms produced are dysenteric and a peculiar form of cirrhosis of liver. It is followed by a condition known as intestinal schistosomiasis.
   c. *Schistosoma japonicum*: It gives rise to oedema and excites dysenteric symptoms, emaciation and in later stages cirrhosis of liver. The adult lives in the veins of the large intestines.

Schistosoma or Bilharzia haematobium: The male is ½ inch (12.7 mm) long and the female is ¾ inch (19.05 mm) long. They are generally lodged in the veins of intestines, bladder, ureter or kidney. They give rise to a chronic disease called Bilharziasis characterised by cystitis, haematuria and other symptoms due to blockage of the urinary passages producing a papillomatous growth. These are common in Africa and Palestine. An endemic centre has recently been discovered in Ratnagiri district of Maharashtra. The males are narrow, flat, leaf-like worms and look cylindrical from the folding in the side of the skin, forming the gynaecophoric canal, where the female is partially enclosed.

The eggs are oval or spindle-shaped with a stout spine at the posterior end. These are forced through walls of the vessel and eventually appear in the bladder or rectum and escape either through urine or the faeces, as the case may be. They find their way into water, develop into a ciliated embryo or miracidium, which becomes attached to its intermediate host, viz. fresh water molluscs and develops into a cercaria form. They infect man through the skin. They enter the veins where they gradually develop. They are able to pass through and, therefore, any one bathing or even putting an arm in water infected by these organisms easily gets infected.

Incubation period: Systematic manifestations usually begin when the worms are reaching maturity about 3–6 weeks after infection. Usually the eggs are found in urine and faeces a week or two after the appearance of symptoms.

Control

Control efforts usually focus on:
   a. Reducing the number of infections in people and/or
   b. Eliminating the snails that are required to maintain the parasite's life cycle.

For all species that cause schistosomiasis, improved sanitation could reduce or eliminate transmission of this disease.

Control measures can include mass drug treatment of entire communities and targeted treatment of school age children. Some of the problems with control of schistosomiasis include:

1. Chemicals used to eliminate snails in freshwater sources may harm other species of animals in the water and, if treatment is not sustained, the snails may return to those sites afterwards.

2. For certain species of the parasite, such as *S. japonicum*, animals such as cows or water buffalo can also be infected. Run off from pastures (if the cows are infected) can contaminate fresh water sources.

Treatment: Praziquantel is the drug of choice for both intestinal and urinary schistosomiasis.

Epidemiology of Communicable Diseases

With the advance of civilisation, more and more diseases are coming into light. These are being investigated and classified into communicable or non-communicable diseases. A communicable disease is one in which the causative organism may pass or is carried from one person to another either directly or indirectly. Only a few important ones are discussed here, keeping in view the limitations of the book.

DISEASES CARRIED BY INSECTS

16.1 MALARIA

Malaria is a mosquito-borne infectious disease of humans caused by parasitic protozoa belonging to the genus *Plasmodium*. Malaria causes symptoms that typically include fever with chills and rigor, fatigue, vomiting and headaches. In severe cases, it can cause yellow skin, seizures, coma and death. It may result in anaemia and spleen enlargement among the sufferers in the long run. Globally, there were about 198 million cases of malaria in 2013 and an estimated 584,000 deaths. In India, it continues to be major public health problem, mostly due to *Plasmodium falciparum* which is more prone to complications. About 22% Indian population live in malaria high transmission areas. There are around 1.07 million reported confirmed cases and 535 reported deaths. Nearly, 128 million tests were being conducted on the suspected cases, with *P. falciparum* causing 53% and *P. vivax* causing 47% of the infections. The incidence of malaria in India accounted for 58% of cases in the South-East Asia Region of WHO. No other disease in India has caused in the aggregate more sickness or greater loss of life than malaria. Its social and economic effects are extremely deplorable.

Besides these statistics, other social implications of the disease were:

1. Illness of the wage-earner, especially in families under the marginal income groups, resulted in dislocation of the family of the worker.

2. Lowering of vitality due to attacks of malaria led to the victim becoming an easy prey to many diseases such as tuberculosis, etc. This ended in a loss to the nation as a whole.

3. Deaths caused by malaria amongst the age groups, which otherwise would have provided efficient labour for many years resulted in a loss of production to the nation.

4. Lowering of vitality of industrial or agricultural workers due to attacks of malaria led to inefficiency of the Indian labour and consequently lowered both the industrial and agricultural production.

5. It was well established that wherever malaria prevailed and almost in direct proportion to its prevalence, the population was generally physically, mentally, and economically subnormal.

Aetiology

The causal organism or the malarial parasite is a protozoan named Plasmodium which was discovered by Charles Laveran in 1880. Man acquires infection naturally only through the bite of an infected female Anopheles mosquito, which injects the malarial parasites in the form of sporozoites. Fatality in untreated cases varies from 1–10% depending upon the character of parasite and degree of resistance of the host. The malarial parasites are of the following types:

1. *Plasmodium vivax (benign tertian malaria):* It has a cycle of 48 hours causing fever, recurring after every two days.

2. *Plasmodium malariae (quartan malaria):* It has a cycle of 72 hours causing fever, recurring after every three days.

3. *Plasmodium falciparum (malignant tertian malaria):* The fever is very irregular with chills and rigor and may occur after every 48 hours. The symptoms are very severe and of malignant type, e.g. high fever, delirium and sometimes coma.

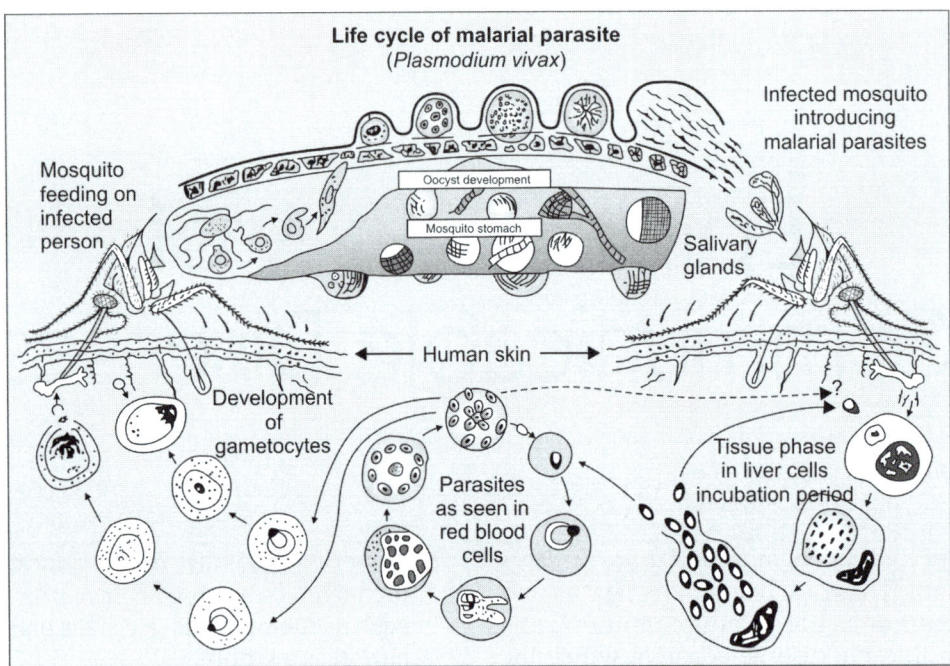

Fig.16.1: Life cycle of malarial parasite (*Plasmodium vivax*)

4. *Plasmodium ovale,* a parasite, which produces a mild form of tertian malaria. This is now found in Baroda district of Gujarat and Koraput district of Odisha in India.

Developmental Cycles

The life history of all the parasites is the same. The mosquito is a definitive host and man is the intermediate host. There are two cycles:

1. *Asexual or human cycle or schizogony*: When an infected female anopheline mosquito bites a healthy person and sucks blood, she injects salivary fluid containing *sporozoites* in the circulation system. Sporozoites enter the parenchymal cells of the liver and are called *cryptozoites,* where they undergo developmental changes. During this period, the patient does not show any symptoms or signs, nor any parasite in the blood. After the incubation period, which ranges from 10 to 14 days, *pre-erythrocytic merozoites* are released, which enter red blood cells of peripheral blood and give rise to clinical attack of malaria. They pass through the stages of trophozoite, schizont and merozoite. Each trophozoite assumes a round shape and continues to enlarge and the pigment appears. After sometime, chromatin begins to divide and then it is known as *schizont* or a rosette body, which divides into small bodies called *merozoites.* These, on breaking down of blood corpuscles escape into blood plasma and enter fresh red blood corpuscles. This constitutes the asexual cycle and is called *schizogony.* This may be continued indefinitely until checked by proper treatment.

2. *Sexual or mosquito cycle or sporogony*: After a certain number of asexual generations, some of the young trophozoites, instead of becoming schizonts, grow into male and female forms called *gametocytes* in the red cells. They are incapable of further development unless they are taken by a female Anopheles mosquito. In the stomach of the mosquito, the male and the female form escape from the red blood corpuscles and undergo exflagellation which are known as *gametes.* One of the male gametes (*micro-gamete*) fertilises a female gamete (*macro-gamete*) and forms a body known as a *zygote,* which lengthens and matures into ookinete within next 24 hours. Then, it burrows itself into the stomach wall of anopheline mosquito and grows there, where a cyst is formed around it. It is called *oocyst.* This increases in size and is packed with *sporozoites.* The oocyst ruptures, discharging *the sporozoites* into the body cavity of the insects and ultimately they find their way into the salivary glands of mosquito, from where they are transferred to a healthy person.

It takes about 36 hours after feeding on blood of an infected person, for the zygote to develop in the stomach wall of the mosquito. The sporozoites reach the salivary glands on the 10th to 12th days. The whole development in the mosquito takes about 12 days. It is infective from the 12th day onwards and remains infective for the rest of its life.

Incubation period: On an average, incubation period is 12 (9 to 14) days for *P. falciparum,* 14 (8 to 17) days for *P. vivax,* 30 (18 to 40) days for *P. malariae* and

17 (16 to 18) days for *P. ovale*. It is the period from the bite of an infected mosquito and the first appearance of fever.

Malaria Index

It means the degree of prevalence of malaria in a locality or a district. It can be ascertained in the following ways:

1. *Infant parasite rate*: It is defined as the percentage of infants below one year of age showing malarial parasites in their blood films. It is the most sensitive index of recent transmission of malaria in a locality.

2. *Spleen rate*: This term refers to the percentage of children between 2 and 9 years of age who are suffering from enlarged spleen. Generally children under 10 years of age are examined for the following reasons: (a) They are easily available for the purpose. (b) Adults are excluded due to frequent occurrence of malaria in causing splenic enlargement.

   If splenic index is less than 10%, the locality is considered having low endemicity or is healthy. If it is between 11 and 50%, the locality is considered as mesoendemic. If it is between 50 and 75%, the locality is considered as hyperendemic. If it is above 75%, the locality is considered as holoendemic.

3. *Average enlarged spleen*: It denotes average size of enlarged spleen. Thus, the percentage of people having enlarged spleens and the degree of enlargement correlate with risk of infection in a community.

4. *Parasitic rate*: It represents the percentage of children between the ages of 2 and 10 years showing malarial parasites in their blood films.

5. *Proportional case rate*: It is the number of clinically diagnosed malaria cases per 100 patients attending hospitals, dispensaries and health centres.

6. *Sporozoite rate*: It is calculated by determining the percentage of female anopheline mosquitoes, who show malarial parasites in their bodies after capturing and dissecting them. In a place highly infected with malaria, this index may range from 5 to 10%.

7. *Human blood index*: It is the proportion of freshly fed female anopheline mosquitoes whose stomach contains human blood. It indicates the degree of anthrophilism.

8. *Mosquito density*: It is usually expressed as the number of mosquitoes per man hour catch.

9. *Man biting rate*: It is defined as the average incidence of anopheline mosquito bites per day per person.

10. *Annual parasite incidence (API)*

$$API = \frac{\text{Confirmed cases during one year}}{\text{Population under surveillance}} \times 1000$$

It is based on intensive active and passive surveillance, and cases are confirmed by blood examination.

11. *Annual blood examination rate (ABER)*

$$ABER = \frac{\text{Number of slides examined}}{\text{Population}} \times 100$$

It is an index of operational efficiency which depends upon the annual blood collection and examination rates.

12. *Annual falciparum incidence*: Data are collected regarding total facliparum cases, since the emergence of falciparum problem in India.

Surveillance in Malaria

It aims at the detection of malaria cases through laboratory tests and provide facilities for proper treatment. There are three types of surveillance in malaria—active, passive and sentinel.

1. *Active surveillance*: It is carried out through the agency of paid workers known as "surveillance workers", who are now being replaced by multi-purpose workers (MPWs). Each worker is allotted a population of about 10,000 or 1500 to 2000 houses. To supervise their work, for every four workers, a surveillance inspector called "health assistant" is also appointed.

2. *Passive surveillance*: The process of searching malaria cases by hospitals, dispensaries, primary health centres, etc. is called passive surveillance. These agencies collect blood smears from the patients suffering from malaria and also from those having recent history of fever. The blood slides are collected and sent by the surveillance workers/ MPWs to the laboratory for microscopic examination. The results of blood examination are sent by the laboratory back to the surveillance worker/MPW for administration of proper medicine, if found positive.

3. *Sentinel surveillance*: There is one weakness in the current malaria surveillance system. It is the lack of articulation with hospitals for which severe malaria cases are not reported separately and very few malaria deaths are reported. That is why sentinel surveillance is being established in highly endemic districts.

Methods of Prevention and Control

These can be discussed under the following heads:

a. To do away with the conditions which render possible the breeding of mosquitoes.

b. To destroy mosquitoes at some period of their life, i.e. during adult and larva stage.

c. To prevent mosquitoes from biting man.

d. To attack the parasite as it circulates in the blood of man, i.e. adoption of antiparasitic measures.

a. To do away with conditions which render possible the breeding of mosquitoes

i. To provide drainage in the country on a large scale so as to drain properly the swamps and lakes. The drains should be narrow and deep rather than broad and shallow. Sometimes, subsoil drains are also provided. They are more effective in dealing with hill streams. However, their maintenance cost is high.

ii. To provide drainage on a small scale around the town, so as to prevent rainwater collection in the pools, and in the compounds of houses. All the depressions and small pools, where water may collect should be filled up.

iii. To keep clean, straight and free from weeds, the edges of canals and small water courses. This makes the water run quickly and by removing the weeds from the banks, there remains no shelter or hiding place for the larvae.

iv. To avoid having burrowpits along the roads, railway lines, tanks and pools, where water can stagnate.

v. To properly maintain irrigation channels and exercise proper control on the supply of canal water so that water is not supplied in excess of actual requirements of the locality concerned.

b. To destroy mosquitoes at some period of their life

1. *Destruction of mosquito larvae or antilarval measures* These are as follows:

i. *Malariol, kerosene oil, diesel or fuel oil, etc.*: It is sprayed on the surface of water with a knaspack spray once a week or by soaking gunny bags, lump of tow or cottonwaste in it and throwing them into water; say 2 oz (56.70 gm) of kerosene oil for 30 sq ft (2.78 sq metres). It asphyxiates the larvae, as they cannot breathe. Vegetation in water should be removed to render it fully effective.

ii. *Pyrethrum extract*: Pyrethrum is an insecticide of vegetable origin, which is extracted from the flowers of *Chrysanthemum cineraria folium*—a plant cultivated in Kashmir. It is used in the following form:

	Pyrethrum extract 2%	0.5 gallon (2.27 litres)
A	Pine oil	0.5 gallon (2.27 litres)
	Kerosene	9.5 gallons (43.13 litres)

All the three are mixed together.

	Liquid soft soap containing	
B	40% actual soap	5 pints (2.83 litres)
	Water	5 gallons (22.70 litres)

Now both A and B solutions are mixed together with thorough stirring.

This forms a concentrated stock solution. It is diluted with 10 times of water and stirred thoroughly just before spraying.

iii. *Paris green or acetoarsenite of copper*: It is mixed with 100 parts of fine road dust, slaked lime, soapstone, sawdust, etc. and blown either by a machine or manually. It is very toxic to anopheline larvae but it does not kill culicine and aedes larvae. It is effective even in presence of dense vegetation. It does not kill fish or spoil water for domestic purposes. ½–1 lb (0.226–0.453 kg) of Paris green is used per acre (0.4 hectare).

iv. *Dichlorodiphenyltrichloroethane (DDT)*: It is a white amorphous powder having a mild smell. It is insoluble in water, but dissolves in most organic solvents. The technical grade contains about 80% of pp isomer. It is an efficient larvicide. It is effective even in very small quantities and thus there is a great saving, if it is used for the purpose. It is used as, 5 to 10%, oily solution for spraying or 10% if used as a dust.

v. *Larvicidal fish*: These eat larvae of mosquitoes. There are many species of small fish in India. *Gambusia affinis* or water minnows, etc. are ideal for this purpose. They multiply rapidly, and feed voraciously on larvae and pupae. They are surface feeders and are especially effective against Anopheles larvae.

vi. *Gammexane WDP*: To control mosquito breeding in wet crops like paddy fields, where use of malariol is contraindicated on account of its charring effects on plants, gammexane has been found useful and economical. For stagnating water, in such fields two ounces (56.70 gm) of gammexane WDP mixed in a gallon (4.54 litres) of water is used at a rate of 15 gallon (68.19 litres) of suspension per acre. It destroys mosquito larvae but has no effect on eggs and pupae.

vii. *Observance of dry day*: In cantonments, one day in a week is fixed when all cisterns, cess pits, stores of water, gharras, etc. are emptied, kept dry for some time and then refilled. In this way, if there is any breeding in these waters, it is destroyed. Similar 'dry days' should be observed in the rest of malaria prone places in the country.

2. *Destruction of adult mosquitoes*

i. *DDT or dichlorodiphenyltrichloroethane,* a residual insecticide, is largely used these days in the form of emulsion or oily solution for spraying. After the evaporation of the solvent, minute crystals of insecticide remain on the surface of the walls. When the mosquitoes rest on the wall for 10–20 minutes, they absorb some of the DDT through their legs, feet, get themselves poisoned and die. Generally an emulsion of 5% strength is sprayed at such a rate that it will be sufficient to give protection against one mosquito breeding season. Dosage is 100 to 200 mg per square foot (0.092 sq m). It is used in the following forms:

a. *DDT aromax emulsion*

DDT technical	110 lb (49.89 kg)
Aromax	36 gallons (163.65 litres)
Soap Lux flakes	8 lb (3.63 kg)
Water	32 lb (14.51 kg)

110 lb (49.89 kg) of DDT is placed in a 45-gallon (204.57 litres) capacity barrel with an open top. Its lumps are thoroughly broken. About 4-gallon (18.18 litres) of aromax is then added to DDT and thoroughly macerated to make a paste which is constantly stirred. Soap and water solution is prepared separately in a container. This resultant mixture forms 25% DDT concentrate and is diluted in the ratio of 1 in 10 with water to obtain 2.5% DDT emulsion. It is sprayed with a stirrup pump or knapsack sprayer, on the walls.

b. *50% DDT kerosene oil solution*

DDT technical	8 oz (0.226 kg)
Kerosene oil (grade 3)	1 gallon (4.54 litres)

The required quantity is added into a container and stirred thoroughly to make a 5% DDT kerosene oil solution.

c. *Geigy's (50% DDT water wettable powder) suspension*: Geigy's malaria spray

Powder	8 oz (0.22 kg)
Water	1 gallon (4.54 litres)

A paste of the Geigy's powder with a small amount of water is made and then more water is added to obtain the suspension of requisite consistency.

d. *Pyrethrum DDT kerosene oil mixture of flit*: Pyrethrum extract

Liquid 4%	3 oz (85.05 gm)
DDT technical	1 oz (28.35 gm)
Kerosene oil	1 gallon (4.54 litres)

DDT is dissolved in kerosene oil and then pyrethrum extract liquid is added. It is sprayed with a flit pump.

e. *DDT in aerosols*: The aerosol bomb contains 0.40% of pyrethrin, 3% DDT, 5% cyclohexanone, 5% sesame or some other oils in freon. Its pressure forces the combination to disperse into the room. It is widely used against mosquitoes and other insects.

ii. *Gammexane or benzene hexachloride or BHC*: It is effective against mosquitoes as a residual spray, but its lasting properties are not quite good. Gammexane P520 contains 50% BHC and is soluble in water forming suspension.

Gammexane P520 (water dispersible powder)	12 oz (0.33 kg)
Water	1 gallon (4.54 litres)

With a small amount of water, a paste of gammexane is made and then the balance water added to make a milky suspension. It is sprayed by a pressure sprayer.

iii. *Dieldrin*: The insecticide is better than DDT and BHC and unlike BHC whole weight of dieldrin in a formulation is insecticidally active. It is said to be more effective against flies and mosquitoes than other insecticides. 4 ounces (113.40 gm) of dieldrin. 50% water wettable powder is used in a gallon (4.54 litres) of water for surface spraying of 2000 sq ft (185.8 sq metres). The normal dose is 25 mg per sq ft (0.09 sq metre).

iv. *Traps* of various types are available in the market. The mosquitoes are caught in the traps and subsequently killed.

v. *Cutting* down of jungles and other useless vegetations, where mosquitoes conceal during the daytime, is of great value in a campaign launched against adult mosquitoes.

vi. Bats, birds, lizards and dragon flies are natural enemies of mosquitoes, but they themselves are a nuisance.

c. **Protection against the bite of mosquitoes:** The use of mosquito nets, repellents, fumigants, household screens and electrical devices is beneficial, but these devices are not foolproof in effectiveness. Ointments on various exposed parts of the body repel the mosquitoes by the smell, e.g. dimethylphthalate (DMP), citronella oil, eucalyptus oil, sandalwood oil (plain or cream), etc. which if applied to the skin, remain effective as a repellent for several hours.

d. **Adoption of antiparasitic measures:** It signifies giving treatment to patients.

Radical treatment: It is given to those patients, whose blood film is positive for the presence of malarial parasites.

i. *P. vivax malaria*: The treatment consists of a 14-day course, which is recommended as under:

   a. 25 mg/kg body weight of chloroquine in three divided doses over 3 days, i.e. 10 mg/kg on day 1, 10 mg/kg on day 2 and 5 mg/kg on day 3 plus

   b. 0.25 mg/kg primaquine daily for 14 days.

ii. *P. falciparum malaria*: Artemisinin-based combination therapy (ACT) is used to treat falciparum cases.

a. In states other than North Eastern states, artesunate is given 4 mg/kg body weight daily for 3 days along with sulphadoxine (25 mg/kg)—pyrimethamine (1.25 mg/kg) on day 1 and primaquine 0.75 mg/kg in a single dose on day 2.

b. In North Eastern states, artemether (20 mg) and lumefantrine (120 mg) combinations are used. For 5 to 14 kg, 1 tablet twice daily, for 15 to 24 kg, 2 tablets twice daily, for 25 to 34 kg, 3 tablets twice daily and lastly for >34 kg, 4 tablets twice daily are given for 3 days plus 0.75 mg/kg primaquine is given on day 2.

c. In case of mixed infections (vivax + falciparum), all are treated with full course of ACT as per the guidelines of different states written above along with 0.25 mg/kg body weight of primaquine daily for 14 days.

16.2 KALA-AZAR (DUMDUM FEVER OR BLACK FEVER)

It is an infectious disease that is caused by unicellular eukaryotic obligatory intracellular protozoa, i.e. *Leishmania donovani* which primarily affects reticuloendothelial system. It produces a wide variety of clinical syndromes ranging from self-healing cutaneous ulcers to fatal visceral disease. There are mainly 3 categories: Visceral leishmaniasis (VL), cutaneous leishmaniasis (CL) and mucosal leishmaniasis (ML). It had been named in 1903 after their discoverers Sir William Leishman and Donovan. It is transmitted by sandflies. In the beginning, fever may be very severe and the patient is emaciated, anaemic, with black pigmentation of the skin (kala-azar black sickness), advanced emaciation of limbs/chest, and with hepato-splenomegaly. The patient loses weight, becomes lean and weak. If not treated, the disease is highly fatal.

Etiology (*Leishmania donovani*): Exists in two forms, i.e. amastigote occurs in man and promastigote occurs in gut of sandfly. In human, it has a small round or oval body and is found in cells of reticuloendothelial system, i.e. in spleen, liver and bone marrow.

Prevalence: In India, it is prevalent in Uttar Pradesh, Bengal, Assam, Odisha, Tamil Nadu, Jharkhand and Bihar.

Incubation period: It varies from 1 to 3 months.

Mode of transmission: It is transmitted to man by the bite of infected female sandfly, i.e. *Phlebotomus argentipes*. The fly is infected by sucking the peripheral blood or by ingesting parasites present in the skin of an infected individual. It remains infected for 6–9 days after an infected blood meal. Transmission of kala-azar has also been recorded by blood transfusion.

Prevention: Following measures need to be adopted:
1. Early diagnosis and notification
2. Isolation of sick

3. Regular house to house survey and mass survey to detect cases in endemic areas
4. Elimination of breeding places of sandflies
5. Use of repellents gives a temporary protection
6. Destruction of sandflies with spraying DDT at regular intervals.
7. Keeping the houses and their surroundings clean and filling all the pits on the walls of the houses with earth.

Treatment: Sodium stibogluconate (SSG) is used in areas where SSG sensitivity is >90%. It is given as IM or IV injection with a dose of 20 mg/kg body weight for 20 days. In areas with SSG sensitivity <90%, amphotericin B (1 mg/kg body weight) is given IV infusion daily or alternate day for 15–20 infusions. In areas with high level of SSG resistance (>20%), miltefosine 100 mg daily in two divided doses for 4 weeks is given.

16.3 YELLOW FEVER

It is an acute febrile viral haemorrhagic disease associated with severe hepatic and renal involvement. It is characterised by toxic jaundice (yellowness of skin), albuminuria, haemorrhages from the stomach, nose and mouth, shock, agitation, stupor and coma.

Distribution: It is a disease of tropical climates. There are an estimated 2,00,000 cases of yellow fever, causing 30,000 deaths, worldwide each year, with 90% occurring in Africa. Forty-four endemic countries in Africa and Latin America, with a combined population of over 900 million, are at risk. In Africa, an estimated 508 million people live in 31 countries at risk. The remaining population at risk are in 13 countries in Latin America, with Bolivia, Brazil, Colombia, Ecuador and Peru at greatest risk. The jungle type or "jungle yellow fever" occurs in America due to viral infection from monkeys, since the disease is transmitted from animal to animal and the man is accidentally infected through *Aedes* moquitoes.

Aetiology: Yellow fever is caused by the Flavivirus fibricus, a 40- to 50 nm-wide enveloped RNA virus, member of family Flaviviridae. In forest areas, the main reservoirs are monkeys and forest mosquitoes. The blood of patients is infective for 3 to 4 days. In case of mosquito, it becomes infective 8 to 12 days after the extrinsic incubation period.

Mode of spread: The disease is spread through the bites of infected female *Aedes aegypti* mosquito within first three days of illness. Hence, the importance of early diagnosis and preventing an individual from being bitten by mosquitoes especially during the incubation period is stressed. The mosquitoes are not infective for 12 days after bite due to extrinsic incubation period, but after that period they remain infective throughout their life. These mosquitoes bite both during day as well as night.

Incubation period: 3 to 6 days.

Fatality rate: It varies from 5 to 50%

Immunity: Its recovery from one attack gives lifelong immunity. Infants born from immune mothers have maternal antibodies, which remain active up to 6 months.

Preventive measures: These are:

1. Immediate notification

2. Isolation of the case and the patient must be screened from the bite of mosquitoes for the first 4 to 5 days of illness

3. Measures against mosquitoes
   These are:
   i. Elimination of their breeding places
   ii. Antilarval measures
   iii. Antiadult mosquito measures
   iv. Protection from bites of mosquitoes.

4. Disinfection of the houses with a residual insecticide such as DDT chlordane, dieldrin or benzene hexachloride.

5. *Protective inoculation*: (a) Inoculation with yellow fever vaccine, which consists of attenuated virus grown in chick embryo and dried in vacuum should be done. It is issued in sealed ampoules and reconstituted with distilled water. The injection does not have any reaction. Immunity is established after 10th day and lasts for 10 years.

6. *Quarantine*: Non-immunized persons, coming from endemic areas either in an aircraft, a ship or a train are placed in quarantine for 6 days on arrival at a place, where the disease is unknown.

If the traveller arrives before the international certificate of vaccination becomes valid, he is isolated till the certificate becomes valid. YF is a notifiable disease as per IHR (revised) 2005.

Measures against importation of yellow fever in India by aerial navigation. The aircraft which has started from or transited at any airport in a yellow fever endemic country within 30 days of its arrival in India, provided such aircraft has not been disinfect in accordance with the procedure laid down by WHO, shall be required to properly disinfected before landing in any airport in India. No person may land in India by aircraft either as a passenger or a member of crew during the six days following his departure from or landing in a similar region as detailed above, unless he has been protected by vaccination, which is considered efficacious or by a previous attack of the disease. The airport health officer shall coordinate with concerned agencies to keep a distance of at least four hundred meters around the perimeter of every airport free of vectors of yellow fever.

Treatment: No specific antiviral therapy is available. Treatment is directed toward symptomatic relief and management of complications. Associated bacterial infections can be treated with antibiotics.

16.4 DENGUE OR "BREAK BONE" FEVER

It is an acute febrile infectious disease sometimes with or without haemorrhagic manifestations. It has a sudden onset with malaise, skin rash, intense frontal headache, severe pain in bones and joints and retro-orbital pain. Fever lasts for about five days and a slow convalescene begins with skin rashes covering up to 50% of the body. The disease is spread by the bite of infected mosquitoes *Aedes aegypti*, and *Aedes albopictus*. The virus is acquired by the mosquito by sucking blood from a patient from the day before onset to the 50th day. It becomes infective 8 to 10 days after biting and remains a lifelong carrier of the virus. Some 2.5 billion people are at risk of developing the disease in tropical and subtropical countries. An estimated 50 million dengue infections occur worldwide annually and 500,000 people with dengue haemorrhagic fever require hospitalization every year. In India, dengue is endemic in 31 states/UTs. During 2013, about 74,168 cases were reported with 168 deaths. The population of Aedes mosquito fluctuates with rainfall and water storage.

Incubation period: It is from 3 to 15 days, but usually it ranges from 5 to 8 days.

Prevention: The methods of prevention which depend upon control of *Aedes aegypti* mosquitoes are same as used against yellow fever, e.g. screening of rooms, use of mosquito repellents, preventing breeding in and around premises by avoiding accumulation of water in pots, barrels, drums, etc. by emptying them once a week. Treatment is directed towards symptomatic relief and management of complications.

16.5 SANDFLY FEVER

This is a 3-day fever accompanied with frontal headache, pyrexia, sharp articular and muscular pains, flushing of face, fast heart rate and occasionally rash. The incubation period is 3 to 6 days. The vector is *Phlebotomus pappataci* which must bite a patient of sandfly fever within first 36 hours. It becomes infective after 6 to 7 days and remains so for life.

Preventive measures: These are:

1. Isolation of the sick

2. Control of breeding of sandflies and their destruction.

3. Prevention of sandfly bites—by anointing the skin with citronella oil, etc.

4. Disinfestation of the premises with, DDT or BHC.

Treatment: It is symptomatic.

16.6 RELAPSING FEVER

These are of two kinds:

1. Louse relapsing fever.
2. Tick relapsing or tick fever.

1. Louse Relapsing Fever

Definition: It is an acute infectious bacterial disease characterised by an attack of high fever of sudden onset lasting for 2 to 9 days terminating in a crisis and by a series of relapses, if the person is not treated. It is associated with chills and rigor, muscle or joint aches and nausea. A rash may also occur.

Aetiology: The infection is due to *Rickettsia prowazekii*, *Bartonella quintana* and *Borrelia recurrentis* which are generally found in peripheral blood during the attack of the fever but are absent in apyrexial stage.

Predisposing factors: They are overcrowding, and insanitary conditions of life. Spread of disease is greatly enhanced when persons sleep closely huddled together, using common beddings, cots, etc. Infection may directly occur through clothes and use of common combs.

Mode of spread: It is not communicable from man to man. It is carried from the sick to the healthy by blood sucking insects, i.e. body lice and possibly bugs. When a louse bites an infected person, it swallows the rickettsia, which at first disappear but a week later, will be found in large numbers in the body fluids of the louse. When this infected louse bites a healthy person, he feels irritation and scratches the place with his finger nales where louse has bitten. In doing so he crushes the louse incidentally and thus infection is transmitted through the skin. The rickettsia enter the body through the abrasion caused by scratching.

Incubation period: It is from 5 to 15 days.

Mortality: 1% with treatment and 30 to 70% without treatment.

Seasonal prevalence: The disease is most prevalent in cold season and early part of hot weather. In famine and war, this disease generally spreads and so it is sometimes called *famine fever*.

Class of people affected: In rural areas, poor classes are generally affected while in towns it has so far been confined to sweepers, shoemakers, coolies, etc. So the disease is mainly due to poverty and unclean conditions.

Preventive measures: These are as follows:

1. Early diagnosis and notification of the disease.
2. Isolation of the patient in an isolation hospital or at home.
3. *Destruction of lice*: Disinfestation of the clothings, beddings, cots, etc. of the patients and contacts, are done by dusting 5–10% DDT powder (mixed with talcum powder). In head lice, 3 applications of DDT at weekly intervals should be made. It should be dusted preferably before bedtime and rubbed vigorously. One should avoid getting the powder in eyes, nostrils or mouth by covering these parts with a cloth. A cloth should be tied around the hair and the powder left on the scalp for the night. The hair should not be washed for at least 24 hours after the application of the powder.

Before the discovery of DDT or other insecticides with residual effect, following measures were carried out:

a. Boiling of clothes in a solution of soap and crude potassium hydrate or *Sajji* for half an hour in an empty kerosene oil tin. This was particularly carried out in villages.

b. Improvement of living conditions with provision for frequent bathing and washing of clothes.

c. *Specific treatment*: Tetracycline-class antibiotics are most effective. It is easily treated with a one- to two-week-course of antibiotics, and most people improve within 24 hours.

2. Tick Relapsing Fever

It is caused by *Borrelia* species, i.e. *mainly Borrelia crocidurae, Borrelia duttoni and Borrelia hermsii,* which are transmitted by various species of ticks from infected persons to healthy ones. It is not communicable from man to man. The disease is non-existent in India except in Kashmir. It is also found in North Western parts of Pakistan. It is widely spread throughout tropical Africa, Spain, Saudi Arabia, Canada and America.

The disease is difficult to control on account of difficulty in destroying all the ticks particularly those hiding in the burrows of rodents.

Incubation period: It varies from 3 to 6 days. The interval for relapse between fever episodes is 4 to 14 days.

Prevention: As a preventive measure, one should avoid the bite of the ticks by not going in the houses or places infested with ticks. However, if exposure is unavoidable, tick repellents like DEET, i.e. N, N-diethyl-m-toluamide (for skin or clothing) and per-methrin (applied to clothing and equipment) should be used. DDT or gammexane powder should be freely dusted on the floors, crevices and other hiding places of the ticks be promptly removed by applying a drop of kerosene oil or turpentine oil to its body.

16.7 RICKETTSIAL DISEASES

This group of diseases, except Q fever, are transmitted through arthropod vectors and caused by specific rickettsial organisms.

1. Classification

Disease	Causative organisms	Arthropod vectors
1. Typhus group		
a. Epidemic (louse-borne) typhus	*R. prowazekii*	Body louse flea
b. Endemic (flea-borne) typhus	*R. typhi*	
2. Spotted fever group		
a. Rocky Mountain spotted fever	*R. rickettsii*	Tick
b. Indian tick typhus	*R. conorii*	Tick
c. Rickettsial pox	*R. akari*	Mite
3. Scrub typhus	*R. tsutsugamushi*	Mite
4. Q fever	*Coxiella burnetii*	Nil
5. Trench fever	*R. quintana*	Body louse

2. Epidemic Typhus

It was the most formidable rickettsial disease in the past. Recrudescent form of epidemic typhus is called Brill-Zinsser disease.

Causative agent is *Rickettsia prowazekii*. Vector is louse (*P. corporis* and *P. capitis*).

Symptoms: Onset is sudden with headache, vomiting, high temperature and delirium. The eyes become pink and watery. A characteristic maculopapular rash appears around the fifth day firstly on the upper trunk and spreads to the rest of the body but usually not to the face, palms of the hands or soles of the feet which frequently become petechial. The case fatality rate is up to 40% in the absence of specific treatment. Louse-borne typhus fever is the only rickettsial disease that can cause explosive epidemics.

Mode of spread: A louse bites an infected person, with febrile disease and takes intrinsic period of 10 to 14 days before it becomes infective for another human being. It excretes rickettsia in its faeces and usually defaecates at the time of feeding. Man is not infected by the bite of louse but is infected by rubbing infected louse faeces or crushed lice into the wound made by the bite or superficial abrasion of the skin.

Diagnosis

1. Western blot (test to identify presence of typhus bacteria).
2. Immunofluorescence test (using fluorescent dyes to detect typhus in sputum samples).
3. Blood test (results can indicate infection).

Season: It is mainly a disease of temperate climates and occurs in colder areas of the world, where people live under unhygienic conditions and are louse infected.

Prevalence: Typhus fever occurs in colder (i.e. mountainous) regions of Central and Eastern Africa, Central and South America, and Asia. In recent years, most outbreaks have taken place in Burundi, Ethiopia and Rwanda. Typhus fever occurs in conditions of overcrowding and poor hygiene, such as in prisons and refugee camps.

Preventive measures

1. Notification
2. *Isolation*: Patient should be stripped of all clothings before being admitted to the isolation hospital and should receive a bath and have all body hair shaved. He should be thoroughly dusted with 5% DDT powder.
3. Delousing of patient and delousing or destruction by fire of his clothings should be done.
4. Disinfestation of the infested house. It should be done by DDT emulsion or malathion or lindane.
5. *Clothing*: These are disinfested and disinfected with steam. DDT powder, i.e. 5–10% DDT with French chalk or talcum powder, is sprayed or dusted on clothings.
6. Improvement of living conditions with a provision for frequent bathing and washing of clothes should be aimed at.

Treatment: Treatment is symptomatic. Antibiotics such as chloramphenicol, ciprofloxacin and tetracycline have given good results. Primary treatment is doxycycline 200 mg once followed by 100 mg bid until the patient improves, has been afebrile for 24 to 48 h, and has received treatment for at least 7 days. Chloramphenicol 500 mg or IV qid for 7 days is second-line treatment.

16.8 PLAGUE

Plague is a highly infectious and highly fatal systemic zoonosis disease characterised by high fever, inflammation of lymphatic glands, formation of buboes and sometimes by pneumonia or septicaemia. The onset is sudden. The patient is obviously severely toxic with rapid irregular pulse, marked headache, tremor, restlessness, unsteady gait, mental confusion, prostration, delirium, coma, etc. Haemorrhages may also sometime occur.

Cause

The specific cause of the disease is *Yersinia pestis*. It is present in large numbers in the buboes of all cases of bubonic plague, in sputum of pneumonic cases and blood of septicaemic cases. It is also present in the spleen, intestines, lungs, kidneys, liver, viscera, and blood in small numbers. The virulence is related to its ability to produce exotoxin, endotoxin and fraction 1 and many other antigens and toxins.

Incubation period: It is 3–6 days in bubonic plague but is shorter in pneumonic plague, which varies from 2 to 3 days.

Varieties of Plague

1. *Bubonic plague:* It is most common type. The lymph glands draining the site of orginal inoculation are enlarged, which develop on about the 3rd day and are painful. The buboes are tender and the surrounding tissue is swollen from periganglionic oedema. The buboes are formed most commonly on inguinal but can also be on the neck, axilla depending on the site of bite. Abdominal pain can occur from intra-abdominal node involvement. Suppuration is common. Bacilli are obtained by puncture of glands.

2. *Pneumonic plague:* It is conveyed by droplet infection during coughing by another person or an animal with primary or secondary plague pneumonia and not by ratfleas. Sputum contains a large number of *Y. pestis.* Bilateral alveolar infiltrates are seen on chest X-ray, and diffuse interstitial pneumonitis with scanty sputum production is typical. The case mortality is 98 to 100%.

3. *Septicaemic plague:* A minority (10–25%) of infections with *Y. pestis* presents as gram-negative septicaemia (hypotension, shock) without preceding lymphadenopathy. It is proved by blood smear or blood culture. It is rare.

Mortality

In untreated plague, there is 50–60% mortality rate. Modern medical therapy has materially reduced the fatality rate.

Epidemiology

There are two groups:
a. Urban or domestic form occurs in densely populated localities. It spreads along trade routes and is transmitted from rats.
b. Sylvatic or rural plague: It is characterised by sporadic cases scattered over extensive country area through epizootic infection. Sylvatic plague is most commonly found in prairie dog colonies and some mustelids like the black-footed ferret.

Seasonal prevalence: It shows a well-marked seasonal prevalence. Its intensity being at its lowest ebb in July, gradually increasing till it reaches its zenith in March and declining during next four months. It depends upon rodent factors as they commence aestivation from May onwards. A relative humidity of 60% and a mean temperature of 20–25°C are considered favourable for the spread of plague.

Diseases spread by rats

1. *Through the bite of a rat flea*
   a. Flea typhus.
   b. Plague.

2. *Through the bite of rats*
   a. Rat bite fever.
3. *Through contamination of human food by rats and their excreta and urine.*

Role or the part played by rats: Plague is actually an epizootic in rats and to a less extent in other animals like guinea pigs, but under certain circumstances it attacks human beings. There are two varieties of rats:
1. Black domestic rat or *Rattus rattus* is a comparatively small animal living in the dwellings and houses. It lives in close association with man and does not migrate to any distance. It is not associated with plague as once thought.
2. *Tatera indica:* It is a wild rat, that has been incriminated as main reservoir, which has become immune to plague subsequently.

The rat plague is disseminated primarily by the *Tatera indica* to black domestic rat or *Rattus rattus.* The epizootic among rats is followed after about a fortnight by the outbreak of human plague.

Rat flea: It is a small-sized bright-coloured flea which loves darkness and is very sensitive to light. Three important species of rat fleas are:
1. *Xenopsylla cheopis,* which is the main vector of plague.
2. *Xenopsylla brasiliensis.*
3. *Pulex irritans:* Both sexes of the flea bite and transmit the disease.

Total flea index: It is the average number of fleas of all species found on a rodent. The average flea index is 5.5. The flea index is highest during latter part of winter and lowest in the monsoon months.

Specific percentage of flea: It is the percentage of a particular species of fleas found on a rodent.

Cheopis index: It is the average number X cheopis per rat. If the index is more than one, then it indicative of potential explosiveness of the situation, should a plague outbreak occurs.

Mode of spread: It is contracted from (a) infected rat flea bite, (b) direct contact with infected animals, and (c) by droplet infection from a case of pneumonic plague:
1. Commensal rats → rat flea → man
2. Wild rodents → wild rodents fleas → man
3. Wild rodents, commensal rats, domestic rats → fleas → human
4. Man → man, it results when a primary case of bubonic plague develops secondary pneumonic plague and infects the contacts by droplet infections.

Blocked flea: Xenopsylla cheopis ingests the infected blood on biting. The proventricullus of the flea gets blocked with mass of bacilli pestis growing on the ingested blood. The flea is called blocked flea. It cannot fill the midgut with blood and, therefore, it is in a starved condition. When it makes efforts to suck more blood it causes injection of the bacilli into the skin of the host.

Partially blocked flea: When the flea is feeding, it not only draws blood from the wound made by the mouth parts but also draws forward the contents of midgut; the regurgitated blood from the midgut mixing with the blood in the oesophagus may then readily infect the wound with plague bacilli. It is a serious danger to the community. It lives longer as it is able to ingest small quantities of blood as compared to a completely blocked flea.

Prevention and Control

The preventive measures are as follows:

1. *Early diagnosis*: During epidemic situations, early diagnosis can be made readily on clinical backgrounds. Subsequently, plague-suspected individuals and rodents should be examined bacteriologically to confirm the plague.

2. **Notification:** Prompt and compulsory notification of the incidence of plague cases as well as of the abnormal mortality among rats be enforced.

3. **Isolation:** The person suffering from plague into an infectious disease hospital, if practicable, or in any segregated room of the house particularly in case of pneumonic plague.

4. **Evacuation of the infected premises:** As soon as the disease is recognised in an epizootic form, the inmates of infected houses are isolated to segregation camps and huts.

5. **Disinfection:** Disinfection by sputum, discharges and articles soiled by patient should be carried out. Dead bodies should be handled with aseptic precautions.

6. **Prophylactic antiplague inoculation:** Haffkine's anti-plague vaccine modified by Sokhey: Vaccine is given subcutaneously 0.5 ml and 1.0 ml at an interval of 7–14 days (2 doses). It confers immunity for 6 months. Booster dose is recommended after 6 months.

7. **Campaign against rats**
   a. *Via construction of ratproof houses*: The grain stores and grain markets should be situated away from the residential area and should never be utilised for the purpose of human habitation. Rat burrows should be eliminated by blocking them with cement and concrete. The lower part of the outer doors should be protected with metal plates to prevent rats from gnawing through. Windows should be screened and doors provided with springs.
   b. *Rat destruction*: The public should be educated that the rats are their greatest enemies and they

should be destroyed at all costs. The methods employed are as follows:
   i. *Poisonous baits*: Baits consist of an inner base to which is added some poisons. The common bases used are atta, bread mash, sugar meal, etc. The most common poison used is barium carbonate. It is a cheap, tasteless powder and is safe to handle. One great disadvantage of this method is that these operations are sometimes followed by an offensive smell in some of the houses due to decomposition of dead rats in places from where they cannot be removed easily. This can be usually prevented by closing the rat holes with concrete to entomb them.

   The other common poisons used for this purpose are strychnine, white arsenic, phosphorus, zinc phosphide, alpha-naphthylthiourea, antu 1 to 3.5% and red squill 10%. A mixture of antu 20%, DDT 8% and 72% of inert powder may be used to kill the rats and rat fleas. Recently, highly effective rodenticides as sodium fluoroacetate (1080) and dicoumarine (warfarin) have come into the market. Only trained personnel should be engaged to distribute them since they are very dangerous to human beings also. The workers should use rubber gloves, while handling these chemicals.

   ii. *By fumigation*: It is a very effective method. It should be carried out by a trained squad. All openings of the burrows except one should be closed. The nozzle of the pump is introduced into the burrow and fumigation is done. Consequently all the rats along with their fleas are killed. Calcium cyanide also called "cyanogas A" dust or cymag is blown by cyanogas apparatus which is very commonly used and is very effective.

   The other gases which are used carbon monoxide, carbon dioxide, sulphur dioxide, etc. An ideal fumigation should be toxic to both rat and fleas. It should have a great penetrative power and must be non-combustible and non-explosive. It should be easily available in the market and should preferably be cheap.

   iii. *By trapping*: Generally wire cage traps are used for this purpose. There is a great advantage of killing rats by trapping over baiting in the sense that it can be carried out as a more or less permanent measure. It is relatively inexpensive and requires good supervision. To be effective, it should be carried out continuously with sufficient energy to ensure that more rats are removed than replenished by breeding. For systematic trapping, a number of traps equal to 5% of human population will be found sufficient. The traps are placed in adjoining houses for 20–30 days and then removed to the next block. Trapped rats are transferred everyday to the collecting cage, which is taken to the disposal station where the rats are drowned by immersing whole cage in a tub containing water and phenyl or any other suitable disinfectant or pulicide. Traps should be cleaned with boiling water and smeared with sweet oil once a week to keep clean and attract the rats and prevent their rusting. Attention must be paid in varying the baits. Stale, useless vegetables and fruits are good for the purpose. Onions, rice, chapaties, and melons are excellent baits.

8. **Destruction or extermination of rat fleas:** This is a most important measure adopted these days for the prevention of plague. Pulicides like DDT or gammexane are the chief insecticides used for the destruction of rat fleas. The floors are dusted with 10% DDT powder and the walls are sprayed with 5% DDT emulsion in kerosene oil. Similarly, gammexane dust 8 oz (226.80 gm) for every 100 sq ft (9.29 sq metres) may be used. Since fleas are found in cracks and crevices, so the floors and walls up to 4 ft (1.21 metres) should be specially attended to.

The standard kerosene oil and soap emulsion or pyrethrum extract in kerosene oil in ratio of 1 in 20 may be used as a spray. Naphthalene may be sprinkled on floor.

In clothing and beddings, the fleas are killed by means of exposing them to sun's rays. It has experimentally been shown that a temperature of 116°F (41.6°C) for 45 minutes will kill fleas in clothing and quilts.

9. **Disinfection of room with 5–10% DDT** in talcum powder or prophylite or gammexane emulsion should be done in bubonic plague. Spraying with pestrine or kerosene oil or naphthalene and cresol fumigations is also carried out. In pneumonic plague, fumigation with formaldehyde should be done.

10. **Personal protection** of field workers should be done against fleas by weekly dusting of their clothing with an insecticide powder. Daily application of insect repellents is a valuable adjunct. In presence of pneumonic or suspected pneumonic plague, physicians, nurses and attendants must be protected against the bite of rat fleas by wearing complete overalls, gloves and hoods equipped with face masks of three-tailed bandage with a pad of cotton wool. This face mask should be burnt after each exposure to infection. Moreover, in chemoprophylaxis, the drug of choice is tetracycline. For adults, the dose is 500 mg 6 hourly for 5 days. it has been useful for all nursing, public health and medical personnel exposed to the risk of infection may be considered, if they cannot be kept under close observation to detect the presence of disease, in its earlier stages.

11. **Education** should be imparted to general public by means of lectures, handbills, films and slides to show how infection occurs and to teach them how to guard against rats and fleas.

Treatment

Streptomycin is the drug of choice for the treatment of all forms of plague, provided therapy is begun within 24 hours of its onset. Streptomycin (30 mg/kg body weight daily) should be given intramuscularly in two divided doses for 7 to 10 days. Tetracycline orally (30–40 mg/kg body weight daily) is alternative choice of treatment. It should be administered intramuscularly in the following doses: 0.5 gm every 3 or 4 hours given until the temperature becomes normal, thereafter 1 gm of the medicine is given daily in divided doses until a total of 15 gm has been administered. In severe cases, aureomycetin, terramycin or chloromycetin should be used additionally.

DISEASES CONVEYED BY INGESTION

16.9 ENTERIC FEVER

Enteric fever is a clinical syndrome characterized by constitutional and gastrointestinal symptoms and headache. It can be caused by any *Salmonella* species. *Salmonella typhi* is the major cause of enteric fever. *S. paratyphi* A and *S. paratyphi* B are less common. These are acutely infectious and highly communicable fevers of long duration found all over the world affecting middle age groups, prevalent more in males, than in females. The annual incidence of typhoid is estimated to be about 17 million cases worldwide. In 2013, it resulted in about 161,000 deaths. Typhoid fever is endemic in India. In 2013, there were about 1.53 million cases and 361 deaths.

Incubation period: It is variable, but general average is about 2 weeks. It is some what longer for paratyphoid A than for B and C.

Symptoms: Onset is insidious. The patient complains of severe frontal headache and backache. Slow fever starts which goes on rising by step ladder pattern. The disease is characterised by continued fever of 2–4 weeks duration accompanied by pea soup diarrhoea, and enlargement of spleen. Tongue is dry and coated. Pulse is slow in comparison to high

temperature. If not treated, it sinks into typhoid stage. The diagnosis is confirmed by:
1. Blood culture.
2. Widal reaction.

Typhoid and paratyphoid bacilli are found in blood, during the first two weeks and in urine and faeces of the patient after two weeks. Besides, they are present in faeces and urine of the carriers also. Bacilli remain alive in faeces and water for a considerable period, when not exposed to sunlight, but do not multiply in them. They multiply in milk. They are destroyed by heat at 60°C. They are killed by phenyl having a strength of 2.5.%. They may live for many weeks even in ice. In the upper layers of the soil, they retain their vitality for a long time.

Mode of spread: The disease is chiefly spread by the discharges from the bowel and urine through the medium of contaminated water, milk, articles of food, drink, etc. and also through the agencies of flies, fomites and dust. Typhoid carriers are one of the important causes of spread of the disease, which the faecal carriers are more common than the urinary ones. Carriers are more common among persons over 40 years of age, especially females. There are different type of carriers:
1. Incubatory carriers
2. Convalescent carriers excrete the bacilli for 6 to 8 weeks.
3. Chronic carriers are those who excrete bacilli for more than a year after a clinical attack. They persist in the gall bladder and the billiary tract.

The infection enters through mouth and reaches intestines where the organisms attack the lymphoid follicles (Peyer's patches) and enter the systematic circulation causing the bacilli to be found in it first week. Later on, the bacilli are discharged in the faeces and urine.

The infection may be direct or indirect. The former is due to lack of observance of proper precautions in handling patients and their discharges. The latter is through contaminated articles of food and drink such as water, milk, vegetables, oyster, shellfish, etc. Soil plays an important part in the spread of the disease.

Prevention: Following measures should be adopted:
1. Arrangements should be made for thorough con-current disinfection. The attendants should dip their hands in some strong disinfectant solutions. Rooms and gutters should be sprayed with carbolic acid or phenyl lotion.
2. *Prophylactic inoculation.*
   a. *TAB inoculation is done in two phases:* An initial dose of 0.5 cc and subsequent dose comprising 1 cc is given after a week or 10 days. It confers immunity for six months.
   b. *Typhoral (live oral Ty21 a) vaccine:* It contains >10^9 viable organism of attenuated *S. typhi.* One capsule is given in days 1, 3, 5 (booster of 3 doses, once in every 3 years). Immunity is up to 3 years.
   c. *Typhim Vi vaccine:* Vi polysaccharide containing vaccine is given as single dose intramuscular or subcutaneous. Not given in age <2 years.
3. *General sanitary precautions:* These consist of:
   a. Efficient conservancy arrangements, leaving no refuse for breeding of flies.
   b. Purified and safe water supply. Public water supplies must be chlorinated.
   c. Pure and wholesome supply of milk and milk products. Only boiled, pasteurised milk and dairy products including cheese, should be taken.
   d. Proper supervision of articles of food, places where they are manufactured and offered for sale. They should be protected from dust and flies. The milk should be boiled or pasteurised.
   e. Adoption of adequate antifly measures.
   f. Discovery and proper control of carriers. Training of convalescents and chronic carriers in personal hygiene, particularly about sanitary disposal of excreta, thorough washing of hands after defaecation and before eating and also exclusion from becoming food handlers.
   g. Proper licensing of food handlers in restaurants and public eating establishments.
4. Education of the public through leaflets, posters, filmstrips and cinema slides, particularly about the role of **5 Fs,** viz. **f**ingers, **f**ood, **f**lies, **f**aeces and **f**omites.

Treatment: Fluoroquinolones such as ciprofloxacin 750 mg orally twice daily or levofloxacin 500 mg orally once daily, 5–7 days for uncomplicated enteric fever and 10–14 days for severe infection is the agent of choice for treatment of salmonella infections. Ceftriaxone, 2 g intravenously for 7 days, is also effective. Case fatality rate varies from 5 to 20% in typhoid and 2.5–3.5% in paratyphoids.

16.10 CHOLERA

Cholera is an actue diarrhoeal infectious disease, characterised by sudden onset of severe watery diarrhoea, vomiting, cramps in legs, great thirst, suppression of urine followed by rapid dehydration and collapse. The stools are like rice water and there may be griping pain. Every year, there are an estimated 3–5 million cholera cases and 100 000–120 000 deaths due to cholera. In 2013 alone, there were 1,29,060 cases, notified from 47 countries including 2,012 deaths. In India, about 1,127 cases are detected with 5 deaths.

Season: It occurs in summer and autumn and generally fades away with the appearance of cold weather.

Warmth and moisture are important predisposing factors for the prevalence of the disease.

Aetiology: The organisms considered responsible for causations of cholera are *Vibrio cholerae,* which are gram-negative, actively motile, comma-shaped organisms. There is two types, i.e. *V. cholerae* 01 (Classical or El Tor) and O139, mainly affecting alimentary canal.

Cholera carriers: Four types of cholera carriers are reported, (i) preclinical or incubatory carrier is of short duration as incubatory period is only 1–5 days, (ii) convalescent carrier may persist for 2–3 weeks after the disease. These are those carriers who may have recovered from the disease, but still excrete vibrios, (iii) contact carrier may be a household carrier, i.e. carrier in contact with a case in a house or a community carrier, i.e. in a community affected with cholera. Their duration of excretion is usually 10 days or so. Contact carriers probably play a leading role in transmission of infection, (iv) chronic carriers are persons who excrete organisms for more than 3 months cases of chronic carriers for as long as 10 years duration have been reported. Chronic carriers may serve as a reservoir of infection especially during inter-epidemic period.

Mode of Spread

1. *Faecally contaminated food:* When polluted water, infected milk or food are taken.
2. *From person to person:* Person to person transmission occurs through contaminated fingers or contaminated linens or fomites while attending the cholera patient.
3. *Indirectly:* Through flies which carry infection both mechanically and vitally.

Incubation period: It is very short, ranging from a few hours to 5 days but usually 1–2 days.

Period of communicability: 7–14 days when cholera vibrios are present in faeces and vomits.

Immunity: One attack confers a mild grade of immunity which appears to afford some protection for several years.

During the epidemic period, the proportion of deaths to the attack is greatest during the period of maximum intensity of the epidemic. When it begins to subside, the recovery rate may considerably exceed the number of deaths.

Preventive Measures

These are as follows:

1. *Notification:* The case should be notified promptly even if it is a doubtful one. Under International Health Regulations, cholera is notifiable to WHO by national government within 24 hours.
2. *Isolation:* Isolation of the case in an isolation hospital or at home. The contacts should be segregated and treated.

3. *Local measures*
   a. All excreta should be received in a basin and they should be mixed with an equal quantity of 5% cresol solution or 30% of freshly prepared bleaching powder solution. It should be then buried or burnt away at a great distance from the town.
   b. Lime should be sprinkled on the floor of the room in which the patient is being treated.
   c. Anti-fly measures should be adopted. They should be destroyed by fly traps, tangle foot papers, formalin solution, etc.
   d. Disinfection of solid linen should be done, by soaking in 2% solution of cresol for about 1/2 to 1 hour before it is sent for washing.
   e. Some suitable disinfectant like Dettol or 1% cresol solution be kept at the door for washing hands after attending and nursing the patient.
   f. Protection of articles of food and drink from flies and dust.
   g. All latrines, drains, etc. should be cleaned with phenyl or any other disinfectant lotion or sprinkled with lime or bleaching powder.
   h. Licencing of food handlers in restaurants and public eating places.

4. *Immunisation in cholera:* Vaccines now used are oral which are of two types:
   a. *Dukoral (WC-rBS):* It is a monovalent vaccine containing formalin and heat killed whole cells of *V. cholerae* 01 (classical and el Tor, Inaba and Ogawa) and recombinant cholera toxin B. The vaccine is provided as 3 ml single dose vials. Primary immunization consists of 2 oral doses given ≥7 days apart (but <6 weeks apart) for adults and children above 6 years of age. Children aged between 2 to 5 years, receive 3 doses ≥7 days apart
   b. *Shanchol and mORCVAX:* It is closely related to bivalent oral cholera vaccines. Unlike dukoral, it does not contain recombinant cholera toxin B. According to the manufacturer, Shanchol should be administered orally in 2 liquid doses 14 days apart for individuals aged ≥1 year. A booster dose is recommended after 2 years..

5. *Sterilisation of water supplies:* Provision of a properly filtered water supply has been in itself sufficient in stamping out cholera in Europe. It has also reduced the incidence of this disease in India. During incidence of infection, immediate disinfection of supplies (which are exposed to risk of infection) is carried out by the following methods:
   a. *Chlorination:* Bleaching powder or chlorinated lime is commonly used.
   b. Permanganate of potash treatment.

c. Boiling of water in houses to remove the danger of infection.

6. *Supervision of food*: Food should be well cooked, properly protected from flies and dust. Taking of uncooked or raw food should be avoided:

Sprinkling of lime or bleaching powder of slaughter houses, meat shops, sweetmeat shops or other shops, where food is prepared, should be done.

7. *Health education*: The following instructions should be given on the posters or the handbills:

   a. Taking of raw vegetables, unripe or overripe fruits, shellfish and stale food should be avoided, as they give rise to indigestion and so predispose to cholera infection.

   b. As cholera is a filth disease, so extreme cleanliness should be observed in the house. There should be no flies.

   c. Milk and water should be boiled shortly before use.

   d. The use of bazar-made aerated waters, cold drinks, ice creams, etc. should be avoided.

   e. Taking of purgatives should be avoided.

8. *Anti-cholera propaganda*: By means of lectures, films and slides should be carried out.

9. *Special measures in melas and fairs*: Besides adopting the aforesaid measures following precautions should also be taken:

   a. Protection of water supply.

   b. Special accommodation and kitchen arrangements.

   c. Special bathing places.

   d. Proper disposal of night-soil.

   e. Free inoculation, at least one week before the arrival of pilgrims.

Treatment

The treatment consists of rehydration and antibiotics. For rehydration, a standard intravenous solution of Ringer's lactate solution or diarrhoea treatment solution (sodium chloride 4 gm, sodium acetate 6.5 gm, potassium chloride 1 gm and glucose 10 gm in one litre) is given. If nothing is available, normal saline can be given.

Age	30 ml/kg	70 ml/kg
Infants (<12 mon)	1 hour	5 hours
Older	30 minutes	2 ½ hours

Low osmolar oral therapy has also been emphasized upon. The oral rehydration solution as recommended by WHO consists of 2.6 gm of NaCl, 2.9 gm NaHCO$_3$, 1.5 gm of potassium chloride and 13.5 gm of glucose in one litre of previously boiled water. The solution thus prepared should be used within 24 hours and should never be kept for more than 24 hours. Besides intravenous and oral rehydration, doxycycline, tetracycline or chloramphenicol are the drug of choice.

Furazolidone and septran have also been recommended in pregnancy and children, respectively.

16.11 POLIOMYELITIS

Poliomyelitis or infantile paralysis is one of the main crippling diseases of childhood. It is an acute viral disease affecting the central nervous system (brain, spinal cord and nerves) and infrequently resulting in paralysis of voluntary muscles; most commonly of lower extremities. It attacks children of all ages, but most vulnerable age group is in between 6 months and 3 years.

Cause

It is due to poliovirus, which is found in nasopharyngeal secretion, faeces, urine of patients and carriers. The virus is of three serotypes, i.e. PV1, PV2 and PV3. PV1 is the most common cause of epidemic. PV2 is most antigenic and easily eradicable. PV3 is the most common cause of vaccine-associated paralytic polio (1 per 1 million chance). The carriers play an important part in the spread of the disease. Faecal carriers are more dangerous than the nasopharyngeal ones. There are no chronic carriers. Most infections are subclinical. The cases are most infectious 7 to 10 days prior and after onset of infections. There are several risk factors to precipitate an attack such as fatigue, trauma, intramuscular injections, operative procedures (tonsillectomy) and administration of alum containing DPT vaccines. The causative agent invariably involves the nervous system, especially nerve cells of spinal cord and medulla oblongata. The seriousness of disease and its aftereffects depend upon the extent of damage that the virus does to the nerve cells. If they are only slightly damaged complete recovery is possible. But if a nerve centre is completely destroyed by the virus infection, then the muscles controlled by it are permanently paralysed. When nerves controlling breathing are affected, breathing stops and death occurs. The disease may be conveyed through water or milk. Approximately 60% cases are recorded during June to September.

Incubation period: It is usually 7–12 days but sometimes it may vary from 3 to 30 days.

Symptoms

There are four clinical spectrums:

a. *Inapparent (subclinical) infections*: This occurs approximately in 95% cases. There are presenting symptoms. It is recognized by isolation or rising antibody titres.

b. *Abortive polio or minor illness*: It occurs in 4 to 8% of infections. Mild or self-limiting illness occurs due to viraemia. Recognition is only by virus isolation or rising antibody titre.

c. *Non-paralytic polio*: It occurs in 1% of all infection. There is symptoms like aseptic meningitis such as stiffness and pain of the neck and back. The disease lasts for 10 days.

d. *Paralytic polio*: It occurs in <1% of infections. There is descending asymmetric flaccid paralysis due to involvement of CNS. A history of fever at the time of onset of paralysis is suggestive of polio.

Symptoms appear in two stages:

1. *Pre-paralytic stage*: The attack of poliomyelitis begins with high fever, coryza, headache, chilliness, pain all over the body and occasionally epistaxis. Children are drowsy but the adults are restless. It is followed by irritability and rigidity of neck. Cerebrospinal fluid remains clear in this stage.

2. *Paralytic stage*: After the first stage, there is recovery for 2–3 days and then second stage follows, with its characteristic implication of group of muscles. The *"spinal sign "* of this stage is the pain produced when an attempt is made to bend the spine forward. The paralysis is of a flaccid type and shows great variation in degree and range. The limbs seem to be loose and like a flake. Foot drop, irritability to raise the arm and straighten the legs, facial paralysis and squinting of eye, are the result of this disease. If muscles of larynx and pharynx are involved, it proves fatal.

Mortality: One in 200 infections leads to irreversible paralysis. Among those paralysed, 5 to 10% die when their breathing muscles become immobilized.

Prevention and Control

Following measures should be adopted:

1. Prompt notification of the case to the health authorities.

2. The patient should be isolated. He/she should be given complete rest and symptomatic treatment.

3. Since poliovirus has been found in human faeces and in sewage, indiscriminate disposal of night-soil particularly of patients suffering from this disease is dangerous.

4. All sources of water supply should be protected.

5. Poliomyelitis vaccine discovered by Jonas Salk is a preparation of formalin killed virus combining antigens of 1, 2 and 3 and is said to be effective in preventing paralytic poliomyelitis in about 75% of persons who are vaccinated. The vaccine is administered in 4 injections of 0.5 ml each; the first three doses are given at intervals of 1 to 2 months apart and 4th dose 6–12 months after the third dose.

6. Active immunisation, with a live-attenuated oral polio vaccine (Sabin) is used which is included in National Immunisation Schedule. A total of 4 doses are given; the first 3 doses are given at 4 weeks interval started from 6 weeks along with a booster dose at 18 to 24 months.

7. For residual paralysis, ambulance treatment, massage and muscle re-education without fatigue are the proper measures during the stationary stage, which begins about 2 years after the acute attack. Deformities may require to be corrected by the use of plaster, forcible stretching, tenotomy or by adopting similar surgical procedures.

Treatment

It is symptomatic, as there is no specific treatment. Use of antibiotics has been found of service in prevention and treatment of respiratory and aural complications. Treatment by way of fomentation and massage, which must be given for a long duration of time, help temporarily weakened muscles to grow strong and useful again.

Polio Eradication and Endgame Strategic Plan 2013–2018

The Polio Eradication and Endgame Strategic Plan 2013–2018 is a comprehensive, long-term strategy that addresses what is needed to deliver a polio-free world by 2018.

The plan was developed by the Global Polio Eradication Initiative (GPEI) in consultation with national health authorities, global health initiatives, scientific experts, donors and other stakeholders, in response to a directive of the World Health Assembly.

The Polio Eradication and Endgame Strategic Plan 2013–2018 addresses the eradication of all polio disease, whether caused by wild poliovirus or circulating vaccine-derived poliovirus, while planning for the backbone of the polio effort to be used for delivering other health services to the world's most vulnerable children.

The plan has four objectives:

1. Detect and interrupt all poliovirus transmission.

2. Strengthen immunisation systems and withdraw oral polio vaccine.

3. Contain poliovirus and certify interruption of transmission.

4. Plan polio's legacy.

Global polio eradication initiative (GPEI): Global polio eradication initiative (GPEI) is the largest and most far-reaching public health initiative of all time. This global initiative has a single goal—a polio-free world for all children. The national governments, the World Health Organization, Rotary International, UNICEF and the US Centers for diseases control and prevention are partners in the GPEI.

Since the GPEI was launched in 1988 during the World Health Assembly, the number of global polio cases has decreased by 99%, from over 3,50,000 in 1988 to fewer than 1,000 in 2003. However, two major challenges to the initiative emerged. First, wild polio transmission continues in two endemic countries and second, the polio virus continues to re-infect previously polio-free areas. Consequently, 2005–2006 was a period of unprecedented innovation to address these challenges. New tools such as monovalent vaccines (mOPV) were developed, and refined laboratory procedures allowed the confirmation of poliovirus 50% faster than before.

The current status is that no wild poliovirus (WPV) cases have been detected in the African continent since 11 August 2014. In addition, almost 30 months have passed without detection of wild poliovirus type 3 anywhere in the world. Persistent circulating vaccine-derived poliovirus type 2 (cVDPV2) circulation has been detected only in Nigeria and Pakistan during 2014. However, the continued spread of WPV1 from Pakistan to Afghanistan at the end of 2014 led the International Health Regulation Emergency Committee to conclude in February 2015 that the international spread of poliovirus continues to be a Public Health Emergency of International Concern.

DISEASES CAUSED BY INHALATION

16.12 DIPHTHERIA

It is an acute infectious and communicable disease characterised by involvement of the respiratory system, formation of false membrane of a soluble exotoxin, peculiar inflammation of the surface membrane of the nose, throat and tonsils, enlargement of regional lymph nodes and signs and symptoms of toxaemia. If this membrane spreads to the air passage, it may block entry of air and cause difficulty in breathing. It may also choke the patient, if adequate treatment is not given. Besides this membrane, its bacteria produce toxin, which if untreated, is absorbed into the blood, causing serious complications in the nervous system and heart. It occurs chiefly in 3 clinical forms, i.e. nasal, tonsillar and laryngeal diphtheria. The disease is caused by a gram-positive, non-motile organism known as *Corynebacterium diphtheriae* (Klebs-Loeffler bacillus) which grows chiefly in the throat, larynx and other portions of the upper respiratory passages. It is found in the secretions of mouth, nose, throat and in shreds of mucous membrane. Nasal diphtheria is commonly characterised by one-sided nasal discharge and excoriated nares. Occasionally, it forms membranes on the eyes and rarely in infected wounds.

The bacillus is killed by direct exposure to sunlight and heat. It is comparatively a hardy micro-organism.

Severity of the condition depends upon: (i) amount of the membrane, (ii) colour of the membrane, (iii) amount of adenitis, and (iv) amount of nasal discharge and presence of haemorrhage.

Geographical Distribution

It is a widely spread infection and is more prevalent in temperate regions. Improving socioeconomic conditions are changing the epidemiology of diphtheria. These epidemics are largely due to: (i) decreasing immunization coverage among infants and children, (ii) weaning immunity to diphtheria in adults, (iii) movement of large group of populations worldwide in the last few years, and (iv) an irregular supply of vaccines. In 2012, about 4490 diphtheria cases were reported globally. In India, there are 4090 cases and 64 deaths during the year of 2013.

Age: Although no age is exempted from its attack, yet it is common in children between the age of 1 and 5 years. Newborn infants are not affected due to inherent immunity received from the mother.

Seasonal prevalence: The epidemic commences with the beginning of the cold season and its maximum intensity reaches in November and December. Fatality of the disease varies but generally it ranges from 2 to 5%.

Predisposing causes: Lowered vitality due to overcrowding, insanitary surroundings, sore throat, nasal catarrh, laryngitis and unhealthy conditions of mouth and throat.

Incubation period: It is short and usually varies from 2–6 days but occasionally, it may be longer.

Mode of spread: The most common way is by personal communication chiefly through the carriers, which is 95% of total disease transmission. Nasal carriers are more dangerous than throat carriers. In majority of cases, the disease is spread by droplet infection and droplet nuclei, the bacilli being expelled from the mouth and nose by coughing, sneezing, spitting, speaking or kissing.

It may be indirectly transmitted through infected articles such as handkerchiefs, toys, slates, pencils, etc.

Fomites may also spread infection. Cross-infection in hospitals is common. Infection can spread over patient's own body; thus a child may infect his fingers by picking his nose, or his eyes, by wiping his eyes after picking his nose, etc.

Nasal, laryngeal, pharyngeal, and cutaneous forms of diphtheria occur. Nasal infection produces a few symptoms other than a nasal discharge. Laryngeal infection may lead to upper airway and bronchial obstruction. In pharyngeal diphtheria, the most common form, a tenacious grey membrane covers the tonsils and pharynx. Mild sore throat, fever, and malaise are followed by toxaemia and prostration. Myocarditis and neuropathy are the most common and most serious complications. Myocarditis causes cardiac arrhythmias, heart block, and heart failure. The neuropathy usually involves the cranial nerves first, producing diplopia, slurred speech, and difficulty in swallowing.

Immunity: One attack of diphtheria is not known to confer immunity. A large proportion in developing countries seem to acquire active immunity through inapparent infections. A herd immunity of over 70% of children is considered necessary to prevent any epidemic, but some believe the critical level may be as high as 90%.

Schick test: It is a test by which presence of diphtheria antibodies in the body of a person are detected. The test consists of giving an intradermal injection into the skin of the forearm of diphtheria toxin, 1/50 of a minimum lethal dose for a guinea pig, diluted to 0.2 ml. A control test is made on the other forearm with similar amount of toxin, which has been previously heated to 75°C to destroy the toxin. A positive reaction is shown by the appearance of a circumscribed area of redness of 10 to 50 mm diameter within 24–48 hours and indicates that the person is susceptible to diphtheria. A negative reaction is shown by the absence of reaction in either arm and indicates that the person is immune to diphtheria. Schick test surveys in India have shown that about 70% of children over the age of 3 years, and 99% over the age of 5 years are already immune to diphtheria.

Pseudo reaction: Persons who are sensitive to these proteins, will (irrespective of the presence or absence of antitoxin in their sera) show on both forearms a red flush within 24 hours, which fades away completely within 4 days.

Preventive Measures

These are as follows:

1. *Early detection:* Efforts should be made for an early detection of diphtheria carriers. Swabs should be taken from nose, throat and examined for the presence of diphtheria bacilli.

2. *Isolation:* The patient should be isolated either in an isolation hospital or at home in a well-ventilated room until he is free of infection or at least 14 days or until proved free of infection.

3. *Prophylactic immunisation:* Educational measures should be taken to inform the public, particularly the parents of infants and children about the hazards of diphtheria, and the necessity and advantages of active immunisation.

    For immunizing infants, the preparation of choice is DPT. According to National Immunisation Schedule, the vaccine should be given at 6, 10 and 14 weeks along with booster doses at 18 to 24 months and at 5 years completion.

    Recently pentavalent vaccine has been launched that contains five components (diphtheria, pertussis, tetanus, hepatitis B and *Haemophilus influenzae* and has replaced DPT in VIP at the age of 6, 10, 14 weeks.

Active immunisation gives more durable and permanent immunity. The underlying principle is that *C. diphtheriae* produces an exotoxin which stimulates the production of antibodies when injected.

Td is a tetanus-diphtheria vaccine given to adolescents and adults as a booster shot every 10 years, or after an exposure to tetanus under some circumstances. Tdap is similar to Td but also containing protection against pertussis. Adolescents 11–18 years of age (preferably at age 11–12 years) and adults 19 and older should receive a single dose of Tdap. Women should receive Tdap during each of their pregnancies (preferably in the third trimester between the 27th and 36th week). Tdap should also be given to 7–10 years old who are not fully immunised against pertussis. Tdap can be given no matter when Td was last received.

4. *Passive immunisation:* It is given by injecting in doses ranging from 20,000 to 1,00,000 units of anti-diphtheria serum, to the susceptible exposed child, which gives immunity after 24 hours, and which lasts for 2–3 weeks. The disadvantages are that the immunity lasts for only 2–3 weeks and the patient is rendered hypersensitive to serum.

5. *Institutional control:* When diphtheria has broken out in a community or an institution, the whole community should be Schick tested and swabs from throats should also be examined. From the results of Schick test and swab test of virulence, following classification is adopted.

   a. Schick positive (+), swab negative (–) (harmless and susceptible).

   b. Schick positive (+), swab positive (+) bacilli avirulent (harmless and susceptible).

   c. Schick positive (+), swab positive (+), bacilli virulent (watch and treat with antitoxin).

   d. Schick negative (–), swab nagative (–), bacilli avirulent (harmless and immune).

   e. Schick negative (–), swab positive (+), bacilli avirulent (harmless but susceptible).

   f. Schick negative (–), swab positive (+), bacilli virulent (dangerous carriers. Isolate from the onset).

Treatment

Antitoxin, which is prepared from horse serum, must be given in all cases when diphtheria is suspected. For mild early pharyngeal or laryngeal disease, the dose is 20,000–40,000 units; for moderate nasopharyngeal disease, 40,000–60,000 units; for severe, extensive, or late (3 days or more) disease, 80,000–100,000 units. Removal of membrane by direct laryngoscopy or bronchoscopy may be necessary to prevent or alleviate airway obstruction. Either penicillin, 250 mg orally four times daily, or erythromycin, 500 mg orally four times daily for 14 days, is effective therapy, although erythromycin is slightly more effective in eliminating the carrier state. Azithromycin or clarithromycin is probably as effective as erythromycin. The patient should be isolated until three consecutive cultures at the completion of therapy have documented elimination of the organism from the oropharynx. Contacts to a case should receive erythromycin, 500 mg orally four times daily for 7 days, to eradicate carriage.

Age of the patient	Mild	Moderate	Severe	Very severe
Children under 15 years of age	3–5	5–10	10–20	15–30
Above 15 years and adults	5–10	10–15	2040	30–60

16.13 SMALLPOX OR VARIOLA

It is a highly communicable and an acutely infectious disease caused by *Variola virus*. The disease is chara-cterised by a sudden onset of high fever ranging from 100° (37.8°C) to 105°F (40.6°C) accompained with backache, headache, vomiting and sometimes even convulsions, especially in children. On the 3rd day of onset of fever, a rash appears on the body of patient, which passes through successive stages of macule (3rd day), papule (5th day), vesicle (7th day), pustule (9th day), and finally a brown crust or scab (14th day). The scab ultimately dries up and falls around 21st day leaving behind permanent scars on the body of the patient.

History

The disease had been considered once as a major killer disease throughout the world, but thanks due to consistent efforts of various countries of the world, under the expert guidance and financial/technical assistance from WHO, it has been completely eradicated now. India was declared free from this dreadful disease in April, 1977 by an International Commission for Assessment of Smallpox Eradication. WHO also formally declared in May, 1980 that smallpox has been completely eradicated amongst the entire population of the world.

Case Definition for Notification of Smallpox Under the International Health Regulation 2005

State parties to the IHR (2005) are required to immediately notify to WHO of any confirmed case of smallpox. The case definition for a confirmed smallpox case includes the following:

Confirmed Case of Smallpox

An individual of any age presenting with acute onset of fever (≥38.3°C/101°F), malaise, and severe pro-stration with headache and backache occurring 2 to 4 days before rash onset.

And

Subsequent development of a maculopapular rash starting on the face and forearms, then spreading to the trunk and legs, and evolving within 48 hours to deepseated, firm/hard and round well-circumscribed vesicles and later pustules, which may become umbilicated or confluent.

And

Lesions that appear in the same stage of development (i.e. all are vesicles or all are pustules) on any given part of the body (e.g. the face or arm).

And

No alternative diagnosis explaining the illness.

And

Laboratory confirmation.

16.14 CHICKENPOX OR VARICELLA

It is a highly communicable disease of sudden onset with slight fever, mild constitutional symptoms and rash which passes through the stages of macule, papule and crust. It occurs mostly in children in an epidemic form. It very often coincides with an epidemic of smallpox. The rash is most abundant on the trunk usually appearing first on the chest without prodromal rashes or systematic disturbances and it advances quickly through following stages of macule, papule, vesicle and scab. Scabbing begins 4 to 7 days after the rash. The vesicular stage is noticed later.

Complications: They are bronchopneumonia otitis media, conjunctivitis, panophthalmitis and encephalitis, acute cerebellar ataxia and Reye's syndrome.

Aetiology: The causative virus is called varicella zoster virus [human (alpha) herpesvirus 3] which is conveyed by droplet infection or by air or by personal contact. Source of infection is always a case. The period of communicability of patients with varicella is estimated to range from 1 to 2 days before the appearance of rash, and 4 to 5 days thereafter. Fomites convey infection in rare cases.

Immunity: One attack generally confers immunity for the rest of life; subsequent attacks are rare.

Incidence: It is greatest during the first ten years of age. It occurs rarely in adults.

Incubation period: About 14 to 16 days.

Prevention

1. Notification of the case to the medical officer of health. The diagnosis should be confirmed.
2. *Isolation of patient*: Isolation of cases for at least 6 days after the onset of rash.

Treatment: There is no specific treatment. But anti-virals like acyclovir can prevent the development of systemic disease in varicella-infected immunosuppressed patients.

Table 16.1: Comparison between smallpox and chickenpox

S. no.		Smallpox	Chickenpox
1.	Prodromal symptoms	Rash appears after the temperature comes down	Rash appears simultaneously with fever
2.	Incubation period	About 12 days	About 17 days
3.	Distribution of rash	i. More profuse on face and limbs ii. Axilla involved only rarely iii. Palms and soles also affected	i. More profuse on the trunk ii. Axilla involved iii. Palms and soles are not affected
4.	Characteristics of rash	i. Deep seated and firm ii. There is no inflammation iii. Vesicles are multilocular and umbilicated	i. Superficial, ruptures easily ii. There is inflammation around the vesicles iii. Vesicles are unilocular and not umbilicated
5.	Evolution of rash	i. Rash is slow and systematic passing through distinct stages of macule, papule, vesicle and pustule ii. Scabs begin to form within 10–14 days from the day of appearance of rash iii. Scabs fall off within 14–28 days after beginning of rash iv. Scars are deep seated and permanent	i. Appearance of rash is sudden and rapid Different stages of rash may be present at the same time ii. Scabs begin to form within 4–7 days from the day of appearance of rash iii. Scabs fall off within 14 days after the beginning of rash iv. Scars are superficial
6.	Fever	When rash appears, fever subsides, but it again rises upon the onset of pustular stage	Fever rises with every fresh crop of rash

Vaccine: A live attenuated varicella virus vaccine is safe and currently recommended for children between 12 and 18 months of age who have not had chickenpox.

16.15 MEASLES (RUBEOLA)

Measles is one of the most common infectious diseases of childhood. In India, few other diseases cause as much morbidity and mortality as measles does among young children. The disease has a worldwide distribution. It is endemic but tends to occur in epidemic form every years because of accumulation of susceptibles reaches about 40%. In the year 2010, world's two most populous countries made promising advances in measles control: China held the largest ever SIA, vaccinating >103 millon children, and India started implementation of a 2-dose vaccination strategy. In the year of 2012, 1,22,000 measles death occurred globally. In 2010, World Health Assembly, targets are endorsed to be met by 2015 as milestones towards an eventual global measles eradication.

Global Measles Rubella Strategic Plan (2012–2020)

The strategy focuses on the implementation of five core components:

1. Achieve and maintain high levels of population immunity by providing high vaccination coverage with two doses of measles and rubella containing vaccines.
2. Monitor disease using effective surveillance, and evaluate programmatic efforts to ensure progress.
3. Develop and maintain outbreak preparedness, respond rapidly to outbreaks and manage cases.
4. Communicate and engage to build public confidence and demand for immunization.
5. Perform the research and development needed to support cost-effective operations and improve vaccination and diagnostic tools.

Clinical Features

The clinical course of the disease can be divided into two stages, viz. (a) pre-eruptive or catarrhal stage, and (b) eruptive or exanthematous stage. During the catarrhal stage (duration about 3–4 days), the disease is characterised by acute febrile onset with nasal catarrh, sneezing, redness of conjunctiva, photophobia, watering of the eyes, cough and hoarseness of voice due to laryngitis. During this stage, appearance of eruptions (Koplik's spots) on the buccal mucous membrane confirms the diagnosis.

The exanthematous stage starts after 3–4 days of initial symptoms of the disease and is characterised by the appearance of dark red, pink or maculopapular rash first on the back of ears and forehead, to be rapidly followed by rash all over the body. The rashes are caused by the multiplication of blood-borne virus in the skin. The rashes fully appear in about 2–3 days and tend to become confluent and blotchy. Fever and malaise disappear as the rashes fade in a couple of days leaving a brownish discolouration of skin, which may persist for quite a long time even after the disappearance of the rash from the body.

Complications

The most common complications are otitis media, pneumonia, measles-associated diarrhoea and other respiratory complications. Secondary bacterial infection is the most common cause of mortality, e.g. infection by haemolytic streptococci leading to pneumonia or bronchopneumonia. The most serious are neurological complications which include febrile convulsions, encephalitis and subacute sclerosing panencephalitis. Complications of measles are usually more common and severe in infants, young children and under conditions of overcrowding, malnutrition and poor hygiene.

Treatment

The patient should be nursed in a well-ventilated room or in a verandah to avoid secondary infection. Antibiotic therapy is needed in unequivocal secondary bacterial infections only. It is, however, advisable to provide antibiotic cover, if the child is young, e.g. below 3 years or in persons with a debilitating disease, e.g. bronchitis, rheumatic fever, tuberculosis and malnutrition because of chances of complications.

Epidemiology

Agent Factors

i. *Infectious agent*: The disease is caused by measles virus which belongs to paramyxovirus group.

ii. *Reservoir of infection*: Man is a reservoir of infection. Cases are most important in this respect as subclinical attacks are rare.

iii. *Source of infection*: The only source of infection is a case only. Secretions of nose and throat constitute the source of infection.

iv. *Period of communicability*: This is usually 4 days before to 4 days after the appearance of rash. However, the disease is most infectious during pre-eruptive stage and at the stage of eruption of rash. The infectivity declines rapidly thereafter.

Host Factors

i. *Age*: The disease is most common during childhood. The median age of the disease in India has been observed to be 6 months–5 years. This is in contrast to the finding in developed countries where measles affects higher age group children.

ii. *Resistance*: Susceptibility to measles is universal, sex, race or economic status notwithstanding. Babies born of immune mothers are ordinarily immune during the first 6 months of life. An attack of measles produces lifelong immunity. It is also considered that subclinical infection may be important in boosting the level of antibodies.

iii. *Pregnancy*: An attack of measles during pregnancy may lead to abortion or premature delivery. Foetus, in late pregnancy attack, may show rashes.

iv. *Incubation period*: It is usually 10 days (7–21 days) from exposure to infection till appearance of rash.

Environmental Factors

i. *Season*: Like most other acute respiratory infections, measles shows higher incidence during winter months.

ii. *Overcrowding*: In overcrowded communities, the infection usually affects children at an early age because of a greater chance of transmission of the infection.

iii. *Social factors*: Measles in India is believed to be a variety of pox (Mata) infection and as such its treatment and nursing is rigidly governed by beliefs and customs. These may result into deprivation of food and fluids, poor hygiene and nursing care during illness and reluctance to seek medical aid when threatened with serious complications and ultimately even death.

iv. *Mode of transmission*: Measles is one of the most readily transmitted communicable diseases. The disease is principally transmitted by droplet infection and droplet nuclei. Direct contact with an infected person or indirect contact with fomites freshly soiled with secretions of nose and throat may also be responsible for transmission of infection.

Prevention and Control of the Disease

i. *Isolation*: However, isolation is advised to reduce transmission of infection as much as possible as also to prevent secondary bacterial infection in the patients. The usual period of isolation is from the date of diagnosis till 7 days after the appearance of rash.

ii. *Concurrent disinfection*: Concurrent disinfection of articles soiled with throat and nasal secretions is recommended to limit the transmission of infection.

Prevention of Measles

Measles can be prevented by either active immunisation with a live or killed vaccine or by passive immunisation with immune gammaglobulin.

1. **Live-attenuated vaccine:** Various studies have shown that a single injection of live-attenuated vaccine containing Edmonston strain induces antibody formation and gives protection to about 95% of children inoculated. The protection appears to be long-lasting like after a natural infection.

   It is given as 0.5 ml subcutaneous in the right arm. There are two doses, i.e. one is given at 9 completed months and second dose is given at 15 months either singly or in combination such as MMR.

Contraindications: Pregnancy, leukaemia, lymphomas, resistance depressing drugs, e.g. steroids, irradiation, etc. severe illnesses like tuberculosis, hypogamma-globulinaemia, and immunocompromised individuals are the contraindications of live-attenuated measles vaccination. The vaccine should also not be given within 3 months after large dose of measles immuno-globulins or before 9 months of age (because of maternal antibodies) as these will interfere with immunity production.

2. **Combined vaccine:** Measles can be combined with other live-attenuated vaccines such as MMR (measles, mumps and rubella), MMRV (measles, mumps, rubella and varicella) and such combinations are highly effective.

3. **Passive immunisation:** The dose of immunoglobulin according to WHO to prevent measles early in incubation period, is 0.25 ml/kg body weight.

Outbreak control measures: The following control measures has been recommended: (i) isolation for 7 days after onset of rash, (ii) immunisation of contacts within two days of exposure, and (iii) prompt immunisation at the beginning.

16.16 GERMAN MEASLES (RUBELLA)

German measles is a highly infectious communicable disease caused by an RNA virus. It is accompanied by low grade fever, lymphadenopathy and a maculo-papular rash. Although mildest of all eruptive fevers, it is of significant interest from the point of view of community health because of its tendency to cause foetal malformations in children born of mothers, who had an attack of rubella in early pregnancy.

Clinical Features

There may be a prodromal phase lasting for 1–2 days and characterised by mild catarrhal symptoms, viz. fever, and enlargement of lymph glands. In children, these symptoms are very mild and the disease may be noticed after appearance of the rash only. The rash, which is pink and mascular in character usually appears first behind the ears and the forehead but spreads rapidly to trunk and limbs. Lymphadenopathy is a common and significant feature and helps differential diagnosis. The glands usually affected are posterior cervical, specially the mastoid and occipital. Other glands may also be involved sometimes. They are small, shotty and tender. Rubella in adults may be more severe than in children with features of joint and muscle pain, tonsillitis, generalised lymphadenopathy and conjunctivitis. Complications following rubella are only conjunctivitis and comprise polyarthritis, specially of small joints, encephalomyelitis and thrombocytopenic purpura.

Treatment: No treatment is needed. Bed rest for 1–2 days, ample amount of fluid and light diet is indicated.

Epidemiology

Agent Factors

i. *Infectious agent:* The disease is caused by RNA virus of a Togavirus family.

ii. *Reservoir of infection:* Reservoir of infection is cases of rubella. Subclinical cases in rubella are also common. Infants with congenital rubella must also be considered as reservoir of infection as they have been found to harbour infection for a long time. In fact secondary cases of rubella have occurred in susceptible persons in contact with these patients.

iii. *Source of infection:* The nasopharyngeal secretions of cases of rubella contain virus and, therefore, are a source of infection.

iv. *Period of communicability:* The period of com-municability is considered to be short, usually one week prior to appearance of rash to about one week thereafter.

Host Factors

i. *Age:* Rubella is principally an infection of older children and young adults. Many persons, who escape infection during childhood are liable to acquire infection in later adolescence.

ii. *Resistance:* Susceptibility to rubella infection is universal. An attack of rubella confers long-lasting immunity but some second attacks have been reported. Intrauterine rubella infection does not cause immune tolerance but results in persistence of virus with production of active immunity by foetus and infants.

iii. *The incubation* period of the disease is 14–21 days with an average of 17 days.

iv. *Rubella during pregnancy and foetal malformation:* Rubella infection in pregnant mothers may cause foetal malformation. This was first shown by Gregg in 1941 and has since been confirmed by various retrospective as well as prospective enquiries. In India, approximately 40% of women of childbearing age are susceptible to rubella. The probable risk of an abnormal baby following maternal rubella within the first 12 weeks of pregnancy appears to be 15–18%, i.e. seven to eight times more than usual. Various congenital defects, viz. cataract, patent ductus arteriosus, microcephaly, deaf mutism, mental retardation, cleft palate, club foot, etc. may occur singly or in combination and are known as "rubella syndrome". Rubella virus is also responsible for abortion, stillbirths, low birth weight and increased mortality during the first year of life. The pathogenesis of congenital malformation following maternal rubella is believed to be that the rubella virus circulating in maternal blood crosses and infects the placenta and then localises in the developing and differentiating embryonic cells, specially cells of the eye, ear, heart, brain and teeth.

Environmental Factors

i. *Season:* Like in most other acute respiratory tract infections, the incidence of rubella is highest in winter and spring, although cases occur throughout the year.

ii. *Transmission:* Rubella is transmitted by droplet infection from both acquired and congenital cases. Direct contact with cases or indirect contact with freshly soiled fomites with nasopharyngeal discharges may also play a role in transmission of infection. Airborne spread or infection within certain limits is also possible.

16.17 MUMPS (INFECTIOUS PAROTITIS)

Mumps is an acutely infectious disease of sudden onset, characterised by fever, general malaise, enlargement and tenderness of one or both parotid glands and occurrence of *orchitis*. It lifts the ears and gives the face a whimsical appearance. It is first unilateral, passing later onto the other side. Trismus is well marked and pain may be felt at the angle of the jaw before swelling appears and mouth cannot be opened properly. Involvement of ovaries and testicles in aged persons is also common.

Cause: It is caused by *Myxovirus parotitis* of para-myxovirus group, which is present in saliva, blood and cerbrospinal fluid. For its spread, a close contact is necessary. Indirectly, the disease may spread through articles freshly soiled with saliva of the patients.

Incubation period: It is from 2 to 3 weeks, usually 18 days.

Age: The disease is more prevalent in children in the age group of 5–9 years.

Complications: These are orchitis in males, pancreatitis, meningoencephalitis, thyroiditis, neuritis, hepatitis, myocarditis, mastitis and oophoritis in small pro-portion in females. It may cause deafness in rare cases.

Prevention: Following measures should be adopted:

1. Vaccination: Highly effective live-attenuated vaccine is now available. Widely used live attenuated mumps vaccine strains include the Jeryll Lynn, RIT 4385, Leningrad-3, L-Zagreb and Urabe strains. A single dose (0.5 ml) intramuscularly produces detectable antibodies in 95% of vaccines.

2. Contacts should be kept under surveillance.

Treatment: It is symptomatic. In orchitis, surgical relief of pressure has been of much use. The use of steroids has also shown some success.

16.18 CEREBROSPINAL FEVER

It is an acutely infectious disease characterised by nasopharyngeal infection, followed by sudden rigor, fever, severe headache, nausea, vomiting and symptoms of meningitis that is rigidity of neck or retraction of head. *Kerning's sign* is present and pulse is slow. Patient becomes apathetic.

Etiology: The disease is caused by the organism known as *Neisseria meningitidis or meningococcus* and is found in cerebrospinal fluid of patients and nasopharynx of carriers of the disease. Up to 5,00,000 cases of meningococcal disease are thought to occur worldwide each year, and around 10% of the affected die.

Incubation period: It is from 2 to 10 days.

Mode of spread: The disease is spread through healthy carriers rather than by droplets and direct contact. Patients themselves are doubted as the source of infection. They are mildly infectious during the course of disease. The person attending the patient often becomes a carrier. He rarely contracts the disease. Carriers play a most important part in the spread of this disease. An epidemic of cerebrospinal fever is heralded by an excessive increase in the number of carriers. Adults act as carriers and children suffer from the disease.

Incidence: It is mostly prevalent in children and young adults. No age is exempted from its attack.

Seasonal prevalence: The highest prevalence of the disease is from February to April. It is common in jails, barracks, schools, army, etc.

Complications: These are paralysis of the face/other parts of body, blindness or deafness.

Mortality: It is high. It may be from 20 to 75% among infected persons.

Prevention

1. *Isolation of cases:* Contacts should be segregated for 3 weeks.

2. Efforts should be made to prevent overcrowding in living quarters and working places. Fresh air and sunlight should be provided.

3. The most effective way to protect you and your child against certain types of bacterial meningitis is to complete the recommended vaccine schedule. There are vaccines for three types of bacteria that can cause meningitis:

   a. *Neisseria meningitidis* (meningococcus)

   b. *Streptococcus pneumoniae* (pneumococcus)

   c. *Haemophilus influenzae* type b (Hib).

Treatment: Empirical antibiotic therapy for suspected cases consists of a third-generation cephalosporin such as ceftriaxone (75–100 mg/kg per day in one or two divided IV doses). Cefotaxime (200 mg/kg per day in four divided doses IV) to cover various bacteria. Dehydration should be prevented by giving fluid by mouth or by injecting normal saline.

16.19 ACUTE RESPIRATORY INFECTIONS (ARIs)

ARI is an acute, highly communicable disease. While they are the source of discomfort, disability and loss of time for most adults, they are a substantial cause of morbidity and mortality in young children and the elderly. ARI may cause inflammation of the respiratory tract anywhere from nose to alveoli. The upper respiratory tract infections include include common cold, pharyngitis and otitis media. The lower respiratory tract infections include epiglottitis, laryngitis, laryngotracheitis, bronchitis, bronchiolitis and pneumonia. Every year ARI in young children is responsible for an estimated 3.9 million deaths worldwide. On an average, children below 5 years of age suffer about 5 episodes of ARI per child per year, thus accounting for about 238 million attacks. In India, during the year of 2013, about 31.7 million cases of ARI were reported. During 2013, about 3,278 people died of ARI and 2.597 died of pneumonia.

Causes: The microbial agents causing ARI are numerous and include bacteria and viruses.

Bacteria

1. *Bordetella pertussis*
2. *Corynebacterium diphtheriae*
3. *Haemophilus influenzae*
4. *Klebsiella pneumoniae*
5. *Streptococcus pneumoniae*, etc.

Virus

1. Adenoviruses
2. Enteroviruses
3. Influenzae
4. Measles
5. Respiratory syncytial virus
6. Rhinovirus, etc.

There are factors which make one more susceptible, such as dry over heated rooms, sudden changes in temperature, draughts, improper food, obstructions of the nose, fatigue, exposure to cold and dampness; and other conditions which produce lower vitality.

Mode of transmission: It occurs by direct contact or by droplet infection or through fomites.

Symptom: It manifests itself by the mucous membrane of the nose becoming swollen, the secretions copious and the eyes watery. The nose becomes obstructed and thus in turn produces a temporary loss of smell and taste. Sometimes at the onset of disease, fever, backache and pain in limbs becomes prominent:

a. Count breathes in one minute: Fast breathing is present when the respiratory rate is:
   - 60 breathes per minute or more in case of a child less than 2 months
   - 50 breathes per minute or more in case of a child aged between 2 and 12 months
   - 40 breathes per minute or more in case of a child aged between 12 months and 5 years.
b. Look for chest indrawing
c. Look and listen for stridor
d. Look for wheeze
e. See if the child is abnormally sleepy or difficult to wake
f. Check for fever or low body temperature
g. Check for severe malnutrition.

Treatment: Cotrimoxazole is the drug of choice of treating pneumonia. In children less than two months, cotrimoxazole is not recommended. In case of severe pneumonia, penicillin or ampicillin or chloramphenicol has to be used. In case of mild cases, symptomatic treatment and care at home is generally enough for such cases.

Immunization holds promise of saving millions of children from dying due to pneumonia. Measles vaccine, Hib vaccine and pneumococcal pneumonia vaccine (PPV 23 and PCV) are used to prevent mainly bacterial pneumonia.

16.20 INFLUENZA

It is an acute highly communicable febrile disease of the upper respiratory tract, which is caused by influenza virus, of which there are 3 types—A, B and C. It is characterised by abrupt onset of fever, headache, chills, great prostration, pain in limbs and back, frequent inflammation of the respiratory and gastrointestinal tract and vomiting. Fever may rise up to 104°F (40°C). Distressing symptoms and development of serious complications may arise if proper care of the sick is not taken. Frequent complications are acute sinusitis, otitis media, purulent bronchitis and pneumonia. The most dreaded complication is pneumonia which should be suspected, if fever persists beyond 4 or 5 days or recurs abruptly during convalescence.

It assumes a pandemic form after certain intervals and spreads in all parts of the world, e.g. influenza of 1918–19. It affected about 3–5 million, out of which more than 2,00,000 to 5,00,000 people died. India had reported 937 cases and 218 deaths from swine flu in the year 2014. By mid-February 2015, the reported cases and deaths in 2015 had surpassed the previous numbers. The total number of laboratory confirmed cases crossed 33000 mark with death of more than 2000 people.

Aetiology: It is an Orthomyxoviridae family virus, of which there are three strains, i.e. A, B and C. These three strains are antigenically distinct. There is no cross-immunity. Influenza types A and B are responsible for epidemics. Until last epidemic Pfeiffer bacillus was believed to be its cause. One view is that Pfeiffer bacillus is only a complicating agent like *Streptococcus haemolyticus*, puemococcus, etc.

Incubation period: It is short and varies from 1 to 3 days.

Mode of spread: The virus is present in the nasal discharges and the sputum of the patient. The infection usually spreads from one person to another directly, i.e. minute particles of sputum contain the virus and may be present in fomites also, is highly contagious and occurs in all seasons, affects all ages and thus the disease spreads through droplet infection. The disease is most infectious during its first 3 days. Carriers probably play a part in its spread. It is usually a self-limited disease with recovery in 48–72 hours.

Fatigue, overcrowding, ill-ventilation, exposure to dusty and chilly atmosphere, etc. are important predisposing causes. Railways, cinemas, etc. also play a great part in the spread of disease.

Immunity: It does not confer immunity and subsequent attacks are comparatively more severe.

Prevention: Isolation of cases should be rigorously enforced. At the outbreak of an epidemic, the cinemas, theatres, etc. should be closed as there is a risk of getting chill, on suddenly coming out of these congested places. Overcrowding of rooms should be avoided. Well-ventilated rooms and avoidance of draught should be encouraged. Hygienic living, taking of good nourishing diet. Moreover, sneezing, spitting and coughing in public places should be avoided.

N 95 face-mask should be used while attending a patient. The clothes, beddings, handkerchiefs and the room used by the patient should be thoroughly disinfected. Secretions from nose and throat of the patient should be received in a spittoon containing some disinfectant. As there is a risk of conveying infection by hand, they should be immediately washed after their coming in contact with a patient. Inclusion of hygienic practices during handling of poultry products, like hand washing and prevention of cross-contamination, as well as thorough cooking, to more than 70°C of poultry products should be practiced.

Prophylactic vaccination: Most influenza vaccination programmes make use of killed vaccines. A single inoculation administered by subcutaneous route or intramuscular route. The protective value of vaccine is 70–90% and immunity lasts for only 6–12 months. Attempts have been made to prevent or modify the disease by giving injections of living attenuated virus. A trivalent live-attenuated influenza vaccine administered as a single dose intranasal spray.

Treatment: Some antiviral drugs have been tried for prophylaxis and therapy of seasonal influenza infections. Chemoprophylaxis against influenza A and B is traditionally accomplished with a single daily dose of the neuraminidase inhibitors oseltamivir (75 mg/d, oral) or zanamivir (10 mg/d, inhaled).

16.21 WHOOPING COUGH OR PERTUSSIS

Pertussis is an acute respiratory infection, caused by *Bordetella pertussis* involving the trachea, bronchi and bronchioles and characterised by an initial catarrh with insidious onset and irritating cough lasting for a few days to several weeks.

Emerging into a stage—the chief feature which is a series of paroxysmal cough accompanied by sudden indrawing of breath producing the characteristic 'whooping sound' in which the face becomes suffused, the tongue protrudes, the saliva is blood stained and finally vomiting takes place. However, in milder cases of infection, whoop may be absent. During the year 2012, about 2.49 lakh cases were reported to WHO globally. In India, 36,661 cases were reported during 2013.

Incubation period and period of communicability: The incubation period is often about 7 to 14 days. The period of danger of the spread of disease extends from 7 days after exposure to three weeks after the onset of typical paroxysm.

Mode of spread: It is most infectious, before it is diagnosed, i.e. in the early catarrhal stages and the infection spreads directly from person to person by droplet infection and direct contact. The main sources of infection are nasopharyngeal, laryngeal and bronchial discharges. Most children contract the infection from playmates, who are in the early stages of the disease before the 'whoop' has developed. The germs are present in the nose and throat of the patient and each time an infected person talks, sneezes or coughs, these germs are sprayed in the air.

Age: Whooping cough occurs in all ages, but is predominantly a disease of children under 5 years of age. It is extremely dangerous, if it affects infants under six months of age. The case mortality in the first year of life is about 70%. Of the total deaths, about 90% occur under the age of 5 years.

Sex: A peculiar feature of the disease is that female children are affected comparatively more frequently than the male and that deaths are more common among the females.

Seasonal incidence: It varies but cases are highest in the later part of winter and spring, i.e. during March and April due to overcrowding.

Complications: These are epistaxis and subconjunctival and other haemorrhages, convulsions, hernia, bronchitis, bronchopneumonia, bronchiectasis and ulcer of frenulum linguae in children. Bronchopneumonia occurs in about 5.2% of cases. It is the most prominent problem, with relatively high mortality.

Treatment: Antibiotic treatment should be initiated in all suspected cases. Treatment options include erythromycin, 500 mg four times a day orally for 7 days; azithromycin, 500 mg orally on day 1 and 250 mg for 4 more days; or clarithromycin 500 mg orally twice daily for 7 days. Trimethoprim sulfamethoxazole, 160–800 mg orally twice a day for 7 days, also is effective. Treatment shortens the duration of carriage and may diminish the severity of coughing paroxysms. These same regimens are indicated for prophylaxis of contacts to an active case of pertussis that are exposed within 3 weeks of the onset of cough in the index case.

Control: Whooping cough like other infectious diseases can be avoided, if due precautions are taken at the right time. The first and the foremost important item in prevention of spread of the disease is early diagnosis in the individual patient and his subsequent isolation. She/he should be excluded from school for a period of about 6 weeks.

Several pertussis vaccines are available for prophylactic purposes. The vaccine is usually administered in the national immunisation programme as DPT pentavalent or DTaP vaccine. Five doses of vaccine are recommended to be given between the age of 6, 10, 14 weeks with booster doses at 18 to 24 months and at the age of 5 years.

16.22 TUBERCULOSIS

It is a specific communicable bacterial disease and constitutes an important cause of death in most parts of the world. It is rather an insidious and deceptive disease. It is caused by *Tubercle bacillus (Mycobacterium tuberculosis)* which was first discovered by Robert Koch, a German scientist in 1882. It attacks both pulmonary as well as non-pulmonary tissues.

It is a facultative intracellular microorganism and can live in dry state for about six months. When exposed to direct sunlight, it is killed after eight hours. It is also destroyed by boiling for 10 minutes. TB affects all ages. Males are affected more than females. Malnutrition is widely believed to predispose to TB. Man has no inherited immunity against it. It is prevalent both in tropical as well as temperate climates and is more prevalent in large overcrowed cities and towns. It is spread by droplet infections.

Symptoms of Pulmonary Tuberculosis

The onset may be insidious or acute. A common mode of onset is an acute transient febrile illness accompanied by respiratory catarrh and malaise. The most outstanding of these early manifestations are haemoptysis and pleurisy. Three stages (minimal, moderately advanced and far advanced) are distinguished according to the extent of lung damage and intensity of the disease. Activity is determined by progression as detected in reoentgenograms, by presence of tubercle bacilli, various symptoms, etc. The characteristic symptoms are:

1. *Excessive fatigue*: Patient is exhausted in ordinary work. He has a general feeling of weakness and disinclination to work.
2. Loss of weight.
3. Failure of appetite.
4. *Amenorrhoea in females*: Menstruation may become scanty or absent as a result of the tuberculosis.
5. Slight rise of temperature, in the evening.
6. Husky cough and hoarseness of throat.
7. Night sweating.
8. Slight palpitation.
9. Rapid pulse.
10. Chest pain and haemoptysis.

Later symptoms: The toxaemia is shown by swinging of temperature. The body is wasted, the cheeks are flushed, the eyes bright and sunken, and the lips are dry. The breath has peculiar odour, the sputum is copious and purulent. There is often an unnatural sense of wellbeing and hopefulness of recovery. Besides, the retraction of the upper part of the thoracic wall and displacement of mediastinum, immobility over the diseased areas of the lung will be noted. Overextensive infiltration, air entry and movements are often restricted and rales and rhonchi are heard. Consolidation is characterised by impaired resonance.

Incubation period: The time from receipt of infection to the development of a positive tuberculin test ranges from 3 to 6 weeks. It may vary from a few weeks to a few years depending upon the host parasite relationship and the severity as well as frequency of infection.

Modes of Infection

These are:

1. Infection by inhalation of droplets expelled by tubercular patients, through coughing, sneezing, yawning and loudly speaking up to a distance of 3 feet (0.91 metre) is called droplet infection.
2. Inhaling fine dust containing tubercle bacilli derived from dried sputum and other infected discharge thrown on floor, walls, furniture, clothes, etc. which disintegrate into fine atomised particles.
3. Infection may occur by handling sputum or other discharges of a tubercular patient and therefrom articles of food and drink may get contaminated.
4. Through the ingestion of articles of food and drink contaminated with tubercle bacilli.
5. Children sometimes get the infection by taking unpasteurised milk infected with tubercle bacilli, i.e. milk derived from a tubercular cow.

Infection depends on several factors such as

   i. The virulence of the tubercle bacilli introduced in the body.
   ii. Dose or the number of bacilli introduced.
   iii. Frequency of infection.
   iv. Path of infection, whether through susceptible tissues or not.
   v. The immunity of the individual.

Problem of tuberculosis in the world: **During the year 2013, an estimated 9 million people developed TB, which is equivalent to 126 cases per 1,00,000 population. Most of the cases occurred in Asia (56%) followed by the African region (29%). It is estimated that about 1.5 million people died of TB, of these 3,60,000 were HIV positive and 2,10,000 were MDR-TB cases.**

Tuberculosis problem in India: **India is the highest TB burden country. It accounts for one-fourth of the estimated global incident TB cases. As per WHO estimation, TB prevalence per lac population was 211 in 2013. TB mortality had reduced to 19 per lac population as on 2013. HIV among estimated incident cases of TB was about 5%. MDR-TB among notified new pulmonary TB patients was about 2.2%, and among retreatment cases was about 15%.**

Tuberculosis Control

It means reduction in the prevalence and incidence of disease in the community. The fundamentals of tuberculosis control are: (a) early detection of cases, (b) chemotherapy, (c) chemoprophylaxis, (d) BCG, and (e) rehabilitation. The Revised National Tuberculosis Control Programme (RNTCP) in India comprises: (a) BCG vaccination, (b) establishment of district TB centres with expansion of domiciliary treatment, (c) setting up of training and demonstration centres, (d) isolation and treatment of cases in hospitals and sanatoria in special circumstances, (e) rehabilitation, and (f) research.

The objectives of RNTCP are

1. Achievement of at least 85% cure rate in TB
2. Case detection rate should be at least 70% of estimated cases through quality sputum microscopy.

DOTS strategy adopted by RNTCP initially had the following five main components

1. Political will and administrative components
2. Diagnosis by quality assured sputum smear microscopy
3. Adequate supply of quality assured drugs
4. Directly observed treatment
5. Systematic monitoring and accountability.

Organisation: **The profile of RNTCP in a state is as follows:**

1. State TB office—state TB officer
2. State TB training and demonstration centre—director
3. District TB centre: District TB officer
4. TB unit—medical officer—TB control
   a. Senior treatment supervisor
   b. Senior TB laboratory supervisor
5. Microscopy centres, treatment centres
6. DOTS providers.

In India, RNTCP has established a nation wide laboratory network, encompassing over 13,309 designated microscopy centres (DMCs), which are being supervised by intermediate reference laboratories (IRL) at state level, and national reference laboratories (6 NRLs) and central TB division at the national level. There are around 51 RNTCP certified C and DST laboratories in the country which includes IRLs and medical colleges, private sector and operate by NGOs.

New initiatives

1. RNTCP has completed the feasibility study of introducing Gene Xpert in 18 TB units in 12 states.
2. *Nikshay*: TB surveillance using case-based web-based IT systems.
3. *TB notification*: According to the Government of India notification dated 7th May 2012, it is now mandatory for all health care providers to notify every TB case to local authorities.
4. Ban on TB serology.

Standardized treatment regimens are one of the pillars of the DOTS strategy. Isoniazid, rifampicin, pyrazinamide, ethambutol, and streptomycin are the primary antitubercular drugs used. Most DOTS regimens have thrice-weekly schedule and typically last for 6 to 9 months, with an initial intensive phase and a continuation phase.

Based on the nature/severity of the disease and the patient's exposure to previous anti-tubercular treatments, RNTCP classifies tuberculosis patients into two treatment categories.

New	Previously treated
New sputum smear-positive	Sputum smear-positive relapse
New sputum smear-negative	Sputum smear-positive failure
New extrapulmonary tuberculosis, others	Sputum smear-positive treatment after default, others
$2H_3R_3Z_3E_3 + 4H_3R_3$	$2H_3R_3Z_3E_3S_3 + 1H_3R_3Z_3E_3 + 5H_3R_3E_3$
2 months intensive phase + 4 months continuation phase. Four drugs at thrice-weekly schedule for 2 months intensive phase and two drugs at thrice-weekly schedule for remaining 4 months continuation phase	3 months intensive phase + 5 months continuation phase. Five drugs at thrice-weekly schedule for initial 2 months followed by: Four drugs for next 1 month intensive phase. Three drugs at thrice-weekly schedule for remaining 5 months continuation phase

H: Isoniazid (300 mg), R: Rifampicin (450 mg), Z: Pyrazinamide (1500 mg), E: Ethambutol (1200 mg), S: Streptomycin (750 mg)

1. Patients who weigh 60 kg or more receive additional rifampicin 150 mg.

2. Patients who are more than 50 years old receive streptomycin 500 mg. Patients who weigh less than 30 kg receive drugs as per pediatric weight band boxes according to body weight.

Regimen for MDR TB: The treatment is given in two phases, the intensive phase (IP) and the continuation phase (CP). This regimen comprises six drugs—kanamycin, levofloxacin, ethionamide, pyrazinamide, ethambutol and cycloserine during 6–9 months of the intensive phase and four drugs—levofloxacin, ethionamide, ethambutol and cycloserine during the 18 months of the continuation phase. All drugs should be given in a single daily dosage under supervision. Pyridoxine should be administered to all patients on the regimen for MDR-TB.

Regimen for extensively drug-resistant tuberculosis: All XDR-TB patients should also be subject to a repeat full pretreatment evaluation, but also including consultation by a thoracic surgeon for consideration of surgery. Identification must be done for the site (tertiary centers) with such surgical facilities. The "intensive phase" will consist of seven drugs—capreomycin (Cm), PAS, moxifloxacin (Mfx), high-dose INH, clofazimine, linezolid and amoxiclav. The "continuation phase" will consist of six drugs—PAS, moxifloxacin (Mfx), high-dose INH, clofazimine, linezolid and amoxiclav.

BCG Vaccination or Prophylactic Immunisation

Bacillus Calmette-Guérin (named after their discoverers—the French bacteriologists Calmette and Guérin) is a living bovine strain of tubercle bacillus which has been rendered avirulent and is used for the preparation of vaccine for immunisation. BCG vaccination confers definite though partial protection. Under NIP, BCG is given 0.1 ml ID over the left deltoid of the infant. The dose is 0.05 ml in newborn aged below 4 weeks. Two to three weeks after a correct ID injection of a potent vaccine, a papule develops at the site of injection. It then subsides into a shallow ulcer. Healing occurs spontaneously within 6 to 12 weeks. The duration of protection is 15 to 20 years. If there is a local abscess formation, it should be treated by aspiration or it should be incised and treated with daily local application of PAS or INH powder.

a. Individual Measures

1. The patient should not spit everywhere. He should spit in a sputum cup containing some disinfectant, say carbolic acid 1 to 20 solution. When he is going about, he should spit in his handkerchief which may be boiled afterwards, if a paper handkerchief is not used by him.
2. While coughing, he should keep the handkerchief before his mouth.

b. Contacts

1. They should avoid frequent unnecessary visit to patient's room. Contacts should visit a tuberculosis dispensary and get themselves thoroughly examined periodically.
2. They should live under hygienic conditions.
3. A physiological balanced diet is essential.

DISEASES OF ANIMALS CONVEYED TO MAN (ZOONOTIC DISEASES)

16.23 RABIES

Rabies is an acutely infectious disease communicated from the rabid animal to a susceptible animal usually through a wound produced by biting or even licking of a rabid animal on a scratch or an abraded surface. Dogs, jackals, wolves, cats, etc. are common carriers; the former being the most common one. It is a disease caused by a virus highly fatal in acute stage. Its infection is localised in the central nervous system and salivary glands. When it affects man, the most characteristic symptom produced is *hydrophobia*, i.e. fear of water. This symptom is not found in dogs or other animals. The patient complains about pain and itching at the site of wound. Temperature is raised, pulse is more frequent and saliva runs from the mouth. He becomes maniacal and dies after 2–4 days either due to resultant paralysis or during one of the convulsions, when the severity of disease reaches its highest level. He is infective during this stage. Once the disease sets in, it is fatal and there is no treatment of hydrophobia. So its mortality rate is 100%.

Aetiology

The casual agent of rabies is Lyssavirus type 1. It occurs in salivary glands, central nervous system and medulla of an infected animal. In the nerve cells of central nervous system, Negri bodies are seen histologically which greatly vary in size; their diameter vary from 5 to 20 microns. All mammals are susceptible to rabies but the disease is contracted by man from infected animals, through the bite of a mad dog or a wild animal, like jackal, bear, monkey, etc. It occurs in more than 150 countries and territories. Infection causes thousands of deaths every year, mostly in Asia and Africa. 40% of people who are bitten by suspect rabid animals are children under 15 years of age.

Incubation Period

It is extremely variable. It can be 7 days to several years.

Average for man: 10 days, up to a year or even longer period.

Average for dog: 21 to 90 days.

The incubation period depends upon:

1. Site of the wound and its distance from the brain.
2. Relation of wound to nerves.
3. Degree of virulence of the virus.
4. Immunity of the person.
5. Depth of the wound, the number of bites, the species of biting animals and intervention of clothing, etc. are the main factors, which influence the magnitude of the infection risk.
6. Load of virus into the wound.

Bites by infected wild animals are more severe and dangerous than bites of domestic animals.

Prophylactic Treatment

This may be considered under the following heads:

Immediate treatment of the wound: The wound should be carefully and thoroughly washed with soap and water and rinsed with plenty of water for at least 15 minutes. This simple procedure is extremely important and is useful as it reduces mortality to a great extent.

Whatever residual virus remains in the wound, after cleansing, should be inactivated by irrigation with virucidal agents—either alcohol (400–700 ml/litre), tincture or 0.01% solution of iodine or povidone iodine

Suturing is contraindicated in bite wound. If suturing is necessary, it should be done 24 to 48 hours later, applying minimum possible stitches, under the cover of rabies immunoglobulin locally.

The application of antibiotics and anti-tetanus procedures when indicated should follow the local treatment recommended above.

The patient suffering from rabies should be kept in a separate quiet room, free from all sorts of noise, light, cold draught and other stimuli, which may be conducive to aggravating the spasms and convulsions in the patient. Sedatives and morphine may be administered to the patient to control his excitability and unrest. Intake of fluids should be avoided since they have a tendency to produce spasms.

Pasteur's anti-rabies kasauli vaccines: Since their development more than four decades ago, concentrated and purified cell culture vaccine and embryonated egg-based vaccine have proved to be safe and effective in preventing rabies.

Categories of contact with suspect rabid animal	Post-exposure prophylaxis measures
Category I: Touching or feeding animals, licks on intact skin	None
Category II: Nibbling of uncovered skin, minor scratches or abrasions without bleeding	Immediate vaccination and local treatment of the wound
Category III: Single or multiple transdermal bites or scratches, licks on broken skin; contamination of mucous membrane with saliva from licks, contacts with bats	Immediate vaccination and administration of rabies immunoglobulin; local treatment of the wound

Regimen of vaccine

1. 5 dose intramuscular regimen prescribes one dose 0.5 ml on each of days 0, 3, 7, 14 and 28.
2. The 2-site intradermal regimen prescribes injection of 0.1 ml at 2 sites on days 0, 3, 7 and 28.

Guidelines for pre-exposure prophylaxis

It requires IM doses of 0.5 ml or ID administration of 0.1 ml volume per site is given on 0, 7, 21 or 28 days. In adults the vaceine should be adminished in the deltoid are of the arm whereas for children <1 year of age, anterolateral aspect of thigh is preferred.

Human rabies immunoglobulin (HRIg) or equine rabies immunoglobulin line should be used for category III and some category II animal bites (as per the table given above).

Igs are administered in a dose of 20 IU/kg wt for equine Ig. It should be administered just before or shortly after the first dose of vaccine. It can be given until seventh day of initiation of the primary senses of post-exposure prophylaxis.

The full dose of rabies immunoglobulin, or as much as feasible, should be administered in and around the wound site and rest injected IM at a site distant from the site of active vaccine administration.

Diagnosis of Rabies in Dogs

The course of the disease may be divided into 3 stages:

1. *Premonitory stage:* There is a change in disposition of the animal. It is easily excited.
2. *Stage of excitement:* It is restless and may become furious and even show signs of delirium. Eyes are red, barking is hoarse and harsh. There may be profuse salivation. It rushes about attacking every object and dogs, biting and inoculating men and animals. It runs straight.
3. *Stage of paralysis:* It soon sets in, first starting in the hind limbs and then becoming general. The progress of the disease is always rapid.

A guide for specific post-exposure treatment of rabies has been adopted from World Health Organization Technical Report Series 1957, No. 121.

If all these stages are noticed, then it is a case of *furious* rabies. If the first two stages are transient or absent then it is a *dumb or paralytic* rabies. Death occurs in 2 or 3 days. Presence of Negri bodies in the brain of a rabid dog is the most important evidence. So whole of the head packed in ice should be sent to the laboratory for examination.

Table 16.2: Condition of biting animal

Nature of exposure	At the time of exposure	During observation period of 10 days	Recommended treatment (in addition to local treatment)
I. No lesions: Indirect contact	Rabid	–	None

II. Licks:
  a. Unabraded skin
  b. Abraded skin and abraded or unabraded mucosa
	Rabid
	a. Healthy
	b. Signs suggestive of rabies
	c. Rabid, escaped, killed or unknown
		–
		Clinical signs of rabies or proven rabid
		Healthy
			None
			a. Start vaccine at first signs of rabies in the animals
			b. Start vaccine immediately. Stop treatment, if animal is normal on 5th day after exposure
			c. Start vaccine immediately

III. Bites: a. Mild exposure	a. Healthy b. Healthy c. Signs suggestive of rabies d. Rabid, escaped, killed, or unknown, or any bite by wolf, jackal, fox, bat or other wild animals	Healthy Clinical signs of rabies or proven rabid Healthy	a. None b. Start vaccine at first sign of rabies in the animal c. Start vaccine immediately. Stop treatment, if animal is normal on 5th day after exposure
b. Severe exposure (multiple, or face, head or neck bites)	a. Healthy b. Healthy c. Signs suggestive of rabies d. Rabid, escaped, killed or unknown. Any bite by wild animal	Healthy Clinical signs of rabies or proven rabid Healthy	a. Hyperimmune serum immediately, no vaccine as long as animal remains normal b. Hyperimmune serum immediately start vaccine at first signs of rabies c. Hyperimmune serum immediately, followed by vaccine; may be stopped if animal is normal on 5th day after exposure d. Hyperimmune serum immediately, followed by vaccine

Notes

1. Hyperimmune serum is most effective when given within 72 hours of exposure, but there is no time limit as to when the serum may be given. Dose 0.5 cc per kg of body weight.
2. Nowadays, HDC (Mericux inactivated rabies) vaccine and human diploid OH vaccine are also being progressively used with great success.

Control of Rabies in Dogs (TRS 931, WHO 2008)

It consists of:

1. *Destruction of all ownerless, stray dogs*: This may be used as a supplementary measure to mass vaccination.
2. *Registration and licencing* of all pet dogs in a municipality or a district board.
3. *Muzzling and restraint* of dogs during control campaign. Quarantine of all dogs brought into the country should be imposed.
4. *Compulsory notification* of all cases of rabies.
5. *Prophylactic treatment* of pet dogs should be given with antirabic vaccine, preferably with an attenuated live vaccine.
6. *Education* of the public regarding rabies and its prevention through publicity campaigns should be resorted to.
7. Mass canine vaccination.
8. Surveillance of rabies.

16.24 TETANUS

Tetanus or lock-jaw, may follow a wound, induced by the toxin of tetanus bacillus, when infected by dirt, horse or cow dung, etc. is carried into the tissues especially if the dirt is picked from barns or from road. The chief wounds, which give rise to it, are deep stabs or penetrating wounds or those with much confusion or wounds received on roads, gardens or on agricultural lands. During 2012, a total of 10.392 cases of tetanus and 4,650 cases of neonatal tetanus were reported to WHO worldwide. In India, about 528 cases of neonatal tetanus were reported in 2013.

The tetanus bacilli called *Clostridium tetani* are commonly found in the intestinal tract of horses and cattle. They are gram-positive, anaerobic and spore-producing, generally remaining in soil, dust or dirt. The incubation period is from 6 to 10 days.

The most common symptom of the disease is a painful spasm (contraction) of the back muscle, bending the back on spine like a bow and the jaw muscles. This accounts for the common name "lock-jaw".

The first symptoms of tetanus usually appear from 3 days to 3 weeks, after the infection finds access into the wound. The duration of the incubation period is dependent, to some extent, on the character, extent and location of the wound. The first indications of the trouble are irritability and restlessness together with headache and occasional chills. Gradually the neck becomes stiff and there is difficulty in chewing and swallowing. Subsequently, spasms of the muscles of the jaw and face take place and thus "lock law" occurs. The temperature in the early stages ranges from 100° to 105°F (37.7° to 40.5°C) or even higher. There is a severe pain and a large percentage of the cases die after a few days. The patient should be kept in a dark and calm room, free from noise.

The disease is highly dangerous and accounts for up to 80% mortality rate. Neonatal tetanus has a marked seasonal incidence in India which occur in the months of July, August and September. The natural habitat of organism is in soil and dust. Males are more sensitive to tetanus toxins. Agricultural workers are at higher risks. No age is immune unless protected by previous immunization.

Prevention: All wounds should be treated carefully especially if there is a fear of contamination with refuse from stables.

It is also included in NIP as monovalent vaccines or combined vaccines, e.g. DPT. DPT is given on 6, 10, 14 weeks, with booster at 18 to 24 months and at 5 years of age. TT is given at 10 and 16 years. In order to prevent neonatal tetanus, the pregnant ladies get immunized with 2 doses of TT vaccines at 4 weeks intervals as early as pregnancy is detected. In case of repeated pregnancy within 3 yrs, one booster dose of TT is given.

In case an individual is frostated against tetanus as per the NIP Schedule, there is no need to give tetanus toxoid everytime, incase of uninfected wounds.

16.25 ANTHRAX

Anthrax is a disease caused by *Bacillus anthracis*. It is primarily an epizootic of hoofed animals especially of goats, sheep and cattle but transmissible to men. It is usually contracted from working with infected animals or animal products, e.g. hair, wool, hides, contaminated shaving brushes, flesh of infected animals, etc. Human anthrax occurs in the following three forms:

1. **Cutaneous anthrax:** This occurs within 2 weeks after exposure to spores; there is no latency period for cutaneous disease as there is with inhalational anthrax. The initial lesion is an erythematous papule, often on an exposed area of skin that vesiculates and then ulcerates and undergoes necrosis, ultimately progressing to a purple to black eschar. The eschar typically is painless; pain indicates secondary staphylococcal or streptococcal infection. The surrounding area is oedematous and vesicular but not purulent. Regional adenopathy, fever, malaise, headache, and nausea and vomiting may be present. The infection is self-limited in most cases, but haematogenous spread with sepsis or meningitis may occur.

2. **Inhalational anthrax:** Illness occurs in two stages, beginning on average 10 days after exposure, but may have a latent onset 6 weeks after exposure. Nonspecific viral-like symptoms such as fever, malaise, headache, dyspnoea, cough, and congestion of the nose, throat, and larynx are characteristic of the initial stage. Anterior chest pain is an early symptom of mediastinitis. Within hours to a few days, progression to the fulminant stage of infection occurs in which symptoms or signs of overwhelming sepsis predominate. Delirium, obtundation, or findings of meningeal irritation suggest an accompanying haemorrhagic meningitis.

3. **Gastrointestinal anthrax:** This form was recently reported in the United States. Fever, diffuse abdominal pain, rebound abdominal tenderness, vomiting, constipation, and diarrhoea occur 2–5 days after ingestion of meat contaminated with anthrax spores. The primary lesion is ulcerative, producing emesis that may be blood-tinged or coffee-ground and stool that may be blood-tinged or melenic. Bowel perforation can occur. The oropharyngeal form of the disease is characterized by local lymphadenopathy, cervical edema, dysphagia, and upper respiratory tract obstruction.

Incubation period: It is within 7 days, but usually less than 4 days.

Treatment: Strains of *B. anthracis* (including the strain isolated in the bioterrorism cases) are susceptible *in vitro* to penicillin, amoxicillin, chloramphenicol, clindamycin, imipenem, doxycycline, ciprofloxacin (as well as other fluoroquinolones), macrolides, rifampin, and vancomycin. *B. anthracis* may express β-lactamases that confer resistance to cephalosporins and penicillins. For this reason, penicillin or amoxicillin is no longer recommended for use as a single agent in treatment of disseminated disease. Based on results of animal experiments and because of concern for engineered drug resistance in strains of *B. anthracis* used in bio-terrorism, ciprofloxacin is considered the drug of choice for treatment and for prophylaxis following exposure to anthrax spores. Other fluoroquinolones with activity against gram-positive bacteria (e.g. levofloxacin, moxifloxacin) are likely to be just as effective as ciprofloxacin. Doxycycline is an alternative first-line agent.

Prevention: The workers who deal in wool, bristle, hides and animal products should take the following precautions:

1. All workers should wear overalls and respirators. Gloves may be used, which must be disinfected after use.
2. No one with a cut or abrasion on his body should be allowed to work and all workers should wash their hands thoroughly before taking meals.
3. The bales of wool, bristles, hides, etc. particularly those received from countries where the disease is common should be soaked in water, and disinfected by saturated steam or boiling for half an hour or by a suitable powerful disinfectant, before handling.
4. Mechanical exhausts should be provided beneath the sorting benches for the removal of dust.
5. Dust and sweepings should be destroyed by burning.
6. The floor of the sorting room should be impermeable and washed regularly with a suitable disinfectant.
7. All manipulations should be carried out through machinery.
8. Anthrax in man can be best prevented by controlling the disease among animals. Animals suspected of anthrax should be promptly isolated and treated. In enzootic areas, they should be inoculated annually with anti-anthrax vaccine. Prompt diagnosis and slaughtering of infected animals has rendered the disease rare in some countries. The bodies of animals which have died of anthrax should be buried in a pit 6–7 feet (1.82–2.13 metres) in depth after plugging all the natural openings of the animal with a tow of cotton saturated with disinfectants, surrounded by quicklime, and no postmortem examination should be made as the blood contains a large number of bacilli, which when exposed to air produce spores. It is still better to burn the animal, if sufficient fuel is available.
9. Shaving brushes should be thoroughly disinfected before sending to market for sale. They should not be used, if they happen to be of unknown origin.
10. Under no circumstances, the skin of an animal who has died of anthrax, should be cut off and removed.

16.26 MALTA FEVER OR UNDULENT FEVER

The causative organism is *Brucella melitensis, B. abortus, B. suis* and *B. canis. B. melitensis* is the most virulent and invasive species among the all. It is a disease with long pyrexial periods, many relapses, very varied features like continued, intermittent or irregular fever of variable durations, and a few deaths. There are three types of causative organisms, those affecting goats, pigs and cows, all of which can cause human disease.

Malta or Mediterranean fever (also called brucellosis) is usually contracted as a result of drinking infected milk of goats suffering from chronic form of disease in which the health of the animal is little affected. It may also be conveyed to man, by direct contact with the animal as it happens in the case of goat herds. Most commonly infection occurs by direct contact with infected tissues, blood, urine, vaginal discharge, aborted fetuses especially placenta. It very rarely spreads from man to man.

Incubation period: It is highly variable. This is approximately about 14 days but may be as long as 6 months or more.

Prevention: Following measures should be adopted:

1. Prevalence of disease in the animals should be diagnosed. The infected animals should be isolated and treated or slaughtered, to stamp out the disease.
2. The milk especially goat's milk, should not be taken raw, but should be boiled or pasteurised before use.
3. Vaccine of *B. abortus* 19 is commonly used for young animals.
4. There should be clean sanitary environment for animals.
5. Early diagnosis and treatment: In uncomplicated cases, the drug of choice is tetracycline with a dose of 500 mg every 6 hours for 3 weeks.
6. In case of humans, live vaccine of *B. pertussis* strain 19-BA is available.

16.27 GLANDERS

Glanders is a widespread communicable disease of solipeds (horses, mules, asses). Cattle are immune. It is caused by *Burkholderia mallei* which is non-spore bearing. It is readily communicable to man and is characterised by the occurrence either in nasal mucous membrane or the skin of the inflammatory nodules, which breakdown forming ulcers. The mortality is about 50%. It occurs both as an acute and in chronic forms.

Incubation period: It is variable but usually varies from 1 to 5 days.

Prevention: It is done by eradication of the disease in animals. This is carried out by early diagnosis by the mallein and serological tests, isolation, slaughtering and disinfection. Streptomycin + tetracycline is the drug of choice. Alternative combination is chloramphenicol + streptomycin. Other measures include abolition of common feeding and drinking troughs and sanitary supervision of stables where horses are kept. The personal prophylaxis of glanders in man depends upon education and care of those, who have to handle horses. Rubber gloves may be used while handling horses.

DISEASES SPREAD BY CONTACT INFECTION

16.28 LEPROSY

Leprosy is an ancient communicable disease, but organised effort of leprosy control work were not known until the beginning of last century. It is estimated that 2.15,656 new cases of leprosy were detected during 2013, and the registered prevalence at the beginning of 2014 was 1,80,618 cases. Among the new cases detected in 2013, 71.68% was the multibacillary leprosy cases. In SEAR countries, it ranged from 43.9% in Bangladesh to 83.4% in Indonesia. The proportion of new cases with grade 2 disability was 7.36%. In India, registered prevalence at the start of 2014 was 86,147. During 2013, no. of new cases detected were 1,26, 913, out of which 63,337 cases were new cases of multibacillary leprosy. There were 5,256 new cases with grade 2 disabilities. As on 1st April 2014, the prevalence rate was 0.68/10,000 population. India has achieved the phase of elimination as the prevalence rate is <1/10,000. Males are more affected than females as there are about twice as many cases of leprosy in men as there are in women. It is a chronic granulomatous disease, characterised by lesions of the skin and by involvement of peripheral nerves with consequent anaesthesia, muscle weakness, paralysis and trophic changes in the skin, muscles and small bones of hands and feet. Leprosy is caused by *Mycobacterium leprae* and was discovered by a Norwegian leprologist named Armaur Hansen in purulent discharges from nose, ulcers, etc. The disease develops slowly after a long exposure. Children are more susceptible to it than adults. There are two forms of the disease:

1. **Paucibacillary:** Leprosy occurs more often in a benign form called paucibacillary or PB leprosy. It has some tendency to heal spontaneously.
2. **Multibacillary:** It occurs in malign form called multibacillary or MB leprosy. It harbours large numbers of bacteria which are the principal source of transmission of infection from one person to another.

Signs of Leprosy

1st stage: Initially, there is an appearance of a small patch on the skin. It has less sensation than the surrounding area of the skin. There is a thickening of the ulnar nerve and feeling of tingling sensation when nerves are pressed. The patient is seldom infectious, in this stage.

2nd stage: Skin of the face becomes thick and wrinkled, ears are swollen and skin of the whole body is thickened and covered with nodules. The nodules affect the nose and throat which consequently discharge a fluid containing acid-fast lepra bacilli. The stage is infectious and lepra bacilli are passed even in urine and faeces of the patient.

3rd stage: In this, there are very few lepra bacilli and the patient is less dangerous. Patient develops deformities of hands and feet. The fingers and toes become bent, ulcerated or drop and disappear altogether. The patient is sometimes unable to shut his eyelids. There may be foot drop. This is the most painful and loathsome stage of the disease and it is difficult to do anything at this stage.

Leprous or lepra reaction: This is observed during treatment and is specially marked in second stage. When it occurs, the diseased part, i.e. patches and nodules swell up suddenly and become red, the patient may develop fever which may reach 104°F (40°C) and he appears to be much worse. The leprous reaction may continue for 10–14 days. Some patients appear to have improved following a reaction, while others may get worse. There may be one reaction after another for many months.

Incubation period: It is prolonged and rather undermined varying from a few months to 15 or even up to 20 years.

Prevention

1. Compulsory notification.
   a. *Stop stigmatizing:* Treat leprosy patients with kindness and dignity. Do not turn them away from jobs and social events.
   b. *Spread awareness:* The best solution to reduce stigma is to talk openly about the condition. Emphasize the fact that leprosy is an infectious disease, and not a curse. It can be cured completely with appropriate treatment.
   c. *Encourage detection:* Take the individuals with suspected leprosy to the nearest primary health care centre or alert health workers who may be able to visit the individual and carry out tests.
2. Isolation and segregation of infectious cases in ones own home, hospitals and institutions.

A number of leprostatic agents is available for treatment. For paucibacillary (PB or tuberculoid) cases, treatment with daily dapsone and monthly rifampicin for six months is recommended. While for multibacillary (MB or lepromatous) cases, treatment with daily dapsone and clofazimine along with monthly rifampicin for twelve months is recommended.

Multidrug therapy (MDT) remains highly effective, and people are no longer infectious after the first monthly dose. It is safe and easy to use under field conditions due to its presentation in calendar blister packs. Relapse rates remain low, and no resistance to the combined drugs is seen.

It is estimated that approximately 25% of the patients who are not treated at an early stage of disease develop anaesthesia and/or deformities of the hand and feet. According to WHO, community-based rehabilitation measures are taken which require planned and systematic actions such as medical, surgical, social, educational and vocational.

16.29 TRACHOMA

Trachoma is a major eye disease in some of the states of India. According to recent estimates, about 2.2 million people currently suffer from visual impairment due to trachoma, of these 1.2 million are irreversibly blind, and about 324.85 million are at risk of infection. It is estimated to be responsible for 0.2% of visual impairment and blindness in India. Trachoma is a contagious follicular conjunctivitis with characteristic 'SAGO' granulations. It is generally preceded by some other abnormal eye condition following the acute state of granulation; there is a chronic state of cicatrization as a result of which the lids may become deformed. The disease is serious because it may lead to scarring of the eye tissues and even blindness.

It is caused by a virus called *Chlamydia trachomatis* that invades the mucous membrane covering the surface of the eyeball and lining of the lids. Its incubation period varies from 5 to 12 days. Persons with active or chronic disease act as reservoirs. Typically, seen in 2 to 5 years children. Direct sunlight, dust, smoke, kajal or surma can predispose to infection.

The disease may be spread from person to person by direct contact or from indirect contact through handling of towels, handkerchiefs and other linen, which has been handled by a person suffering from the disease.

The spread of trachoma is favoured by malnutrition, overcrowding and inadequate personal cleanliness.

The antibiotic of choice is 1% ophthalmic ointment or oily suspension of tetracycline. Erythromycin and rifampicin have also been used in the treatment. Deformity of the eyelids requires a surgical treatment. Attention should be paid to personal hygiene.

16.30 SEXUALLY TRANSMITTED DISEASES (VENEREAL DISEASES)

These diseases pose as one of the most acute public health problems in the world today. They constitute a group of communicable diseases, which are transmitted predominantly by sexual contact/intercourse and caused by a variety of viral, bacterial, ectoparasites and fungal agents. The list is expanded from 5 "classical" diseases to (syphilis, gonorrhoea and chancroid or soft sore and granuloma inguinale and lymphogranuloma venereum) to include more than 20 agents which are all important from public health point of view.

Bacterial

- Chancroid (*Haemophilus ducreyi*)
- Chlamydia (*Chlamydia trachomatis*)
- Gonorrhoea (*Neisseria gonorrhoeae*), colloquially known as "the clap"
- Granuloma inguinale or (*Klebsiella granulomatis*)
- *Mycoplasma genitalium*
- Syphilis (*Treponema pallidum*)

Fungal

Candidiasis (yeast infection)

Viral

- Viral hepatitis (hepatitis B virus)
- Herpes simplex (herpes simplex virus 1, 2)
- HIV (human immunodeficiency virus)
- HPV (human papillomavirus)
- Molluscum contagiosum (molluscum contagiosum virus—MCV)

Parasites

- Crab louse, colloquially known as "crabs" or "pubic lice" (*Pthirus pubis*)
- Scabies (*Sarcoptes scabiei*)

Protozoal

Trichomoniasis (*Trichomonas vaginalis*), colloquially known as "trich".

More than 1 million people acquire a sexually transmitted infection (STI) everyday. Each year, an estimated 500 million people become ill with one of 4 STIs: Chlamydia, gonorrhoea, syphilis and trichomoniasis. More than 530 million people have the virus that causes genital herpes (HSV2). More than 290 million women have a human papillomavirus (HPV) infection. The majority of STIs are present without symptoms. Some STIs can increase the risk of HIV acquisition three-fold or more. STIs can have serious consequences beyond the immediate impact of the infection itself, through mother-to-child transmission of infections and chronic diseases. Drug resistance, especially for gonorrhoea, is a major threat to reducing the impact of STIs worldwide.

1. **Syphilis:** It is quite common throughout the world but in Western countries its incidence has been lowered to a great extent. It is caused by a corkscrew or spiral shaped germ called *Spirocheta or Treponema pallidum*, which passes through cracks in skin or mucous membrane. The germ has 8–15 spirals. It survives easily in most surroundings, but it dies readily outside the body. The entry occurs directly during sexual intercourse or congenially by foetus *in utero*. Primary sore may also be formed on mouth or lips after kissing an infected part. Man is the only reservoir of infection.

   Incubation period: It varies from 10 days to 10 weeks. Average is about 3 weeks.

2. Gonorrhoea: It is an acutely infectious venereal disease characterised by inflammation of the urethra, painful micturition, purulent discharge and a liability to certain complications such as ophthalmia, endocarditis and arthritis. Unlike syphilis it is difficult to diagnose the disease especially in females. It is a very delicate organism and is easily destroyed by drying and even with weak disinfectants. The disease is contracted by sexual intercourse. In a few cases, it may be caused indirectly by infected towels, beds clothes, etc. But it is rare since the germs die readily outside the body.

Incubation period: It varies from 2 days to 2 weeks. Average is about one week.

3. Soft chancre (also called soft sore or chancroid): It starts as a small painful sore or ulcer on the sex organs, accompanied by swelling of the glands in the groins. It is thus localised and may heal spontaneously but vaccine of *Haemophilus ducreyi* will hasten recovery, and sulphonamides (sulphanilamide, sulphadiazine or sulphathiazole) are also used as a remedy. It may be of interest to note that often the sore of chancroid, is mistaken for the sore formed in early stages of syphilis. Sometimes both syphilis and chancroid may be found in the same patient.

Syndromic Approach to STD

Many different agents cause sexually transmitted diseases. However, some of the agents give rise to similar or overlapping clinical manifestation. The traditional method of diagnosing STD is by laboratory tests. Since 1990, WHO has recommended syndromic management of STDs in patients presenting with consistently recognised signs and symptoms of STDs.

Control of STDs

The aim of the control programme is the prevention of ill health resulting from the above conditions. It may be considered under the following heads:

1. Initial planning: Control programmes have to be designed to meet the unique needs of each country and to be lined with what country's health care system, its resources and priorities.

2. Intervention strategies

   a. Case detection is an essential part of any control programme. The usual methods to early detection in a STD control programme are screening, contact tracing and cluster testing.

   b. Adequate treatment of patients and their contacts is the mainstay of STD control.

   c. Epidemiological treatment or otherwise called as contact treatment has become a key stone of the control programme.

   d. Personal prophylaxis through barrier contraceptives and vaccines.

16.31 AIDS/HIV

AIDS means acquired immunodeficiency syndrome. It is a fatal disease caused by a human-immunodeficiency virus (HIV) which is responsible for destroying human body's immune system leaving the patient vulnerable to various infections, malignancies and neurological disorders. A person; if once infected with HIV, will remain infected throughout his life till the disease advances, ultimately causing death to the patient.

According to a rough estimate of World Health Organization, HIV continues to be a major global public health issue, having claimed more than 39 million lives so far. In 2013, 1.5 (1.4–1.7) million people died from HIV-related causes globally. There were approximately 35.0 (33.2–37.2) million people living with HIV at the end of 2013 with 2.1 (1.9–2.4) million people becoming newly infected with HIV in 2013 globally. Sub-Saharan Africa is the most affected region, with 24.7 (23.5–26.1) million people living with HIV in 2013. Also sub-Saharan Africa accounts for almost 70% of the global total of new HIV infections. HIV infection is usually diagnosed through blood tests detecting the presence or absence of HIV antibodies. There is no cure for HIV infection. However, effective treatment with antiretroviral (ARV) drugs can control the virus so that people with HIV can enjoy healthy and productive lives. In 2013, 12.9 million people living with HIV were receiving antiretroviral therapy (ART) globally, of which 11.7 million were receiving ART in low- and middle-income countries. The 11.7 million people on ART represent 36% (34–38%) of the 32.6 (30.8–34.7) million people living with HIV in low- and middle-income countries. Paediatric coverage is still lagging in low- and middle-income countries. In 2013, less than 1 in 4 children living with HIV had access to ART, compared to over 1 in 3 adults.

Agent Factors

In May 1986, the virus responsible for spreading AIDS was named as "Human immunodeficiency virus (HIV)". This virus is very destructive and infective in nature being capable of spreading throughout the body. Besides it is so powerful that it can easily destroy human T4 helper cells. The virus is capable of passing through blood–brain barrier and can destroy even brain cells. It is generally found in greatest concentration in blood and semen, but it has been also found to be present in saliva, breast milk, mouth, urine and vaginal secretions, in lesser concentration occasionally. HIV 1 is the more commonly known virus. In Africa, another type HIV 2 has been lately isolated, which is less lethal than HIV 1. HIV 1 and HIV 2 also have different strains/sub-types. Presently nine sub-types have been isolated for HIV 1 and four for HIV 2. Sub-types A, B, C, and E of HIV 1 are commonly found in India. In fact, those pathogenic viruses completely ravage the entire immune system of the human body thus rendering it practically defenceless against any infection.

Modes of Transmission

a. **Sexual transmission:** The HIV is most frequently transmitted from person to person through sexual route, since in fact, it is mostly a sexually transmitted disease spreading through infected vaginal and anal secretions during intercourse. About 60–70% of infected cases were found to be in men who were homosexual men having sex with men (msm) or bisexual (attracted sexually to both the sexes).

But in India and some other developing countries, infection has also spread through heterosexual contact (through infected woman to man and *vice versa*). Multiple sexual acts of intercourse, anal intercourse and male homosexual acts increase the risk of transmitting infection. Evidently, infection spreads mainly through infected partners.

b. **Blood contact:** The disease can be transmitted through the use of infected needles, while giving intravenous injections or during blood transfusion process or even through contaminated blood, viz. by transfusion of whole blood and cell platelets and factors VIII and IX derived from human plasma.

c. **Maternal-foetal transmission:** The HIV infection can be transmitted from an HIV-infected mother to her child during pregnancy through the placenta or during delivery of the child.

Symptoms

The symptoms of HIV vary depending on the stage of infection. The patients may remain asymptomatic for quite sometime after acquiring the infections.

As the infection progressively weakens the person's immune system, the individual can develop other signs and symptoms such as swollen lymph nodes, weight loss, fever, diarrhoea and cough. Without treatment, they could also develop severe illnesses such as tuberculosis, cryptococcal meningitis, and cancers such as lymphomas and Kaposi's sarcoma, among others.

Incubation period: It has not been defined clearly as yet since the virus can remain dormant or inactive in the body for many years. In fact, it is fairly long (in some cases it may be up to 10 years or even more) from contacting HIV infection and actual development of AIDS disease.

WHO Case Definition

Adults and children 18 months or older: HIV infection is diagnosed based on: positive HIV antibody testing (rapid or laboratory-based enzyme immunoassay). This is confirmed by a second HIV antibody test (rapid or laboratory-based enzyme immunoassay) relying on different antigens or of different operating characteristics; and/or; positive virological test for HIV or its components (HIV-RNA or HIV-DNA or ultrasensitive HIV p24 antigen) confirmed by a second virological test obtained from a separate determination.

Children younger than 18 months: HIV infection is diagnosed based on: positive virological test for HIV or its components (HIV-RNA or HIV-DNA or ultrasensitive HIV p24 antigen) confirmed by a second virological test obtained from a separate determination taken more than four weeks after birth. Positive HIV antibody testing is not recommended for definitive or confirmatory diagnosis of HIV infection in children until 18 months of age.

Prevention and Control

No specific cure or vaccine for curing the disease has been developed so far. The treatment is simply symptomatic.

The HIV sentinel surveillance (HSS) system in India involves carrying out cross-sectional facility and targeted intervention (TI) based HIV sero-prevalence surveys at regular intervals among selected population groups. These populations are also referred to as "sentinel groups". HIV sentinel surveillance is carried out once a year in designated sentinel sites for twelve weeks.

Testing strategies: The safety of blood and blood products is of paramount importance because of the enormous risk involved in the transmission of HIV through blood. Since the PPV is low in populations with low HIV prevalence, the WHO/Government of India have evolved strategies to detect HIV infection in different population groups and to fulfil different objectives. The various strategies, so designated, involve the use of categories of tests in various permutations and combinations.

1. ELISA/Rapid test (E/R) used in strategy I, II, and III.
2. Confirmatory tests with high specificity, like WBs and line immunoassays, are used in problem cases, e.g. in cases of indeterminate/discordant result of E/R.

Testing Approaches

i. *Unlined anonymous testing*: This testing approach is used for HIV surveillance purposes. All the identifiers are removed for the specimen before they are sent to the laboratory of testing, so that the test results cannot be linked to the individuals.

ii. *Voluntary confidential counselling and testing*: This approach is followed for the diagnosis of HIV infection in an individual. This testing is done after per test counselling is provided and after obtaining informed consent for the individual. The test result is disclosed to the individual only after post test counselling. Confidentiality needs to be maintained throughout the process.

iii. *Mandatory testing:* Mandatory testing is recommended in India, only for the screening of donated units of blood, blood products, and donors of semen, organs, or tissues in order to prevent the transmission of HIV to the recipient. The national HIV testing policy reiterates the following: No individual should be made to undergo a mandatory testing for HIV. No mandatory HIV testing should be imposed as a precondition for employment or for providing healthcare services and facilities. Any HIV testing must be accompanied by pre test and post test counselling services and informed consent. Confidentiality of result should be maintained.

The National AIDS Control Programme (NACP), launched in 1992, is being implemented as a comprehensive programme for prevention and control of HIV/AIDS in India. In the **first phase** of the programme, the focus was on awareness generation, setting up surveillance system for monitoring HIV epidemic, measures to ensure access to safe blood and preventive services for high risk group populations.

The second phases of National AIDS Control Project (NACP II) launched in November 1999, with the support of World Bank. The key objectives of the second phase were:

i. To reduce the spread of HIV infection in India, and

ii. To increase India's capacity to respond to HIV/AIDS on a long-term basis.

The **major initiatives** that were taken during NACP II were adoption of National AIDS Prevention and Control Policy (2002); scaling up to targeted interventions for high risk groups in high prevalence states; Adoption of National Blood Policy: A strategy for greater involvement of people with HIV/AIDS (GIPA); launch of National Adolescent Education Programme (NAEP); introduction of counseling, testing and PPTCT programmes; launch of National Anti-retroviral Treatment (ART) Programme; formation of an inter-ministerial group for mainstreaming; and setting up of the National Council on AIDS, chaired by the Prime Minister; and setting up of State AIDS Control Societies in all states.

The **third phase** of the national programme (NACP III) was launched in July 2007 with the goal of halting and reversing the epidemic over its five-year period by scaling up prevention efforts among high risk groups (HRG) and general population and integrating them with care, support and treatment services. Thus, prevention and care, support and treatment (CST) for the two key pillars of all the AIDS control

efforts in India. Strategic Information Management and Institutional Strengthening activities provide the required technical, managerial and administrative support for implementing the core activities under NACP-III at national, state and district level.

*The **fourth phase** (NACP IV) was launched in 2014 with the following components*

1. Intensifying and consolidating prevention services with a focus on high risk groups (HRG) and vulnerable populations. The two sub-components under this are:

   1.1 *Scaling up coverage of TIs among HRG by*

   i. The provision of behaviour change interventions to increase safe practices, testing and counselling, adherence to treatment, and demand for other services.

   ii. The promotion and provision of condoms to HRG to promote their use in each sexual encounter.

   iii. Provision or referral for STI services including counselling at service provision centres to increase compliance of patients with treatment, risk reduction counselling with focus on partner referral and management.

   iv. Needle and syringe exchange for IDUs as well as scaling up of opioid substitution therapy (OST) provision.

   1.2 *Scaling up of interventions among other vulnerable population by*

   i. Risk assessment and size estimation of migrant population groups and truckers at transit points and at workplaces.

   ii. Behaviour change communications (BCC) for creating awareness about risk and vulnerability, prevention methods, availability and location of services, increase safe behaviour and demand for services as well as reduce stigma.

   iii. Promotion and provisioning of condoms through different channels including social marketing.

   iv. Development of linkages with local institutions, both public and NGO owned, for testing, counselling and STI treatment services.

   v. Creation of "peer support group" and "safe spaces" for migrants at destination.

   vi. Establishment of need-based and gender-sensitive services for partners of IDUs.

   vii. Strengthening networks of vulnerable populations with enhanced linkages to service centres and risk reduction interventions, specifically condom use.

2. Expanding IEC services for (a) general population and (b) high risk groups with a focus on behaviour change and demand generation.

3. Comprehensive care, support and treatment for all those who are in need of such services and facilitate additional support systems for women and children affected and infected with HIV/AIDS. The comprehensive care, support and treatment of HIV/AIDS will include:
   i. Anti-retroviral treatment (ART) including second line
   ii. Management of opportunistic infection.
   iii. Facilitating social protection through linkage with concerned departments/ministries. The program will explore avenues of public–private partnerships. The program will enhance activities to reduce stigma and discrimination at all levels particularly at healthcare settings.
4. *Strengthening institutional capacities*: Programme planning and management responsibilities will be strengthened at state and district levels to ensure high quality, timely and effective implementation of field level activities and desired programmatic outcomes.

HIV treatment: Antiretroviral therapy (ART) is the use of medicines to treat HIV infection. People on ART take combination of HIV medicines (called HIV regimen) everyday. Selection of an HIV regimen depends on several factors, including possible side effects of HIV medicines and potential drug interactions between medicines. The HIV medicines are grouped into six drug classes according to how they fight HIV. A Person's initial HIV regimen usually includes three or more HIV medicines from at least two different HIV drug classes. ART cannot cure HIV but help people with HIV live a longer life with better quality along with reduced risk of HIV transmission.

Currently, the national programme provides the following combinations for first-line regiments
   i. Stavudine (30 mg) + Lamivudine (150 mg)
   ii. Zidovudine (300 mg) + Lamivudine (150 mg)
   iii. Stavudine (30 mg) + Lamivudine (150 mg) + Nevirapine (200 mg)
   iv. Zidovudine (300 mg) + Lamivudine (150 mg) + Nevirapine (200 mg)
   v. Efavirenz (600 mg)
   vi. Nevirapine (200 mg)

Fixed-dose combinations (FDCs) are preferred because they are easy to use, have distribution advantages (procurement and stock management), improve adherence to treatment and thus reduce the chances of development of drug resistance. The current national experience shows that twice a day regimens of FDCs are well tolerated and complied with. At present, second-line drug regimens are not available under the national programme.

When HIV multiplies in the body, the virus sometimes mutates (changes for) and makes variations of itself. Variations of HIV that develop while a person is taking HIV medicines can lead to drug-resistant strains of HIV. HIV medicines that previously controlled a person's HIV are not effective against the new, drug-resistant HIV. In other words, the person's HIV continues to multiply. Poor adherence to an HIV regimen increases the risk of drug resistance and treatment failure.

PPTCT: The prevention of parent to child transmission of HIV/AIDS (PPTCT) programme was launched in the country in the year 2002 following a feasibility study in 11 major hospitals in the five high HIV prevalence states. As on 31st August 2016 in India there are 20,756 Integrated Counselling and Testing Centers (ICTC), most of these in government hospitals, which offer PPTCT services to pregnant women.

In case of HIV infected pregnant women requiring ART, the recommended first-line regimen is Tenofovir (TDF) (300 mg) + Efavirenz (EFV) (600 mg). The recommended first-line regimen for pregnant and breastfeeding women, is available as a fixed dose combination (FDC) which is safe for both pregnant and breastfeeding women and their infants and is well tolerated.

Surveillance

The Government of India has established four regional surveillance centres, where special facilities are available for record keeping, diagnosis and prevention of this dreadful disease. These are All India Institute of Medical Sciences, New Delhi, National Institute of Communicable Diseases, Delhi, National Institute of Virology, Pune and Christian Medical College, Vellore. Government has also opened a National AIDS Research Institute at Pune, which is doing a good work for this disease. Besides WHO has also launched a "Global Programme on AIDS" in 1987 to provide guidance and assistance about the problem to various countries in the world.

16.32 RINGWORM (TINEA)

This is an infection of skin caused by a sporing fungus which is a very minute form of vegetable plant life. The disease is primarily caused by dermatophytes in the *Trichophyton* and *Microsporum* genera that invade the hair shaft. It penetrates into hair follicles and destroys hair; these break off leaving stumps scattered over ring shaped scaly patches which soon become yellow and crusted. There are different types of the fungus affecting the scalp, body, beard area, feet, nails and also the skin of animals. The affected hairs are highly infectious, since they are loaded with innumerable spores. It may appear as thickened, scaly, and sometimes boggy swellings, or as expanding raised red rings (ringworm). Common symptoms are severe itching of the scalp, dandruff, and bald patches where the fungus has rooted itself in the skin. It often presents identically to dandruff or seborrhoeic dermatitis. The disease is more annoying than dangerous and becomes serious only when the skin breaks up due to scratching when secondary infection takes place.

The infection begins as a small papule and spreads peripherally leaving scaly patches of alopecia (baldness).

Ringworm of the scalp affects mostly children. Ringworm of the body generally affects the face and the neck but in some persons it is also common around the waist, because of excessive perspiration in these areas. Ringworm of the feet, also known as "athlete's foot" is more prevalent in summer in persons who have to keep their feet wet for the greater part of the day, e.g. dhobies, bhishties (water carriers), etc. Likewise, it is common among those who do not change socks often or those who use public baths, swimming pools, etc.

Incubation period: It varies from 10 to 14 days.

Treatment of Ringworm of Scalp

1. *Shampoos:* The hair is cut short all over the scalp so that the shampoo can be applied on the affected area. Antifungal shampoos like ketoconzole and selenium sulphide twice a week will cure the infection.

2. *Treatment of the scalp:* It should be washed every-day either with painting with tincture of iodine or ketoconazole shampoo.

   The drug of choice is griseofulvin: The recommended paediatric dosage is 10 mg/kg/day for 6–8 weeks. Other oral antifungal treatments for tinea capitis also frequently reported in the literature include terbinafine, itraconazole, and fluconazole; these drugs have the advantage of shorter treatment durations than griseofulvin.

3. *Isolation and disinfection:* The child is isolated from others and everything else which he uses or plays with is kept separate. Hats, brushes', combs and toilet articles should be destroyed since it is impossible to free them from spores; all articles not boiled or destroyed should be steam sterilised. Other fungicidal agents like cresol, etc. can also be used with advantage, for proper disinfection of contaminated towels, floors, benches, shower stalls, etc.

EMERGING AND RE-EMERGING INFECTIOUS DISEASES

Emerging infectious diseases are newly identified and previously unknown infectious agents that cause public health problems either locally or internationally. Re-emerging infectious agents are the ones that have been known for some time, had fallen to such low levels that they were no longer considered public health problems and are now showing an upward trend in incidence or prevalence worldwide. Emergence of infectious disease is the result of dynamic interactions between rapidly evolving infectious agents, changes in the environment and changes in host behaviour that provide such agents with favourable new ecological niches. The factors contributing to emergence or re-emergence of the infectious diseases are:

1. **Agent factors:** Resistance of vectors to pesticides, mutations *de novo* or as a consequence to development of resistance to drugs, microbial adaptation and change leads to evolution of pathogenic infectious agents.

2. **Host factors:** Increased urbanisation and population movements lead to inhabitation of new areas and changes in human demography and thus transmission of infection from one area or country to other, e.g. influenza. Unsafe sexual practices and use of drugs and intoxicating agents predisposes individuals to infections like HIV, gonorrhoea, syphilis. Poverty and social inequality leads to malnutrition thus increasing the human susceptibility to infections due to immunosuppression. Uncontrolled urbanization and population displacement causes growth of densely populated cities leading to substandard housing, unsafe water, poor sanitation, overcrowding, indoor air pollution thus predisposing to ARI, diarrhoea and intestinal parasitic diseases, that form >10% preventable causes of ill health.

3. **Environmental factors:** Changing climate and ecosystems, economic development leading to urbanisation and deforestation for land use, food processing and handling, International travel and commerce, breakdown of public health measure due to war, unrest, overcrowding, lack of political will leading to deterioration in surveillance systems are some important factors that brings animals into closer human contact thus causing the infectious agent to breach species barrier between animals and humans, e.g. global warming leads to spread of malaria, dengue, leishmaniasis, and filariasis. Changes in ecology, increasing deer populations, and suburban migration of population can lead to Lyme disease (*B. burgdorferi*). Poor populations serve as a major reservoir and source of continued transmission of infections due to poverty, neglect and weakening of health infrastructure. Lack of funding, poor prioritization of health funds towards curative rather than preventive services/ infrastructure, failure to develop adequate health delivery systems, wrong prescribing practices of drugs can lead to changes in the disease patterns and trends due to inadequate or ineffective implementation of control programmes, antimicrobial drug resistance, etc.

16.33 EMERGING INFECTIOUS DISEASES

Some of the infections/diseases of public health importance that are emerging infections are as follows:

a. **Hepatitis C:** First identified in 1989, its estimated global prevalence was 3% in mid-90s.

b. **Hepatitis B:** It was identified several decades earlier but has an upward trend in all countries with prevalence rate of more than 90% in high-risk population.

c. **Emerging zoonoses:** Due to human animal interface like Ebola, avian influenza, Nipah virus, Marburg virus, hantavirus pulmonary syndrome, Lyme's disease (*Borrelia burgdorferi*), Lyssa fever through Mostomyes rodents, Ixodes scapularis or deer ticks, SARS (severe acute respiratory syndrome), novel swine origin influenza A or swine flu (H1N1).

i. Viral Haemorrhagic Fever

Emerging infectious diseases classified as VHFs include the conditions caused by the Ebola, Marburg, and Yellow fever viruses. Fatality rates average 5–20% for all of these viral infections. The Ebola death rate is between 50 and 90%. Outbreaks of VHF are often in small remote areas. There is currently no successful therapy for VHF infection. These viruses are transmitted in diverse ways including both arthropod and rodent vectors. All of the haemorrhagic viruses can be transmitted directly from human to human. Symptoms include fever, bleeding, and circulatory shock.

Ebola

Previously known as Ebola haemorrhagic fever, is a rare and deadly disease caused by infection with one of the Ebola virus species. Ebola can cause disease in humans and non-human primates (monkeys, gorillas, and chimpanzees). Ebola is caused by a virus of the family *Filoviridae*, genus *Ebolavirus*. There are five identified Ebola virus species. Four of the five have caused disease in humans: Ebola virus (*Zaire ebolavirus*); Sudan virus (*Sudan ebolavirus*); Taï Forest virus (*Taï Forest ebolavirus*, formerly *Côte d'Ivoire ebolavirus*); and Bundibugyo virus (*Bundibugyo ebolavirus*). The fifth, Reston virus (*Reston ebolavirus*), has caused disease in non-human primates but not in humans. Ebola viruses are found in several African countries, four of the five subtypes occur in an animal host native to Africa. Ebola was first discovered in 1976 near the Ebola river in what is now the Democratic Republic of the Congo. Since then, outbreaks have appeared sporadically in Africa.

The natural reservoir host of Ebola viruses remains unknown. However, on the basis of evidence and the nature of similar viruses, researchers believe that the virus is animal-borne and that bats are the most likely reservoir. Only a few species of mammals (e.g. humans, bats, monkeys, and apes) have shown the ability to become infected with and spread Ebola virus. It is believed that the first patient becomes infected through contact with an infected animal, such as a fruit bat or nonhuman primate. Ebola is spread through direct contact (through broken skin or unprotected mucous membranes in, for example, the eyes, nose, or mouth) with blood or body fluids (including but not limited to faeces, saliva, sweat, urine, vomit, breast milk, and semen) of a person who is sick with Ebola, objects (like needles and syringes) that have been contaminated with the virus, infected fruit bats or primates (apes and monkeys), and possibly from contact with semen from a man who has recovered from Ebola (e.g. by having oral, vaginal, or anal sex).

A person infected with Ebola virus is not contagious until symptoms appear. Common signs and symptoms of Ebola include fever, severe headache, fatigue, muscle pain, weakness, diarrhoea, vomiting, stomach pain and unexplained bleeding or bruising. Symptoms may appear anywhere from 2 to 21 days after exposure to the virus, but the average is 8 to 10 days.

Healthcare providers and the family and friends in close contact with Ebola patients are at the highest risk of getting sick because they may come in contact with infected blood and body fluids. During outbreaks of Ebola, the disease can spread quickly within healthcare settings (such as a clinic or hospital). Exposure to Ebola virus can occur in healthcare settings where hospital staff are not wearing appropriate protective clothing including masks, gowns, gloves, and eye protection.

Early symptoms such as fever are non-specific to Ebola, thus its diagnosis in early disease is difficult. Ebola virus is detected in blood only **after** onset of fever which accompany the rise in circulating virus within the patient's body. It may take up to three days after symptoms start for the virus to reach detectable levels.

There is no specific treatment for Ebola, only symptoms and complications are treated as they appear. Stabilization of patients by providing intravenous fluids for balancing electrolytes, maintaining oxygen status and blood pressure and treating other co-infections are the basic interventions to improve the survival of patients. Good supportive care and the patient's immune response can increase the chances of survival after Ebola infection. People who recover from Ebola develop antibodies that last for at least 10 years, possibly longer, however some patients have developed long-term complications, such as joint and vision problems.

Prevention

Since there is no vaccine available for prevention from Ebola, careful hygiene measures like handwashing with soap and water or an alcohol-based hand sanitizer, avoiding contact with blood and body fluids, avoiding handling items that may have come in contact with an infected person's blood or body fluids (such as clothes, bedding, needles, and medical equipment) and funeral or burial rituals that require handling the body of someone who has died from Ebola are few simple measures for prevention of infection. In case of suspected contact, the person should monitor health for 21 days and seek medical care immediately in case he develops symptoms of Ebola.

Healthcare workers who may be exposed to patients of Ebola are advised to:

a. Wear appropriate personal protective equipment (PPE).

b. Practice proper infection control and sterilization measures.

c. Isolate patients with Ebola from other patients.

d. Avoid direct contact with the bodies of people who have died from Ebola.

e. Notify health officials if you have had direct contact with the blood or body fluids of a person sick with Ebola.

ii. SARS

SARS became readily transmissible in the 1990s. First documented case was identified in mainland China. It is transmitted by droplet aerosol and fomites deposited on the respiratory mucosal epithelium. It causes pneumonia-like disease. 2002–2003 outbreak infected 8400+ with 916 confirmed dead. SARS is an infection of the lower respiratory system and its symptoms include fever, malaise, and T cell lymphopenia. Twenty to thirty per cent of patients infected with SARS require intensive care and approximately 10% will die. The pathogenesis of SARS is due to a high viral load in the lower respiratory tract. Therapy includes antiviral drugs but they are only effective if given during the first few days of the infection.

iii. Middle East Respiratory Syndrome Coronavirus (MERS-CoV)

Middle East respiratory syndrome (MERS) is a viral respiratory disease caused by a novel coronavirus (MERS-CoV) that was first identified in Saudi Arabia in 2012. Symptoms of MERS include fever, cough and shortness of breath. Pneumonia is common, but not always present. Gastrointestinal symptoms, including diarrhoea, have also been reported. About 36% of reported patients of MERS have died.

The virus passes easily from person to person in close contacts such as during providing unprotected care to a patient. Thus, the transmission of MERS has been primarily human-to-human, however, camels are likely to be a major reservoir host for MERS-CoV and an animal source of MERS infection in humans. However, the exact role of camels in transmission of the virus and the exact route(s) of transmission are unknown. Majority of cases (>85%) have been reported since 2012 primarily in Saudi Arabia and several cases have been reported outside the Middle East. The ongoing outbreak in the Republic of Korea is the largest outbreak outside of the Middle East, and while

concerning, there is no evidence of sustained human-to-human transmission in the Republic of Korea. No secondary or limited secondary transmission has been reported in countries with exported cases.

No specific treatment is available currently, only supportive is indicated based on the patient's clinical condition. There is no vaccine available for prevention, however, practice of general hygiene measures should be used by people visiting farms, markets, barns, or other places where camels and other animals are present, i.e. regular handwashing before and after touching animals, avoiding contact with sick animals and consumption of raw or undercooked animal products, including milk and meat. Animal products that are processed appropriately through cooking or pasteurization are safe for consumption, but should also be handled with care to avoid cross-contamination with uncooked foods. Camel meat and camel milk are nutritious products that can continue to be consumed after pasteurization, cooking, or other heat treatments.

People suffering with diabetes, renal failure, chronic lung disease, and immunocompromised persons are considered to be at high risk for severe disease thus should practice strict preventive measures.

Transmission of the virus has been reported to have occurred in healthcare facilities from patients to healthcare providers and between patients in a health care settings. However, identification of patients may not always be without testing because of non-specific symptoms and clinical features.

Prevention and control measures are critical to prevent the possible spread of infection in the healthcare facilities by educating and training the health workers to take appropriate measures to decrease the risk of transmission of the virus from an infected patient to other patients, healthcare workers, or visitors.

WHO is working to gather and share scientific evidence to better understand the virus and the disease it causes, to determine outbreak response priorities, treatment strategies, and clinical management approaches. The organization also aims to develop public health prevention strategies to combat the virus.

Countries irrespective of the MERS cases reported in them, should maintain a high level of surveillance, especially those with large numbers of travellers or migrant workers returning from the Middle East. Infection, prevention and control procedures in healthcare facilities should be in place. All the countries should report confirmed and probable cases of infection along with information about their exposure, testing, and clinical course to WHO so that effective international preparedness and response can be done.

iv. West Nile Fever

West Nile virus is caused by an arbovirus (arthropod-borne, RNA viruses). The virus is carried in the saliva of mosquitoes and is transmitted through bites. Birds, like crows and cardinals are, the primary hosts. Infection is spread from bird to bird by mosquitoes. Most infected people are asymptomatic unless the infection causes an invasive neurological disease called West Nile fever. Symptoms include fever, headache, myalgia, and anorexia. Severe infection can cause profound fatigue, myocarditis, pancreatitis, and hepatitis. Particularly severe cases can result in encephalitis or meningitis and death. The illness can also be transferred through blood transfusions and transplantation.

16.34 RE-EMERGING INFECTIOUS DISEASES

Diphtheria—early 1990s epidemic in Eastern Europe (1980–1% cases; 1994–90% cases).

- Cholera—100% increase worldwide in 1998 (new strain eltor, 0139).
- Human plague—India (1994) after 15–30 years absence.
- Dengue/DHF—over past 40 years, 20-fold increase to nearly 0.5 million (between 1990 and 98).

In India, plague re-emerged in August 1994, when it was detected in the Beed district of Maharashtra. This was followed by pneumonic plague in Surat in Gujarat state, resulting in over 50 deaths and inducing a mass exodus of people. Eventually plague was reported from 12 Indian states.

Avian Influenza (Swine Flu—H1N1)

Avian influenza ("bird flu") is an infectious disease of birds caused by type A strains of the influenza virus. The infection can cause a wide spectrum of symptoms in birds, ranging from mild illness, which may pass unnoticed, to a rapidly fatal disease that can cause severe epidemics. Avian influenza viruses do not normally infect humans, however, A(H5N1) and A (H7N9) have caused serious infections in humans. In most cases, the people infected had been in close contact with infected poultry or with objects contaminated with their faeces. Nevertheless, there is concern that the virus could mutate to become more easily transmissible between humans, raising the possibility of an influenza pandemic.

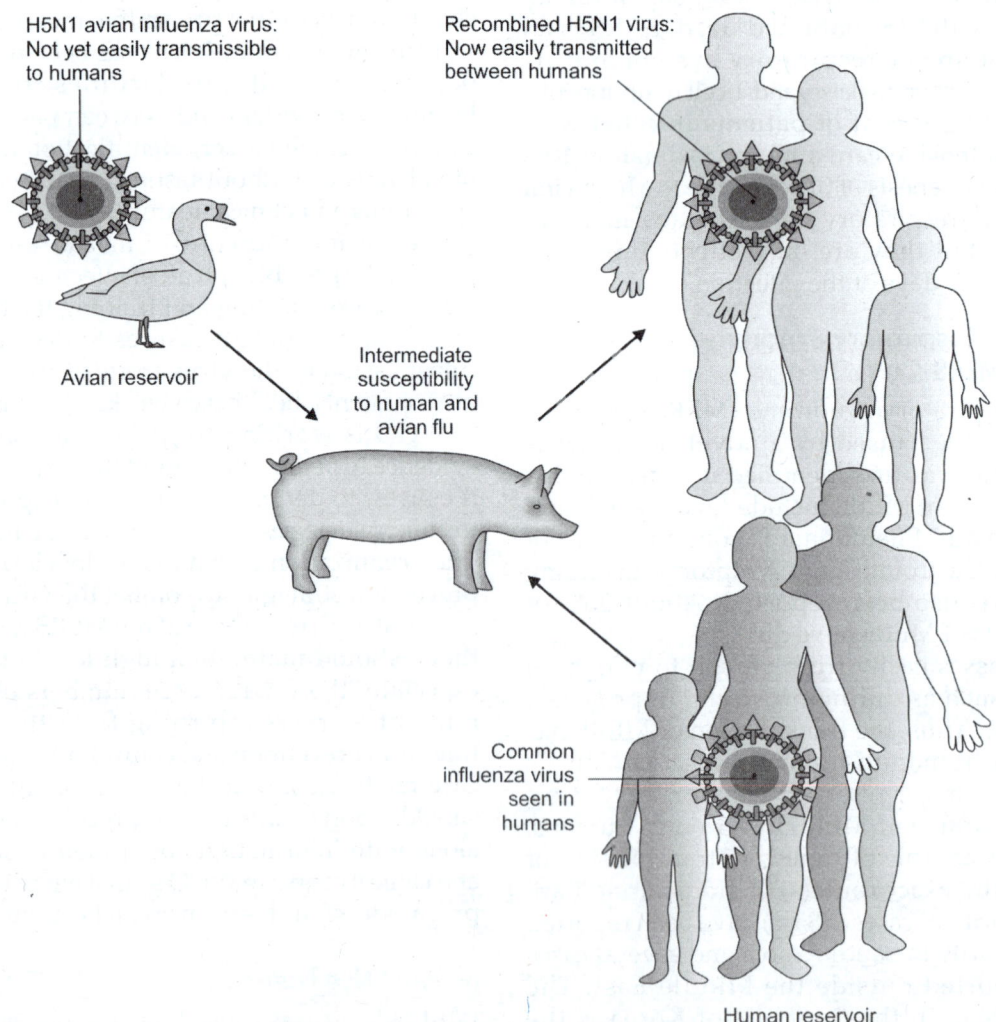

H5N1 avian influenza virus: Not yet easily transmissible to humans

Recombined H5N1 virus: Now easily transmitted between humans

Avian reservoir

Intermediate susceptibility to human and avian flu

Common influenza virus seen in humans

Human reservoir

Fig. 16.2: Microbiology: A clinical approach

Since Nov 2003, avian influenza H5N1 in birds affected 60 countries across Asia, Europe, Middle East and Africa. More than 220 million birds killed by AI virus or culled to prevent further spread. Majority of human H5N1 infection occurred due to direct contact with birds infected with virus.

Influenza is caused by an RNA virus that contains eight separate segments of RNA. High mutation rates continuously change viral characteristics. There are two surface glycoproteins hemagglutinin (H) and neuraminidase (N) and both occur in several subtypes 16H and 9N. H (1, 2, 3) and N (1 and 2) are most common in humans. The virus has a stable reservoir in aquatic birds. The severity of infection depends on the viral virulence and the host's overall health. Virulence factor genes keep on mutating constantly. H and N also mutate affecting immune recognition which influence virulence, i.e. there is always a potential for increased virulence in future strains.

The incubation period for A(H5N1) avian influenza is around 2 to 3 days. Current data for A(H5N1) infection indicate an incubation period ranging from 2 to 8 days and possibly as long as 17 days. Current data for A (H7N9) infection indicate an incubation period ranging from 2 to 8 days, with an average of five days. Thus, WHO currently recommends that an incubation period of 7 days be used for field investigations and the monitoring of patient contacts.

Initial symptoms include high fever, usually higher than 38°C along with other influenza-like symptoms (cough or sore throat). Diarrhoea, vomiting, abdominal pain, chest pain, and bleeding from the nose and gums have also been reported as early symptoms in some patients. Respiratory distress, a hoarse voice, and a crackling sound when inhaling are commonly seen. Complications of A(H5N1) and A(H7N9) infection include hypoxaemia, multiple organ dysfunction, and secondary bacterial and fungal infection.

In suspected cases, oseltamivir should be prescribed preferably within 48 hours following onset of symptoms which can reduce the duration of viral replication and improve prospects of survival.

An influenza pandemic occurs when an influenza virus emerges with the ability to cause sustained human-to-human transmission, and the human population has a little to no immunity against the virus. With the growth of global trade and travel, a localized epidemic can transform into a pandemic rapidly, with little time to prepare a public health response. In addition to A(H5N1) and A(H7N9), other animal influenza virus subtypes reported to have infected people include avian H9, and swine H1 and H3 viruses. H2 viruses may also pose a pandemic threat.

Novel Swine Origin Influenza A (H1N1): Swine flu causes respiratory disease in pigs with low mortality and high level of illness. Pigs can get infected by human, avian and swine influenza virus, however, human swine infection is reported occasionally. 12 cases of human infection with swine flu were reported in US from December 2005 to February 2009.

Prions and Prion Diseases

They are caused by infectious proteins called prions and not by microorganisms. The diseases are called transmissible spongiform encephalopathies (TSE).

Prions are proteins normally found on nerve cells and are known as PrPc (prion protein cellular). Infectious prions are routinely found in scrapie (a neurological disease of sheep) and are prions that are folded improperly and are known as PrPsc (prion protein scrapie). Infectious PrPsc prions aggregate into fibrous structures in the brain and are referred to as a plaque. These plaques disrupt the cell membrane causing cell death and have potential to convert normal prions into abnormal prions.

The infection is transmitted by ingestion of infective prions with prion-containing material. These prions can move through the intestinal wall rapidly and enter lymph nodes where they incubate. They are picked up by peripheral nerves and move to the spinal cord and brain. Infectious prions can be transmitted between species, however, the incubation time is significantly longer when they cross between species.

Prions cause transmissible spongiform encephalitis (TSE), which is a neurodegenerative disease and can affect cattle and humans. There is no test for it in live organisms and the condition is incurable. The symptoms usually include lack of coordination, staggering, slurred speech, dramatic mood swings and paralysis. Death usually occurs within one year of the onset of symptoms.

"Mad cow disease" was first seen in Britain in 1984. There were 1,80,000 confirmed cases in cattle in Britain by the year 2000. The cause of infection in cattle was found to be sheep brain supplement included in cattle feed. First human case was reported in 1996 in Britain. Till date, more than 120 cases have been documented in humans and the toll is expected to vary from a few hundred to 150,000 in the next few decades.

Since there is a possibility that human blood and plasma could be a vehicle for the transmission and spread of the disease, there have been new regulations for blood donations to prevent the transmission of infections.

16.35 CONTROL AND PREVENTION OF EMERGING AND RE-EMERGING INFECTIONS

There is a need for robust public health surveillance and response systems to rapidly detect unusual, unexpected, unexplained disease patterns, track and exchange information in real-time, response effort that can quickly become global and contain transmission swiftly and decisively. The best strategy for defense would be multipronged: (a) coordinated, well-prepared, well-equipped public health systems; (b) partnerships—clinicians, laboritarians and public health agencies; (c) improved methods for detection and surveillance; (d) effective preventive and therapeutic technologies; (e) strengthened response capacity; (f) political commitment and adequate resources to address underlying socioeconomic factors; and (g) international collaboration and communication.

The Global Outbreak Alert and Response Network (GOARN): It is a technical collaboration of existing institutions and networks who pool human and technical resources for the rapid identification, confirmation and response to outbreaks of international importance. The network provides an operational framework to link this expertise and skill to keep the international community constantly alert to the threat of outbreaks and ready to respond. The Global Outbreak Alert and Response Network contributes towards global health security by combating the international spread of outbreaks ensuring that appropriate technical assistance reaches affected states rapidly contributing to long-term epidemic preparedness and capacity building.

International health regulations (IHR): WHO member countries in 2007 signed a formal code of conduct for public health emergencies of international concern (PHEIC) for collective protection against spread of serious public health threats with potential to spread beyond a country's borders, to other parts of the world. The IHR outlines assessment, management, and information sharing for PHEICs on a large scale. The IHR defines a PHEIC as an extraordinary event which constitutes a public health risk to other countries through international spread of disease and potentially need a coordinated international response.

The "old" IHR requirements mandated notifying WHO of cholera, yellow fever, and plague (and smallpox at one time, until its elimination).

The "new" IHRs have a decision algorithm to assess if a PHEIC exists, so it involves a new paradigm for reporting and (potentially) might include chemical spills or radiological events. Following a notification, the WHO member country is expected to communicate detailed public health information about the event. At the request of the WHO member country, WHO will collaborate in the public health response by providing technical guidance and assistance in assessing the potential for international disease spread and by assessing the effectiveness of control measures in place. In addition, WHO may offer to mobilize international teams of experts for on-site assistance when necessary.

The IHR sets out the basic public health capacities WHO member countries must develop and maintain in order to detect and report a PHEIC. WHO Secretariat is required to collaborate with member countries in order to evaluate, assess, and strengthen their core capacities. The assistance includes supporting member countries in identifying resources to develop and maintain these capacities. The WHO Secretariat also provides technical and logistical assistance to member countries in order to facilitate effective compliance with the IHR. The minimal core capacities for detection and reporting are described at three health levels—local, intermediate, and national. WHO member countries must develop, strengthen, and maintain the capacity to detect, report, and respond to health events. This includes the capacity to report events involving disease or death above expected levels or urgent events that meet defined criteria. Core capacities also include routine inspection and control activities at international airports, ports, and some ground crossings to prevent international disease transmission.

Diseases like poliomyelitis, human influenza, new subtype and SARS are always notifiable whereas cholera, pneumonic plague, yellow fever, viral haemorrhagic fever, West Nile fever and biological, radiological, or chemical events may fit the decision algorithm and be reportable.

16.36 BIOTERRORISM

Bioterrorism is the unlawful use or threatened use of microorganisms or toxins derived from living organisms to produce death or disease in humans, animals and plants. The act is intended to create fear and intimidate governments, societies in pursuit of political, religious or ideological goals. Biological agents are attractive instruments of terror as they are easy to produce but are difficult to detect and can cause mass casualties along with widespread panic and civil disruption. Aerosol dissemination is the likeliest route for widespread transmission of infection. The agents with highest potential for bioterrorism are *B. anthracis*, *C. botulinum* toxin, *F. tularensis*, *Y. pestis*, variola virus, viral haemorrhagic fever viruses. The bioterrorism agents are classified into following categories by Centre of Disease Control (CDC), Atlanta in 2004 to accordingly put in public health efforts to prevent and control diseases.

Category A: The disease agents that are highly contagious, and their infection leads to high death rates and a high health impact on the public, e.g. anthrax, botulism, taluremia, plague and smallpox.

Category B: The disease agent is moderately easy to spread and causes some illness and death rates in the population where they have been used, e.g. cholera, typhoid, typhus and other water safety threats.

Category C: The disease agents can be easily produced and spread. These have high potential for high death rates, e.g. hantavirus, yellow fever, tick-borne fever and multidrug resistant tuberculosis.

The key indicators of a bioterrorism attack are occurrence of a vector-borne disease with no vector, atypical seasonality, abnormal geographical location of disease, cluster of sick or dead animals and more of respiratory presentation.

Public health measures in case of a suspected bioterrorist attack

i. Hospital infection control
ii. Isolation of cases

iii. Laboratory control: Public health labs should be able to identify the agent either in-house or through referrals to the higher labs.

Hospital Administration

Role of Local Public Health Department

a. Assess environment, i.e. water and sanitation safety and health impact in the community.
b. *Media handling*: Health officer should coordinate information for the public and healthcare providers.
c. Public health nurses should ensure activities like isolation, shelter operations.

Chapter 17

Noncommunicable Diseases

Noncommunicable diseases (NCDs), also known as chronic diseases, are not transmitted from person-to-person. They are of long duration and generally slow progression. These constitute the largest global share of death and disability, accounting for almost 60% of all deaths worldwide. Almost three quarters of NCD deaths—28 million occur in low- and middle-income countries. Sixteen million NCD deaths occur before the age of 70; 82% of these "premature" deaths occurred in low- and middle-income countries.

The 4 main types of noncommunicable diseases are cardiovascular diseases (like heart attacks and stroke), cancers, chronic respiratory diseases (such as chronic obstructed pulmonary disease and asthma) and diabetes, that account for 82% of all NCD deaths. About 18 million deaths annually are contributed by cardiovascular diseases, followed by cancers (8.2 million), respiratory diseases (4 million), and diabetes (1.5 million).

In developed countries, noncommunicable diseases are leading health problems after the control of communicable diseases. For example, in affluent countries, cardiovascular diseases, cancer, diabetes, accidents, mental illnesses, osteoarthritis and other degenerative conditions are leading problems of public health. However, the developing countries are bearing a double burden of diseases. With poor standard of living, overcrowding, nutritional problems and inadequate sanitary conditions, these countries are struggling with very high rates of morbidity and mortality due to communicable diseases, the noncommunicable diseases have already started rising. Recent researches have shown that India is currently fighting a double burden of nutritional problems, i.e. undernutrition and overnutrition (obesity).

In nutshell, NCDs are dependent on the lifestyle problems that may range from unhealthy diets, physical inactivity, exposure to tobacco smoke or the effects of the harmful use of alcohol. These may show up in individuals as raised blood pressure, increased blood glucose, elevated blood lipids, and obesity. These are called 'intermediate risk factors' for cardiovascular diseases.

The risk factors for the NCDs can be

a. **Modifiable behavioural risk factors:** Tobacco use, physical inactivity, unhealthy diet and the harmful use of alcohol increase the risk of NCDs. Tobacco consumption, both active and passive, account for around 6 million deaths every year and is projected to increase to 8 million by 2030. About 3.2 million deaths annually can be attributed to insufficient physical activity alone. More than half of the 3.3 million annual deaths from harmful drinking are from NCDs. These behaviours lead to **four key metabolic** changes that increase the risk of NCDs: Raised blood pressure, overweight/obesity, hyperglycaemia (high blood glucose levels) and hyperlipidaemia (high levels of fat in the blood). In terms of attributable deaths, the leading metabolic risk factor globally is elevated blood pressure (to which 18% of global deaths are attributed) followed by overweight and obesity and raised blood glucose.

b. **Nonmodifiable/physiological risk factors:** Gender predisposition and family history are two important nonmodifiable risk factors for noncommunicable diseases.

Thus, noncommunicable diseases are multifactorial in aetiology that can be prevented by incorporating lifestyle changes early in life, e.g. diet modification for weight management and prevention of hyper-cholesterolaemia, prevention of smoking, etc. Genetic factors may play an important role in conditions, like bronchial asthma, diabetes mellitus, etc. However, environmental factors, especially social or cultural factors, attitudes and practices continuously interact with genetic factors for manifestation of a disease, e.g. a child born to diabetic parents may be able to prevent and delay the onset of diabetes by modifying his food and exercise habits. Preventive health examinations have important role to play in early detection, prevention and effective management of noncommunicable diseases. Some important noncommunicable diseases and conditions are discussed hereunder.

17.1 ACCIDENTS

An accident is an "occurrence in a sequence of events which may produce unintended injury, death or property damage". A recent data from WHO highlights that more than 5 million people die each year as a result of injuries, resulting from acts of violence against oneself or others, road traffic accidents, burns, drowning, falls, and poisonings, among other causes. Injuries account for 9% of the world's deaths, nearly 1.7 times the number of fatalities that result from HIV/AIDS, tuberculosis and malaria combined. In addition, tens of millions of people suffer non-fatal injuries which require treatment. As per the data from National Crime Records Bureau 2013, about 1500 deaths are reported per day due to accidents and suicides. Road traffic accidents are the major preventable cause of accidents contributing 377 deaths and 1287 injuries per day.

Few common types of accidents are road accidents. Rate in Indian is one of the highest in the world, accidents at home and workplace, industrial accidents, e.g. mines accidents, railways, air accidents and suicides (about 40,000 per year in India). Regarding the epidemiology of accidents, following points may be highlighted. Extremes of age are more commonly affected. Infants are exposed to the risk of suffocation. Pre-school children are exposed to falls and risk of foreign body obstruction. School children and adolescents are exposed to the risks of falls, injuries, drowning, burns, etc. The elderly are prone to risk of falls often leading to fracture of neck or femur. Drivers indulging in drinking and driving are exposed to road accidents much more than those who do not drink. There are factors that make a place more prone for accidents like environmental defects and emotional problems are responsible for accidents at workplace and in industries. Slippery bathroom floors, defective ladders, defective or poorly designed machines, defective vehicles, unprotected safety belts, lack of safety devices, e.g. seat-belts in high-speed cars, planes, etc. are a few factors conducive for accidents. Environmental factors: Heat, noise, defective lighting arrangements, poor visibility, high humidity, etc. are the environmental factors conducive for accidents.

Accidents are preventable to a large extent as they happen owing to a sequence of events. For every fatal accident, there are at least 100 accidents with serious injuries and several hundred accidents with minor injuries. Still further there would be several thousand potential situations where accidents might have been just avoided. Legislative measures, environmental control, personal protection and health education are some of the very important primary preventive measures for prevention of accidents. Strengthening of emergency medical and trauma services along with rehabilitation is needed to deal with serious accident cases.

17.2 BLINDNESS

WHO defines 'low vision' as visual acuity less than 6/18 but equal to or better than 3/60, or a corresponding visual field loss to less than 20°, in the better eye with the best possible correction. 'Blindness' is defined as visual acuity of less than 3/60, or a corresponding visual field loss to less than 10°, in the better eye with the best possible correction. 'Visual impairment' includes both low vision and blindness as per the available data, 285 million people are estimated to be visually impaired worldwide, of which 39 million are blind and 246 have low vision. India shoulders the largest burden of global blindness, about 3.5 million across the country with 30,000 new cases being added each year. The causes of blindness can be classified into following categories: (a) Communicable diseases like inflammatory ophthalmias of various etiologies, trachoma, venereal diseases and (b) noncommunicable diseases like cataract, glaucoma, malnutrition (vitamin A deficiency), injuries, diabetes, congenital abnormalities like childhood cataract, optic atrophy, ill effects of faulty posture, glare, poor lighting and refractory errors. In India, cataract has been considered to be responsible for 62.6% of blindness. Estimated national prevalence of childhood blindness/low vision is 0.80 per thousand.

The global initiative known as **'VISION 2020'**: 'The right to sight' is an established partnership between the World Health Organization (WHO) and the International Agency for the Prevention of Blindness (IAPB). It was launched in 1999 with the twin aims of eliminating avoidable blindness by the year 2020 and preventing the projected doubling of avoidable visual impairment between 1990 and 2020. The ultimate goal of the initiative is to integrate a sustainable, comprehensive, high quality, equitable eye care system into strengthened national healthcare systems.

National programme for control of blindness (NPCB) was launched in the year 1976 as a 100% centrally sponsored scheme with the goal to reduce the prevalence of blindness from 1.4 to 0.3%. As per data procured from Rapid Survey on Avoidable Blindness conducted under NPCB during 2006–07 showed the prevalence of blindness as 1%. Various activities/initiatives were undertaken during the Five-Year Plans under NPCB that were targeted towards achieving the goal of reducing the prevalence of blindness to 0.3% by the year 2020. The (Goals and Objectives of NPCB in the XII Plan:

a. To reduce the backlog of blindness through identification and treatment of blind at primary, secondary and tertiary levels based on assessment of the overall burden of visual impairment in the country.

b. Develop and strengthen the strategy of NPCB for "Eye health" and prevention of visual impairment; through provision of comprehensive eye care services and quality service delivery.

c. Strengthening and upgradation of regional institute of ophthalmology (RIOs) to become centre of excellence in various subspecialities of ophthalmology.

d. Strengthening of the existing and developing additional human resources and infrastructure facilities for providing high quality comprehensive eye care in all districts of the country.

e. To enhance community awareness on eye care and lay stress on preventive measures.

f. Increase and expand research for prevention of blindness and visual impairment.

g. To secure participation of voluntary organizations/ private practitioners in eye care.

17.3 CANCER

Cancer is the abnormal division of cells that grow beyond their usual boundaries, invade adjoining parts of the body and spread to other organs, the latter process referred to as metastasis. Metastases are the major cause of death from cancer. Cancers figure among the leading causes of morbidity and mortality worldwide, with approximately 14 million new cases and 8.2 million cancer-related deaths reported in 2012. The number of new cases are further expected to rise by about 70% over the next 2 decades. The 5 most common sites of cancer diagnosed amongst men in 2012 were lung, prostate, colorectum, stomach, and liver. Among women the 5 most common sites diagnosed were breast, colorectum, lung, cervix, and stomach cancer.

The transformation from a normal cell into a tumour cell is a multistage process, typically progressing from a pre-cancerous lesion to malignant tumours. These changes are the result of the interaction between a person's genetic factors and of external agents that include: (a) *physical carcinogens*, such as ultraviolet and ionizing radiation; (b) *chemical carcinogens*, such as asbestos, components of tobacco smoke, aflatoxin; (c) *food contaminant* and *arsenic*; (d) *drinking water contaminant*; and (e) *biological carcinogens*, such as infections from certain viruses, bacteria or parasites. Viral infections, such as HBV/HCV and HPV, are responsible for up to 20% of cancer deaths in low- and middle-income countries.

The behavioural and dietary risk factors for cancers are high body mass index, low fruit and vegetable intake, lack of physical activity, tobacco use, alcohol use.

Ageing is another fundamental factor for the development of cancer due to risk accumulation over the years with impaired tendency for cellular repair mechanisms.

Prevention and Control

Personal protection and health education are the two main interventions for prevention of cancers. Prevention and control of cancers include:

A. **Modifying and avoiding risk factors**
   i. Environmental measures include prevention from exposure to chemical carcinogens.
   ii. Lifestyle modification, e.g. increased intake of fruits and fibre in diet, avoidance of use of tobacco chewing and cigarette smoking, improving genital hygiene, etc. Prevention strategies include avoidance of the risk factors listed above, vaccinate against human papillomavirus (HPV) and hepatitis B virus (HBV), control exposure to occupational hazards, reduce exposure to nonionizing radiation by sunlight (UV) or due to medical diagnostic imaging.

B. **Early detection and treatment:** Early detection includes early diagnosis and screening. The awareness of early signs and symptoms about various types of cancers can help in early detection especially for those cancers when there is no effective screening method or in low-resource settings when no screening and treatment interventions are implemented.

Screening aims to identify individuals with abnormalities suggestive of a specific cancer or precancer and refer them promptly for treatment or when feasible for diagnosis and treatment. Screening programmes are especially effective for frequent cancer types for which cost-effective, affordable, acceptable and accessible screening tests are available to the majority of the population at risk. For, example, PAP cytology test for cervical cancer and mammography screening for breast cancer.

Mass screening camps may serve the dual purpose of awareness generation and early detection for prompt management.

Treatment of cancers may involve one or more of the following modalities—surgery, radiotherapy, hormone therapy and chemotherapy. The primary goal of treatment is to cure cancer or to considerably prolong life along with improving the patient's quality of life. Some of the most common cancer types, such as breast cancer, cervical cancer, oral cancer and colorectal cancer have high cure rates when detected early and treated according to best practices whereas leukaemias and lymphomas in children, and testicular seminoma, have high cure rates, if appropriate treatment is provided.

C. **Palliative care:** Supportive or palliative care and psychological support are important for improving the quality of life of the patient. Effective public health strategies comprising of community- and home-based care are essential to provide pain relief and palliative care for patients and their families in low-resource settings. Improved access to oral morphine is mandatory for the treatment of moderate to severe cancer pain, suffered by over 80% of cancer patients in terminal phase.

Based on these principles of management and control of cancers, National Cancer Control Programme was launched by Government of India which has now been made a part of National Programme for Prevention and Control of Cancer, Diabetes, CVD and Stroke (NPCDCS) in 12th Five-Year Plan (2012–2017).

17.4 HYPERTENSION (HIGH BLOOD PRESSURE)

Blood pressure is the pressure, which the blood exerts against the walls of the arteries through which it flows. Hypertension, also known as high or raised blood pressure, is a condition in which the blood vessels have persistently raised pressure. Blood is carried from the heart to all parts of the body in the vessels. Each time the heartbeats, it pumps blood into the vessels. Blood pressure is created by the force of blood pushing against the walls of blood vessels (arteries) as it is pumped by the heart. The higher the pressure the harder the heart has to pump, thus can lead to heart failure and coronary artery disaese due to increased workload and other associated conditions like stroke, paralysis, etc.

The arteries are flexible and elastic in nature and can withstand a great amount of pressure exerted by blood when it is pumped into arteries by the heart.

Sometimes due to the deposition of fatty plaques and cholesterol in the walls, the arterial walls thicken and become hard leaving the arteries inflexible. This condition is known as "arteriosclerosis". In this condition, the heart pumps the blood to the body through these hardened arteries exerts an extra pressure, causing hypertension. While measuring blood pressure by means of a blood pressure measuring apparatus (sphygmomanometer), two types of readings are recorded, viz. *systolic* (arterial pressure when the heart is contracting) and *diastolic* (arterial pressure when the heart is relaxing). As per the recommendations of seventh report of the Joint National Committee on prevention, detection, evaluation, and treatment of high blood pressure (JNC-VII), HT can be classified as follows:

Classification of Blood Pressure for Adults (JNC VII)

Category	Systolic mm Hg		Diastolic mm Hg
1. Normal	120	and	80
2. Prehypertensive	120–139	or	80–89
3. Stage I hypertension	140–159	or	90–99
4. Stage II hypertension	>160		>100

All the patients in stage I and stage II of hypertension should be treated whereas people with blood pressure in prehypertensive category must begin with lifestyle modification in order to reduce their risk of developing hypertension in future. The treatment goal for individuals with hypertension is <140/90 mm Hg whereas for individuals with prehypertension is to lower BP to normal levels with lifestyle changes, and prevent the progressive rise in BP using the recommended lifestyle modifications.

Symptoms

Hypertension can occasionally cause headaches, irritability, palpitations, vision problems, dizziness, or shortness of breath, but most people with hypertension have no symptoms. This is why hypertension is referred to as the "silent killer". Hypertension is usually discovered at a regular medical check-up.

Causes

Primary (or essential) hypertension is when the cause is unknown. The majority of hypertension cases are primary. When there is an underlying problem such as kidney disease or hormonal disorders that is causing hypertension, it is called *secondary hypertension*. Other risk factors that can contribute to hypertension include age (blood pressure usually increases with age since the arteries get hardened by gradually losing elasticity thereby resulting in the onset of high blood pressure), diet with high salt and fat and low fibre, excessive alcohol consumption, lack of exercise, obesity, sleep apnea and stress. Similarly emotional upsets, worry, anxiety, tension, etc. are other contributing factors for causing and aggravating high blood pressure. Hypertension is one of the main risk factors for heart disease, stroke, and kidney failure.

Prevention

The key elements of effective control of the hypertension in the community include an improvement of the awareness of hypertension among health professionals and the population at large, and, more specifically, among the individuals with hypertension.

Diet and nutrition have been extensively investigated as risk factors for major cardiovascular diseases and their risk factors like diabetes, high blood pressure and obesity. Diet comprising of low sodium and high potassium, regular frequent intake of fruits and vegetables and polyunsaturated fatty acids are protective against hypertension. Composite diets such as DASH (dietary approaches to stop hypertension) diet (focuses on increasing intake of foods rich in nutrients that are expected to lower blood pressure, mainly minerals like potassium, calcium, magnesium, protein, and fibre) has been demonstrated to reduce the risk of hypertension and CHD.

Lifestyle modification including stress management techniques, like meditation, should be practiced besides dietary modification. Cigarette smoking, and alcohol intake should preferably be avoided. Regular exercise like brisk walking, cycling, jogging should be done at least five times a day for 35–40 minutes per session. Salt intake should preferably be kept low and not more than 5 gm per day from all the sources.

Early diagnosis and treatment of hypertension can prevent the occurrence of related cardiovascular complications.

17.5 CARDIOVASCULAR DISEASES

Cardiovascular diseases (CVDs) are a group of disorders of the heart and blood vessels and they include:

a. *Coronary heart disease*: Disease of the blood vessels supplying the heart muscle.

b. *Cerebrovascular disease*: Disease of the blood vessels supplying the brain.

c. *Peripheral arterial disease*: Disease of blood vessels supplying the arms and legs.

d. *Rheumatic heart disease*: Damage to the heart muscle and heart valves from rheumatic fever, caused by streptococcal bacteria.

e. *Congenital heart disease*: Malformations of heart structure existing at birth.

f. *Deep vein thrombosis and pulmonary embolism*: Blood clots in the leg veins, which can dislodge and move to the heart and lungs.

Heart attacks and strokes are usually acute events and are mainly caused by a blockage that prevents blood from flowing to the heart or brain. The most common reason for this is atherosclerosis; a build-up of fatty deposits on the inner walls of the blood vessels that supply the heart or brain. Strokes can also be caused by bleeding from a blood vessel in the brain or from blood clots. The common risk factors for these events are tobacco use, unhealthy diet and obesity, physical inactivity and harmful use of alcohol, hypertension, diabetes and hyperlipidaemia.

As per the available data for the year 2012, about 17.5 million people died from CVDs, representing 31% of all global deaths. Of these deaths, an estimated 7.4 million were due to coronary heart disease and 6.7 million were due to stroke.

CVDs are the leading cause of death in India and affect a relatively younger age group. About 2.25 million deaths have been reported in India due to CVDs in 2010 excluding stroke and the figures are projected to 2.94 million in 2015 as per the estimates of National Commission on Macroeconomics and Health.

Another data from a meta-analysis in 2008 has shown that CVDs accounted for around one-fourth of all deaths in India. CVDs are the chronic illness growing at the rate 9.2% annually from 2000 onwards

with a significant increase in the incidence for people between ages 25 and 69 to 24.8%. There is an evidence that an average mortality due to CVD in 20–49 years age group is 4% and is 6% in those above 50 years. According to a WHO report, the current age standardised CVD mortality rates among males and females in India (per 100,000) are 363–443 and 181–281, respectively.

Each cardiovascular disease has its own epidemiological characteristics. Congenital heart disease is associated with (a) viral infections like German measles, measles and mumps, (b) exposures to radiations or radioactive or cytotoxic drugs, antimetabolites and other drugs like thalidomide, etc. Rheumatic carditis is considered as a manifestation of type A streptococcal infections. Cardiovascular syphilis, toxic myocarditis owing to diphtheria and subacute bacterial endocarditis owing to *Streptococcus viridans* are other infections leading to cardiovascular diseases.

Coronary heart disease or ischaemic heart disease: It is the "impairment of heart functions due to inadequate blood supply to the heart as per its needs, caused by distractive changes in the coronary circulatory system". It is the cause of about 25% of deaths in developed countries. About two-thirds of these cases are known smokers and almost 50% are either diabetic or hypertensive. Also persons with high blood cholesterol and high blood pressure have four times the risk of ischaemic heart disease as compared to persons with normal blood pressure and normal blood cholesterol level. The disease is also 4 to 10 times more common in males than females.

Risk Factors

The most important behavioural risk factors of heart disease and stroke are unhealthy diet, physical inactivity, tobacco use and harmful use of alcohol. The effects of behavioural risk factors may show up in individuals as raised blood pressure, raised blood glucose, raised blood lipids, and overweight and obesity. These "intermediate risk factors" can be measured in primary care facilities and indicate an increased risk of developing a heart attack, stroke, heart failure and other complications. There are also a number of underlying determinants of CVDs or "the causes of the causes". These are a reflection of the major forces driving social, economic and cultural change—globalization, urbanization and population ageing. Other determinants of CVDs include poverty, stress and hereditary factors.

The aetiological factors for coronary heart disease are:

a. Familial predisposition

b. *Personality type*: Individuals with type A personality are predisposed.

c. *Personal*: Habits like sedentary lifestyle, smoking, excess intake of alcohol and saturated fats.

d. Hypercoagulability of blood.

e. High blood cholesterol level.

f. Hormonal imbalances, e.g. women are predisposed after menopause.

g. Other diseases like hypertension, diabetes, atherosclerosis, etc.

Symptoms

Often, there are no symptoms of the underlying disease of the blood vessels. A heart attack or stroke may be the first warning of underlying disease. Symptoms of a heart attack include pain or discomfort in the centre of the chest, pain or discomfort in the arms, the left shoulder, elbows, jaw, or back. The person may also experience difficulty in breathing or shortness of breath; vomiting; feeling light-headed or faint; breaking into a cold sweat; and becoming pale.

The most common symptom of a stroke is sudden weakness of the face, arm, or leg, most often on one side of the body. Other symptoms include sudden onset of numbness of the face, arm, or leg, especially on one side of the body; confusion, difficulty speaking or understanding speech; difficulty seeing with one or both eyes; difficulty in walking, dizziness, loss of balance or coordination; severe headache with no known cause; and fainting or unconsciousness.

The intervention strategies for control and/or prevention of cardiovascular conditions can be population-based and individual level, which are recommended to be used in combination to reduce the greatest cardiovascular disease burden.

1. *Population-based interventions:* These are cost effective in resource constraint settings. These include (a) comprehensive tobacco control policies, (b) taxation to reduce the intake of foods that are high in fat, sugar and salt, (c) building walking and cycle paths to increase physical activity, (d) strategies to reduce harmful use of alcohol, and (e) providing healthy school meals to children.

2. *Interventions at individual level:* At individual level, healthcare interventions need to be targeted to those at high total cardiovascular risk or those with single risk factor levels above traditional thresholds, such as hypertension and hypercholesterolaemia.

   a. Prevention and treatment of conditions like obesity, diabetes, stress management along with periodic checkups and therapeutic management of early cases are needed.

   b. Dietary and lifestyle modification for prevention of hypercholesterolaemia and atherosclerosis. Restriction of dietary fats to less than 20% of total calorie intake with dietary cholesterol consumption to be less than 100 mg per 1000 kcal per day. Curtailing or even total avoidance of alcohol consumption and reduction of daily salt intake to less than 5 gm.

   c. Avoid exposure to radiations, antimetabolites and cytotoxic drugs, viral infections and immunisations by living viral vaccines during first trimester of pregnancy for prevention of congenital heart diseases.

   d. Treat all streptococcal infections by chemotherapy and if needed give chemoprophylaxis especially to children with chronic infections and those living in overcrowded damp houses of pencillin and/or long-acting sulpha drugs for prevention of rheumatic heart conditions.

   e. Periodic check up for screening and early detection of risk factors.

Use of aspirin, beta-blockers, angiotensin-converting enzyme inhibitors and statins for secondary prevention of cardiovascular disease in those with established disease, including diabetes. Strengthening the public health facilities and accreditation of private health facilities for surgical interventions like coronary artery bypass, balloon angioplasty, pacemakers, prosthetic valves, etc.

17.6 DIABETES MELLITUS

Diabetes mellitus is a chronic disease, which occurs due to insufficiency of pancreas leading to decreased production of insulin, or when the body cannot effectively use the insulin it produces. Insulin controls the metabolism of glucose, fats and amino acids. Insufficiency of insulin in amount or functioning leads to an increased concentration of glucose in the blood; a condition known as hyperglycaemia which over time leads to serious damage to many of the body's systems, especially the nerves and blood vessels. There are two types of *diabetes mellitus*. Type 1 diabetes (previously known as insulin-dependent or childhood onset diabetes) is characterized by a lack of insulin production and type 2 diabetes (formerly called non-insulin-dependent or adult onset diabetes) is caused by the body's ineffective use of insulin. It often results from excess body weight and physical inactivity. Gestational diabetes is hyperglycaemia that is first recognised during pregnancy.

In 2014, the global prevalence of diabetes was estimated to be 9% among adults aged 18+ years. Globally, an estimated 346 million people have diabetes and 3.4 million die annually due to high blood sugar. Three out of four people with diabetes live in low- and middle-income countries. Nearly 71 million were estimated to be living with diabetes in 2010 in the South-East Asia (SEA) region, and an equal number had impaired glucose tolerance. Approximately 1 million people die from consequences of high blood sugar in SEA region every year.

The aetiology of two types of diabetes is different. The causes of type 1 diabetes, while not known, may be diverse such as autoimmune, genetic or environmental. However, the risk factors for type 2 diabetes are overweight/obesity, family history of diabetes, tobacco use, excess alcohol intake, prior history of gestational diabetes, impaired glucose tolerance and physical inactivity. Diabetes has a wide-spectrum with a state of prediabetes at one end and overt diabetes at the other end. Prediabetes is the period of life from conception to first appearance of carbohydrate metabolism abnormality. Impaired glucose tolerance (IGT) and impaired fasting glycaemia (IFG) are intermediate conditions in the transition between normality and diabetes. People with IGT or IFG are at high risk of progressing to type 2 diabetes, The GTT with 50 gm glucose load orally is the standard test recommended by WHO for diagnosis of diabetes.

Gestational diabetes is hyperglycaemia with blood glucose values above normal but below those diagnostic of diabetes, occurring during pregnancy. Not only women with gestational diabetes are themselves at an increased risk of complications during pregnancy and at the time of delivery, but their baby is also prone to have a spectrum of complications in the intrauterine life. Such mother and babies born to these mothers are also at increased risk of type 2 diabetes in the future. Gestational diabetes is diagnosed through prenatal screening, rather than reported symptoms.

The common symptoms of diabetes include excessive excretion of urine (polyuria), excessive thirst (polydipsia), constant hunger, weight loss, vision changes and fatigue. These symptoms may occur suddenly. However, one should investigate for diabetes in case of peripheral neuritis, repeated and uncontrolled boils, balanitis, delayed healing of wounds, undue fatigue, sudden loss of weight, diminution of vision and unconsciousness. There is a tendency for ketoacidosis with poor prognosis in type 1 or juvenile onset diabetes. Type 2 or adult type, mostly affects adult obese persons more than 40 years of age and is neither insulin-dependent nor prone to develop ketoacidosis. Thus adult diabetes can be controlled with dietary restrictions and oral antidiabetic drugs.

The complications of diabetes contribute higher to the mortality than the disease per se. Prolonged diabetes can damage the heart, blood vessels, eyes, kidneys, and nerves.

i. It increases the risk of heart disease and stroke. Almost 50% of people with diabetes die of heart disease and stroke.
ii. There are increased chances of foot ulcers and non-healing infections due to reduced blood flow and neuropathy (nerve damage) in the feet which may lead to eventual need for limb amputation.
iii. Long-term accumulated damage to the small blood vessels in the retina may lead to blindness due to diabetic retinopathy. About 1% of global blindness can be attributed to diabetes.
iv. Diabetes is among the leading causes of kidney failure.

Prevention

Simple lifestyle measures have been shown to be effective in preventing or delaying the onset of type 2 diabetes. To help prevent type 2 diabetes and its complications, people should achieve and maintain healthy body weight (about 10% less than optimum for their age and sex). Physical activity like brisk walking for 30 minutes a day on most the days of week can delay the onset of diabetes. Healthy diet should constitute of at least 3 to 5 servings of fruit and vegetables a day and reduced sugar and saturated fats intake.

Diagnosis and Treatment

Early diagnosis can be accomplished through blood testing, such as fasting or random blood glucose test, oral glucose tolerance test, or glycated haemoglobin (HbA1c) test.

Treatment of diabetes involves lowering blood glucose and the levels of other known risk factors that damage blood vessels. People with type 1 diabetes require insulin whereas type 2 diabetes can be treated with oral medication and diet modification but may at times also require insulin. Control of blood pressure and hygiene and care of feet is important for prevention of complications.

Other cost-saving interventions include generating awareness and health education to the patients and their caretakers about the warning signs of retinopathy or renal disease. The patient should be regularly screened for early signs of retinopathy and diabetes related renal disease. Blood levels of lipids should be monitored regularly to ensure regulated cholesterol levels. These measures should be supported by a healthy diet, regular physical activity, maintaining a normal body weight and avoiding tobacco use.

17.7 NATIONAL TOBACCO CONTROL PROGRAMME

India is the second largest consumer (after China) of tobacco products in the world. As per Global Adult Tobacco Survey (GATS), India, 2009–10, conducted in the age group of 15 years and above, 47.8% men and 20.3% women consume tobacco in some form or the other. The Global Youth Tobacco Survey (GYTS), 2009 indicates that nearly 15% children in the age group of 13–15 years are consuming tobacco in some form. Govt. of India enacted the "Cigarettes and other Tobacco Products (Prohibition of Advertisement and Regulation of Trade and Commerce, Production, Supply and Distribution) Act (COTPA), 2003" to discourage the use of tobacco. The specific provisions under COTPA are:

1. Prohibition of smoking in a public place (Section 4).
2. Prohibition of direct and indirect advertisement, promotion and sponsorship of cigarette and other tobacco products (Section 5).
3. Prohibition of sale of cigarette and other tobacco products to a person below the age of eighteen years [Section 6(a)].
4. Prohibition of sale of tobacco products near the educational institutions [Section 6(b)], and
5. Mandatory depiction of statutory warnings (including pictorial warnings) on tobacco packs (Section 7).

The ministry co-hosted 'The International Conference on Public Health Priorities in the 21st Century: The Endgame for Tobacco' in New Delhi in September 2013. National level public awareness campaign was also launched as a key activity under the National Tobacco Control.

17.8 NATIONAL PROGRAMME FOR PREVENTION AND CONTROL OF CANCER, DIABETES, CARDIOVASCULAR DISEASES AND STROKE (NPCDCS)

NPCDS was launched in 2008 by Government of India in pilot phase in 100 districts which was later in 2013 expanded to cover the entire country. The objectives of the programme in pilot phase were risk reduction for prevention of NCDS (diabetes, CVD and stroke) and early diagnosis for appropriate management of diabetes, cardiovascular diseases and stroke.

The target groups under the programme are—healthy general population and high-risk groups.

a. *Health promotion* has been targeted for the general population that are apparently healthy population. This involves development of an effective communication strategy to modify individual, group and community behaviour through media. It also focuses on community mobilization and participation to mainstream the agenda of health promotion till the village level. The interventions involve at various settings of community, school and workplace.

   i. Community-based interventions involve health education regarding benefits of physical activities, dietary changes, mainstreaming the agenda of health promotion into the activities of village health and sanitation committees (VHSCs), Gram Panchayats, self-help groups and faith-based organisations.
   ii. Workplace interventions to introduce health promotion for their respective organisations by identifying peer educators and providing initial training.
   iii. School-based interventions by evaluation of the existing school health programme components, viz. physical education, nutrition and food services, health promotion for school personnel, health education and health services followed by activities to make health promotion, a defined agenda in the school curriculum.

b. *Disease prevention for the high-risk groups*: Interventions are aimed at early diagnosis and appropriate management for reducing morbidity and mortality targeting people who are at an higher risk due to risk factors like hypertension, obesity, high blood lipid and glucose levels and also those who have suffered from a previous cerebral or coronary event. The interventions include:

   i. Strengthening public health delivery system at the primary, secondary and tertiary levels. Capacity building of healthcare providers at all levels for risk detection and screening, viz. blood pressure checks, recommending lifestyle modifications, dissemination of information and referring for further management.
   ii. Special clinic for diabetes/cardiovascular disease/stroke have been established at the district hospital for screening, management and referral.
   iii. The services of private sector have been explored to correct the imbalance towards care using high cost, low yield technologies and use of more cost-effective interventions.
   iv. Specific interventions have been made at the tertiary level to established the prompt intervention to manage a cardiac event to reduce mortality to a large extent. Establishing and strengthening referral linkages have been done besides strengthening of the centre through provision of necessary infrastructure and manpower.
   v. Specific activities for creation of public awareness, reorientation of primary healthcare providers for early detection and referral of rheumatic fever and rheumatic heart disease.

17.9 GLOBAL ACTION PLAN FOR THE PREVENTION AND CONTROL OF NCDS 2013–2020

In 2013, WHO launched the Global Action Plan for the Prevention and Control of Non-communicable Diseases 2013–2020 that aims to reduce by 25% premature mortality from cancer, cardiovascular diseases, diabetes and chronic respiratory diseases by 2025. Some of the voluntary targets are most relevant for cancer prevention, including target 5 aimed at reducing the prevalence of tobacco use by 30%.

Sanitation and Water Supply in Rural Areas

As per census 2011, about 69% of population are rural in India. With rapid urbanisation, it is estimated that by 2025, more than 50% of the country's population are expected to be living in cities and towns. This would lead to likely increase in demand for infrastructural facilities, notably declining per capita water availability/quality and sanitation.

18.1 CURRENT STATUS

- More than 50% households hvae access to improved sanitation facilities in all 1st phase states
- 2/3rd households have access to improved source of drinking within every state/UT.

As per census 2011, the facility of sanitary toilets is available to only 30% of the rural population, 22.17% of rural households have their drinking water source beyond 500 metres. Also 11.8% of rural households obtain drinking water from uncovered wells and 4% from other sources (other than handpump/tubewell, tap water or well water).

Need for Safe Drinking Water and Sanitation Programme in Rural Areas

Water supply and sanitation were added to the national agenda during the first five-year planning period (1951–1956). In 1954, the first national water supply programme was launched as part of the government's health plan.

Rural sanitation came into focus in India in the World Water Decade of 1980s. The Central Rural Sanitation Programme (CRSP) was started in 1986 to provide sanitation facilities in rural areas. It was a supply-driven, high subsidy and infrastructure-oriented programme. The experience of community-driven, awareness—generating campaign-based programmes in some states and the results of evaluation of CRSP, led to the formulation of the Total Sanitation Campaign (TSC) approach in 1999.

18.2 MASS EDUCATION

Health, especially preventive health, is a subject of low prioirity and importance. Less is known to people about role of hygiene and sanitation in prevention of diseases. Health education using mass media, role plays and interpersonal communication (IPC) can communicate the importance of sanitation and hygiene in prevention of transmission of diseases like cholera, typhoid, diarrhoeas and saving the treatment cost and a number of lives annually by observing simple precautions.

The dangers of insanitary environmental conditions and poor hygiene, overcrowding, ill-ventilation, unhygienic surroundings and pollution of water supply should be impressed upon the community. This can be best done through lantern slides, lectures, films, posters, pamphlets in different local languages, etc. A primer in simple language for imparting knowledge on sanitation, hygiene and preventable diseases should be introduced right from the school level in rural areas.

18.3 ACTIVITIES UNDER NATIONAL HEALTH MISSION (NHM)

The Village Health Sanitation and Nutrition Committee (VHSNC) have been constituted involving of Panchayati Raj representatives and other local committee members, ANM and Accredited Social Health Activist (ASHA). These committees act as an important tool for community empowerment and participation at the grassroots level.

Untied grants of ₹10,000 are provided annually to each VHSNC under NHM, which are utilized for capacity building of the VHSNC members with regards to their roles and responsibilities for maintaining the health status of the village is being done. Till date, more than 5 lakh VHSNCs have been set up across the country that facilitate convergence with ICDS/drinking water/sanitation and PRIs. These are also being involved in dealing with disease outbreak.

ASHAs are also trained to generate awareness amongst the community regarding importance of sanitary toilets and are incentivised, if they are able to facilitate building of sanitary toilets in the households.

18.4 TOTAL SANITATION CAMPAIGN (TSC)

TSC was launched with objective to bring about an improvement in the general quality of life in the rural areas through:

a. Accelerated sanitation coverage in rural areas using cost-effective and appropriate technology.
b. Awareness generation and health education to create felt demand for sanitation facilities.
c. Cover schools/anganwadis in rural areas with sanitation facilities and promote hygiene education and sanitary habits among students.
d. Eliminate open defaecation and manual scavenging practices to minimize risk of contamination of drinking water sources and food. Ensure availability of pour flush latrines instead of dry latrines.

TSC is 'community-led' and 'people-centered' where 'demand-driven approach' is adopted with increased emphasis on awareness creation and demand generation for sanitary facilities in houses, schools and for cleaner environment. Incentive is being given to the poorest of the poor households for sanitation measures.

Rural school sanitation: It is the entry point for wider acceptance of sanitation by the rural people. Technology improvisations to meet the customer preferences and location-specific intensive IEC campaign involving Panchayati Raj institutions, cooperatives, women groups, self-help groups, NGOs, etc. are other important components of the strategy. The strategy addresses all sections of rural population to bring about the relevant behavioural changes for improved sanitation and hygiene practices and meet their sanitary hardware requirements in an affordable and accessible manner.

Under the campaign, there is a financial provision of ₹1500 for individual household latrines in plains and ₹2000 in case of hilly and difficult areas respectively to BPL households after they construct and use toilets. APL households are motivated to construct toilets with their own funds or by taking loans. The cost for provision of toilets in schools and Anganwadis is shared by central and state governments in the ratio of 70:30. Community sanitary complexes are being constructed and the assistance is being provided to the production centres of sanitary material and rural sanitary marts. Management of solid and liquid waste using latest technology is another important component of the programme.

TSC is being implemented in phases, for which the project has to be approved by Ministry of Rural Development, Government of India as it is passed through the state authorities after emanating from the district. At the first instance, funds are made available for preliminary IEC work with a synergistic interaction between the government agencies and other stakeholders, and advocacy with participation of NGOs/Panchayati Raj institutions and resource organizations to bring about the desired behavioural changes for relevant sanitation practices.

Some new financial initiatives have been undertaken by provision of ₹35000 for school toilet block (38500 for hilly and difficult areas) and 8000 for anganwadi toilet (₹10000 for hilly and difficult areas).

18.5 RURAL TOWN PLANNING

The houses in rural areas should be build as per the standards to ensure the healthy environment with due emphasis on the sanitation measures. Cattle sheds and shelters should be made at a distance from the house that is inhabited by the family. Government should construct some model villages and provide some agency for giving advice to the villagers on the planning of villages and construction of houses. As per the guidelines of planning commission 2014, the houses in rural areas should be built on a plinth having a height of at least 1 ft. (0.3 metre) with each of the rooms should be at least 15 ft. (4.57 metres) × 12 ft. (3.65 metres) with 12 ft. (3.65 metres) height. Each house should contain at least two rooms, a kitchen, a bath room, a courtyard and a verandah. The kitchen should be provided with a smokeless *chullah* or other smokeless fuel for cooking. The room should be provided with windows and ventilators; the floors should be made of bricks or some other impermeable material. The privy should be constructed in the courtyard away from the living rooms and kitchen.

Indira Awas Yojana (IAY): It is a cash subsidy-based programme, under which assistance is provided to rural BPL families for constructing dwelling units on their own. Sixty percent of the funds provided under IAY are meant for SC and ST beneficiaries and the subsidy is sanctioned either in the name of the female member of the household or jointly in the names of both spouses. The present per unit assistance is ₹25,000 in plain areas and ₹27,500 in hilly and difficult areas. Funding under IAY is provided by the centre and the state in the ratio of 75:25. The beneficiary is expected to construct a house of at least 20 sqm plinth area with a sanitary latrine and a smokeless chullah. Government departments can give technical assistance or arrange for coordinated supply of raw material such as cement, steel and bricks if beneficiaries so desire.

The Prime Minister announced Bharat Nirman Programme on August 15, 2005 to build irrigation, roads, housing, telecommunications, power and water supply in the rural areas. It is an ambitious plan of the Government of India for expansion of rural infrastructure and bridging the rural-urban divide.

18.6 SANITARY DISPOSAL OF WASTE

Arrangements should be made for the provision of privies in every house. If this is not possible, public latrines should be provided at suitable places and the people should be encouraged to use them. In areas where water carriage system of disposal of human excreta is not possible, bored hole latrines or dugwell latrines can be useful and, therefore, their use is especially advocated. Trench latrines are also quite useful and inexpensive, however, septic tank latrines must be build where water is available.

Disposal of dry refuse is very important, which consists of refuse from stables, cowdung, food wastes, dust, etc. This is used by the villagers as a manure in their fields. Proper manure pits should be provided at a suitable distance from their residential houses. The refuse should be covered with earth so that the flies may not breed in them which should then be removed to fields in due course of time. Incineration of refuse particularly when mixed with night soil also makes its disposal sanitary.

The liquid waste, rainwater and waste water should be drained through pucca drains with a proper gradient and cleaned periodically. This water should be utilised for irrigation purposes for the agricultural land. Incineration of the refuse is also suggested particularly when it is mixed with night-soil as its disposal becomes more sanitary, when subjected to incineration.

The removal of waste water, rainwater and other liquid wastes is generally affected through surface drains. They should be made pucca with a proper gradient and should be cleaned periodically. Arrangements should be made for utilising this water for irrigation purposes over agricultural land.

18.7 SANITATION IN FAIRS AND FESTIVALS

The fairs and religious festivals sometimes can be a source of outbreak of epidemic diseases like typhoid, diarrhoea and cholera. Thus, it is important to carry out the planning to implement the preventive measures. The responsibility of hygiene, sanitation and other related issues should be handed over to some person. A team of paramedical workers must be made under the administrative and financial control of medical officer, who would be responsible for all the arrangements.

For efficient prevention and control of outbreak of epidemics during these fairs, following points should be attended to:

a. **Planning for the arrangements:** The organisers of the fair along with the medical officer of health and other members of the advisory committee should chalk out a plan. It is for him to see that the ground is cleared of all vegetation, levelled and demarcated into different blocks with well-planned roads. The layout plan should be fixed, at a prominent place for the information of the public. In fact long before opening of the fair/festival, the pilgrims should be advised through posters and newspaper advertisements of their obligations vis-à-vis the arrangements made.

b. **Accommodation:** It is to be provided for the organisers, police, health and medical authorities in the first instance. For the pilgrims, dharamsalas or residential blocks along with sanitary conveniences should be arranged. Each room or temporary camp, or hut should be at least 10 feet (3 metres) high and should have windows equivalent to 10% of floor area. The land selected should have natural drainage and should be well-shaded and watered. If there are any depressions, cesspits or pools, they should be filled up. The main road approaching the Mela ground should be metalled or otherwise made smooth and firm.

c. **Medical and sanitary arrangements:** The fair should be under the charge of a medical officer of health and the whole area should be divided into blocks placed under the charge of sanitary inspectors. Moreover, accommodation and stretchers should be provided for infectious diseases' cases, if need be. Adequate quantity of disinfectants drugs and vector control measures should be available. Temporary hospitals and dispensaries with qualified doctors should be arranged for the treatment of sick persons. Arrangements should be made beforehand for the stretchers for removal of sick and badly hurt persons in case of an stampede, outbreak of fire, accidents, etc.

d. **Water supply:** Efficient arrangements for the supply of wholesome water (filtered/chlorinated) should be made available from some waterworks which is very safe or deep tube wells. All these sources should be thoroughly disinfected beforehand so as to avoid the danger of an outbreak of any water-borne epidemic. The amount of water provided should be about 20–25 litres per capita per day. The residents of the village should be advised to drink boiled water during epidemics. The water of tanks and wells should be sterilised by means of bleaching powder. Washermen should not be allowed to wash dirty and infected clothes in the tanks or well water used for drinking purposes.

e. **Efficient conservancy:** Adequate whole-time con-servancy staff should be engaged for sweeping the roads and residential blocks, cleaning the latrines, urinals or other sanitary conveniences.

i. *Sweeping*: The roads should be properly swept and watered. At least one sweeper for every 2,000 participants/pilgrims must be provided. Covered dustbins should be placed at suitable sites in the ground for collection of rubbish and sweepings, from where they should be removed by carts or trucks to the place of disposal.

ii. *Latrines*: Suitable sites should be selected and different types of latrines constructed both for males and females separately. Female sweepers should be employed for latrines meant for use by women. The number of seats of latrines must be 2 seats for 1,000 people in case the fair is to last for one day and one seat for 100 persons, if their stay is longer than a day.

iii. *Urinals*: Adequate number of urinals should be provided at suitable places all over the Mela ground which should be separate for both sexes. In ordinary soil, a pit, 4 feet (1.22 metres) square and 5 feet (1.52 metres) deep, filled with broken bricks and covered with sand should be made.

These latrines and urinals should be kept in a clean and sanitary condition and they should not be too far away, otherwise there is a likelihood that people will not use them. No latrine should be situated at a distance of more than 100 yards (91.44 metres) away from the fair area. There should be a proper lighting arrangement at night. Picture boards indicating the sex for which they are meant should be fixed near the entrance. Satisfactory arrangement for removal and disposal of refuse and night-soil should be made. The refuse may be dumped and incinerated. In the latter case, beehive pattern or an open incinerator may be more useful.

f. **Food supply:** Strict supervision on the sale of food supply should be exercised. No unhealthy or stale articles of food and drink, overripe fruits and decaying vegetables should be allowed to enter the fair ground. They should be immediately seized and destroyed as a preventive measure. Particularly at the time of outbreak of epidemics, people should be taught to protect their foodstuffs from dust and flies. Milk should be boiled before use.

g. **Vaccination:** Vaccination during the festival or fair has no significant role. However, people intending to attend these fair and festivals should be immunised against cholera, tetanus and typhoid beforehand and must carry a certificate for the same while attending the fair.

h. **Provision of inspection or checkposts:** They are provided on the roads, before entry into the ground where the fair or festival has been organised, to keep a check on the emerging or upcoming infections or diseases.

18.8 WATER SUPPLY

Rural areas need water for agriculture purposes besides human consumption. The agriculture sector accounts for between 90 and 95% of surface and ground water in India, while industry and the domestic sector accounts for the remaining. Wide regional disparities in water availability also exist.

About 26–31% of India's rural population is unserved for safe drinking water as per the assessment report of Planning Commission in 2002. More than 65 million people across 17 states are estimated to be at risk for Fluorosis, nearly 14 million people in 75 blocks are at an increased risk of health problems due to excess arsenic in ground water, and other health issues due to varying iron levels, presence of nitrates and heavy metals, bacteriological contamination and salinity in drinking water.

Provision of pure water supply for drinking and cooking purposes is the most important problem in villages. Water quality is affected by various factors like sewage discharge, discharge from industries, agrochemicals, run-off from agricultural fields and urban run-off. Water quality is also affected by lack of awareness and education among users. The need for user involvement in maintaining water quality and looking at other aspects like hygiene, environment sanitation, storage and disposal are critical elements to maintain the quality of water resources (Fig. 18.1).

Model deep wells or tube wells should be provided and they should be guarded against all possible sources of pollution. In some places, model tanks are provided. They should also be supervised on similar lines. Wherever possible, water pumps should be provided to wells and tanks for drawing water. If this is not possible, a metal bucket and a chain may be used. In no case, steps should be provided in the wells as the

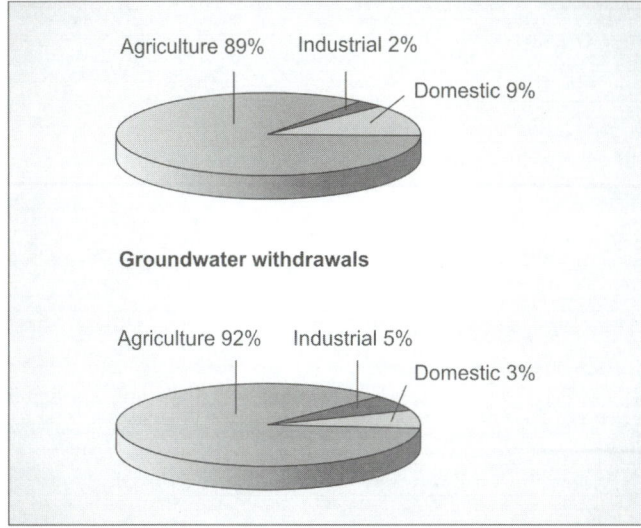

Fig. 18.1: Source of water for various purposes (*Source*: Earth Trends 2001, World Resources Institute)

danger of water getting polluted therefrom is considerably enhanced. This polluted water may prove to be a potent source of water-borne infection. Regular disinfection by bleaching powder should be carried out.

Government initiatives: A national water policy was drafted in 1987 which was subsequently revised in 2002. For ensuring sustainability of the systems, steps were initiated in 1999 to institutionalise community participation in the implementation of rural drinking water supply schemes through the sector reforms project. Target 7C under Millennium Development Goals (MDGs) is to halve, by 2015, the proportion of the population without sustainable access to safe drinking water and basic sanitation.

Since 2000, water quality monitoring has been accorded a high priority and institutional mechanisms have been developed at national, state, district, block and panchayat levels accordingly. The government has also outlined requisite mechanisms to monitor the quality of drinking water and devise effective information, education and communication (IEC) interventions to disseminate information and educate people on health and hygiene.

The Government of India launched the National Rural Drinking Water Quality Monitoring and Surveillance Programme in February 2006 which envisages institutionalisation of community participation for monitoring and surveillance of drinking water sources at the grassroots level by Gram Panchayats and village water and sanitation committees, followed by checking the positively tested samples at the district and state level laboratories.

In 2009, the Accelerated Rural Water Supply Programme was modified as the National Rural Drinking Water Programme (NRDWP) with major emphasis on ensuring sustainability of water availability in terms of potability, adequacy, convenience, affordability and equity, on a sustainable basis, while also adopting decentralized approach involving PRIs and community organizations. The XIIth Five-Year Plan approach of focus on piped water supply, increasing household tap connections and raising drinking water supply norms from 40 to 55 lpcd.

Department of Drinking Water, Ministry of Rural Development has come up with a strategic plan 2011–22 ensuring drinking water security in rural India. The target is that at least 50% of rural population in the country should have access to 55 lpcd within their household premises or within 100 metres radius, with at least 30% having individual household connections by 2017.

Sanitation at Fairs and Festivals

Many a times, fairs and other religious festivals have been a source of outbreak of epidemic diseases, chiefly cholera. So it is very essential that arrangements should be made for their successful control beforehand. For carrying on these measures, some person or persons should be made responsible for the organisation of the fair. There should also be appointed a medical officer of health with executive powers, who should be put in-charge of the sanitary arrangements. Adequate funds will be needed by him to make himself effective.

For efficient control of epidemics during these fairs, following points should be attended.

19.1 PLANNING OF THE ARRANGEMENTS

The organisers of the fair along with the medical officer of health and other members of the advisory committee should chalk out a plan. It is for him to see that the ground is cleared of all vegetation, levelled and demarcated into different blocks with well-planned roads. The layout plan should be fixed at a prominent place for the information of the public. In fact long before opening of the *mela*, the pilgrims should be advised through posters and newspaper advertisements of their obligations vis-à-vis the arrangements made.

19.2 ACCOMMODATION

It is to be provided for the organisers, police, health and medical authorities in the first instance. For the pilgrims, dharamsalas or residential blocks along with sanitary conveniences should be arranged. Each room or temporary camp, or hut should be at least 10 feet (3 metres) high and should have windows equivalent to 10% of floor area. The land selected should have natural drainage and should be well-shaded and watered. If there are any depressions, cesspits or pools, they should be filled up. The main road approaching the *mela* ground should be metalled or otherwise made smooth and firm.

19.3 MEDICAL AND SANITARY ARRANGEMENTS

The fair should be under the charge of a medical officer of health and the whole area should be divided into blocks placed under the charge of sanitary inspectors. Moreover, accommodation should be provided for infectious diseases' cases, where patients should be removed on stretchers. Adequate quantity of disinfectants and patent medicines should be provided. Temporary hospitals and dispensaries, with qualified doctors, should be arranged for the treatment of sick persons. Arrangements should be made for the provision of stretchers for the removal of sick and badly hurt persons in the case of an outbreak of fire, accidents, etc.

19.4 WATER SUPPLY

Efficient arrangements for the supply of wholesome water should be made available from any one or more of the following sources:

a. Filtered and chlorinated water from some water-works which is very safe.
b. Deep tube wells.
c. Wells.
d. Galvanised iron cisterns.

All these sources should be thoroughly disinfected beforehand so as to avoid the danger of an outbreak of any water-borne epidemic. The amount of water provided should be about 20–25 litres per capita per day.

19.5 EFFICIENT CONSERVANCY

Adequate whole time conservancy staff should be engaged for:
a. Sweeping of the roads, residential blocks, etc.
b. Cleansing of latrines, urinals or other sanitary conveniences.

Sweeping: The roads should be properly swept and watered. One sweeper for every 2,000 pilgrims is the standard aimed at. Covered dustbins should be placed at suitable sites in the *mela* ground for collection of rubbish and sweepings, from where they should be removed by carts or trucks to a place of disposal.

Latrines: Suitable sites should be selected and different types of latrines constructed both for males and females, separately. Trench latrines are recommended. Female sweepers should be employed for latrines meant for use by women. The number of seats of latrines aimed at is as under:

1. 2 seats for 1,000 people, if the fair is to last for one day.
2. One seat for 100 persons, if their stay is longer than a day.

Urinals: Adequate number of urinals should be provided at suitable places all over the *mela* ground which should be separate for both sexes. In ordinary soil, a pit, 4 feet (1.22 metres) square and 5 feet (1.52 metres) deep, filled with broken bricks and covered with sand should be made.

These latrines and urinals should be kept in a clean and sanitary condition and they should not be too far away, otherwise there is a likelihood that people will not use them. No latrine should be situated at a distance of more than 100 yards (91.44 metres) away from the fair area. There should be a proper lighting arrangement at night. Picture boards indicating the sex for which they are meant should be fixed near the entrance. Satisfactory arrangement for removal and disposal of refuse and night soil should be made. The refuse may be dumped and incinerated. In the latter case, beehive pattern or an open incinerator may be more useful.

19.6 FOOD SUPPLY

Strict supervision on the sale of food supply should be exercised. No unwholesome or stale articles of food and drink, overripe fruits and decaying vegetables should be allowed to enter the *mela* ground. If these are found out, they should be immediately seized and destroyed as a preventive measure.

19.7 VACCINES

During *mela* days, all the persons attending the fair/ *melas*/festivals should be inoculated with cholera and typhoid vaccine. People at risk should also be given hepatitis A and B vaccine.

19.8 PROVISION OF INSPECTION OR CHECKPOSTS

They are provided on the roads, before entry into *mela* ground, where the staff is instructed to see that no person suffering from an infectious disease visits the *mela* ground. The certificates of anticholera inoculation may also be checked by them.

Health Education and Communication

WHO defines health as a "state of complete physical, mental and social wellbeing and not merely absence of any disease or infirmity". Health education has been defined by World Health Organization (1998) as consciously constructed opportunity for learning involving some form of communication designed to improve health literacy, including improving knowledge and developing life skills that are conducive for individual and community health. Thus, it aims for promoting health and bringing about a behaviour change towards positive health.

Thus, before actually understanding the concept of health education, it is important to understand what do we mean by 'health literacy' and what are the behavioural factors that influence the decision-making of an individual and community towards seeking health. The degree to which people are able to access, understand, appraise and communicate information to engage with the demands of different health contexts in order to promote and maintain good health across the course of life is health literacy.

Health literacy: It is important for enabling people to increase control over and improve their health *(health promotion)*.

Awareness, information, knowledge and skills are the interventions that act on the behavioural attributes that influence the process of decision-making for seeking health by an individual or community, i.e. beliefs, attitude and values. *Beliefs* are statements of perceived fact or impressions about the world. Whereas relatively constant feelings, predispositions and set of beliefs directed towards an idea, object, person or situation is *attitude*. And a collection of beliefs and attitude comprises *value system*. Thus, the role of health literacy is to bring about a change by acting on beliefs and attitude.

The theories derived from behavioural or social sciences help to design more effective and efficient health education programmes. The study of human behavioural and social sciences helps in practice of health education and health promotion by facilitating developing programme objectives that are measurable, identifying the method of choice and a right mix of strategies, timing of intervention and communication aids to be used for health education. Health education, thus is a process of communication or dissemination of scientifically correct information in individuals or community to bring about a desired change on promotion of health, healthy living and prevention of diseases through the help of an expert. It enables people to acquire knowledge and skill to solve their own health problems. So community health is increasingly concerned with the behaviour of an individual in relation to various health practices, viz. dietary practices, drug addiction, pollution of water, soil, air, family planning, etc.

The aims of health education are: (a) To inform the general public about the principles of physical and mental health and methods of preventing diseases, (b) empower them with correct knowledge and information so that they are able to make technically and scientifically right choice for maintaining health, and (c) to facilitate the acceptance and proper usage of medical measures.

20.1 PRINCIPLES OF HEALTH EDUCATION

a. **Interest:** The health education programme must be prepared as per the interest of the audience as per their 'felt needs'.

b. **Participation:** Ensuring participation of the people for whom the programme is being designed through group discussions, etc. helps in better acceptance of the programme.

c. **Comprehension:** The messages should be simple and in a language that the audience is able to understand. Use of complex scientific and technical jargon should be avoided.

d. **Motivation:** Fundamental desire for learning is motivation. There can be Primary Motive for inborn desires, i.e. food, housing, clothing and secondary motive for outside forces, i.e. rewards, praises and achievements.

e. **Reinforcement:** Repetition of the information intending to bring a desired change is reinforcement. It is important to bring about a change as per some new information.

f. **Known to unknown:** The issues known to people should be discussed first to build the interest of the people and then newer subjects should be introduced subsequently.

g. **Learning by doing:** Learning is better, if doing an activity succeeds the knowledge of theoretical concepts.

h. **Information, media and receiver:** The information to be transmitted, media and audience are in dynamic relationship with each other. This relationship is important to bring about a desired change.

i. **Leaders:** Community health leaders can influence the recipients' behaviour for decision-making towards health promotion.

j. **Good human relations:** The empathetic and polite behaviour of the health educator increases his acceptability among the audience and thereby increases the effectivity of the message communicated by him to the audience.

20.2 METHODS OF APPROACHES IN HEALTH EDUCATION

a. **Legal or regulatory approach:** It makes use of the law to protect health of the public, e.g. Epidemic Disease Act, Pollution Act, etc. The limitations of this approach are that it is applicable in specific situations and does not alter the behaviour of an individual or community.

b. **Administrative or service approach:** This is based on 'felt needs' of individuals and intends to provide all the health facilities that are needed by people.

c. **Educational approach:** It is the most effective method and works through communication for motivation leading to the process of decision-making. It results in slow but permanent and enduring change. The individuals get sufficient time for learning the new and correct facts and unlearning the uncorrect ones.

Thus, the government uses educational approach to provide health education under all the public health programmes.

20.3 EDUCATIONAL AIDS USED IN HEALTH EDUCATION

i. **Auditory aids:** These are based on the principle of sound, electricity and magnetism. These include microphones, tape recorders, sound amplifiers, public addressing systems, etc.

ii. **Visual aids:** These include a group that does not require projection like black boards, posters, models, specimens, flannel graphs, newspapers, pamphlets, magazines, puppet shows, etc. and others that require projection are film strips, slides, epidiascopes, video cassettes, etc.

iii. **Combined audiovisual aids:** These utilize modern media for educating people. The impact produced by picture and sound combined together makes a better impact. These include movies, television, multimedia computers, etc. and are more interesting and informative than other methods.

Mass media is the best method to provide health education for general public when a large group has to be addressed. This is a cost-effective method where one message can be sent to a large number of audience/beneficiaries in a single go. However, the efficacy of this method is low since all the audience receiving the message may not have a felt need for the subject. The modes of communication used are television, hoardings, radio, newspapers, etc.

Educational media have, therefore, been extensively used in educating the public in various fields of infant and child care, nutrition, personal hygiene, family planning, etc.

The methods used for individuals are interpersonal communication (IPC) and counselling. Lectures, groups and panel discussion and workshops and seminars are used for group education. Radio, TV, Internet, printed material and newspapers are used for mass education.

20.4 COMPONENTS OF HEALTH EDUCATION

While promoting any programme on health education, great emphasis is laid on various branches of hygiene, viz. general hygiene, personal hygiene, environmental hygiene and other aspects like nutrition, family planning, prevention of accidents and occurrence of disease, etc. US Department of Health and Human Services, have identified 38 areas of focus in *Healthy People 2020* which underscore the importance of health promotion (Table 20.1).

Health education embodies several components under its ambit. The essential components of health education programmes and services aimed at enhancing an individual's and a community's health are:

a. **Community involvement:** Community members must be involved in all stages of programme development from needs assessment to evaluation of results.

b. **Planning:** It involves identifying community health problems that are preventable, setting goals, identifying intervention behaviour, deciding on stakeholders and making the cohesive group.

Table 20.1: Healthy people 2020

1. Access to health services
2. Adolescent health
3. Arthritis, osteoporosis and chronic back
4. Blood disorders and blood safety
5. Cancer
6. Chronic kidney disease
7. Dementias, including Alzheimer's disease
8. Diabetes
9. Disability and health
10. Early and middle childhood
11. Educational and community-based programs
12. Environmental health
13. Family planning
14. Food safety
15. Genomics
16. Global health
17. Healthcare-associated infections
18. Health communication and health information technology
19. Health-related quality of life and well-being
20. Hearing and other sensory or communication disorders
21. Heart disease and stroke
22. HIV
23. Immunization and infectious disease
24. Injury and violence prevention
25. Lesbian, gay, bisexual, and transgender health
26. Maternal, infant, and child health
27. Medical product safety
28. Mental health and mental disorders
29. Nutrition and weight status
30. Occupational health
31. Older adults
32. Oral health
33. Physical activity
34. Preparedness
35. Public health infrastructure
36. Respiratory diseases
37. Sexually transmitted diseases
38. Sleep health
39. Social determinants of health
40. Substance abuse
41. Tobacco use
42. Vision

c. **Needs and resource assessment:** It is important to assess the health needs of the community that may need an intervention and then assess the resources available.

d. **Comprehensive programme:** Comprehensive programmes ensure better results, i.e. the one that targets multiple risk factors and intervenes at multiple levels, i.e. individuals, families, community. These are designed to change not only risk behaviour but also the factors and conditions that sustain this behaviour (e.g. motivation, social environment).

e. **Long-term change:** Health education programmes should be designed to produce stable and lasting changes in health behaviour.

f. **Research and evaluation:** An evaluation and research plan is integral to a plan, not only to document programme outcomes and effects but also to describe its formation and process and its cost-effectiveness and benefits.

20.5 BARRIERS IN COMMUNICATION

a. **Physical or environmental:** Excessive noise, difficulty in vision and congested noise.

b. **Physiological:** Emotional disturbances, neurosis and depression.

c. **Psychological:** Difficulties in self-expression, hearing and understanding.

d. **Cultural:** Persistent patterns of behaviour, beliefs, customs, attitudes, habits, religion, etc.

20.6 BASIS OF HUMAN BEHAVIOUR

Human behaviour patterns have important roles to play in aetiologies, diagnosis, as well as management including organisation of medical or health care patterns. Thus, any health education programme targeted to bring a change at individual or community level must bring a behavioural change in the target population. Research shows that those interventions most likely to achieve desired outcomes are based on a clear understanding of targeted health behaviours, and the environmental context in which they occur.

The human behaviour has multifactorial aspects like biological, psychodynamics, economical, political, religious and sociocultural forces and thus has to be studied through multiple disciplines of social sciences—sociology, social psychology, anthropology, economics, political science, and biological science including human physiology in its various components. The equation $B = f(P, E)$ can help us to comprehend human behaviour (B) at any point in time by taking into consideration the genetically developed (with physiological needs) and socially trained (with social drives) person (P) in his ecological settings (E). It is beyond the scope of this chapter or book to discuss all the components individually which are essential for scientific comprehension.

There is a long list of human activities commonly thought as 'instinctive' which conform to the ethological (science of animals behaviour) scheme of instinctive behaviour, e.g. food, water, shelter, procreation, etc. but it is from the culturally approved menu of values that he is expected to develop his norms of behaviour. The secondary drives or motives represent learned (behavioural) ways of satisfying, experiencing or interpreting primary biological drives.

Various models or theories that attempt or predict to explain the effect of interventions on the human behaviour focus on three areas: (a) Individual capacity such as knowledge, attitudes, beliefs and personality traits, (b) interpersonal that focuses on interpersonal relationships and supports; including family, friends and peers that provide social identity, support and role definition, and (c) examine environmental supports and contexts. Health education mainly focuses on the first two.

a. Theories that influence behaviour in individual capacity

i. *The rational model*: Also known as KAP model, it is based on the premise that increasing a person's knowledge will prompt a behaviour change by bringing a change in attitudes and beliefs. However, the weakness of this model is that knowledge may not be a sufficient factor in changing individual or collective behaviour, motivation may come from some other factors.

ii. *Health belief model*: This model is based on the principle that people's beliefs about the severity of a disease and their susceptibility to it influences their willingness to take preventive action.

iii. *Extended parallel process model (EPPM)*: This model proposes that people, when presented with a risk message, their decision-making is influenced by their perception about the susceptibility and severity to the risk factor. Thus, behaviour change will come only if they believe that they are susceptible to a severe threat that arouses their level of fear which motivates them to assess whether the recommended action can reduce that threat (i.e. response efficacy) and if they can perform the recommended action (i.e. self-efficacy).

iv. *Transtheoretical model of change*: Behaviour change is viewed as a progression through a series of five stages: precontemplation, contemplation, preparation, action and maintenance. Need for specific information, self-efficacy and balanced decision-making are central to the theory.

v. *Theory of planned behaviour*: The theory holds that intent is influenced not only by the attitude toward the behaviour but also the perception of social norms (the strength of others' opinions on the behaviour and the person's own motivation to comply with those significant others) and the degree of perceived behavioural control.

vi. *Activated health education model*: This is a three-phased model—experiential, awareness and responsibility. The first phase actively engages the individuals in assessment of their health. The second phase generates awareness about the health behaviour which is translated into change, identification of personal health values and develop plan for behaviour change occurs in the third phase (Fig. 20.1.).

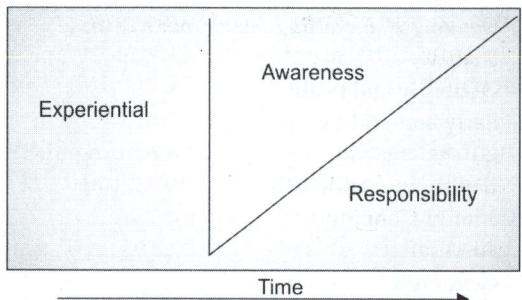

Fig. 20.1: The activated health education model

b. Interpersonal support

i. *Social learning theory*: This is based on the concept of 'reciprocal determinism' which means that opinion, thoughts, advice, behaviour and support of the people surrounding an individual influence his or her feelings and behaviour and the individual has a reciprocal effect on those people.

ii. *Social cognitive theory*: It adds the principles of observational learning and vicarious reinforcement (watching and learning from actions of others) to social learning theory. Self-efficiency here is considered as the most important personal factor in behaviour change (Fig. 20.2).

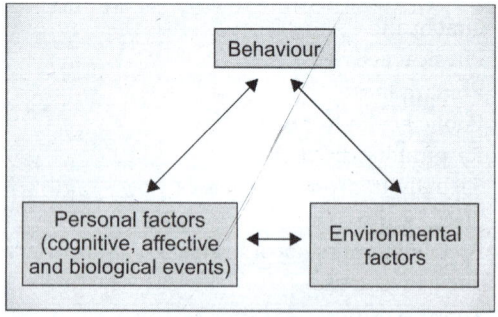

Fig. 20.2: Social learning theory: Concept model

20.7 HEALTH EDUCATION AND BEHAVIOUR

Health education essentially aims at behaviour change: (a) To ensure that health is valued as an asset in a community, (b) to equip people with skills, knowledge and attitudes to enable them to solve their health problems by their own actions and efforts, and (c) to promote development and utilisation of health services. Thus, health education aims at training an individual or group of individuals for a positive change behaviour by understanding of the holistic concept of the disease prevention and health promotion. Thus, the term health education is not only imparting knowledge but also to study the effect of the knowledge in terms of change in behaviour. This, is now recently more accepted as behaviour change communication (BCC).

a. **Environmental context of behaviour change:** The environmental context falls mostly within the realms of health promotion, however, communication theory and diffusion innovation theory are the two concepts that have a role in health education.

  i. *Communication theory:* Communication has its central interest in those behavioural situations in which the communicator (originator of health message) transmits the message to the communicant, i.e. the recipient. Three levels of learning usually occur, i.e. verbal level, attitudinal or appreciation level and effective action level. Communication theory believes that repeated exposure to the same message especially when it is delivered through multiple channels intensifies its impact on the audience. The audience may show immediate learning or delayed learning. There may be generalised learning about the concepts secondary to the message, social diffusion through discussion amongst the social groups and institutional diffusion.

  ii. *Diffusion innovation theory:* Community organisation and utilisation of leaders for *diffusion of innovation* or new ideas and practices through mass media are other essential components for effective communication by health educators. Whenever a new practice is introduced, the process of adoption passes through five stages, i.e. (a) awareness, i.e. knows about practices but lacks details, (b) interest, i.e. tries to learn details, (c) evaluation for effectiveness in one's own situations, (d) trial of practice, and (e) adoption if found useful, otherwise rejection. Accordingly people adopting are also classified into five categories—innovators, early adopters, early majority, late majority and laggards (Fig. 20.3).

20.8 METHODS AND MEDIA OF HEALTH EDUCATION

Those methods which provide only one way communication, e.g. lectures, etc. are known as didactic methods. Those methods which are characterised by questions, answers and discussions are described as socratic (two way) methods. Media are the tools which are used in health education, e.g. charts, posters, pamphlets, etc. Some of the methods used for health education are given below.

1. Lectures

In a lecture, contents are systematically presented and in a minimum time as compared to discussions. During lecture, only the lecturer is active while listeners are passive participants. Talks are usually divided in four groups: (a) Extempore talk, i.e. when the talks are delivered without previous preparation, (b) impromptu talk, i.e. speaker takes advantage of any unexpected opportunity and uses the same for talk, (c) memorised speech, i.e. when speaker speaks from a prepared speech which was previously memorised, and (d) read speech, i.e. which is read out—this can be delivered tactfully and successfully.

Since it is a one way communication, it may not be very effective in bringing a change in behaviour.

2. Discussions
Group Discussions

  i. *Informal group discussions:* Informal group discussions are good as group exerts pressure on individual members for behaviour change. A discussion group ideally should be of 6–20 people. The members should be of the same economic, social or educational level and should share common interests or same goals for group discussion. A leader, a recorder, an observer and a resourceful person may be selected or designated. They should know their roles and all members of the group should actively participate in discussions to reach common agreed norms or values.

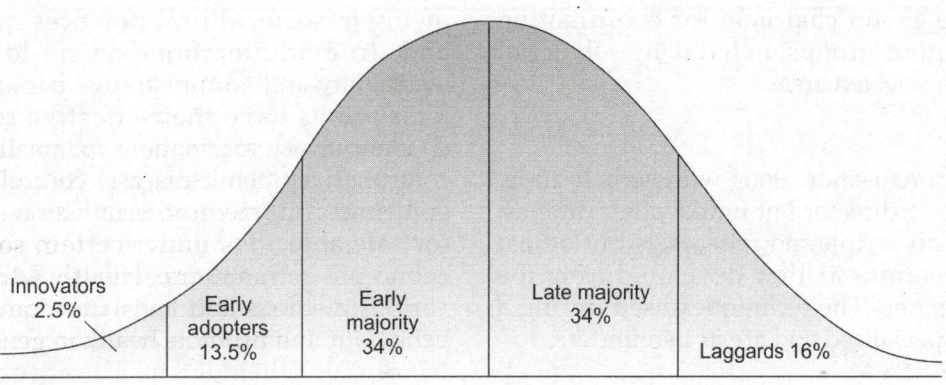

Fig. 20.3: Diffusion of innovations: Process of adoption

ii. *Formal discussions*

    a. *Panel discussion*: A panel consists of 4–8 qualified persons with a moderator or a chairman. The panel sits in front of an audience and conducts the discussions among themselves. There are no set topics. The chairman introduces the members and their respective areas of interest. The characteristic of the panel is spontaneity of discussions. When the main aspects of the subject are explored, a pattern of thinking is established, the audience is invited to participate by raising questions or by making contributions of their own.

    b. *Symposium*: In contrast to panel discussions, in a symposium, there is a set programme of prepared speeches on selected topics by selected speakers. These may be followed by questions from the audience. There are no discussions among symposium members (unlike panel discussions). The speeches are used to supply information, judgement and interpretations which serve as a basis of consultations by the audience. The chairman makes a comprehensive summary at the end.

    c. *Debate*: A debate is a highly structured form of discussion with speakers sharing their opinion 'for' or 'against' the proposition before the house. In the end, the proposition is accepted or rejected by the house.

    d. *Open forum*: This method consists usually of a lecture followed by a brief discussion period in which the audience participates.

    e. *Institute*: Institute is a series of meetings and utilises a variety of techniques, e.g. lectures, panels, informal group discussions and symposia.

    f. *Workshop*: Workshop is a method in which consultants as well as groups of experienced persons get together for solving problems. It is recognised as one of the most effective ways of learning and problem solving. It consists of a series of meetings usually 4 or 5. There are periodic presentations of progress reports by the respective group chairman for coordination among various groups undertaking solving of problem in selected areas.

3. Sociodrama

Sociodrama is dramatisation along with verbalisation. It is played under a director but unlike other dramas, the actors have no scripts, no rehearsals but adjust according to situations as they develop during the course of discussions. The techniques used during a sociodrama are specialised and are as hereunder:

    i. *Role taking*: Assuming or carrying out or developing an assigned role.

    ii. *Actualisation*: Acting out spontaneously the roles which grow out of the problem.

    iii. *Interaction*: Making necessary adjustments as the individual feels that he should.

    iv. *Auxiliary coaching*: During the proceedings to bring conflicts into focus.

    v. *Discussions*: An analysis of the performance by the audience, actors and director.

4. Programmes or Self-instruction

The device is also known as teaching machine. The material is presented to the learner in systematic steps known as 'instructional frame'. Each frame presents a problem or a question. The learner records his answer and gets a check for correct answer. Failing that, he gets referred back. Each learner proceeds at his own pace.

20.9 DEMONSTRATION

A practical demonstration leaves a visual impression on the minds of participants. Various health practices (like infant feeding, cooking), health processes (like blood circulation), health objectives (e.g. causative organisms) can be demonstrated. Result demonstrations are very effective, e.g. immunisations of healthy babies.

20.10 MISCELLANEOUS METHODS

Other miscellaneous methods, e.g. interviews, counselling, seminars, brainstorming, field trips, radio talks, health fares and cultural programmes are also used.

20.11 HEALTH EDUCATION VS HEALTH LEGISLATION FOR BEHAVIOURAL CHANGES

For effective behavioural changes, the health educational approach is more effective than short-term changes implemented through legislation, though it is slow, steady and gradual. Many laws remain ineffective for various reasons, e.g. child marriages in rural areas owing to sociocultural practices, widespread food and drug adulterations owing to socioeconomic, availability and administrative parameters. However, legislations have their effective role to play, e.g. (i) compulsory vaccinations for smallpox eradication/control, (ii) epidemic diseases control act for control of epidemics, (iii) medical termination of Pregnancy Act for safe abortions under certain social, health and economic parameters. Health education through various methods and legislation can reorient human behaviour and promote health in general.

Chapter

21

Public Health System in India

India is a union of 29 states and 7 union territories with largely independent states under its constitution. Every state has its own system of public healthcare delivery since health is mainly a state subject, however, centre has its executive role. So far as centre is concerned, the functions of centre are policy-making, guiding, assisting, evaluating and general coordination between the states. It establishes and maintains food and drug standards and administers, central institutes. It coordinates and supervises various national health programmes and interstate quarantine for control and spread of communicable diseases. Besides, it supplies states with vital information on medical subjects in close coordination with various national and international health organisations like World Health Organization, United Nations International Children's Emergency Fund, Ford Foundation, Rockefeller Foundation, International Red Cross and Indian Red Cross Society.

The health system in India has three main levels—central, state and local or peripheral.

21.1 AT THE CENTRE LEVEL

The Ministry of Health and Family Welfare, Directorate General of Health Services (DGHS) and Central Council of Health and Family Welfare are the three official organs.

a. **Ministry of Health and Family Welfare:** The ministry is headed by a cabinet minister, minister of state and deputy health minister. The ministry is directly responsible for the health of centrally administered areas. The ministry has two independent departments for health and family welfare. Secretary to Government of India is the head of the Department of Health and is assisted by Joint Secretaries, Deputy Secretaries and other Administrative Staff. In 1966, Department of Family Welfare was separately created established under the Secretary to Government of India, Ministry of Health and Family Welfare assisted by

Additional Secretary and Joint Secretary. It maintains international health through regulations at the port, controls the central health institutes, and regulates medical and allied professions in the country. It promotes research, establishes and maintains drug standards. The ministry also collects and publishes health-related data and coordinates with states and other ministries for promotion of health.

b. **Directorate General of Health Services** has three main units (medical care and hospitals, public health and general administration) and functions under Director General of Health Services (DGHS), who is assisted by Additional, Deputy and Assistant Directors and other administrative staff, who deal with different branches. DGHS is the chief advisor to the government in the matters of health.

Its general functions are surveys, planning, coordination and appraisal of all health-related matters in the country. It is also involved in regulating international health, medical education, drug standards and medical stores depots in the country. It plays lead role in planning and implementation of National Health Programmes, and Central Government Health Scheme (CGHS). Institutions, like Central Health Education Bureau (CHEB), Central Bureau of Health Intelligence (CBHI) and National Medical Library (NML), are actively involved in providing health education, health intelligence and information management across the country under its jurisdiction.

c. **Central Council of Health (CCH):** The Union Health Minister is the chairperson whereas the ministers of state are the members of the CCH. It promotes the coordinated and concerted actions between centre and state for implementation of programmes and measures pertaining to health in the country. This body is mainly involved in health policy recommendations and propose health legislations regarding the medical and public healthcare in the country.

21.2 STATE HEALTH SYSTEM

The states are autonomous in respect of medical relief and public health. In all the states, the health system comprises of State Ministry of Health and Directorate of Health Services. The State Ministry of Health is headed by an elected minister, who is assisted by a secretary along with deputy and under-secretaries. There is a Director of Health Services, who is an administrative officer and incharge of medical education, medical and public health administration. He has a Deputy Director of Health (Medical), Deputy Director of Health (Public Health) and Assistant Directors incharges of various sections. In most of the states, the medical and public health departments have been integrated. The Director of Health Service (DHS) is the chief advisor to the State Government in medical and public health-related matters. In few states, with the advent of family planning as a separate programme, the designation of DHS has now been changed to Director of Health and Family Welfare (Fig. 21.1).

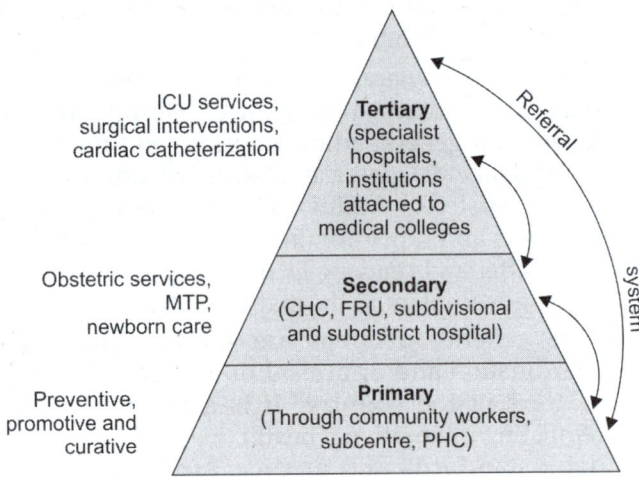

Fig. 21.1: Levels of healthcare

21.3 DISTRICT LEVEL

Each district has been divided into various administrative units, i.e. subdivisions, tehsils (talukas) comprising of 200–600 villages, community development blocks in the rural areas comprising about 100 villages with a population of about 80,000 to 1.2 lakhs, municipalities and corporations, villages and panchayats.

The main unit of administration is the district under a collector. The urban areas of district are organized into following:

a. Town area committees over a population of 5,000–10,000 to mainly involved in providing sanitary services.

b. Municipal boards over population ranging from 10,000 to 200,000. These are headed by a chairman, elected usually by the members for a term of 3–5 years. These are involved in construction and maintenance of roads, water supply, sanitation, education, registration of vital events and maintenance of hospitals and dispensaries.

c. Corporations with population above 2 lakhs are headed by Mayor. The Mayor is an elected member with the councilors, who are representatives of various wards.

The health at the **district level is under** chief medical officer with three deputy chief medical officers, with each of them being incharge of one-third of the district for integrated health, family welfare and implementation of national health programmes. However, since health is a state subject, the models may vary from state to state. The state government is responsible for providing health services at hospitals, dispensaries, health centres, clinics, public health measures regarding control of infectious diseases, establishment of training centres for medical and paramedical staff, maternity and child welfare services, sanitation projects, etc.

In the states, where there has not been any integration, there are still two separate directors—director of medical services and director of public health. Under them at district level, there are civil surgeons and district medical officers of health on curative and preventive sides, respectively.

In the rural areas, the principle administrative unit is Panchayati Raj, which is local self-government. It is also the basic unit of decentralized planning. The Panchayati Raj is a three-tier system constituting Panchayat at village level, Panchayat Samiti at block level and Zila Parishad at district level.

a. **Panchayat**
   i. *Gram sabha*: It elects the members of Gram Panchayat.
   ii. Gram Panchayat is headed by Sarpanch and has 15–30 Panchas as its members. It is constituted over a population of 5,000–15,000 and has a term for 3–5 years.
   iii. Nyaya Panchayat is to resolve disputes and maintain peace among the villagers and local people.

b. **Panchayat samiti:** It is headed by Block Development Officer (BDO) and is constituted over approximately 100 villages or a population of 80,000–1.2 lakhs. It consists of all the Sarpanchs as its members.

c. **Zila Parishad:** Has 40–60 members, these include all the heads of Panchayat Samitis, MPs and MLAs and representatives of scheduled caste, scheduled tribes and women. District collector is a nonvoting member. Zila Parishad mainly has supervisory and coordinating role.

21.4 HEALTHCARE SYSTEM IN INDIA

The healthcare in India is delivered through following facilities:

1. **Public sector or the health services provided by the government**
   a. Primary healthcare
   b. Hospitals/health centres
   c. Indigenous systems
   d. Health insurance schemes
   e. Other agencies
   f. National health programmes

2. **Private sector:** Through corporate or private hospitals, polyclinics, nursing homes and dispensaries.

3. **Voluntary health agencies**

Primary Healthcare

It was launched as a part of Rural Health Scheme 1977 with an aim of placing people's health in people's hand. The first National Health Policy in 1983 aimed to achieve the goal of 'Health for All' by 2000 AD, through the provision of comprehensive primary healthcare services. It stressed the creation of an infrastructure for primary healthcare; close coordination with health-related services and activities (like nutrition, drinking water supply and sanitation); active involvement and participation of voluntary organisations; provision of essential drugs and vaccines; qualitative improvement in health and family planning services; provision of adequate training; and medical research aimed at the common health problems of the people.

Thus, primary healthcare in India is delivered in villages through subcentres and primary health centres.

1. **At the village level:** The community-based care is provided by:
   i. *Accredited Social Health Activist (ASHA):* Under the programme 'National Health Mission', each ASHA is allocated a population of 1,000 in the rural areas and 2000 in the urban areas where she acts as a link worker for them. She is a honorary, voluntary worker who works under the supervision of ANMs. Her basic mandate is to refer the patient for comprehensive health services to the health system. Besides, she provides health education to the community on various health issues and also act as depot holder for Oral Rehydration Salt (ORS) and contraceptives (condoms, oral contraceptives and e-pills. ASHAs are selected by the community

where she is supposed to work as per the standard guidelines under the programme and then subsequently trained periodically.

   ii. *ICDS (Integrated Child Development Services) Scheme:* Under the ICDS Scheme, there is an Anganwadi at the population of 400–800 manned by one Anganwadi worker and one helper. The Anganwadi worker is a part time worker selected from the community where she is supposed to work, trained and entrusted with several responsibilities regarding health, nutrition and child care. The Medical Officers, Auxiliary Nurse Midwife (ANM) and Accredited Social Health Activist (ASHA) form a team with the ICDS functionaries to achieve convergence of different services (Table 21.1).

2. **Subcentre level:** A subcentre is the peripheral outpost of the healthcare system in the rural areas which is the first point of contact of the community with the primary healthcare system. It caters to a population of 5000 in plains and 3000 in hilly, tribals and backward areas and is manned by one multipurpose worker male and female (ANM) each. One female health assistant (lady health visitor) and 1 male health assistant at the PHC level are given the supervision of 6 subcentres.

The services provided by subcentre are
   a. Antenatal, natal, postnatal including family planning and counselling in women.
   b. Prevention of malnutrition and treatment of common illnesses like respiratory tract infections, diarrhoea, fever, worm infestation in children.
   c. Implementation of various national health programmes.

In order to provide quality care through the public health facilities, Indian Public Health Standards (IPHS) have been prescribed for healthcare

Table 21.1: Services provided at the Anganwadi

Services	Target group	Services provided by
Supplementary nutrition	Children below 6 yrs and pregnant/lactating mothers	AWW and helper
Immunization	Children below 6 yrs and pregnant/lactating mothers	ANM/MO
Nutrition and health education	Children below 6 yrs and pregnant/lactating mothers	AWW/ANM/MO
Health check up	Women 15–45 years	AWW/ANM/MO
Referral services	Children below 6 yrs and pregnant/lactating mothers	AWW/ANM/MO
Preschool education	Children 3–6 years	AWW

institutions at all levels to provide basic primary healthcare services to the community and achieve and maintain an acceptable standard of quality of care. These standards also help monitor and improve functioning of the subcentre.

The IPHS for all the public health institutions have been prepared keeping in view the resources available with respect to their functional requirements with minimum standards such as building, manpower, instruments and equipment, drugs and other facilities and desirable standards which represent the ideal situation. The overall objective of IPHS is to provide healthcare that is quality oriented and sensitive to the needs of the community.

3. **Primary health centre (PHC):** Primary health centres are the first level of call to a qualified doctor of the public sector in rural areas for the sick and those who directly report or are referred from subcentres for curative, preventive and promotive healthcare. A primary health centre caters to a population of 20,000 in hilly, tribal, or difficult areas and 30,000 population in plain areas with 4–6 indoor/observation beds. It acts as a referral unit for 6 subcentres and refer out cases to CHC (30-bedded hospital) and higher order public hospitals located at subdistrict and district level. A PHC is manned by a total staff of 15–18 (2 medical officers, one lady MO may be from AYUSH, 1 pharmacist, 3 nurse midwives, I HW female, 1 health educator, health assistant male and female 2 each, 2 clerks, 1 lab technician, 1 driver and 4 class IV workers) to make it facility for 24 × 7 delivery of health facilities.

Minimum assured services cover all the essential elements of preventive, promotive, curative and rehabilitative primary healthcare including implementation of national programmes. This implies a wide range of services that include:

a. *Medical care*: Inpatient (6 beds) and outpatient care, 24 hours emergency and referral services.
b. Maternal and child healthcare including family planning.
c. Medical termination of pregnancy including manual vacuum evacuation.
d. Management of reproductive tract/sexually transmitted infections.
e. Nutrition services in coordination with ICDS.
f. School health.
g. Adolescent healthcare.
h. Promotion of basic sanitation and safe drinking water.
i. Prevention and control of locally endemic diseases like malaria, kala-azar, Japanese encephalitis, etc.
j. Disease surveillance and control of epidemics.
k. Collection and reporting of vital events.

l. Education about health/behaviour change communication (BCC).
m. Implementation of national health programmes including Reproductive, Maternal, Newborn, Child Health + Adolescent (RMNCH + A), HIV/AIDS Control Programme, Communicable and Non-communicable Disease Control Programme.
n. Referral services
o. Basic lab services
p. Training to health manpower
q. Monitoring and supervision
r. Rehabilitation
s. Recording of vital events
t. *Selected surgical procedures*: The vasectomy, tubectomy (including laparoscopic tubectomy), MTP, hydrocelectomy and cataract surgeries as a camp/fixed day approach. Universal precautions must be followed during these surgical procedures to prevent infection.

Universal precautions: All the staff should be adequately trained for the basic elements of universal precautions that include:

i. Handwashing thoroughly with soap and running water before carrying out the procedure, immediately if gloves are torn and hand is contaminated with blood or other body fluids and soon after the procedure, with gloves on and again after removing the gloves.
ii. Barrier precautions: Using protective gloves, mask, waterproof aprons and gowns.
iii. Strict asepsis during the operative procedure and cleaning the operative site. Practise the "no touch technique" which is: any instrument or part of instrument which is to be inserted in the cervical canal must not touch any non-sterile object/surface prior to insertion.
iv. Decontamination and cleaning of all instruments immediately after each use.
v. Sterilisation/high level disinfection of instruments with meticulous attention.
vi. Appropriate waste disposal.

4. **Community health centre (CHC):** The community health centres (CHCs) constitute the secondary level of healthcare and are designed to provide referral as well as specialist healthcare to the rural population. These act both as block level health administrative unit and referral units to higher level of facilities.

As per IPHS, every CHC has to provide services which have been indicated as essential and desirable. Every state/UT must ensure the availability of all essential services and also aspire to achieve desirable services. A CHC should be able to provide following services (Table 21.2):

a. *OPD services and IPD services*: In the specialities of general medicine, surgery, obstetrics and gynaecology, paediatrics, dental and AYUSH services and eye specialist services (at one for every 5 CHCs).

b. *Emergency services*: A CHC is designated as a first referral unit (FRU) for emergency obstetric care (EmOC), if the services are available for round the clock normal delivery, caesarean section, medical termination of pregnancy and a blood storage unit or linkage to a nearby blood bank.

c. Laboratory services

d. School health

e. Adolescent healthcare

f. Blood storage unit

g. Referral

h. Maternal death review

i. Implementation of national health programmes.

Table 21.2: Manpower requirements for a CHC

Doctors	Recommended
Block Health Officer/Medical Superintendent	1
Public health specialist	1
General surgeon	1
Physician	1
Obstetrician and gynaecologist	1
Paediatrician	1
Anaesthetist	1
Eye surgeon	1 for every five CHCs
Dental surgeon	1
General Duty Medical Officer	2
General Duty Medical Officer of AYUSH	1
Total	**10**

Hospitals

The public healthcare delivery system has rural hospitals, subdistrict or subdivisional hospitals, district hospitals, tertiary care at multispeciality hospitals, specialist hospitals, superspeciality and teaching hospitals. Most of the hospitals provide curative services and have less emphasis on the preventive and promotive services.

Medical and health education: Medical colleges were first started in Chennai and Kolkata in 1835, and these were recognised by the Royal College of Surgeons in 1845. In April 1990, there were 148 medical colleges and 54 dental colleges. The total number of hospital beds in country as on 1–4–90 stood at 810,548, and total seats in medical colleges to nearly 11,400.

With a view to provide postgraduate training facilities in teaching and research work in different parts of the country, a scheme for upgrading of certain departments in the medical colleges and research institutes was started in 1948. Medical research is coordinated through the Indian Council of Medical Research, which is an autonomous body.

The rapid increase in the number of medical colleges and their intake capacity has added to the shortage of qualified teachers. Increased emphasis is being laid on postgraduate education.

In a great majority of states, health schools exist for the training of health visitors, midwives, auxiliary nurses and arrangements have been made for the training of sanitary inspectors, vaccinators, nurses, pharmacists, etc.

Indigenous System of Medicine

Ayurveda, Yoga, Unani, Siddha and Homeopathy (AYUSH) have been integrated with the allopathic system of medicine at all the levels to streamline the Indian and alternative systems of medicine into public healthcare system.

Health Insurance

There is growing evidence that the level of healthcare spending in India is currently at over 6% of its total GDP and more than three-quarters of this spending includes private 'out-of-pocket expenses'. As per a data from WHO in 2004, 80% of health expenditure in India is out of pocket expenditure and 24% of all Indians hospitalized fall below poverty line annually (2002). This indicates an emergent need of health insurance for Indians, however, there is no universal health insurance scheme in India. Health insurance in India is limited to industrial workers along with their families and the central/state government servants. Besides a few models of community-based health insurance have also been tried.

i. *Community-based health insurance (CBHI)*: CBHI involves pooling of people's resources to cover the costs of unpredictable health-related events to protect individuals and households from the risk of catastrophic medical expenses. Prepayment (even in the absence of pooling) can facilitate access to expensive medical care, because it spreads costs over time and prevents people having to pay at the time of treatment. By pooling resources, health insurance schemes can improve equity of and access to healthcare and can offer financial protection, e.g. Self-employed Women's Association (SEWA) was started in Ahmedabad in 1972. The Self-employed Women's Association's Integrated Social Security Scheme set up in 1992 provides life insurance, medical insurance and asset insurance to women between 18 and 58 years of age.

ii. *Employees State Insurance Scheme (ESIS)*: This scheme was established in 1948 and provides both cash and medical benefits to the employees, their dependents and retired. This is a scheme under which the insurance premium is shared by the employee and employer in some fixed proportion (*see* details in Chapter on Occupational Health).

iii. *CGHS Scheme*: This scheme provides comprehensive medical care to central government employees. This is again a contributory scheme by contribution from both employer and employees through CGHS dispensaries.

iv. Given the commitment to upscale government expenditure on health, the central and state governments were devising various ways to spend additional resources through "innovative" schemes. The Andhra Pradesh government was the pioneer in launching the **Rajiv Aarogyasri Scheme** in 2007, followed by the central government (the Ministry of Labour and Employment) through the **Rashtriya Swasthya Bima Yojna (RSBY)** in 2008.

The Government has already established IRDA (Insurance Regulatory Development Authority) to regularise the health insurance sector.

Other Agencies

There are multiple agencies that provide health insurance services for its employees like defence medical services, healthcare of railway employees, Delhi Jal Board (DJB), etc.

National Health Programmes

A large number of national health programmes is being run by the Government of India focussing on the major health problems of the country. These programmes are being implemented in coordination with other agencies like municipal bodies through the primary healthcare system to reach the grassroot level. The provision has been made under the programmes to involve the private sector in implementation for better coverage and uniformity in diagnostic and drug policies.

1. *Private Sector*

Private providers which include qualified and alternative private practitioners account for a large share (80%) of healthcare delivered in India. As per the National Health Policy 1983, the healthcare expenditure in India is 6% of GDP of which 1.3% is contributed by the public sector and 4.7% is contributed by private sector.

2. *Voluntary Health Agencies*

There are various types of voluntary health agencies:

1. **National agencies**

a. *Working in the field of MCH*: Family Planning Association of India, Indian Council of Child Welfare and Kasturba Memorial Fund.

b. *Working for specific disease problem*: Hind Kushta Nivaran Sangh, Indian Cancer Society, etc.

c. *Working for general healthcare*: Indian Red Cross Society, Central Social Welfare and All India Women and Appose Conference.

d. *Professional bodies*: INC, IMA, IDA, TNAI, etc.

2. **International NGO/PVO**

Multilateral organizations: These organisations receive funds from multiple governments and non-governmental sources and support developmental effort of governments and organization in less-developed nations of the world. Examples are WHO, UNICEF, World Bank, UNFPA, ILO, UNDP and FAO.

21.5 INDIA AND THE INTERNATIONAL ASSISTANCE

Since India attained independence, a number of health schemes has been launched by the Union Government. In the implementation of these schemes, a number of national and international agencies like WHO, UNICEF, the Colombo Plan, TCM, Rockefeller Foundation, Ford Foundation, CARE, International Red Cross and others has given assistance to India, in the shape of technical know-how, equipment, personnel and other services. India has been a member of the World Health Organization since 1948. India has been receiving striking assistance from the World Health Organization and United Nations International Childrens Emergency Fund. Help from these organisations generally assumes the form of improving existing services, medical literature, fellowships and equipment. They have done a lot to control and cure tuberculosis, venereal diseases, malaria, and improve child health in the country.

World Health Organization

The World Health Organization is a nonpolitical specialised health agency of the United Nations, which came into official existence on April 7, 1948, constituted by the representatives of 61 nations. It is the agency of United Nations with its headquarters at Geneva in Switzerland, i.e. Palais des Nations, for coordinating and directing international health work. Its objective is to promote highest levels of health for all people. Currently more than 150 countries are member signatories of WHO. Their primary role is to direct and coordinate international health within the United Nations' system.

The main areas of work of WHO are health systems, promoting health through the lifecourse, communicable and noncommunicable diseases, corporate services and epidemic preparedness, surveillance and response.

WHO's priority is universal health coverage and accordingly it works together with policymakers, global health partners, civil society, academia and the private sector to support countries to develop, implement and monitor national health plans. In addition, WHO also supports countries to assure the availability of equitable integrated people-centred health services at an affordable price; facilitates access to affordable, safe and effective health technologies; and to strengthen health information systems and evidence-based policy-making.

Promoting good health is one of the basic mandates of WHO, which takes into account the need to address environment risks and social determinants of health, along with gender, equity and human rights.

In the area of communicable diseases, WHO is working with countries to increase and sustain access to prevention, treatment and care for HIV, tuberculosis, malaria and neglected tropical diseases and to reduce the burden of vaccine preventable diseases.

WHO's operational role during emergencies includes leading and coordinating the health response in support of countries, undertaking risk assessments, identifying priorities and setting strategies, providing critical technical guidance, supplies and financial resources as well as monitoring the health situation. WHO also helps countries to strengthen their national core capacities for emergency risk management to prevent, prepare for, respond to, and recover from emergencies due to any hazard that pose a threat to human health security.

Corporate services provide the enabling functions, tools and resources that makes all of this work possible. For example, corporate services encompasses governing bodies convening member states for policy-making, the legal team advising during the development of international treaties, communication staff helping disseminate health information, human resources bringing in some of the world's best public health experts or building services by providing the space and the tools.

For administrative purposes in WHO, the world has been divided into 6 regions:

Region	Headquarters
1. South East Asia, i.e. India, Ceylon, Nepal, Burma, Thailand, Indonesia, Bangladesh, Maldive Islands, Republic of Korea and Mongolia	1. New Delhi (India)
2. America	2. Washington DC (USA)
3. Europe	3. Copenhagen (Denmark)
4. Eastern Mediterranean Muslim Countries including Pakistan.	4. Alexandria (Egypt)
5. Western pacific countries	5. Manila (Philippines)
6. Africa	6. Brazzaville (Congo)

The funds are provided to WHO through the voluntary contributions by various member countries.

They contribute according to their ability to pay, but get aid according to their requirements.

Delegates of WHO: The World Health Assembly is the decision-making body of WHO and is constituted by delegations from all WHO member states and focuses on a specific health agenda prepared by the Executive Board. The main functions of the World Health Assembly are to determine the policies of the Organization, appoint the Director-General, supervise financial policies, and review and approve the proposed programme budget. Its Executive Board consists of 34 technically qualified members for a term of three years who prepare the work of the assembly and give effect to its decisions.

World Health Day: On the 7th April, 1948, Constitution of the World Health Organization officially came into force. Each anniversary is now observed as World Health Day and is used by the national and local authorities to motivate masses for their awareness and cooperation for action in various health issues.

21.6 UNITED NATIONS CHILDREN'S EMERGENCY FUND (UNICEF)

It was started on 11th December 1946, after the Second World War to rehabilitate children in war-ravaged countries. Since 1950, however, the fund is applicable to all underdeveloped countries. Hence, now the words 'international' and 'emergency' have been dropped from the name of the original organisation, viz. United Nations International Childrens' Emergency Fund. It is now called United Nations Children's Fund, but the abbreviation in vogue is still UNICEF. Its headquarter is at New York.

Like World Health Organisation, it is assisting 500 projects in 120 countries. It gives aid to all nations without discrimination of race, colour, political belief, etc. For administrative purposes of UNICEF, the whole world is divided into four regions, viz. (i) Asia with Bangkok as its headquarter, (ii) America, (iii) United Kingdom and Africa, and (iv) Europe, and Eastern Mediterranean countries.

UNICEF is administered by an Executive Director, under policies, including the determination of various programmes, allocation of funds, etc.

UNICEF India recognizes that the health, hygiene, nutrition, education, protection and social development of children are all connected. Targeting efforts for them at all stages of their growth—infant and mother, child and adolescent—and on a range of traditional programme fronts will see that inroads are made to ensure children not only survive, but thrive too.

Various projects aided by UNICEF in India: Under allocation of funds, approved until now, UNICEF is providing equipment and material, for 2,500 primary health centres and 7,000 sub-centres as well as for 163 hospitals and 111 laboratories which support them.

UNICEF is also providing vehicles to enable the staff of primary health centres and the district health teams to travel around their districts while performing their duties. Some of the projects and schemes on public health which had been initiated in India, after having received aid in the form of personnel and material from the UNICEF are the wellknown—BCG Campaign, Venereal Diseases Control Programme, Yaws Control Programme in hilly tracts of Madhya Pradesh, Hyderabad and Andhra, installation of a penicillin factory at Pimpri near Poona, a DDT factory near Delhi, dairy plants at Mumbai and at ten more centres, opening of maternity and child health and nursing training centres at Kolkata, a Paediatric Centre at Chennai, provision for dried skimmed milk to the needy children, nursing bags, etc. for lady health visitors, midwives and other equipment required for maternal and child health centres, etc.

21.6.1 Country Programme Action Plan (CPAP) (2013–2017)

Government of India and the United Nations Children's Fund on the core principle of life cycle approach have come up with CPAP 2013–2017. The programme is based on the acknowledgement that children and women face multiple deprivations at different stages of their life and that multidimensional problems need multipronged, intersectoral solutions. The overall goal is to advance the rights of children, adolescents and women to survival, growth, development, participation and protection by reducing inequities based on caste, ethnicity, gender, poverty, region or religion.

21.6.2 Millennium Development Goals

In September 2000, 189 countries including India signed the United Nations Millennium Declaration, committing to eradicating extreme poverty in all its forms by 2015. A set of time-bound and quantified goals and targets, called the Millennium Development Goals have been developed to track progress toward these commitments like reducing extreme poverty and hunger, disease control, environmental degradation and gender discrimination. The Millennium Development Goals (MDGs) include 8 goals, 21 targets and 60 indicators for measuring progress in the 15 years between 1990 and 2015, when the goals are expected to be met.

The Millennium Development Goals for 2015

Goal 1: Eradicate extreme poverty and hunger
Goal 2: Achieve universal primary education
Goal 3: Promote gender equality and empower women
Goal 4: Reduce child mortality
Goal 5: Improve maternal health
Goal 6: Combat HIV/AIDS, malaria and other diseases
Goal 7: Ensure environmental sustainability
Goal 8: Develop a global partnership for development

India's Progress Against the MDGs

Recognizing the challenges to meeting the Millennium Development Goals, the Government has in recent years implemented national flagship programmes for education, reproductive and child health, child development, child protection, child nutrition, and water and sanitation. Integrated Child Development Services (ICDS) Scheme has been restructured and universalized to respond to the challenges in child development.

Centrally sponsored schemes have increased public resources to key sectors, notably the Sarva Shiksha Abhiyan in education—the national policy to universalize primary education, the RMNCH + A and the National Health Mission. The challenge remains to convert these commitments and resources into measurable results for all children, especially those belonging to socially disadvantaged and marginalized communities to realize the Millennium Development Goals for India.

Current Status in India

Goal 1: Eradicate extreme poverty and hunger: Nearly 1/4th of the world's poor live in India. In 2012, the **Indian** government stated 20.6% of its population is below its official **poverty** limit. The World Bank, in 2011 based on 2005's PPPs International Comparison Program, estimated 21.3% of **Indian** population, or about 276 million people, lived below $1.9 per day on purchasing power parity.

As per the data available for undernutrition in children (NFHS) underweight in <3 yrs—46%, 47%. 51.5% (III, II, I). As per the Global Hunder Index 2009, over 40% of children in India are underweight, with South Asia exceeding in numbers than sub-Saharan Africa. This high percentage is matched by the much poorer African nation of Ethiopia. Only Bangladesh and Nepal have a higher child undernourishment rate at 48%.

Goal 2: Achieve universal primary education: Net enrolment ratio in primary education (% both sexes): 94.2

Percentage of pupils starting Grade 1 and reach Grade 5 (% both sexes): 94%.

Enrolment and completion rates of girls in primary school have improved and are catching up with those of boys, as are elementary completion rates. In light of the Right of Children to Free and Compulsory Education Act (RTE), the challenges now are the quality of education, school results below expectations and completion of upper primary education, particularly among girls, children in rural areas and those belonging to minority groups, and those students in the poorest sections of society.

Goal 3: Promote gender equality and empower women: Gender parity index in primary level enrolment (ratio of girls to boys): 1.0

Literacy rates of 15–24 years old (% both sexes): 82.1.

Goal 4: Reduce child mortality: Mortality rate of children under 5 years old (per 1,000 live births): 48 (2015, world bank) 1-year-old children immunized against measles (%): 74% (2013, undata).

The large scale of undernutrition in expectant mothers and children poses a challenge for India in reaching the Millennium Development Goals on child nutrition, survival and development. On a positive note, recent government efforts in restructuring the Integrated Child Development Services (ICDS) and other initiatives like Janani Shishu Suraksha Karyakram (JSSK), setting up of nutrition rehabilitation corners (NRCs) and sick newborn care units (SNCUs) and other intervention under National Health Mission are evidences of the national commitment to holistic child development.

Goal 5: Improve maternal health: With a maternal mortality ratio (MMR) of 170 deaths per 100,000 live births, India is making progress on Millennium Development Goal 5. One contributing factor has been the introduction of interventions like setting up and functionalization of First Referral Units (FRUs), Indira Gandhi Matritva Sahyogini Yojana (IGMSY) and Janani Suraksha Yojana (JSY) for better access and utilization of emergency and routine obstetric services.

Goal 6: Combat HIV/AIDS, malaria and other diseases: People living with HIV, 15–49 years old (%): 0.26 (2015).

Goal 7: Ensure environmental sustainability: Access to safe drinking water sources (% of total population): 94% (WHO–UNICEF JMP, 2015).

Goal 8: Develop a global partnership for development: Internet users (per 100 people): 10.7.

States have the major role in putting in place programmes to meet the Millennium Development Goals since the responsibility for implementing most of the social sector programmes relating to the goals lies with state governments. A major task for India is the improvement of service delivery and capacity development at district and local levels in order to implement and monitor very large programmes.

Sustainable Development Goals (SDGs)

In September 2015, Heads of State and Government agreed to set the world on a path towards sustainable development through the adoption of 2030 Agenda for Sustainable Development. This agenda includes 17 Sustainable Development Goals, or SDGs, which set out quantitative objectives across the social, economic, and environmental dimensions of sustainable development—all to be achieved by 2030 (Fig. 21.2).

The goals provide a framework for shared action "for people, planet and prosperity," to be implemented by "all countries and all stakeholders, acting in collaborative partnership". As articulated in the 2030

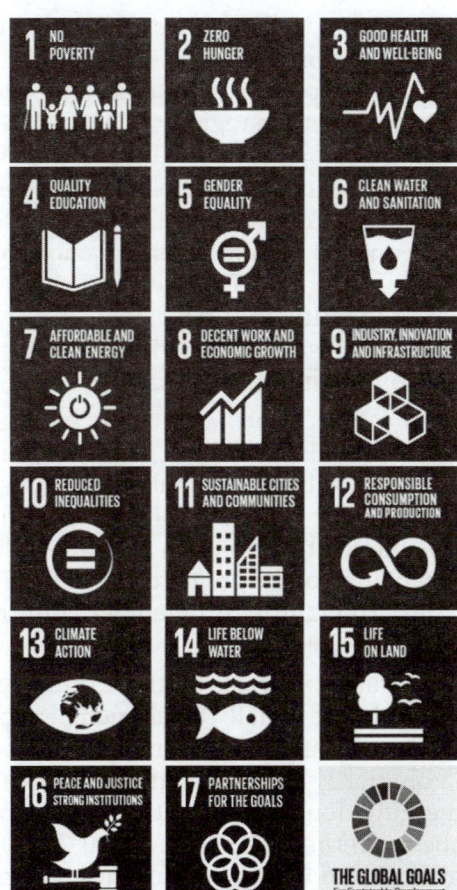

Fig. 21.2: Sustainable development goals—to be achieved by 2030

agenda "never before have world leaders pledged common action and endeavour across such a broad and universal policy agenda". 169 targets accompany the 17 goals and set out quantitative and qualitative objectives for the next 15 years. These targets are "global in nature and universally applicable, taking into account different national realities, capacities and levels of development and respecting national policies and priorities".

21.7 COLOMBO PLAN

The Colombo Plan was established on 1 July 1951 by Australia, Canada, India, Pakistan, New Zealand, Sri Lanka and the United Kingdom and currently has expanded to include 26 member countries including non-commonwealth countries and countries belonging to regional groupings such as ASEAN (Association of South East Asian Nations) and SAARC (South Asian Association for Regional Cooperation). The Colombo Plan is a partnership concept of self-help and mutual-help in development aimed at socioeconomic progress of its member countries.

The organisation structure of Colombo Plan

a. *Consultative Committee (CCM):* Comprising of all member governments, is the highest review and policy-making body of the Colombo Plan. It provides a forum for the exchange of views on current development problems and review of development work in region.

b. *The Colombo Plan Council:* Comprising heads of diplomatic missions of member governments who are resident in Colombo, Sri Lanka. The President of the Council is nominated from among member countries annually. The Council meets every quarter to identify important development issues to ensure the smooth implementation of the Consultative Committee's decisions.

c. *The Colombo Plan Secretariat:* Headed by a secretary-general is located in Colombo, Sri Lanka, since 1951 and functions as the secretariat for the Consultative Committee and the Council. The Secretariat is responsible for the effective administration and implementation of the programmes of the Colombo Plan, in partnership with member countries and collaborating agencies.

The administrative costs of the Council and the Secretariat are borne equally by all member countries. However, the training programmes of the Colombo Plan are voluntarily funded by traditional as well as newly emerging donors among its member countries, nonmember governments and regional/international organizations. The Colombo Plan has 4 permanent programmes: (i) Drug Advisory Programme (DAP), (ii) Programme for Public Administration and Environment (PPA and ENV), (iii) Programme for Private Sector Development (PPSD), and (iv) Long-term Scholarships Programme (LTSP).

The main aim of the Colombo Plan is to achieve a momentum of economic progress which will make it possible for the countries to go forward in self-reliant growth. Under the Colombo Plan, India got financial assistance for the establishment of All India Institute of Medical Sciences, New Delhi. In the field of health also the Plan has rendered valuable assistance in tuberculosis work, antimalarial work, nursing education in the case of crippled, etc. in collaboration with international bodies like WHO, UNICEF, etc.

21.8 OTHER AGENCIES

a. **CARE (Co-operative for American Relief Everywhere):** It was established in 1946 and is a non-governmental American agency. It has been assisting since 1951, state governments in the mid-day meal scheme, for school children and providing equipment, medicines, X-ray plants, etc. to various institutions in India.

Rockefeller Foundation: It was founded in 1913 and is an old philanthropic institution. It started working in India in 1920. It is giving grants for various welfare works. Its main contribution is

rendering of help in the establishment of All India Institute of Hygiene and Public Health at Kolkata.

Ford Foundation: It is an old philanthropic institution. It is working in India to promote rural health service, family planning, research programmes, etc.

b. **Bilateral single government agency:** That provides aid to lesser developed countries. They usually deal directly with other government, e.g. USAID, DANIDA, Colombo Plan and SIDA.

c. **Non-governmental organisations:** They include humanitarian (philanthropic agencies) and professional organizations concerned with global health. These are not under government sponsorships or control, e.g. International Red Cross, Rockefeller Foundation, Ford Foundation, CARE, etc.

Functions of VHA/NGO

1. Direct services or assistance to individual for patient care, nursing, visiting service, provision of consultations. Training and supervision of voluntary workers, preparation and dissemination of public information materials, provides materials for HE and carries on mass health education works.
2. Supplementing the work of official agencies.
3. Contributing the funds for special equipment or other supplementary assistance to service agencies.
4. Financial assistance through scholarships or training grants.
5. Guide the work of official agencies and provides constructive ideas.
6. Advances the health legislation
7. Exhibits demonstration and experimental project. Demonstration of borehole latrine by RF to solve the problem of hookworm in India. RCA latrine has become essential part of environmental sanitation programme.
8. Supplement the efforts of govt. during disasters and emergencies.
9. Effective policy formulation through interpretation of public opinions.
10. Carries on research to explore ways and means of doing new thing, autonomous board helps flexibility to adopt the programme.
11. Channelize human resources and help in efficient programme implementation.
12. VHA take initiation and believes in self-help rather than help from outside, they encourage the local potential leaders to develop as agents of socio-economic change.
13. Creating greater understanding and a positive attitude among the beneficiaries.

21.9 LEVELS OF CARE

Three levels of healthcare are primary, secondary and tertiary and a robust referral system forms the backbone of the three-tier referral system.

Primary level of healthcare: Primary healthcare denotes the first level of contact between individuals and families with the health system. According to Alma Ata Declaration of 1978, primary healthcare was to serve the community and it included care for mother and child which included family planning, immunization, prevention of locally endemic diseases, treatment of common diseases or injuries, provision of essential facilities, health education, provision of food and nutrition and adequate supply of safe drinking water.

In India, primary healthcare is provided through a network of sub-centres and primary health centres in rural areas, whereas in urban areas, it is provided through health posts and family welfare centres. The sub-centre consists of one auxiliary nurse midwife and multipurpose health worker and serves a population of 5000 in plains and 3000 persons in hilly and tribal areas. The primary health centre (PHC), staffed by medical officer and other paramedical staff, serves every 30,000 population in the plains and 20,000 persons in hilly, tribal and backward areas. Each PHC is to supervise 6 sub-centres.

Secondary level of healthcare: Secondary healthcare refers to a second-tier of health system, in which patients from primary healthcare are referred to specialists in higher hospitals for treatment. In India, the health centres for secondary healthcare include district hospitals and community health centres at block level (Fig. 21.3).

Tertiary level of healthcare: Tertiary healthcare refers to a third level of health system, in which specialized consultative care is provided usually on referral from primary and secondary medical care. Specialised intensive care units, advanced diagnostic support services and specialized medical personnel on the key features of tertiary healthcare. In India, under public health system, tertiary care service is provided by medical colleges and advanced medical research institutes (Fig. 21.1).

21.10 PRIMARY HEALTHCARE

As per WHO (2003), primary healthcare is essential healthcare made universally accessible to the community, by means acceptable to them, through their full participation and at a cost the community and country can afford. The key principles of primary healthcare are:

1. **Essential healthcare** which means five components health promotion, disease prevention, restoration, rehabilitation and support.

2. **Equitable distribution and universally accessible:** Healthcare is equally accessible (financially, culturally, functionally and geographically) to all.

3. **Community participation:** Individual, family and community involvement in the needs identification, assessment, planning, implementation and evaluation of healthcare services.

4. **Appropriate technology,** i.e. procedures, techniques and equipment must be scientifically valid, adapted to local needs, and acceptable to clients and providers within available resources.

5. Since health is not a subject in seclusion, other components that are determinants of health such as education, housing, nutrition, and other socioeconomic determinants must be included in comprehensive healthcare delivery system.

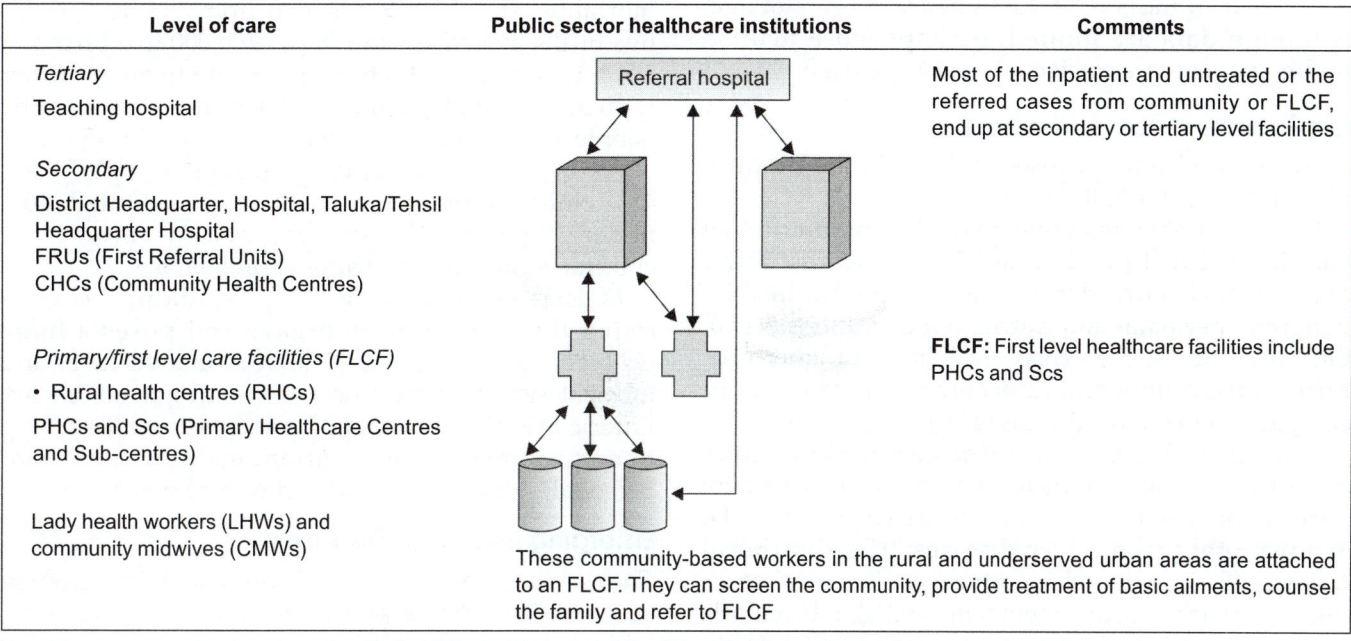

Fig. 21.3: Overview of public healthcare system

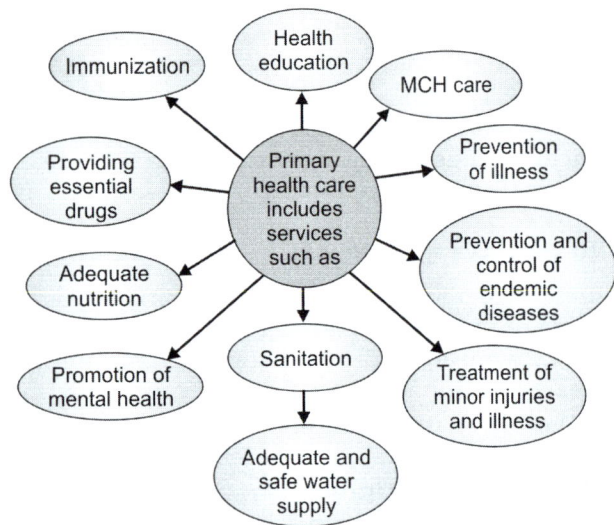

Fig. 21.4: Elements of primary healthcare

21.11 COMMON PUBLIC HEALTH PROBLEMS IN INDIA

India is passing through demographic and environmental transition due to which there is triple burden of diseases, viz. communicable, non-communicable and emerging infectious diseases.

Communicable Diseases

India has the highest number of TB cases in the world. Of the cases of TB that occur in the world every year, about one-fifth occur in India. Experts estimate that nearly 7.6% of the global burden of HIV is contributed by India alone. More than 1.5 million persons are affected with malaria every year, of which almost 50% suffer from falciparum malaria. One-third of global cases infected with filarial disease live in India. More than 300 million episodes of acute diarrhoea occur every year in India in children below 5 years of age. Although data are limited, perhaps more than 35 million persons are carriers of viral hepatitis B.

Non-communicable Diseases

They are the leading causes of death in the country, constituting 42% of all deaths.

Communicable, maternal, perinatal and nutritional conditions constitute another 38% of deaths. Rural areas report more deaths due to communicable, maternal, perinatal and nutritional conditions (41%). On the contrary, the urban areas have a higher proportion from noncommunicable diseases (56%) in comparison to the rural areas (40%).

Overall, the leading cause of death is cardiovascular disease (19%), followed by respiratory diseases (namely chronic obstructive pulmonary disease or COPD, asthma, other respiratory diseases; 9%), diarrhoeal diseases (8%), perinatal conditions (6.3%), respiratory infections such as acute pneumonia (6.2%), tuberculosis (6%), malignant and other neoplasms (5.7%), senility

(5.1%—which is concentrated at ages 70 and higher), unintentional injuries: other (4.9%), and symptoms, signs and illdefine conditions (4.8%).

(*Source*: Report on causes of death in India, 2001–03; Registrar General of India).

Besides, India has an estimated 2–2.5 million cancer patients in India at any point of time with an incidence of more than 7 lakh cases of every year. India has the highest number of blind persons in the world.

National Family Health Survey III has revealed that more than 56% of the women in India have some degree of anaemia and about one-third are undernourished. Similarly, three-fourths of young children are also anaemic.

Prospects of polio eradication in the near future are very bright. Last case of polio in January 2011 in West Bengal, UP and Bihar. The traditional pockets of polio have not reported a case for a long time. India has been declared as polio-free in 2014 and the efforts towards global eradication are ongoing.

Cases of malaria have been reduced to less than 2 million annually from 75 million in early 1950s.

Revised National Tuberculosis Control Programme (RNTCP), launched in 1997, presently covers the entire country and detects over 70% of new sputum cases with treatment success rate of 87%. TB mortality has decreased from over 5 lakh deaths every year at the beginning of programme to about 2.8 lakh deaths presently despite growth in population.

Life expectancy has increased from 36.5 years in 1951 to more than 63.1 years. While crude birth rate declined from 40.8 in 1951 to 21.4 in 2014, crude death rate declined from 25.1 in 1951 to 7 in 2014. Infant mortality rate (IMR) declined from 146 per 1000 live births in 1951 to 44 per 1000 live births in 2014. Maternal mortality ratio (MMR) declined from 398 per 100,000 live births in 1997–98 to 178 per 100,000 live births in 2014. However, India has a long way to go in further reducing mortality among infants, mothers and the people in the most productive age groups (15–45 years).

As per data available from NFHS3 (2005–06), 45% children under 3 years of age are stunted, 40% underweight and 23% stunted, i.e. a vast majority of children suffer from nutritional problems.

Malaria after reaching a point of eradication is again rising through local outbreaks and poses a huge problem again. Leprosy 32 lakh estimated cases and tuberculosis (1.8% prevalence) still claim high morbidities. Enteric infections are claiming increasing tolls owing to environmental insanitation, malnutrition, poor personal, community, food and water hygiene.

Emerging Infectious Diseases

They are a major public health problem in developing countries like India. Because of the existing environmental, socioeconomic and demographic factors, developing countries like India are vulnerable to rapidly evolving micro-organisms. During the past three decades, more than 30 new organisms have been identified worldwide including HIV, *Vibrio cholerae* O139, SARS, corona virus, highly pathogenic avian influenza virus A, and novel H1N1 influenza virus. Many of these organisms emerged in the developing countries of Asia. Infectious diseases, especially the new emerging and re-emerging diseases, result in high morbidity and mortality and affect the public health and economy adversely. For example, plague which was not reported from any part of India for almost a quarter of the century, caused a major outbreak in Beed district in Maharashtra and Surat in Gujarat in 1994 and resulted in huge economic loss to the country.

In the recent times, avian influenza virus A H5N1 created pandemic scare by affecting birds/poultry in more than 60 countries including India and affecting human beings in 15 countries. But pandemic finally occurred due to novel H1N1 virus in 2009. As of 20th of November 2009, more than 0.5 million cases and 6770 deaths due to lab confirmed novel H1N1 infections have been reported to WHO by more than 206 countries, although countries are no longer required to test and report all cases.

A network of national health programmes and peripheral rural services has been developed to control and prevention of diseases of public health importance and ensure health for all.

Control of diseases of public health importance. A few of the health programmes in place that are being implemented for public health problems are:

1. National Malaria Control Programme—launched in 1953 followed by National Eradication Programme in April 1958.
2. National Tuberculosis Programme in 1955 revised in 1994 (Revised National Tuberculosis Programme).
3. Reproductive and Child Health Programme (RCH) now revised to RMNCH + A with additional 'adolescent health component'.
4. National Leprosy Elimination Programme in 1955.
5. National Programme for Control of Blindness (NPCB).
6. National Vector-borne Disease Control Programme (NVBDCP).
7. Applied Nutrition Programme.

The details of these programmes have been discussed with respective diseases/health problems.

HEALTH PLANNING

21.12 COMMUNITY DEVELOPMENT PROGRAMME

Community is a social group in which the individual members have some shared values, attitudes and interests.

Basically, the concept of community development is multidimensional as distinguished from the development relating to particular aspects. Community development is a process of change from the existing traditional way to the modern progressive way. In this efforts of the people themselves are united with those of the government authorities to improve the economic, social and cultural conditions of communities, to integrate these communities into the life of the nation and to enable them to contribute fully to national progress.

In 1952, during the First Five-Year Plan, a beginning was made for the purpose of involving the rural population in the process of planning for their own benefit and welfare schemes. Thus, a programme called Community Development Programme was launched on 2nd October 1952 for the overall development and progress of rural India, which at present covers about 80% of its total population. At that time, the programme was given a wide publicity and was termed as a programme "for the people, by the people and of the people" and was meant to eradicate poverty, ill health, ignorance and disease. In this programme, area to be covered was divided into various blocks, i.e. community development blocks. Each block comprised about 100 villages or even more to cater to the needs of about one lakh population. About 6000 community development blocks were established in the country and each was put under the charge of a block development officer. The programme was considered as a composite multipurpose programme covering almost all the main activities, with which rural population was to come into contact with, i.e. improvement of health, education, sanitation, environment, housing, social welfare, agriculture, industry, etc. But, however, the programme could not achieve its objectives fully due to several factors and its benefits did not reach poor rural population, for whom the programme was initially launched.

21.13 INTEGRATED RURAL DEVELOPMENT PROGRAMME

Subsequently, another programme, i.e. IRDP was launched by Government of India to eradicate rural poverty, ignorance and disease in April 1978. This scheme aimed to improve the lot of rural poor especially small cultivators, landless agricultural labourers, village artisans, craftsmen, etc. granting them subsidy and bank loans on easy terms and imparting them basic training in their respective progessions. The scheme was implemented through District Rural Development Agency (DRDA). Although a huge outlay of ₹2358 crores was provided by Government of India for implementation of this project during the Seventh Five-Year Plan, yet this programme also failed to achieve its targets.

Village worker/gram sewak was identified as the key person to carry out the message about the programme and make them aware about the aims and objectives.

21.14 HEALTH CENTRE APPROACH

In 1858 Danish Act of Parliament introduced Health by law for towns and rural parishads. In 1860, Norway enacted an act under which all local areas were required to establish a board of health. Soon it was followed in Netherlands and Austria. In 1872, Britain divided the whole country in sanitary areas with a locally elected committee.

The concept of comprehensive healthcare, i.e. organised utilisation of medical resources adjusted to needs of the community healthcare, of a preventive and curative nature, to achieve social goals, in health promotion, protection, preservation, and rehabilitation, gained momentum in the beginning of 20th century. Thus, it became necessary to approach the community health problems along integrated rather than fragmented lines.

'Health centre' was identified as functional institution from where all the components of healthcare, viz. curative, preventive and promotive would be delivered to the community, was first conceived in Dawson's report of 1920. It provided the health authorities with a logical approach for extension of health services, particularly in rural areas. After the World War I, Russia, Yugoslavia and Turkey drew fresh plans for public health programmes on the following principles: (i) health centre as a basis of operation, (ii) preponderance of preventive medicine, (iii) complete integration of preventive and curative service, (iv) medicine as a social service, and (v) community participation.

21.15 HEALTH PLANNING IN INDIA

It forms an integral part of national socioeconomic planning and formulates the guidelines for effective execution of decisions in order to achieve the desired results. The Government of India constituted the following committees from time to time to analyse the current situation and suggest changes accordingly:

1.	Bhore Committee	1946
2.	Mudaliar Committee	June 1959
3.	Chadha Committee	1963
4.	Mukherjee Committee	1965
5.	Kartar Singh Committee	1973
6.	Shrivastav Committee	1975

Each of these committees made recommendations from time to time after analyzing the then situation to improve the public health scenario in India. As part of their suggestions, a Family Planning Programme was launched in 1953. During 1963, family planning programme was integrated with, primary health centres. Each committee improved the work done by the previous one. Finally a three-tier programme, consisting of primary health centres, district hospital, and a medical college and hospital, would help and provide the three-tier for the healthcare in any particular region.

Medical Council of India was constituted in 1956 at the centre and was entrusted with the task of regulating and standardising medical education in the country. The state level medical councils, created under state legislation, were then entrusted with registering of qualified medical practitioners and providing a disciplinary from for public grievances against doctors.

21.16 RURAL HEALTH SCHEME

By far the most important recommendation made by Shrivastav Committee was that primary healthcare should be made available in the country itself through the specially trained workers, so that people themselves are directly involved in their health. In 1977, in acceptance of the recommendation of this committee by the Government of India, the Rural Health Scheme was launched.

Under the scheme, necessary steps were taken for the Reorientation of Medical Education (ROME) to meet the needs of the rural people and training of multipurpose workers already engaged in the control of various communicable diseases workers. ROME Scheme was to involve medical colleges in the total healthcare of the community through primary health centres (PHC) of the relevant area.

This plan was adopted for implementation by the joint meeting of Central Council of Health and Central Family Planning Council held in New Delhi in April 1976.

21.17 HEALTH FOR ALL BY THE YEAR 2000 AD

The World Health Assembly in 1977 decided to launch a movement known as "the Health for all by the year 2000 AD". The member countries of WHO defined "Health for All" at the 30th World Health Assembly as "attainment of a level of health that will enable every individual to lead a socially and economically productive life".

The Alma Ata International Conference for Primary Healthcare in 1978 reaffirmed "Health for All" as the major social goal of the government. It was decided to provide primary healthcare to the rural population as well as urban poor so that by the year 2000 AD at least essential healthcare and medical services are provided to the people, which may be conducive for the betterment of their health and longevity.

The Government of India was a signatory to Alma Ata and thus strategically strived to provide "Health for All" to its citizens by 2000 AD. To achieve the desired objective, two reports have been taken into consideration, (i) report of the Study Group on "Health for All—An Alternative Strategy" sponsored by ICMR and (ii) report of the working group on "Health for All by 2000 AD" sponsored by the Government of India, Ministry of Health and Family Welfare. These reports eventually formed the basis of the National Health Policy formulated by Government of India in 1982.

National Health Policy 1983: It was finally approved and adopted by the Indian Parliament in 1983. It had laid down certain specific goals relating to health standards to be achieved by the year 2000 AD as per details given in (Table 21.3).

Table 21.3: As per national health policy

Goals to be achieved by 2005–2015

Goals	Target years
Eradicate polio and yaws	2005
Eliminate leprosy	2005
Eliminate kala azar	2010
Eliminate lymphatic filariasis	2015
Achieve zero level growth of HIV/AIDS	2007
Reduce mortality by 50% on account of TB, malaria and other vector and water-borne diseases	2010
Reduce prevalence of blindness to 0.5%	2010
Reduce IMR to 30/1000 and MMR to 100/lakh	2010
Increase utilisation of public health facilities from current level of <20 to >75%	2010
Establish an integrated system of Surveillance, National Health Accounts and Health Statistics	2005
Increase health expenditure by government as a % of GDP from the existing 0.9 to 2.0%	2010
Increase share of central grants to constitute at least 25% of total health spending	2010
Increase state sector health spending from 5.5 to 7% of the budget	2005
Further increase to 8%	2010

21.18 DECENTRALISED PLANNING

The National Rural Health Mission (NRHM) and RCH Programme proposed the decentralisation of health planning so that the state health plan represents the needs and priorities of respective villages, blocks and districts in the state.

21.19 PLANNING COMMISSION*

The planning commission was set up in March 1950 in pursuance of declared objectives of the Government to promote a rapid rise in the standard of living of the people by efficient exploitation of the resources of the country, increasing production and offering opportunities to all for employment in the service of the community.

Five-Year Plans: After independence in 1947, government realised that nation's health is perhaps the most potent single factor in determining the character and extent of its development and progress and any effort on improving the national health and expenditure of money in respect thereto was an investment, which yielded immediate and steady returns in increased productive capacity. It was also realised to rebuild rural India so as to lay the foundations of industrial progress for the balanced development of all parts of the country. Hence, since 1951 onwards, various Five-Year Plans were announced.

First Five-Year Plan	(1951–56)
Second Five-Year Plan	(1956–61)
Third Five-Year Plan	(1961–66)
3-Year Plan Holiday	(1966–69)
Fourth Five-Year Plan	(1969–74)
Fifth Five-Year Plan	(1974–79)
Plan Holiday	(1979–80)
Sixth Five-Year Plan	(1980–85)
Seventh Five-Year Plan	(1985–90)
Annual Plans	(1990–92)
Eighth Five-Year Plan	(1992–97)
IXth Plan	(1997–2002)
Xth Plan	(2002–07)
XIth Plan	(2007–2012)
XIIth Plan	(2012–2017)

Eighth Five-Year Plan (1992–97): In this plan, a total of ₹798,000 crores was provided by Government of India, as total plan outlay. Out of this a sum of nearly ₹7,576 crores was earmarked for improvement of health and ₹6,500 crores for family welfare programmes. Earlier under the Seventh Plan during 1985, in order to achieve the goal of health for all by 2000 AD, a Health Information Policy was formulated, which recommended the launching of a Plan of "Health

Table 21.4: Goals for some selected fertility/mortality indicators

Indicator	Tenth Plan Goals (2002–2007)	RC-II Goals (2005–2010)	NPP-2000 Goals (by 2010)	Millennium Development Goals
Infant Mortality Rate	<45/1000	<30/1000	<30/1000	–
Under-five Mortality	–	–	–	Reduce by 2/3 from 1990 levels by 2015
Maternal Mortality Ratio	200/100000	<100/100000	<100/100000	Reduce by 3/4 from 1990 levels by 2015
Total Fertility Rate	2.3	2.1	2.1	–
Couple Protection Rate	65%	65%	100%	–

* NITI Aayog has now replaced Planning Commission.

Information for All by 1990" to provide necessary infrastructure for healthcare services.

Broadly speaking, the plan was keeping with certain major policy initiatives taken with the launching of Eigth Five-Year Plan to promote overall growth, industrial development, reinforcement of antipoverty programmes and to give a new direction to the fiscal policy. Besides, it aimed at affecting further improvement in the various public health and other programmes already launched by the Government in the previous plans.

The Twelfth Plan has set a target of 8% growth over the five-year period 2012–13 to 2016–17. The Twelfth Plan seeks to strengthen initiatives taken in the Eleventh Plan to expand the reach of healthcare and work towards the long-term objective of establishing a system of Universal Health Coverage (UHC) in the country. Health services will be delivered with seamless integration between primary, secondary and tertiary sectors. The primary healthcare will be strengthened to deliver both preventive public health and curative clinical services. Publicly funded healthcare would predominantly be delivered by public providers. Private sector will be contracted in only for critical gap filling. In areas where both public and private contracted in providers coexist, patients shall have a choice in selecting their provider. No fee of any kind would be levied on primary healthcare services with the primary source of financing being from general taxation/public exchequer.

Chapter
22

Social Medicine

For a philosophical background of the evolution of social medicine, one should study: (a) the history of the evolution of medicine, (b) the definitions given by various authors to social medicine during various phases of evolution of social medicine, and (c) patterns of health services available in India and over the world.

22.1 MAN, SOCIETY AND SOCIAL MEDICINE

The term social medicine includes two words, i.e. social (pertaining to society) and medicine. Socious means fellow or comrade and society means group or a community of men. Man is a socious in a societas an individual comrade in a group of community. Development begins in the prenatal period followed by natal and postnatal stages. Braodly a man's life can be divided into various stages for convenience to study the problems related to different periods: (a) perinatal, i.e. first seven days and neonatal, i.e. within a month, (b) infant—one month to one year, (c) preschool child or toddler—one to five years, (d) school child—5 to 15 years, (e) adolescence—10 to 19 years, and (f) adulthood—19 years and above.

The social unit of society is the family. A family is a group of individuals related to each other by blood or law and sharing the common kitchen. The biosocial functions of a family begin with marriage followed by:
a. Residence
b. Sharing of responsibilities/division of labour
c. Procreation and child rearing
d. Economic functions
e. Socialization
f. Care to sick and elderly.

A group of families share the same geographical area, values and services of the common organizations, i.e. markets, banks, hospitals constitute a community. Society is a broader term which means an organized system of members that controls and regulates the behaviour of an individual both by customs and laws.

Public health is an essential part of social system because its acceptance and translation into results is influenced by the norms that the society follows.

22.2 SOCIAL MEDICINE

Social medicine is the study of physical, social, economical, environmental, cultural, psychological and genetic factors, which have a bearing on health. Medical sociology (sociology of health and illness) is concerned with all those aspects of contemporary social life which impinge upon well-being throughout the life.

Compared to medicine, social anatomy (structure), social physiology (functions), social pathology (deviations from health), social diagnosis (health statistics) and social therapeutics (management aspects of health services) are to be studied in social medicine.

22.3 SOCIAL STRUCTURE/SOCIAL ANATOMY

Social structure is like the anatomy of the society that comprises the group of major institutions, groups, power structure and status hierarchy. It basically refers to the pattern of inter-relations between persons. The family, school, church, panchayats, etc. are the examples of few social organizations that are important to allocate roles to each individual that are part of that society. Roles are classified as 'ascribed' and 'achieved' by the sociologists, i.e. the roles that a person is required to fulfil by virtue of birth or by virtue of education and social status respectively. Socialization is a process by which an individual is trained gradually to conform to the ascribed social norms and productively contribute to the society.

There are various formal and informal rules that serve as social control mechanisms to control the behaviour of individuals and efficiently play different roles ascribed to them by the society. The laws and enactments are the formal mechanisms whereas the informal pressure may be exerted by the powerful groups, resident welfare associations (RWAs), members of Panchayat, local leaders, etc. The health seeking behaviour of an individual depends upon these formal and informal control mechanisms to an extent.

Social control mechanisms: A norm that is written down and enforced by an official law enforcement agency is the formal social control mechanism.

Informal mechanisms of control have a stronger influence on disease and health seeking. Some informal social control mechanisms that influence the health seeking behaviour of the people are:

a. *Customs:* Customs usually arise out of conventions of a society and are practices accepted and approved by the society. These inspire the laws and are technically divided into "Folklores" and "Mores". Folklores convey a moral lesson and present useful information and everyday life lessons in an easy way for the common people. Whereas 'mores' are strict norms that control moral and ethical behaviour. Individuals who do not follow social mores are often considered social deviants, e.g. women are prohibited from going to temples to worship during menstruation is a 'more'. A norm that society holds so strongly that violating it results in extreme disgust is known as taboo. A taboo can be defined as the social or religious custom prohibiting or restricting a particular practice or forbidden associations with or particular place, person or thing. For example, homosexuality in India, certain professions like hangers executionists, scavangers, etc. are still a taboo in context to Indian society.

b. *Culture:* It is defined as "learned behaviour that has been socially acquired" and lays down norms of behaviour. Cultural factors have deep roots in personal hygiene, immunization, maternal and child care, family planning and nutrition and thus have a significant role in health and disease, e.g. culturally women are restricted with some foods after delivery that might lead to nutritional deficiency in them.

Acculturation is the process of transition and of people into a new cultural environment to adapt to the new culture's behaviours, values, customs and language. Various aspects of the lifestyle of particular cultural groups like dietary habits, patterns of physical activity, etc. may affect the development of specific diseases. Beliefs about causes, treatment, and prevention of illnesses may affect the utilization of health services. People migrating from plains to coastal areas may start eating seafood, which is more readily available in the new settings.

22.4 SOCIAL PHYSIOLOGY

Sociophysiology is a special science that studies the physiological side of interrelations between human. It explores the "intimate relationship and mutual regulation between social and physiological systems that is especially vital in human groups". It encompasses a dynamic system of interpersonal relationships that change continuously during their existence. The interaction between the social factors and health issues is dynamic and depends upon the psychology of the individuals and community.

Social Psychology and Health Behaviour

Social psychology is a discipline that tries to understand the human social behaviour. A change in behaviour and/or belief occurs due to societal influence when the individuals conform to a group norm as a result of real or imagined group pressure.

Health behaviour refers to the activities, people undertake to prevent disease and actions they take to regain health, e.g. regular practice of washing hands before cooking and eating can prevent food-borne and new water-borne infections. Good water storing and drawing practices can also prevent the diseases transmitted by unclean hands and unclean water. Thus, the preventive measures people take depends upon their perception about the cause of illness. Also their treatment seeking behaviour will depend upon their perception of aetiology of the disease. Whether the cause of disease is perceived to be supernatural or rational, the treatment modality is chosen accordingly. Thus, selection of preventive and treatment modality depends upon the **perception** of the community and individuals. There may be errors in perception: (a) Inability to recognise or imperception, (b) false perception or illusion, and (c) imaginary perception or hallucinations.

Attitudes are the complexes of ideas and sentiments. It refers to disposition of men to view an object, subject or concept in a particular manner and act accordingly. Every attitude has three components that are represented in what is called the **ABC model of attitudes where** A is for affective, B for behavioral, and C for cognitive.

The **affective** component refers to the emotional reaction one has toward an attitude, object, or idea. For example, an individual has anxiety and fear of, for some unknown reason, oral polio vaccine to his 2-year-old son. He will not allow his two-year-old son to be vaccinated is the **behavioural** component, which means it refers to the way one behaves when exposed to an attitude. The third and final component of an attitude is the **cognitive** component, which refers to the thoughts and beliefs one has about an attitude object. In this example, cognitive component is 'What does this individual think about oral polio vaccine that makes him avoid allowing his child to be vaccinated'? Thus, attitudes are acquired by social interactions through change in the cognitive component, i.e. correct knowledge will lead to change in attitude.

Beliefs: A belief is an idea which one expects to be true or real. Beliefs are held very strong and are difficult to change. They are socially derived from our parents, grandparents, friends, etc. They can be negative, positive or harmful for the health behaviour. In the above example, the belief could be that oral polio drops will lead to some physical deformity in my child. Thus, this might lead to failure of OPV campaign in that particular area, if this belief is prevalent community wide.

Behaviour: It is the way an individual or community conducts itself to a particular situation. It is important for maintaining and seeking health, thus efforts need to be made to promote and encourage healthy behaviours to achieve goal of 'Health'.

Behaviour Change Communication

Behaviour change communication (BCC) is an interactive process of any intervention with individuals, communities and/or societies (as integrated with an overall programme) to develop **communication** strategies to promote positive **behaviours** which are appropriate to their settings.

The stages in behavior change are

1. **Precontemplation:** In this stage, an individual receives ideas about things he might need to change but has not started accepting the benefits of the intended change in behavior. For example, if we try to tell an individual about the benefits of exercise, he may get the knowledge about the benefits of exercise but may not think of exercising himself.

2. **Contemplation:** The individual actively begins to think about the need to change a behaviour, to fully wrap our minds around the idea. This stage involves the change of an idea (exercise is important) into a deeply held belief (I need to exercise). For example, it may not be the high cholesterol level that gets the overweight women to begin exercising but rather her inability to keep up with her daily routine. This stage comes by finding and activating a *motivating belief*.

3. **Determination:** In this stage, the individual begins preparing mentally and often physically for action. This mustering of a determination is the culmination of the decision to change and fuels an individual towards his goal. This stage is when there begins a change in attitude of an individual towards a desired behaviour.

4. **Action:** This is the stage when the knowledge is translated into action thus desired behaviour takes the shape of 'action' or 'practice'. Knowledge is finally translated into practice through change in attitude.

5. **Maintenance:** This is *continuing* practising the desired behaviour till it becomes a habit, i.e. exercising everyday, watching calories to lose weight and so on.

22.5 SOCIAL PATHOLOGY

Social pathology includes substance abuse, violence, abuse of women and children, crime, terrorism, corruption, criminality, discrimination, isolation, stigmatisation and human rights violations. Social pathologies often lead to social, economic and psychological problems that undermine wellbeing.

Thus it's a social phenomenon that tends to increase social disorganization and unity of a particular society and inhibit personal adjustment. It includes unhealthy, abnormal and generally undesirable social behavioural patterns that interfere with moral, social, civil, political and economic issues and norms.

The study of social pathology is important to the maintenance of social health. Its aim is to identify the causes of social diseases and find ways to remove them.

Besides sociocultural factors, poverty and economy have been identified as one of the major causes of social pathology. Thus, prevention of social pathology needs education, employment, empowerment, strict legislation and ethical awareness.

Socioeconomic status (SES): It is an economic and sociological combined total measure of work experience of an individual's or family's economic and social position in relation to others, based on income, education, and occupation. SES is one of the most important social determinants of health, nutritional status, mortality and morbidity of an individual. It also influences the acceptability, affordability, accessibility and actual utilization of health services. There are various scales used to measure the SES of a family.

a. **BG Prasad Scale** is based on per capita monthly income. Per capita monthly income = Total monthly income of the family/Total members of family. Prasad's classification takes into consideration of income as a variable and it is simple to calculate. This can be applied to assess the socioeconomic status in both rural and urban areas. Depending upon the per capita income of the family, this scale classifies families from I–V.

For 2014	
SES class I	₹6012 and above
SES class II	₹2976–6011
SES class III	₹1762–2995
SES class IV	₹912–1761
SES class V	₹911

(AICI Cin) All India on Sept 2015 = 266)

b. Uday Parekh Scale for Rural Areas has nine characteristics, viz. based on nine characteristics, viz. caste, occupation, education, level of social participation of head of the family, landholding, housing, farm power, material possession and total members in the family is widely used.

Class categorization

Total score	Social class
Above 43	Upper class (I)
33–42	Upper middle class (II)
24–32	Middle class (III)
13–23	Lower middle class (IV)
Below 13	Lower class (V)

c. Modified Kuppu Swamy's Scale for Urban Areas: The social stratification is based on three main variables—education, occupation and income. For each factor, there are seven plausible alternatives which can be selected by the potential subjects. The range of scores which can be obtained is from 3 to 29 (Table 22.1).

Table 22.1: Social stratification scale (modified Kuppu Swamy)

Education	
Profession or honours	7
Graduate or postgraduate	6
Intermediate or post high school diploma	5
High school certificate	4
Middle school certificate	3
Primary school certificate	2
Illiterate	1
Occupation	
Profession	10
Semi-profession	6
Clerical, shop-owner, farmer	5
Skilled worker	4
Semi-skilled worker	3
Unskilled worker	2
Unemployed	1
Family income per month (in ₹)	
≥ 2000	12
1000–1999	10
750–999	6
500–749	4
300–499	3
101–299	2
≤ 100	1
Socioeconomic class	
Upper	26–29
Upper middle	16–25
Lower middle	11–15
Upper lower	5–10
Lower	0 < 5

Class categorization

Total score	Socioeconomic class
26–29	Upper (I)
16–25	Upper middle (II)
11–15	Middle (III)
05–10	Lower middle (IV)
<4	Lower (V)

d. Standard of living index: Standard of living refers to the level of **wealth,** comfort, material goods and necessities available to a certain **socioeconomic class** in a certain geographic area. The standard of living includes factors such as income, quality and availability of **employment,** class disparity, **poverty rate,** quality and affordability of housing, people, hours of work required to purchase necessities, **gross domestic product, inflation rate,** number of holiday days per year, affordable (or free) access to quality healthcare, quality and availability of **education,** life expectancy, incidence of disease, cost of goods and services, infrastructure, national economic growth, economic and political stability, political and religious freedom, environmental quality, climate and safety. The standard of living is closely related to quality of life. In 2013, the **Human Development Index** ranked the top six countries for quality of living as: **Norway, Australia, Switzerland, Netherlands, United States and Germany.**

22.6 SOCIAL WELFARE

The social welfare services are intended to cater to the special needs of persons and groups who by reason of some handicap, social, economic, physical, or mental, are unable to avail themselves of the amenities and services provided by the community. These vulnerable groups include women, adolescents, children, differently abled individuals, aged and infirm, scheduled castes and scheduled tribes.

In the year 1985–86, the Ministry of Welfare was bifurcated into the Department of Women and Child Development and the Department of Social Welfare. Simultaneously, the Scheduled Castes Development Division, Tribal Development Division and the Minorities and Backward Classes Welfare Division were moved from the ministry of Home Affairs and also the Wakf Division from the Ministry of Law to form the then Ministry of Social Welfare. Subsequently, the name of the Ministry was changed to the Ministry of Social Justice and Empowerment in May, 1998. Further, in October, 1999, the Tribal Development Division had moved out to form a separate Ministry of Tribal Affairs. In January, 2007, the Minorities Division along with Wakf Unit have been moved out of the ministry and formed as a separate ministry and the Child

Development Division has gone to the Ministry of Women and Child Development.

Department of Social Justice and Empowerment and Department of Disability Affairs have been **created under the Ministry of Social Justice and Empowerment with effect from May 14th, 2012.** The ministry has been implementing various programmes/schemes for social, educational and economic development of the target groups, i.e. scheduled castes, other backward classes, persons with disabilities and senior citizens and victims of substance abuse.

The Department of Women and Child Development was set up in 1985 as a part of the Ministry of Human Resource Development to give the much needed impetus to the holistic development of women and children which was later upgraded to Ministry (MoWCD) with effect from 2006. The role of MoWCD is to formulate plans, policies and programmes; enact/amend legislation, guide and coordinate the efforts of both governmental and non-governmental organisations working in the field of women and child development. The ministry also designs and implements certain innovative programmes for women and children from time to time. These programmes cover welfare and support services, training for employment and income generation, awareness generation and gender sensitization. All these efforts are directed towards women empowerment. Integrated Child Development Services (ICDS) scheme is one major intervention by the MoWCD providing a package of services comprising supplementary nutrition, immunization, health check up and referral services, preschool non-formal education. The scheme was launched in 1975 with the following objectives:

a. To improve the nutritional and health status of children in the age group 0–6 years.

b. To lay the foundation for proper psychological, physical and social development of the child.

c. To reduce the incidence of mortality, morbidity, malnutrition and school dropout.

d. To achieve effective co-ordination of policy and implementation amongst the various departments to promote child development.

e. To enhance the capability of the mother to look after the normal health and nutritional needs of the child through proper nutrition and health education.

Package of services includes supplementary nutrition, immunization, health check up and referral services, preschool non-formal education, of which immunisation, health check-up and referral services are delivered through public health infrastructure under the Ministry of Health and Family Welfare.

1. **Nutrition including supplementary nutrition:** This includes supplementary feeding and growth monitoring; prophylaxis against vitamin A deficiency and control of nutritional anaemia. Children below the age of six years and pregnant and nursing mothers are given supplementary feeding support for 300 days in a year.

Growth monitoring and nutrition surveillance are two important activities that are undertaken. Children below the age of three years are weighed once a month and children 3–6 years of age are weighed quarterly and their weight-for-age growth cards are maintained. This activity helps to detect children who are severely malnourished that are provided special supplementary feeding and referral to medical services. Children under 72 months of age who are registered with the Anganwadi are given 500 kcal and 12–15 gm proteins per day and 800 kcal and 20–25 gm proteins to severely malnourished children. Pregnant and lactating women are given 600 kcal and 18–20 gm of proteins per day at the Anganwadi centre.

2. **Immunization:** Immunization of pregnant women and infants as per the Mission Indradhanush, Universal Immunization Programme (UIP) to protect children vaccine preventable diseases—hepatitis B, poliomyelitis, diphtheria, pertussis, tetanus, tuberculosis and measles. Immunization of pregnant women against tetanus also reduces maternal and neonatal mortality. The services are provided by the ANM with the help of AWW.

3. **Health checkups:** This includes healthcare of children less than six years of age, antenatal care of expectant mothers and postnatal care of nursing mothers. Services provided by Anganwadi workers and primary health centre (PHC) staff, include regular health checkups, recording of weight, immunization, management of malnutrition, treatment of diarrhoea, deworming, etc.

4. **Referral services:** During health checkups and growth-monitoring, sick or malnourished children, in need of prompt medical attention, are referred to the primary health centre or its sub-centre by the Anganwadi worker (AWW).

5. **Non-formal preschool education (PSE):** The PSE programme is for the three- to six years old children who come to the Anganwadi and is directed towards providing and ensuring a natural, joyful and stimulating environment, with emphasis on necessary inputs for optimal growth and development. It prepares the child for primary schooling along with substitute care to younger siblings.

6. **Nutrition, health and education:** Nutrition, health and education (NHED) is a key element of the work of the Anganwadi worker. This forms part of BCC (behaviour change communication) strategy. This has the long-term goal of capacity-building of women—especially in the age group of

15–45 years—so that they can look after their own health, nutrition and development needs as well as that of their children and families.

ICDS is predominantly centrally funded programme with ratio of 90:10 (centre: state) in North Eastern states and all the other components in rest of the states except supplementary nutrition, where the share of the Central Government is 50% for the other states.

One Anganwadi is set at a population of 400–800 in rural and urban areas whereas over a population of 300–800 in hilly, tribal and difficult areas. The ICDS team comprises the Anganwadi workers, Anganwadi helpers, supervisors, child development project officers (CDPOs) and district programme officers (DPOs). Anganwadi worker is selected from the local community and is the community-based frontline honorary worker of the ICDS programme. She is also an agent of social change, mobilizing community support for better care of young children, girls and women. Besides, the medical officers, auxiliary nurse midwife (ANM) and accredited social health activist (ASHA) form a team with the ICDS functionaries to achieve convergence of different services.

Other important initiatives by MoWCD are **Kishori Shakti Yojana,** launching a nutrition programme for adolescent girls, establishment of the commission for protection of child rights and enactment of **Protection of Women from Domestic Violence Act.**

22.7 SOCIAL SECURITY

The progress and welfare of a society depends upon four important factors, which are as follows:
1. Education
2. Health
3. Social security
4. Production

It has been defined as the security, which the society provides for certain risks to which it's members may be exposed. Through social security, certain benefits are provided to the people at the time of need as a matter of right. The causes that may necessitate social security services can be of the following types: (a) Physical risks, e.g. sickness, invalidity, old age, maternity, accidents, death, etc. and (b) economic risks, e.g. unemployment, sudden loss of job, etc.

There are two approaches to social security
a. **Social assistance** in which the beneficiaries do not make any contributions for various benefits made available to them. The benefits are provided to the people as a matter of right without any means of test, e.g. old age pension, free hospital services, etc.

b. **Social insurance:** Which is based on the principle of compulsory mutual aid, in which the cost of service provided to the beneficiaries is shared by a nominal contribution of the beneficiary and subsidised by his employer and the state, i.e. ESI and CHS schemes.

The word social security is often confused with social insurance. It is an insurance against mishaps in life, like illness, death, disablement, etc. Social insurance is a part of social security. Social security in its modern connotations covers all the contingencies the human beings may come across from the time of birth up to the time of funeral or cremation. According to International Labour Organization (ILO), social security comprises all schemes providing for income security and medical service. A few of the contingencies covered by the social security plan are mentioned below:
1. Medical care in times of illness.
2. Medical care and case allowance during absence of work on account of employment injury.
3. Cash allowance during the time of sickness.
4. Prenatal and postnatal medical benefits during maternity together with case allowance during a period before and after childbirth.
5. Pension during the period of invalidity.
6. Old age pension after attainment of specified age.
7. Dependence benefit, cash allowance to wife or children, in case of death of an earning member of the family.
8. Payment of funeral or cremation expenses.
9. Cash allowance during the period of unemployment.
10. Children's allowance, i.e. payment of cash allowance to each child in a family, so that the children can be brought up.

Social Security in India

India is a country with joint family system which imparts a certain level of social security in the times of crisis. However, social security is the responsibility of the government and thereby various schemes have been launched by the government, however, the government-controlled social security system in India applies to a small portion of the population only. Ministry of Labour and Employment is entrusted with the implementation of social security related schemes in India. Generally, India's social security schemes cover the following types of social insurances: (a) Pension, (b) health insurance and medical, (c) maternity, (d) gratuity, and (e) disability. Most of the schemes are to provide benefit to the **organized labour sector** employed primarily in those establishments which are covered by the Factories Act, 1948, the Shops and Commercial Establishments Act of state governments, the Industrial Employment Standing Orders Act, 1946, etc. This sector already has a structure through which social security benefits are extended to workers covered under these legislations.

The principal social security laws enacted in India are the following:

1. The Employees' State Insurance Act, 1948 (ESI Act) which covers factories and establishments with 10 or more employees and provides for comprehensive medical care to the employees and their families as well as cash benefits during sickness and maternity, and monthly payments in case of death or disablement. (details in Chapter on Occupational Health).

2. The Employees' Provident Funds and Miscellaneous Provisions Act, 1952 (EPF and MP Act) which applies to specific scheduled factories and establishments employing 20 or more employees and ensures terminal benefits to provident fund, superannuation pension, and family pension in case of death during service. Separate laws exist for similar benefits for the workers in the coal mines and tea plantations.

3. The Employees' Compensation Act, 1923, which requires payment of compensation to the workman or his family in cases of employment-related injuries resulting in death or disability.

4. The Maternity Benefit Act, 1961, which provides for 12 weeks wages during maternity as well as paid leave in certain other related contingencies.

5. The Payment of Gratuity Act, 1972, which provides 15 days wages for each year of service to employees who have worked for five years or more in establishments having a minimum of 10 workers.

A separate legislation for provident fund exists for seamen and workers employed in coal mines and tea plantations in the state of Assam.

New initiatives: Prime Minister Sh. Narendra Modi has recently launched three new social security schemes—Atal Pension Yojana, **Pradhan Mantri Jeevan Jyoti Bima Yojana** and **Pradhan Mantri Suraksha Bima Yojana.** All the three schemes are targeted especially to the unorganised sector and economically weaker population but others can get themselves enrolled as well.

22.8 HEALTH INSURANCE IN INDIA

Health is a human right and its accessibility and affordability has to be ensured by the state, i.e. by the government of the country that the health of the people would be protected by the state from ill health and disease. Thus, owing to escalating healthcare costs, coupled with demand for healthcare services, lack of easy access of people from low income group to quality healthcare, health insurance is emerging as an alternative mechanism for financing healthcare in India.

India has about 40 to 50 million people on medication for major sickness at any point of time with public health financing contributing less than 2% of GDP in total healthcare. Over 80% of health financing is private financing, much of which is out of pocket payments and not by any prepayment schemes. Less than 15% of India's population are covered through health insurance, and most of it covers only government employees.

The health insurance schemes available in India can be broadly categorized as:

1. **Voluntary health insurance schemes or private-for-profit schemes:** Here the buyers are willing to pay premium to an insurance company that pools similar risks and insures them for health-related expenses. In the public sector, the General Insurance Corporation (GIC) and its four subsidiary companies (National Insurance Corporation, New India Assurance Company, Oriental Insurance Company and United Insurance Company) provide voluntary insurance schemes.

2. **Mandatory health insurance schemes or government run schemes (namely ESIS, CGHS)**

   a. **Employees' State Insurance Scheme (ESIS):** National Insurance against sickness and injury at work provides a unified and comprehensive scheme and is designed eventually to cover every one. This is the first step towards social security. In 1948, India made a beginning, by introducing Employees' State Insurance Act to provide certain cash and medical benefits to industrial employees in case of sickness, maternity employment injury and disablement (discussed in details under Occupational Health).

   b. **Contributory Health Service Scheme (CHSS):** After launching the Employees' State Insurance Scheme, Government of India introduced Contributory Health Service Scheme for the Central Government employees stationed at Delhi and New Delhi in 1954, based on the principle of a co-operative effort by the employees and the employers, to the mutual advantage of both. The scheme has been extended to Mumbai from November, 1963 and Allahabad from 1968.

   Before the introduction of this scheme, Central Government servants and the members of their families were entitled to free medical aid, but with many reservations. Under the prevailing old system, they had initially to incur the expenditure on their medical treatment under the advice of an authorised medical attendant and they used to get reimbursement of such expenses later on, from the government to the extent admissible under the rules. This system of reimbursement was of course a great handicap, especially for low paid government employees, who could not afford to incur the initial expenditure for getting medical aid at the right time. This system also resulted in delays in the settlement of claims of government servants. The need for better arrangements for medical attendance of Central Government employees was felt by the government, who after steady and thoughtful consideration, decided that a compulsory Contributory Health Service Scheme would be best to serve the purpose.

This scheme seeks to remove the aforesaid defects and to provide an efficient and comprehensive medical service. In the matter of free medical attendance and treatment, it has abolished the distinction between class IV and other classes of government servants. It extends the free medical service, not only to all Central Government employees but to their families as well.

Under this scheme, the standard of medical facilities provided consists of: (i) Free medical attendance for the government servants and their families at the various dispensaries established under the scheme and at their house. The scope of the term "Family" has been extended to include dependant parents who were not earlier covered by the Civil Service Medical Attendance Rules, (ii) supply of all necessary drugs including chemotherapeutics, antibiotics and dressing, (iii) domiciliary visits, (iv) free specialist consultation, (v) laboratory and X-ray investigations, (vi) emergency treatment, (vii) antenatal care, confinement and postnatal care for women, and (viii) advise on family planning, including supply of free subsidised contraceptives, etc.

Functions: Under this scheme, identity cards are issued to the government servants giving the names of the entitled members of their families. The entire area of Delhi and New Delhi has been demarcated into zones with a dispensary in each zone.

An average dispensary with a normal load of approximately 2,000 families or 11,000 beneficiaries, has on its staff 4 medical officers including one lady doctor, four pharmacists, two clerks, two female attendants, two peons, two sweepers and one chowkidar.

The scheme started functioning on 1st July 1954, with 53,000 government servants on its rolls, accounting for 223,000 beneficiaries including family members.

Supply of medicines: The medicines prescribed by the medical officers of the dispensary or the specialist are issued from the dispensaries where most of the items are stocked including special proprietary preparations. A medical storedepot is run for ensuring a regular flow of medicines, the annual expenditure of which is approximately ₹40 lacs for the medicines, not stocked in the dispensaries but prescribed by the medical attendant or the specialist. A special requisition is prepared and passed onto the chemists specifically appointed for this purpose, who deliver the supplies to the dispensary concerned, on the same afternoon.

c. **Universal Health Insurance Scheme (UHIS):** The government announced UHIS in 2003 for providing financial risk protection to the poor. Under this scheme, for a fixed premium of ₹165 per year per person, ₹248 for a family of five and ₹330 for a family of seven, health care for sum assured of ₹30000/- was provided. This scheme has been made eligible for below poverty line families only.

3. **Insurance offered by NGOs/community-based health insurance (CBHI):** Community-based schemes are typically targeted at poorer population living in communities. Such schemes are generally run by charitable trusts or Non-governmental Organizations (NGOs). In these schemes, the members pre pay a fixed amount of premia each year for specified service, which is not income-related. The benefits offered are mainly in terms of preventive, ambulatory and inpatient care. Such schemes tend to be financed through patient collection, government grants and donations. Some of the popular community-based health insurance schemes are: Self-employed Women's Association (SEWA), Tribuvandas Foundation (TF), The Mullur Milk Co-operative, Sewagram, Action for Community Organization, Rehabilitation and Development (ACCORD), Voluntary Health Services (VHS), etc.

4. **Employer-based schemes:** Employers in both public and private sector offer employer-based insurance schemes. These facilities could be through lump sum payments, reimbursement of employees' health expenditure for outpatient care and hospitalization, fixed medical allowance or covering them under the group health insurance schemes. The railways, defense and security forces, plantation sector and mining sector have the employer-based schemes.

22.9 REHABILITATION

WHO defines rehabilitation of people with disabilities as a process aimed at enabling them to reach and maintain their optimal physical, sensory, intellectual, psychological and social functional levels.

Types of Rehabilitation

1. Physical
2. Vocational or occupational
3. Social
4. Mental

Modern medical, surgical science, and modern aid to vocational adjustments have now ensured that physical restoration is now the rule rather than the exception. Vocational preparation for other jobs is accepted as a feasible and successful method of making the people with disability efficient, self-supporting and self-respecting citizens.

Principles

The underlying principles of vocational rehabilitations are based on:

a. The democratic concept of the way of living, demands equality of opportunity for all citizens including the physically handicapped.

b. The society expects the support of each citizen in proportion to his capacity. Vocational rehabilitation offers to the handicapped person, an opportunity for employment and at the same time, makes possible his due contribution to the society.

c. Experience has shown that most disabled persons can work efficiently, if prepared for a job compatible with their physical conditions. A man with a leg amputation can do anything at a bench that a normal man of equal skill can do. A man with an arm amputation may still be a competent salesman, draftsman, artist or a lawyer. A deaf man is handicapped only in communication and can acquire any skill with the use of his hands. Thus, a disabled person has far more vocational assets than that are lost through his impairment.

d. The disabled person has a right to work; his needs do not differ from the need of others. It is a matter of social justice to prepare him for a suitable job and thus place him on economic parity with his fellows.

e. Society benefits by employment of the disabled. The burden on public relief is lessened.

f. A nation's foremost asset is its citizenship. The development of each individual for useful pro-ductiveness is the most sound policy.

g. Vocational rehabilitation is economically sound.

How to Organise Rehabilitation Services

1. Disabled persons are located through an organised case finding programme and offered rehabilitation service, if unemployed or underemployed.

2. An expert diagnosis is made of their employment needs and of their physical, mental and vocational resources.

3. Corrective surgery or therapeutic treatment may be provided or secured, if necessary for employment.

4. Prosthetic devices (limbs, hearing aids, etc.) may be provided or secured, if necessary for employment.

5. Expert counselling or guidance assists them to decide upon a suitable employment objective.

6. A plan is prepared outlining the steps or services needed to enable the disabled person to secure suitable employment.

7. Training, carefully planned and supervised, is provided to those, who need such preparation for employment.

8. Maintenance during training may be provided in case of need.

9. Other necessary services, incident to the solution of personal or family problems are provided or secured.

10. The culminating factor and essential step in every case is entry into suitable remunerative employment. Such placement is followed up to determine its lasting success or to provide any needed adjustment.

Voluntary Organisations in India

For the welfare services of a community in a developing country like India, keeping in view the availability of only limited resources at national level, one has to depend heavily on the contributions made by voluntary organisations. At present, about 2000 such organisations are engaged in India in various medical, educational and other welfare activities, which may be broadly classified as under.

A. Services for Specific Diseases and Disorders

i. *All India Blind Relief Society*: It was established in 1946. It aims at the prevention of blindness by establishing hospitals and dispensaries. It is also responsible for arranging eye camps in rural areas, where cataract operations are performed and other eye ailments are attended to.

ii. *Tuberculosis Association of India*: It was formed in 1939 and it is engaged in research work for prevention and control of tuberculosis and arranges training for the health personnel engaged in the work. It is also responsible for organising every year TB seal campaigns to promote fund collection.

iii. *National Centre for the Deaf*: It has a training centre at Hyderabad and also a school for children, who are partially deaf.

iv. *The Hind Kusht Nivaran Sangh*: It was formed in 1950 with its headquarters in New Delhi. It renders financial assistance to various leprosy homes and clinics in the country. It is also engaged in the process of rendering health education about leprosy through publications, posters, etc.

B. Services for Women and Children

i. *Family Planning Association of India*: It organises family welfare clinics, training for health personnel and research about population and birth control programmes.

ii. *All India Women's Conference*: It was established in 1926. It is responsible for the protection of handicapped women and children, family welfare work, providing handicraft training to women, arranging for day creches for the children of working women.

iii. *Indian Council of Child Welfare*: It was established in 1952. It organises various child welfare activities and arranges for the establishment of minilibraries and playgrounds for the children.

iv. *Kasturba Gandhi National Memorial Trust*: It was created in commemoration of Kasturba Gandhi, after her death in 1944. It generally looks after the welfare of women of rural India through Gram Sevikas. It renders health services to the mothers and children and gives training to village level workers.

v. *Rotary Club*: It contributes for the education of poor school-children by offering monthly stipends and care for the crippled and underprivileged children.

C. Services for Social Work

Indian Conference of Social Work, Bharat Sevak Samaj, Indian Red Cross Society, etc. are responsible for promoting various social welfare activities.

i. *Bharat Sewak Samaj*: It was established in 1952. It is a social welfare organisation with its emphasis on health services and upliftment of rural population.

ii. *Indian Red Cross Society*: It was established in 1920 and is affiliated to the International Red Cross Society. It also runs first aid training centres, etc. It distributes medicines, clothings, milk, etc. to the poor through various voluntary welfare agencies in the country, which it collects through donations and otherwise.

D. Services for Medical Care

Lions Club, Rama Krishna Mission, Marwari Relief Society, etc. are providing medical care by establishing laboratories, dispensaries, hospitals, etc.

Basics of Biostatistics

23.1 MEANING OF STATISTICS

Statistics is the study of the collection, analysis, presentation, organization and interpretation of data. Data is a set of values in unorganized form that represents conditions, ideas or objects. It has to be arranged/organized, presented and analyzed for interpretation and use. There are two types of data:

1. *Qualitative*: Categorical measurement expressed in natural language disruption, e.g. BP low or high.
2. *Quantitative or numeric data*: It can be discrete or continuous.

    a. **Biostatistics:** The branch of statistics that involves with the theory and application of statistical sciences to analyze and interpret public health problems for the course of action and decision-making.

    b. **Health statistics:** It deals with statistical methodologies for the numerical data of health and health related indices in human population. A few example of these are birth and death rates and also diseases in relation to the different factors affecting them. When these numerical data deal with marriages, births and deaths, the statistical methodology used for these factors is called *Vital Statistics*. This is a branch of demography, which deals with the study of human population.

23.2 IMPORTANCE OF STATISTICS

Statistics finds its place whenever numerical facts enter into picture. It adds credibility to an argument or statement. Statistics is an essential component of health and healthcare for planning and management of services and health resources (manpower, material and money). The data also helps in evaluating the services. The importance of statistics data to health workers can be enumerated as follows:

a. As biological observations are variable from one individual to the other or from one group to the other, statistical methodologies are useful to define normal values of variables as well as make comparisons from group to group or within the same group over a period of time.
b. Through various statistical indices, the health status of a community can be measured.
c. Different communities may have different health problems. The differences and then can be analysed through statistics.
d. Planning of health services.
e. The planning and analysis of research investigations in an area.
f. Evaluation of preventive and control measures undertaken.
g. Evaluation of utilization patterns of health services.

Sources of data for health statistics

1. Vital events register.
2. Population census.
3. Routine health services records.
4. Epidemiologic surveillance data.
5. Sample surveys.
6. Disease registers.

23.3 COLLECTION OF DATA

Data can be collected by many methods such as experimentation, surveys or by record maintenance and analysis. While collecting a data by any of the methods, the objectives of data collected should always be kept in mind. Truthfulness, accuracy and clarity should be maintained at the stage of collection. The data should usually collected on pre-designed cards, schedules or registers. Different terminologies used for collection should be well defined, plan of collection including brief instructions for collections should be prepared in advance. The sample for data collection should be statistically planned. All data collection procedures should have a provision for checking the quality of the collected data.

23.4 SURVEY FOR COLLECTION OF DATA

Health surveys are conducted to obtain a wide range of health data such as natalitis, morbidities, mortalities in relation to different biological, social, environmental and economic factors. To collect such information either a general health survey or a specific health survey is conducted. In fact, designing a survey is a dynamic, iterative and interactive process. The usual methods employed in surveys are (i) interview method (ii) health examination method, (iii) record analysis method, and (iv) a combination of all or any of these three methods. Each method has its own advantages and disadvantages. While planning any health survey following points are to be kept in mind.

i. The aims and objectives of the survey should be clearly defined before undertaking the survey.

ii. The variables on which the information is to be collected should be clearly defined.

iii. The methods for data collection, drawing the sample, formulating the question and questionnaire has to be done.

iv. The population and the unit of population from where the information will be collected has to be statistically sampled.

v. The other items such as interview, design, the selection of person from where the information is to be collected, recall periods, etc. should to be properly planned.

vi. The time coverage to elicit the desired information should be planned and depending on this factor the surveys have to be either cross sectional, i.e. pertaining to a particular period of time, or longitudinal, i.e. over a period of time.

vii. Collecting and analyzing the data and writing the report.

23.5 TABULATION OF DATA

The data in the form of a series of numbers will not help in understanding the underlining meanings or trends. Hence, this raw data is arranged in the form of suitable tables. This simple method of arrangement of data into a table is called *frequency distribution*. This table classifies the number of observations into groups according to various values of the variable.

An example of a frequency distribution table is given in Table 23.1. This table gives the number of females adopting family planning practices according to the number of living male children. From the table it can be observed that there are 45.5% and 29.5% females with 2 and 3 alive male children or there are only a few females with either nil or six male living children and so on. Such observations could have been difficult from to comprehend a series of ungrouped data.

When the variable under observation takes a longer range for its values or in the case of continuous type of

Table 23.1: Frequency distribution of females adopting family planning method according to the number of alive male children

No. of living male children	No. of females	%
0	2	0.9
1	17	7.6
2	102	45.5
3	66	29.5
4	30	13.4
5	6	2.7
6	1	0.4
Total	**224**	**100.0**

data, the classification as done in the above table for the values of the variables in terms of each value of the variable is not suitable. In such cases, class intervals corresponding to a range of values of the variable is adopted for classification as indicated in Table 23.2.

Table 23.2: Frequency distribution of population in a community according to their serum cholesterol values

Serum cholesterol in mg %	No. of people	%
Up to 100	130	19.7
101–150	245	37.1
151–200	231	35.0
201–250	48	7.3
251–300	06	0.9
Total	**600**	**100.0**

In Tables 23.1 and 23.2, only quantitative data (where the variable is measured in terms of a quantity) is classified. The variable can also be a qualitative one, i.e. it is enumerated as different alternatives in qualitative terms. The tabular presentation of such a data is shown in Table 23.3.

Table 23.3: Frequency distribution of blood groups of a sample of population

Blood groups	No. of people	%
A	136	19.9
B	239	35.0
AB	67	9.8
O	241	35.3
Total	**683**	**100.00**

Multiple classifications can also be done, if it is required to present more than one variable in the same table. An example of a bivariate distribution table is shown in Table 23.4.

From the above tables, it can be understood that the tabular presentation summarises to a certain extent series of data and makes the data more understandable.

Table 23.4: Bivariate distribution table of serum cholesterol level of population according to their food habits

Serum cholesterol level in mg %	No. of people Vegetarians	Non-vegetarians	Total
Up to 100	75	55	130
101–150	98	147	245
151–200	80	151	231
201–250	16	32	48
251–300	1	5	6
Total	**270**	**390**	**660**

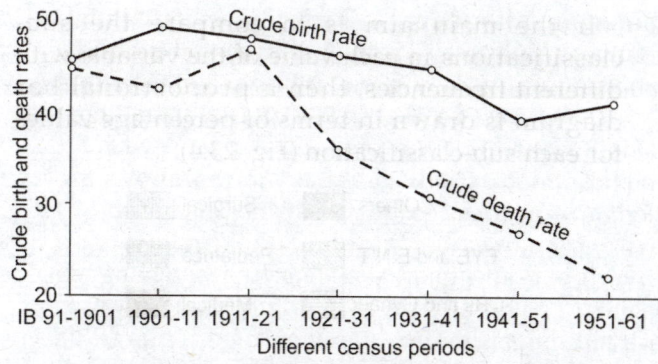

Fig. 23.1: Line diagram showing the crude birth and death rates in India during different census periods

However, to make a table self-explanatory, the table should always contain a clear and a brief title. Each column of the table should be clearly specified as to what is contained in it. Standard symbols should be used and explanatory notes have to be provided, wherever necessary. The beginning and end points of each class interval should not be overlapping with the other class intervals.

Tables are usually prepared by tally marks method, wherein tally marks are put for each observation against the corresponding class interval. The fifth tally mark is usually put diagonally on the four tally marks already put to facilitate counting. Mechanical tabulation procedures are to be utilised when the data is too large or multiple classifications are too many.

23.6 GRAPHICAL PRESENTATION OF DATA

In addition to presentation of data in the form of tables, the statistical data can be depicted in the form of suitable graphs. This will enable a person to grasp the salient features in a better manner though visual appeal diagrams are only preliminary aids in the understanding of the data and is no substitute for further statistical analysis. Because of their visual appeal, greatest care must be taken while interpreting from the graphst. The common graphs of statistical utility are described below.

i. **Line diagram:** It is usually drawn to show the changes in the values of a variable with passage of time. This is drawn by taking the time on the X-axis, i.e. horizontal axis and the corresponding frequencies on the Y-axis, i.e. vertical axis. The line is obtained by joining the points corresponding to the different sets of values of time and the corresponding frequency (Fig. 23.1).

ii. **Bar diagram:** It is a graphic presentation of frequency distribution for a qualitative data or a quantitative discrete type of data. Here a bar is drawn corresponding to the frequency of each value of the variable. Some space is left between each bar. Usually, the width of all the bars will be same unless the class interval are of different sizes (Fig. 23.2).

The height of the bar can be subdivided into various components to show the subclassification

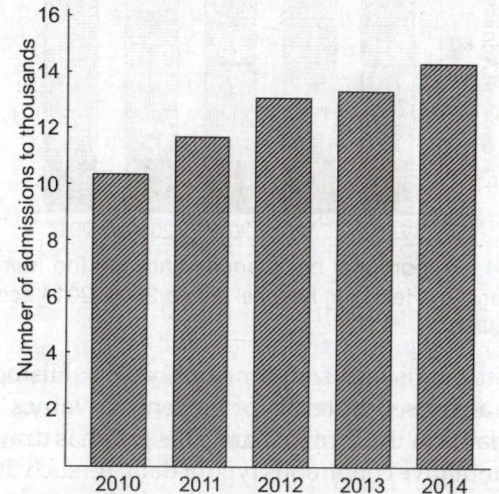

Fig. 23.2: Bar diagram showing the number of admissions in a teaching hospital during any given year (say 2010–2014)

in each value of the variable. Such graphs are called multiple bar diagrams (Fig. 23.3).

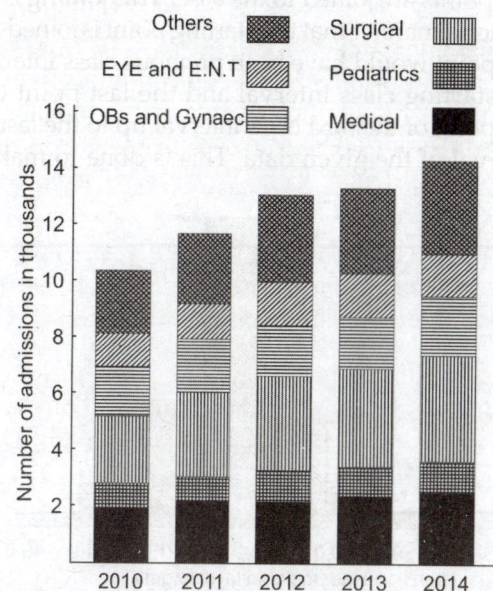

Fig. 23.3: Multiple bar diagrams showing the number of admissions in a teaching hospital during (2010–2014 according to specialists

If the main aim is to compare the sub-classifications in each value of the variable with different frequencies, then a proportional bar diagram is drawn in terms of percentage values for each sub-classification (Fig. 23.4).

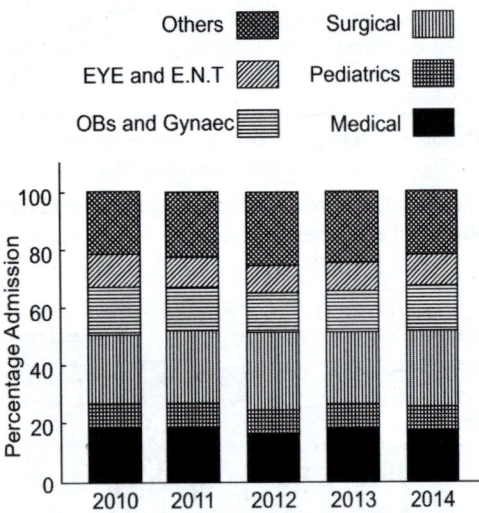

Fig. 23.4: Proportional bar diagram showing the number of admissions in a teaching hospital during 2010–2014 according to specialists

iii. Histograms and frequency polygons: Histograms are also used in terms of presenting values of the variable in the form of bars. This graph is drawn for quantitative continuous type of data. As such the bars are drawn continuously, adjoining to each other, unlike in a bar diagram (Fig. 23.5). Frequency polygons can also be drawn for such type of data. Here points are plotted corresponding to the middle points of the class interval and the frequencies on Y-axis.

These points are all joined by a smooth line and the end points are joined to the base. This joining is done in such a manner that the starting point is joined to the midpoint would have been previous class interval to the starting class interval and the last point to the midpoint of the next class interval up to the last class interval of the given data. This is done to make the

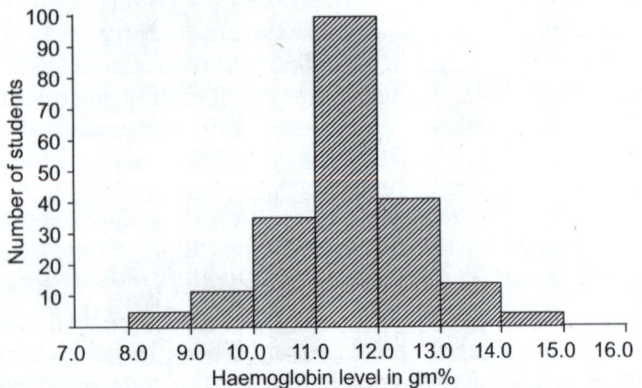

Fig. 23.5: Histogram showing the haemoglobin levels in gm% of students in a class

figure a polygon, whose area is equal to that of the area of the corresponding histogram (Fig. 23.6).

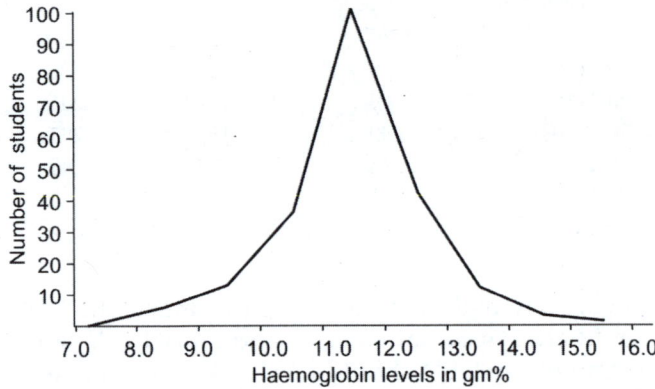

Fig. 23.6: Frequency polygon showing the haemoglobin levels in gm% of students in a class

iv. Pie diagram: This graph is useful for depicting qualitative data. Here the proportion of each item to the total is shown as a sector in a circle (Fig. 23.7). Each sector is given a separate shade. The angle subtended by a sector at the centre is a proportion of 360°, which is equivalent to the proportion of frequency of that particular item to the total frequency. This graph may not be suitable when the number of items are too many.

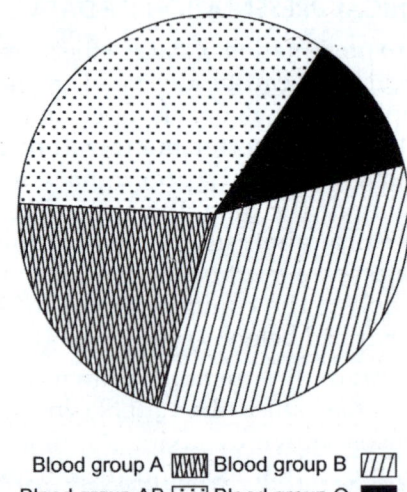

Blood group A · Blood group B
Blood group AB · Blood group O

Fig. 23.7: Pie diagram showing the blood group distribution of a sample of population

v. Scatter diagram: When the relationship between two variables are to be depicted, this type of a graph is drawn (Fig. 23.8). Here points are plotted on a graph corresponding to each set of observations of the two variables, taking each of the two variables on the two axes.

vi. Other types of graphs: There are other variations of the above graph. In all the above graphs, both the axes are in arithmetic scale. But to plot certain types

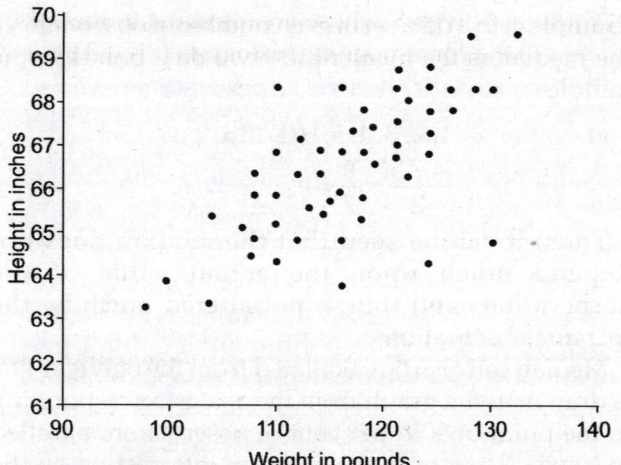

Fig. 23.8: Scatter diagram showing the height and weight of male students in a class

of data like a dose mortality curve, this may not be suitable. In such cases, one axis depicting the dose may be in a logarithmic scale, while the other is in arithmetic scale. Such graphs are said to be in arithlog scale. When both the axes are in logarithmic scale, they are said to be in a log-log scale. If the frequencies are not in arithmetic progression in relation to dose then arithlog graph can be drawn, which makes the curve drawn to be a straight line.

Pictograms and spot maps, which depict the frequencies in the form of pictures or dots in a map respectively, may also be drawn for epidemiological data.

Ogive: It is graph for the cumulative distribution of observations, which can be drawn to understand the value of the variable below or above different percentage of observations (Fig. 23.9). This is drawn by

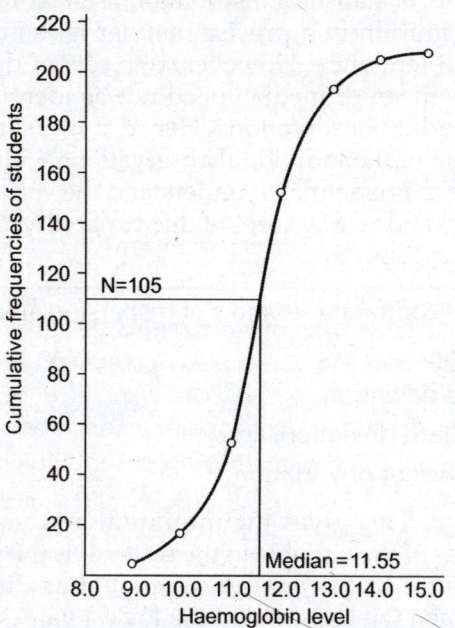

Fig. 23.9: Ogive for the distribution of haemoglobin levels of students in a class

plotting points corresponding to the cumulative frequencies, i.e. the total frequency up to a certain value of the variable, on the Y-axis and the values of the variable on the X-axis. The points so obtained are joined by a smooth curve.

23.7 MEASURES OF CENTRAL TENDENCY

The initial process in the analysis of data is to present it in the form of tables and to visualise the trends in the form of graphs. As the biological observations are subject to great variability it becomes essential to express these observations into a precise estimate on the basis of which these observations can be summarised. One set of such estimates is the measure of central tendency. These measures not only help to summarise the data but also are useful to compare one set of data with the other. These estimates are also called as parameters of the statistical distribution.

The three measures of central tendency are:

i. Mean
ii. Median
iii. Mode.

i. Mean: This is the arithmetic average of observations and expressed as $\bar{x}$, i.e. $\bar{x} = \dfrac{\Sigma x_i}{n}$ where x_i sign denotes the individual observations, Σ means the sum of all values of x_i and n is the total number of observations.

Example 1: If the systolic blood pressure (in mm Hg) of a group of healthy people of a certain age are 118, 122, 118, 119, 120, 122, 118, 123, 120, and 120, their mean systolic pressure is:

$$\bar{x} = \frac{118+122+118+119+120+122+118+123+120+120}{10}$$

$$\bar{x} = \frac{1200}{10} = 120 \text{ mm Hg}$$

If the data is grouped unlike in the above situation, mean

$$\bar{x} = \frac{\Sigma' x_i f_i}{n}$$

where, x_i corresponds to the middle point of each class interval, f_i is the corresponding number of observations in that particular class interval, and n is the total number of observations in a series of data.

To calculate the mean by this method, the steps involved are:

a. To write down the middle points of each of the class interval.

b. To get the product of each of these middle points and the corresponding frequencies and adding these products.

c. To divide the sum by the total number of observations.

Example 2: The haemoglobin levels in gm% of a class of students is tabulated below and the mean is calculated for the data as follows:

Hb in gm%	No. of students (f_i)	Mid-point of class intervals (x_i)	Product $(x_i f_i)$
8.1–9.0	5	8.55	42.75
9.1–10.0	12	9.55	114.60
10.1–11.0	36	10.55	379.80
11.1–12.0	100	11.55	1155.00
12.1–13.0	42	12.55	527.10
13.1–14.0	12	13.55	162.60
		14.55	43.65
Total	210		2425.50

$$\overline{x} = \frac{2425.50}{210} = 11.55 \text{ gm}\%$$

ii. Median: If in a series of data, there are a few extreme values, which are different from most of the other observations then the value of the mean is either inflated or deflated accordingly as the extreme values on the higher side or lower side respectively. If in a ward of a hospital, most of patients have stayed for a period between 1 and 15 days and a few others have stayed for days like 30 to 35, then if the mean is calculated it will be very high which will be different from the true picture of centre of the distribution. To overcome this discrepancy, the exact centre of the distribution, when all the observations are arranged in the ascending or descending order of their magnitude. Median is now the central value in this arranged data for a set of data with odd number of observations. For example, usually the median lethal dosage of the response of a drug is measured instead of the mean dosage in most of the pharmocological experiments.

Example 3. If the number of male living children in a group of families are as follows:
5, 3, 2, 1, 1, 0, 2, 2, 6, 0, 2, 2, 4, the median number of male living children in the families is obtained as follows:
First the data is arranged in the ascending order of the numbers as:

0, 0, 1, 1, 2, 2, 2, 2, 2, 3, 4, 5, 6

The value of the middle observation, i.e. the seventh observation, i.e. 2 is the median for this set of data.
If the total number of observations is even then the average of the middle two observations is taken as the median.

Example 4: In a data set of even number of observations, the median is the mean of the two data points in the middle

1, 2, 3, 4, 5, 6, 17, 18

$$\frac{4+5}{2} = \frac{9}{2} = 4.5$$

Thus, it can be seen that the median does not depend much upon the actual value of the observations and thus is not altered much by the extreme observations.

Median can also be calculated from the ogive. A line is drawn on the graph from the Y-axis corresponding to the point of 50th per cent of observation, paralled to X-axis. Then from this point of intersection on the curve, a line perpendicular to X-axis is drawn. The point where this perpendicular meets, the X-axis is the median value.

iii. Mode: In certain cases, it is neither required to find the average nor the median but the interest will be to see the most frequently occurring value of the variable in the series of the data. This measure of central tendency is known as mode. In the case of study of age of onset of a disease, it is more desirable to see the most common age of onset rather than the mean or the median. In such a case, the value of the variable corresponding to the highest frequency is taken as the mode. In a graph, this is the point on the X-axis corresponding to the point where the curve takes turn from increase to the decrease.

23.8 MEASURES OF DISPERSION

In the previous section, it was seen that one of the parameters of statistical distribution useful for defining the distribution in a precise manner is the measure of central tendency. However, two sets of data with the same mean or median need not be identical with the individual observations. Hence, a measure of the dispersion of the individual observations with respect to the mean is essential to understand the variability of the observations. Measures of this variability are called *measures of dispersion*.

The most common measures of dispersion are:

i. Range
ii. Mean deviation
iii. Standard deviation, and
iv. Coefficient of variation.

i. **Range:** This gives the minimum and maximum values of the variable in the series. It is the simplest measure of dispersion calculated as difference between the highest and the lowest values. It does not provide any information about in between observations but only about the two extreme values, e.g. from the following record of body weights of 10 students of class V in a school:

28, 32, 27, 40.33, 35, 38, 29, 41, 31

It can be seen that the highest value was 41 and the lowest value was 27. The range is expressed as 27 to 41 or by actual difference. In case of a grouped data, range is expressed as the midpoint of extreme categories.

ii. Mean deviation: This is arithmetic average of the difference between the mean and each of the observations. These differences are averaged by taking only their absolute values.

Example 5: The weights of 10 students of a class are as follows: 39, 39, 38, 47, 44, 42, 45, 36, 58, 52. Find the mean deviation.

Weight x	Arithmatic mean x bar	Deviation from mean $x - x$ bar
39	44	−5
39	44	−5
38	44	−6
47	44	3
44	44	0
42	44	−2
45	44	−1
36	44	−8
58	44	14
52	44	8
Total	440	52 (ignoring − sign)

Mean is 440/10 = 44.
Mean deviation = 52/10 = 5.2.

iii. Standard deviation: This is the most widely used measure of the variation of individual observations from the mean. It is calculated as the square root of the mean of the squared deviations of individual observations from the mean. It is also called the *root mean square deviation*. This is one of the important statistical parameters.

Estimate of the standard deviation is calculated from the formula:

For large samples size <30

$$s = \sqrt{\frac{\Sigma'(x_i - \bar{x})^2}{n-1}}$$

For large samples (>30 observations)

$$\sqrt{\frac{\Sigma(x_i - \bar{x})^2}{n}}$$

where, s is the standard deviation
x_i is the individual observations.
$\bar{x}$ is mean.
thus $(x_i - \bar{x})$ is the deviation of each observation from the mean;
n is the number of observations.

Example 6: The calculation of standard deviation for the ungrouped data given in Example 1 is illustrated below:

x	$x_i - \bar{x}$	$(x_i - \bar{x})^2$
118	118−120 = −2	4
122	122−120 = +2	4
118	118−120 = −2	4
119	119−120 = −1	1
120	120−120 = 0	0
122	122−120 = +2	4
118	118−120 = −2	4
123	123−120 = −3	9
120	120−120 = +3	0
120	120−120 = 0	0

$$\Sigma'(x_i - \bar{x})^2 = 30$$

$$s = \sqrt{\frac{30}{9}} = \sqrt{3.333} = 1.83$$

Standard deviation for the grouped data is calculated from the formula

$$s = \sqrt{\frac{\Sigma(x_i - x)^2 f_i}{n-1}}$$

$$= \sqrt{\frac{\Sigma x_i^2 f_i - (\Sigma x_i f_i)^2 / n}{n-1}}$$

where, s, $\bar{x}$ and n have the same meaning as before but x_i is the middle point of each class interval and f_i is the corresponding frequency in that class interval.

Example 7: Standard deviation for the data given in Example 2 is demonstrated below:

Hb. level in gm	No. of students (fi)	Mid paints of class intervals	$x_i^2 (x_i)$	$x_i^2 f_i$
8.1–9.0	5	8.55	73.10	365.50
9.1–10.0	12	9.55	91.20	1094.40
10.1–11.0	36	10.55	111.30	4006.80
11.1–12.0	100	11.55	133.40	13340.00
12.1–13.0	42	12.55	157.50	6615.00
13.1–14.0	12	13.55	183.60	2203.20
14.1–15.0	3	14.55	211.70	635.10
Total	**210**			**28,260.00**

$\Sigma x_i f_i = 2,425.50$ (from Example 1)
$\Sigma (x_i f_i)^2 = 5,883,050.25$
$\Sigma (x_i f_i)^2/n = 28,014.52\ 2$
$\Sigma (x_i f_i)^2 - \Sigma (x_i f_i)^2/n = 28260.00 - 28014.52 = 245.48$

$$s = \sqrt{\frac{245.48}{(210-1) = 209}} = \sqrt{1.17} = 1.08$$

iv. Coefficient of variation: It can be seen that the standard deviation depends on the size of the mean as well as the unit measurement of observations. As such the variability of two groups of observations which are measured in different units and also which have two different means cannot be compared directly with standard deviations. Such comparisons are done through a coefficient of variation which is the percentage standard deviation to the mean.

In other words coefficient of variation

$$= \frac{\text{Standard deviation}}{\text{Mean}} \times 100$$

Coefficient of variation of Hb% level of example is:

$$= \frac{1.08}{11.55} \times 100 = 9.35$$

23.9 SAMPLING PROCEDURES

Both the clinicians and the public health workers need data for patient management, assessing the efficacy of a drug or implementation of a health programme. It is not possible to obtain such data from all the patients suffering from a particular disease or toxicity data from people consuming a particular drug. Thus, the data that is produced from a sample, which is portion of a population from the bigger groups can be used to draw reference for the entire population. The sample selected for the investigation should be representative of the characteristics of the population. Such samples are called as *probability samples.*

Several sampling methods are available depending upon the type and nature of population, objectives of research and type of data required. A few of the important random sampling procedures are enumerated hereunder:

i. **Simple Random Sampling:** In this method, the required number of units are selected at random from the list of entire population. In a random sample, each unit in the population will have a certain preassigned probability of being included in the sample. All statistical methodologies are applicable only to such random samples. Simple random samples can be selected using a random number table or a dice.

ii. **Stratified Random Sampling:** The sample is deliberately drawn in a manner so that each portion of sample is drawn from a corresponding strata of population. This method of sampling is important when the investigator is interested in analyzing the data by certain characteristics of the population, viz. age groups, castewise, genderwise and so on. When the population from which the sample is to be selected is not homogeneous with reference to certain aspects of study then the population is subdivided into homogeneous groups and random samples are taken from each group separately. Usually the number of units to be selected from each group should be proportional to the size of the strata.

iii. **Systematic Random Sampling:** In this method of sampling, the first unit is selected at random and the other units are selected in a systematic manner such as every fourth or fifth unit, etc. is selected from the list of the universe.

iv. **Multi-stage Sampling:** In this procedure, the ultimate sampling unit is selected at different stages. First sampling may be a sample of villages, then in the second stage a few houses in each of these sampled villages may be selected and in the third stage a few individuals in each of these sampled houses may be selected and these individuals constitute the sample.

Sampling error: Sampling error is the error that arises in a data collection process as a result of taking a sample from a population rather than using the whole population. This can be minimised by taking larger samples. As the individual readings vary widely from one another, there is a higher probability of variability arising between various samples.

Non-sampling error: Non-sampling error is the error that arises in a data collection process as a result of factors other than taking a sample, e.g. due to inadequately calibrated instruments, observer variation and so on.

Standard error: It represents the accuracy with which the sample represents the population. In statistical terms, a sample mean deviates from the actual mean of a population; this deviation is the standard error.

23.10 SIZE OF SAMPLE

Usual question an investigator is faced with is that how many units he should include in his sample so that the result of his research on the sample are valid and can be generalized to the population from where the sample has been drawn. The size of the sample is called *adequate sample size.* The calculation for the sample size depends on the following factors:

a. An approximate idea of the estimate of the characteristic under investigation as well as its variability in the population.

b. The precision with which the estimate is to be made.

c. The probability with which the desired precision is to be maintained.

d. The availability of the resources on the basis of which (b) and (c) can be adjusted.

There are several methods used to calculate sample size depending upon the type of data or study design. Generally, the sample size for any study depends on the:

a. Acceptable level of significance
b. Power of the study
c. Expected effect size
d. Underlying event rate in the population
e. Standard deviation in the population.

Some more factors that can be considered while calculating the final sample size include the expected dropout rate, an unequal allocation ratio, and the objective and design of the study.

For qualitative data

Sample size $(n) = 4pq/l^2$ where p is prevalence of that disease or health condition, q is 100-p and l is the allowable error or precision or variability.

Example 8: Calculate the sample size to find out the prevalence of a disease after giving a mass administration of a drug with 10% allowable error. Prevalence of disease before giving the drug was 80%.

$$n = 4 \times 80 \times 20/8 \times 8 = 100 \ (L = 10\% \text{ of } 80 = 8)$$

For quantitative data

$$n : 4\,SD^2/L^2$$

Example 9: Determine the sample size to find out the requirement of vit A, if the mean daily requirement of vit A is documented to be 950 IU with SD of 90 IU. Consider the precision as 9.

$$n = 4 \times 90 \times 90/9 \times 9 = 400$$

23.11 NORMAL DISTRIBUTION

Most of the biological data follows a certain pattern which can be represented through a mathematical formula. This is known as a *statistical distribution*. The commonest distribution of biological data when observed on large samples is the *normal distribution*. The main characteristics of this distribution are:

a. The shape of the curve of distribution resembles a bell.

b. The curve is symmetrical about the centre.

c. Maximum number of observations is at the point of centre of the curve and the number of observations on both sides of this point gradually decrease and there are very few observations at the extremities.

d. The mean, median and mode coincide at the centre.

e. The percentage number of observations included between the mean value of the variable and the various values of the standard deviations are given by the relationship.

Mean ± 1 SD covers 68.3% of the observations.

Mean ± 2 SD covers 95.4% of the observations.

Mean ± 3 SD covers 99.7% of the observations.

23.12 SAMPLING VARIATION AND TESTS OF SIGNIFICANCE

If repeated samples are taken from the same population, they will not yield the same values for the different parameters calculated from the sample. This is because of the inherent variation in biological observations.

Such differences between the estimates from different samples even though they have come out from the same population is called *sampling variation*. The measure of variability of such variation of statistical parameters of different samples from the same population is given by *standard error*. The *standard error* of *mean* tells us how accurate your estimate of the mean is likely to be. This is calculated by the formula:

$$= \frac{\sqrt{\text{Standard deviation of observations in the sample}}}{\text{No. of observations in the sample}}$$

Whenever two sets of observations are to be compared, it becomes essential to find out whether the differences observed between the two groups is because of sampling variation or because of some other factor. The methods by which this is done are known as *tests of significance*. Parametric tests are used when the data is distributed normally and nonparametric tests are used when the data is not distributed normally, usually with small sample size.

In any test, a quantity P is found out which gives the probability that the difference between the two groups is because of sampling variation. If this probability is more than 0.05, the difference is called insignificant and if it is less than or equal to 0.05, the difference is called significant. This value of P is obtained by calculating various tests of significance like standard error test for large samples, χ^2-test for testing association, etc. or F-test for testing variabilities, etc.

23.13 STANDARD ERROR TEST FOR LARGE SAMPLES

Usually when a sample has more than thirty observations it is considered to be a large sample. When the difference between any two large samples estimates in terms of means or proportion are to be tested for knowing whether the difference is because of sampling variation or otherwise, normal distribution probabilities can be used. The probability of the sampling variation as the cause of the difference can be found out from the ratio of the difference between the sample estimate to the standard error. The procedure involved is the calculation of Z (the standard **score**). It allows us to calculate the probability of a **score** occurring within our normal distribution, and (b) enables us to compare two **scores** that are from different normal distributions.

$$Z = \frac{\text{Difference between the estimates of two samples}}{\text{Standard error of this difference (SE)}}$$

A z-score equal to 0 represents an element equal to the mean. A z-score equal to –1 or +1 represents an element that is 1 standard deviation less or more than the mean; a z-score equal to –2, 2 standard deviations less than the mean; etc. If the number of elements in the set is large, about 68% of the elements have a z-score between –1 and 1; about 95% have a z-score between –2 and 2; and about 99% have a z-score between –3 and 3.

The formula for the calculation of standard error of the difference between the two means is:

$$SE = \sqrt{{s_1^2}/{n_1} + {s_2^2}/{n_2}}$$

Where, s_1 and s_2 are the standard deviation of the two samples and n_1 and n_2 the respective sample sizes.

23.14 T-TEST FOR COMPARING MEANS

The usual test is applied to test significance of two means for small samples is t-test. When the investigation is in terms of comparing the observations carried out on the same individuals say before and after a certain experiment, such comparisons are called *Paired comparisons*. When the observations are carried out in two independent samples and their values are compared, it is known as *unpaired comparison*.

1. *t-test for paired comparison*
   a. First the null hypothesis, that the two sets of observations are not different, is set up.
   b. The difference between the before and after experimentation readings are calculated for each individual.
   c. The mean and standard deviations of these differences are calculated.
   d. The standard error of this mean difference is calculated by the formula $S/\sqrt{n}$
   e. t is calculated by the formula

$$t = \frac{\text{Mean difference}}{\text{Standard error of the mean difference}}$$

   f. The degrees of freedom (d.f.) for this calculation t is $(n-1)$ where n is the number of pairs of observation.
   g. From r-distribution table, P is noted down corresponding to $(n-1)$ d.f. and then calculated value of t.
   h. If P is more than 0.05, the mean difference is insignificant and if P is less than 0.05 the mean difference is significant.

2. *The unpaired t-test:*
   a. Set up the null hypothesis that the difference in the two means is zero.
   b. Calculate the means and standard deviations for the two groups separately.
   c. Calculate the standard error of difference of means.
   d. The standard error (smd) of difference between the two means is calculated by the formula:

$$smd = \sqrt{\frac{(n_1+n_2)}{n_1 n_2} \times \frac{(n_1-1)s_1^2 + (n_2-1)s_2^2}{n_1+n_2-2}}$$

Where s_1 and s_2 are the standard deviation of the two samples and n_1 and n_2 the respective sample sizes.

Where s_1 and s_2 are standard deviations of the two groups and n_1 and n_2 are the respective number of observations in the two groups.

   e. *Calculate t by the formula*

$$t = \frac{\text{Difference between the means of two samples}}{\text{Standard error of the difference between the two means}}$$

   f. Compute the pooled degrees of freedom as:

$$n_1 + n_2 - 1$$

   g. Refer to the table of t distribution and find out the probability level P corresponding to the above degrees of freedom and the calculated t
   h. Interpretations are made on the basis of this P, as before.

23.15 CHI-SQUARE TEST

It is the method of testing the significance of difference between two proportions.

When the data is measured in terms of attributes or certain class intervals it becomes necessary to test whether the differences in this distribution of the samples are due to sampling variation or otherwise. As an example, if there are two groups say one healthy group of individuals and another with a particular disease and their social classifications are noted, it may be necessary to test whether the two groups are similar with reference to the social classification or not. In such cases *chi-square test* is applied.

In calculating *chi-square test* statistics, the expected values of the frequencies in each classification is calculated under null hypothesis and the expected and observed values are utilised for calculating *chi-square*.

$$\chi^2 = \frac{\text{Observed frequency} - \text{Expected frequency}}{\text{Expected frequency}}$$

The above sum is taken over all cells of the table. P value is obtained by referring to the χ^2 distribution table corresponding to this calculated value of x at $(c-1)(r-1)$ degree of freedom where c and r are the number of columns and rows in the table. Depending upon this value *of P*, the conclusions are drawn as in other tests of significance.

23.16 VITAL AND MORBIDITY STATISTICS

The previous sections of this chapter have dealt with some aspects of biostatistics applicable in general to the health worker. In the following section, some aspects of vital and morbidity statistics are considered. Major sources of vital and morbidity statistics are:

   i. Census reports and intercensual population projections.
   ii. Records of births, deaths and notifiable diseases.
   iii. Hospital, dispensary and general practitioners, records.

iv. Records of industrial absenteeism, social security programmes and LIC records.
v. Routine survey records.
vi. Special survey records.
vii. Records of recruitment to certain categories of jobs.
viii. Postmortem records
ix. Records of important health institutions.

23.17 POPULATION STATISTICS

Statistics about population is the most important and basic data for the study of health statistics. The population growth of any country constantly undergoes changes in a cyclic manner. This is known as demographic cycle of a population. Details have been discussed in Chapter on Demography and Family Planning.

23.18 CENSUS

Census is a process of complete counting of all individuals in a country on a fixed date in every 10 years. During census, in addition to counting of individuals other subsidiary data pertaining to individuals such as their age, sex, religion, occupation, literacy, housing income, etc. are also collected. Census reports contain the classification of the population according to the above data for each geographical area separately. First census took place in India in 1872 and subsequently it is being conducted once in ten years ending with digit 1. Thus, the last census was taken in 2011. However, in each census there are bound to be some lapses in terms of under-counting. Details discussed under sources of data.

23.19 INTERCENSUAL POPULATION ESTIMATES

If the population of an area is required in between two census periods, it can be estimated by any of the following methods.

1. **Natural increase method:** In this method, all the components of increase or decrease in the population are taken into consideration.

   Thus, estimated population in any year = Previous census population + Number of [(Births–Deaths) + No. of (immigrants—emigrants)] during the period after the last census.

2. **Arithmetical progression method:** In this method, it is assumed that the addition to the population is same from year to year. This rate of addition is calculated on the basis of two previous census estimates.

   Thus, the population of an area in the year 1975 would be:

$$= \frac{\text{Population of the area during 1971 census +} (1971 \text{ census population} - 1961 \text{ census population}) \text{ of the area}}{10} \times 4$$

3. **Geometrical progression method:** Here the increase in the population from year to year is taken as geometrical progression increase, i.e. the population is considered to increase in a constant ratio. This ratio of increase is again estimated from the previous two continuous census. The calculation by this method is done by the formula

$$Pt = Po(1 + r)^t$$

where,

Pt = Population during the year
Po = Population during the last census
r = Geometric rate of growth of population
t = No. of years after census for which the population is to be calculated.

This formula can be evaluated by taking logarithms

$$\log Pt = \log Po + t \log (1 + r)$$

23.20 REGISTRATION OF BIRTHS AND DEATHS

The records of births and deaths are most useful in working out health indices as well as causes of mortality. In India, such registrations were not uniformly done by all the states before independence. The laws governing these registrations were also not uniform. However, an act of parliament was passed for the compulsory registration of births and deaths throughout the country and this has come in force from April 1970.

The channels of registration of births and deaths slightly differ in urban and rural areas.

In urban areas, the whole locality is divided into certain number of wards and each ward has a ward registrar to maintain the records. The hospitals, nursing homes where the delivery is conducted are supposed to report the birth and deaths at the earliest and not later than 21 days of the event. In bigger towns, even burial and cremation grounds contain the registers of deaths. These ward registrars send the returns to the municipal health officer once a week, who in turn forwards the returns to the district medical officer of health. Then these records are also directly sent to the state director of health services by the municipal medical officer.

In rural areas, the primary unit of registration is a *Gaon Sabha*. The Panchyat maintains these registers who get the information from the Pradhans of the village. Pradhans collect the information from the heads of the families. These reports are sent by the Panchayat secretary to the block development officer at the block level. From here, the returns are sent to the district collector. These records are also maintained by the medical officer of a primary health centre who collects the information through the basic health worker. These returns are sent by him to the district medical officer of health who in turn passes on the returns for the whole district to the state director of health services.

The national level report is compiled by the Director General of Health Services and at international level by the World Health Organization.

These statistics are also collected under the sample registration scheme by the Registrar General of India on a sample basis in the whole country. Model registration system for the compilation of information about the deaths and their causes are also undertaken in selected primary health centres.

23.21 LAPSES IN THE REGISTRATION OF BIRTHS AND DEATHS

Only since 1970, a uniform law was enacted for registration of births and deaths and before that each state had its own method of collection of these data. Despite of the enactment of law the under registration ranges from 50 to 60% both in rural and urban areas. Main reasons for lapses are:

i. As the primary responsibility rests with the pradhan of the *Gaon Sabha,* the registration is not given any importance by him due to his lack of interest and knowledge about the utility of the data. Further he is a multipurpose worker.

ii. The law regarding punishment for the nonreporting of the event is rarely followed.

iii. The cause of death and the age at death is seldom recorded accurately.

iv. There is a time lag in the consolidation and onward transmission of records which makes the statements undercompiled.

23.22 HEALTH INDICATORS

Health indicators are required to assess the health status of a community as well as for comparisons of health between the countries, states, communities and also within the same community over a period of time. Usually these indicators are calculated as rates for a particular population base covering a definite period like one calendar year. Health indicators can be broadly classified into four specific groups. These are:

1. Population indicators
2. Morbidity indicators
3. Mortality indicators
4. Health service indicators.

1. **Population indicators:** The different population indicators are enumerated below:

    i. Total population of an area and its breakdown into various aspects like age, sex, socioeconomic status, etc. These are obtained by census reports and intercensual population estimates.

    ii. *Crude birth rate*: It indicates the number of live births taking place in a community in a year and is calculated as:

$$\frac{\text{No. of live births registered or}}{\substack{\text{estimated in an area during a year}}} \times 1000$$
$$\frac{}{\substack{\text{Mid-year estimate of total} \\ \text{population of the area}}}$$

iii. *Fertility rate*: It measures the fertility in a population. A number of indicators for fertility rates are general fertility rate, gross reproduction rate (GRR), net reproduction rate (NRR), total fertility rate (TFR), etc.

Fertility rates can be further calculated as age specific fertility rates corresponding to different age of the reproductive women.

2. **Morbidity indicators:** A morbidity may be broadly defined as any subjective or objective deviation from a state of wellbeing resulting from a disease, an injury or an impairment. A morbidity may be assessed for those prevailing indicators during a period or for those occurring during the period. Keeping these in view the various morbidity indicators are outlined below:

    i. *Incidence rate* of any disease calculated as:

$$\frac{\substack{\text{No. of cases of the sickness starting} \\ \text{during the period in an area}}}{\substack{\text{Average number of persons exposed} \\ \text{to risk during that period in the area}}} \times 1000$$

This rate can be calculated either for the number of persons or spells of the sickness.

ii. *Prevalence rate*: It defines the total prevalence of a disease during a period or at any point in time. Thus prevalence of a disease can be period prevalence or point prevalence as it can be calculated either over a period of time or at any point of time. The prevalence calculated at any point of time is called point prevalence rate and if calculated for a period it is called period prevalence rate. It is calculated as:

$$\frac{\substack{\text{No. of cases of a disease present at} \\ \text{any time or period in the area}}}{\substack{\text{Average number of person exposed} \\ \text{to risk during the point of time or the} \\ \text{period under consideration}}} \times 1000$$

3. **Mortality indicators:** These simply facilitate to understand the extent of mortality as well as their uses in an area. Important mortality indicators are outlined below:

    i. *Crude death rate*: It measures the deaths taking place in an area due to all causes as well as in all age groups. This is calculated as:

$$\frac{\text{Number of deaths during the year}}{\text{Mid-year population}} \times 1000$$

ii. *Age- and sex-specific death rates*: There are calculated to understand the cause and pattern of deaths in different age groups in the two sexes. It is calculated as:

$$\frac{\begin{array}{c}\text{No. of deaths registered or}\\\text{estimated in an age and sex group}\\\text{during a year in an area}\end{array}}{\begin{array}{c}\text{Estimated population of that age and}\\\text{sex group for the year in the area}\end{array}} \times 1000$$

iii. *Infant mortality rate*: It is the age-specific death rate during the first year of life in a population. This is not only an important indicator of health but also Physical Quality of Life Index (PQLI).

Infant mortality rate is calculated as

$$\frac{\begin{array}{c}\text{No. of deaths of children below}\\\text{one year of age during a year in an area}\end{array}}{\begin{array}{c}\text{No. of live births registered or}\\\text{estimated during the year in the area}\end{array}} \times 1000$$

Further break-up of deaths in terms of neonatal (up to 28 days after birth) and early neonatal period (within seven days of birth) can be done and respective rates calculated.

iv. *Disease specific death rate*: It shows the causes of mortality in an area. This will enable to understand the major causes of mortality.

Disease-specific death rate for any disease is calculated as:

$$\frac{\begin{array}{c}\text{No. of deaths registered or}\\\text{estimated during a year due to a}\\\text{specific disease in an area}\end{array}}{\begin{array}{c}\text{Estimated mid-year population}\\\text{of the area}\end{array}} \times 1000$$

v. *Maternal mortality ratio*: It is the ratio of deaths of mothers due to pregnancy and their related causes or complications per hundred thousand live births in an area. This rate is calculated as:

$$\frac{\begin{array}{c}\text{No. of deaths of women due to}\\\text{pregnancy or pregnancy-related causes}\\\text{up to 42 days after delivery}\end{array}}{\begin{array}{c}\text{No. of live births during the year}\\\text{in the area}\end{array}} \times 1,00,000$$

vi. *Case fatality rate*: It gives the extent of fatality of any disease and is calculated as:

$$\frac{\begin{array}{c}\text{No. of deaths reported from a specific}\\\text{disease during a period of time in an area}\end{array}}{\begin{array}{c}\text{No. of cases of that disease reported in area}\\\text{during the period}\end{array}} \times 1000$$

vii. *Expectation of life*: At any age gives an expectation of average number of years of survival for any person at any age. This is calculated from life tables.

4. **Indicators of health service:** These are calculated in terms of availability, and rate of utilization of various health facilities and services.

23.23 STANDARDISATION OF RATES

The fact that the crude death of one place is higher than that of another place is in itself no evidence of one place being worse than the other with regard to health conditions. The population containing a large number of persons in the age group of 10 to 29 must have a lower death rate than that of a population containing many infants or old people. Again a comparison of death rates may also be affected by the sex proportions of the populations considered, for at most ages and from most causes mortality of males and females are not the same.

In comparing the mortality conditions of a number of places, or mortality conditions in the same place at different times the respective crude death rates, should be corrected or standardised to allow for differences in the age and sex distribution of the population.

Two methods of standardisation are commonly used.

i. **Direct method of standardisation:** Standardised death rate by the direct method is obtained by applying the specific death rates in a local population to a standard population. This shows the total death rate in a standard population if it was exposed to death rates of the local population or in other words what would have been the total death rate of the local population, if its age and sex composition was similar to that of the standard population.

Generally the population of the whole country in terms of stationary population of the life table is chosen as the standard population.

The direct method of standardisation requires a knowledge of (a) the number of persons in each age and sex group, and (b) the number of deaths separately in each age or sex group. Sometimes this detailed information is not available. On some occasions, the population at the different ages is so small that the age-specific death rates are subject to large fluctuations through the presence or absence of merely a few deaths. In such instances, the indirect method of standardisation can be applied.

ii. **Indirect method of standardisation:** The first step in the indirect method is the use of a series of age, and sex-specific death rates for the standard population. These rates are applied (by simple proportion) to the population of the local area at various age groups to determine the number of deaths that would have occurred in each sex and age group in that place, if it was exposed to the mortality experience of the standard population. Thus, total number of expected deaths are found. By dividing the expected total deaths by the population of the area under consideration, death rate is obtained. This rate is called the *Index death rate*. It indicates what would the death rate have been for the local area, if it was subjected to the same mortality conditions as prevailed in the standard population.

If the local population had the same age and sex composition as the standard population, then its index death rate would naturally be the same as the crude death rate of the standard population. In that case, no correction to the crude death rate of the locality would be necessary. If, on the other hand the index death rate of the locality is found to be higher or lower than crude death rate of the standard population, then to compensate for the fact that the local population is favourable to mortality, the crude death rate of the locality is to be adjusted. The adjustment consists of diminishing or increasing the recorded crude death rate. The precise degree to which the crude death rate is to be diminished or increased is measured by the ratio of the crude death rate of the standard population to the index deathrate of the locality. This ratio is called the *standardising factor*.

Mental Health

Mental health includes our emotional, psychological, and social wellbeing. It affects how we think, feel and act as we cope with life. It also helps determine how we handle stress, relate to others, and make choices. Mental health is important at every stage of life, from childhood and adolescence through adulthood.

Mental illnesses are serious disorders which can affect our thinking, mood, and behaviour. There are many causes of mental disorders. An individual's genes and family history life experiences, such as stress or a history of abuse biological factors play a note in causation. Through mental disorders are common, then treatments are available.

It is rather impossible to describe a mentally healthy individual or society. However, for practical purposes, we can consider at least three dimensions of a mentally healthy person:

i. **Self image:** A mentally healthy person is supposed to have esteem and a correct image of himself as to what he is and what he is not, neither underestimating nor overestimating himself.

ii. **Universally acceptable humanitarian qualities:** The individual should have genuine interest in others, should love others and be capable of deriving pleasure in helping others.

iii. **Response to stress:** A mentally healthy person is capable of meeting the demands of life and coping with different crisis situations without being unduly shaken.

24.1 MENTAL ILLNESS

Diagnosis and classification of mental illness pose a number of difficulties. However, for practical purposes, mental illnesses can be broadly grouped into following categories (WHO), the details of which are available in psychiatric literature:

i. **Mental retardation or mental deficiency** (including mental subnormality and mental abnormality):

Causes apart from sociocultural and nutritive factors include chromosomal defects (Down's syndrome or Mongolism), trauma and congenital defects.

ii. **Organic brain syndrome:** In which the functioning of brain is impaired either by a physical lesion (trauma, tumour, infection, arteriosclerosis, etc.) or by a toxic process.

iii. **Functional psychosis:** Includes schizophrenia and manic depressive psychosis (MDP).

iv. **Neurosis:** Which represents the most common forms of psychiatric illnesses and includes anxiety states, depression, phobia, obsession and hysteria.

v. **Personality disorders or psychopathy:** Include delinquency, sexual perversions, alcoholism and drug addiction. Psychopathy connotes persistent socially unacceptable behaviour in the absence of demonstrable mental illness or brain pathology.

24.2 SOME SPECIAL CONSIDERATIONS IN THE FIELD OF MENTAL HEALTH

i. Mental symptomatology is so complex that it is difficult to differentiate between normal and abnormal behaviours because the symptoms are often exaggerations of phenomena, which are in other contexts, parts of normal human activities (e.g. bereavement, euphoria, hallucinations, etc.). Moreover, the same symptoms tend to appear in different syndromes, thus the mental illness for the most part is not characterised by pathognomonic symptoms. Classification of the mental illnesses and their diagnosis pose a considerable problem. It is not uncommon to find widely different diagnostic levels on a particular patient by different psychiatrists.

ii. Evolution of psychological science is characterised with diverse schools and approaches to mental phenomena, and there are difficulties in their integration. For example, Pavlovian model emphasises the physiological relationship to frustration. Behaviourism school is built on 'machine model' of man characterised by stimulus-organism-response (S-O-R) relationship. Freudian emphasis goes chiefly to intra-family relationship and Bowlby correlates mental phenomena to exposure, to stimuli, and so on.

iii. Factors influencing mental health include biological factors (genes or brain chemistry), life experiences such as trauma or abuse and family history of mental health problems.

Early warning signs of mental diseases: One or more of the following are the early warning signs of mental disorders.

a. Eating or sleeping too much or too little.

b. Pulling away from people and usual activities.

c. Having low or no energy, feeling numb or like nothing matters.

d. Having unexplained aches and pains.

e. Feeling of helpless or hopeless.

f. Smoking, drinking, or using drugs more than usual.

g. Feeling unusually confused, forgetful, on edge, angry, upset, worried, or scared.

h. Yelling or fighting with family and friends.

i. Experiencing severe mood swings that cause problems in relationships.

j. Having persistent thoughts and memories you can not get out of your head.

k. Hearing voices or believing things that are not true.

l. Thinking of harming yourself or others.

m. Inability to perform daily tasks like taking care of your kids or getting to work or school.

In case of any of the above symptoms, professional help must be sought along with other coping mechanisms like connecting with others, staying positive and getting physically active, helping others, getting enough sleep and developing coping skills.

iv. Mental problems, especially in our country either remain undiagnosed or are often interpreted by laymen in magicoreligious terms. Also due to stigma attached, the patients suffering from mental illnesses fail to reach doctors for professional help.

v. The modern social trends with degradation of human values, loss of social ties, degeneration of intrinsic relationships, lack of opportunities, deprivation, increase in the expectation due to excessive use of mass media, and isolation are leading to an increase in rate of mental illnesses.

24.3 PROBLEM STATEMENT

The mental problems are increasing, and the rate of their increase along with the process of rapid modernisation, is also on the increase.

It is estimated that 6–7% of population suffers from mental disorders. The World Bank report (1993) revealed that the Disability Adjusted Life Years (DALYs) loss due to neuropsychiatric disorder is much higher than diarrhoea, malaria, worm infestations, and tuberculosis if taken individually. Together these disorders account for 12% of the global burden of disease (GBD) and an analysis of trends indicates this will increase to 15% by 2020 (World Health Report, 2001).

World Health Organization estimated that mental and behavioural disorders account for about 12% of the global burden of diseases. In India, the burden of mental and behavioural disorders ranged from 9.5 to 102 per 1000 population. However, burden of mental disorders seen by the world is only a tip of iceberg.

Deprivation, poverty, social exclusion, work and school environment and female gender are the common predisposing factors for mental disorders in India.

With a constantly increasing burden of diseases, it is imperative to study the availability of services for managing these problems. The Central Bureau of Health Intelligence, way back in 1969 brought out that there are only 38 mental hospitals in India employing only 54 psychiatrists. The bed/population ratio is 0.3/10,000 as against the WHO norms of 1/10,000 and the patient turnover rate per year per bed is 1.96.

The situation has improved over the years after coming up of the NMHP and DMHP in the country, however, a lot of inputs in terms of resources are further required in this field.

24.4 HISTORY OF MENTAL HEALTH SERVICES IN INDIA

Though the history of mental health services in world dates back to fourth century in Greece, the mention of mental diseases like schizophrenia and bipolar disorders find place in ancient vedic literature (Atharva veda) much before that. Indian epics like Mahabharata and Ramayana have also made references to disordered state of mind and their coping mechanisms. The Great Indian Epic, Bhagwata Gita is also a classical example of crisis management intervention psychotherapy.

During pre-colonial India also, there is some evidence of presence of mental hospitals in Madhya Pradesh during the times of Mahmud Khilji (1436–1469). During the British rule, under the administrative control of Lord Cornwallis, first mental hospital was made in Calcutta in 1787.

During mid-colonial period (1858–1918), there was a steady growth in the development of mental asylums. First Lunacy Act was also enacted in 1858 whereas Indian Lunacy Act was enacted in 1912.

In 1946, a health survey and development committee, popularly known as the "Bhore Committee," surveyed mental hospitals. The Health Survey and Development Committee report submitted by Col. Moore Taylor in 1946 reported numerical and professional inadequacy and suggested a focus on training of personnel and students in psychiatry, promotion of occupational and diversionary therapies, and separate child psychiatry units. The committee also suggested improvisation and modernization of most hospitals, attachment to medical colleges, and establishment of proper mental health. Thus, a new phase of development of mental hospitals started after India's independence in 1947, when the focus was upon the creation of general health practising units (GHPUs) rather than building more mental hospitals. Emphasis was on improving conditions in existing hospitals, while at the same time encouraging outpatient care through these units. A few new mental hospitals, notably at Delhi, Jaipur, Kottayam and Bengal were also added.

The ICMR study group and the Central Council of Health realised the fact that mental health aspects in the country had been neglected during the three Five-Year Plans. Establishment of a psychiatric clinic in each district and a teaching hospital during the Fourth Plan was recommended. In 1970, the All India Institute of Mental Health, Bangalore, conducted an experiment (Mandya Project) in which a comprehensive mental health team was regularly sent to the district hospital. It then became evident that nearly 73% of the mental cases can be treated in the district hospital itself, if there is a team of specialists available.

In 1971, WHO/SEARO seminar in New Delhi emphasised the need for improvement of training of medical personnel so that they are better equipped to handle mental problems in different situations.

As a follow up to the Health For All by 2000, National Mental Health Programme (NMHP) was formulated in 1982. This led to change in strategy towards decentralization of services, comprehensive community-based care from custodial asylums through District Mental Health Programme, and development of training materials and programmes for practitioners and academicians. The Mental Health Act of India thus came to being in 1987.

National Mental Health Programme

The National Mental Health Programme (NMHP) was formulated in 1982 to develop a national-level initiative for mental healthcare based on the community psychiatry approach. The aim of the programme were to ensure prevention and treatment of mental and neurological disorders by use of mental health technology for application of mental health principles in total national development to improve quality of life.

Objectives

a. To ensure availability and accessibility of minimum mental healthcare for all in the foreseeable future, particularly to the most vulnerable and under privileged sections of population.
b. To encourage application of mental health knowledge in general healthcare and in the social development.
c. To promote community participation in mental health services development, and to stimulate efforts towards self-help in the community.

Strategies

a. Integration of mental health with primary health-care through the national mental health program.
b. Provision of tertiary care institutions for treatment of mental disorders.
c. Eradicate stigmatization of mentally ill patients and protecting their rights through regulatory institutions like the central mental health authority, and state mental health authority.
d. To utilize the existing infrastructure of health services to deliver the minimum mental healthcare services.
e. To provide appropriate task oriented training to the existing health staff.
f. To link health services with the existing community development programme.

District Mental Health Programme (DMHP)

District Mental Health Programme (DMHP) was launched in 1986 based on 'Bellary Model, which is a community-based comprehensive care model. It encompasses the comprehensive preventive, promotive, curative and rehabilitative services for mental illnesses.

Components of the Programme

a. Strengthening of health facilities at all levels (community, primary health facilities, secondary hospitals and tertiary care institutions) for availability of quality services at all levels.
b. Training programmes of all workers in the mental health team at the identified institution.
c. Public education
d. Early detection of illnesses and treatment
e. Providing valuable data and experience at the level of community.

The NMHP was re-strategized in the year 2003 (in Xth Five-Year Plan) with the aim to extend the DMHP to 100 districts, setting up centres of excellence, upgradation of psychiatry wings of government medical colleges/general hospitals, modernization of state mental hospitals, IEC with a component of monitoring and evaluation.

24.5 CURRENT STATUS AND CHALLENGES

Starting with 4 districts in 1996, the programme was expanded to 27 districts by the end of the IXth plan. Presently the DMHP is being implemented in 123 districts of the country. The DMHP envisages a community-based approach for various components under the programme, viz. training of mental health team at identified nodal institutions, increasing awareness and stigma alleviation and early detection and treatment of mental illness in the community (OPD/indoor and follow up). The programme also envisages to provide valuable data and experience at the level of community at the state and centre for future planning and improvement in service and research.

In 2008, new components of School Mental Health Sevices (life skills education and counselling in schools), college counselling services, work place stress management and suicide prevention services have been added besides clinical services, training of general healthcare functionaries, and IEC activities under DMHP. The team of workers at the district under the programme consists of a psychiatrist, a clinical psychologist, a psychiatric social worker, a psychiatry/community nurse, a programme manager, a program/case registry assistant and a record keeper.

Mental Healthcare Bill came into force in 2013 to provide for mental healthcare and services for persons with mental illness and to protect, promote and fulfil the rights of such persons during delivery of mental healthcare and services.

Despite huge interventions and newer initiatives for mental healthcare by the government and a lot of success with DMHP functional over 123 districts, and upgradation of 88 psychiatry wings in medical colleges, the challenges rename in 'Mental Healthcare' in India. Some are:

a. There is a large 'unmet need' for mental healthcare in the community.
b. Lack of or poor understanding of psychological distress as requiring medical intervention in the general population.
c. Limited acceptance of modern medical care for mental disorders among the general population.
d. Limitations in the availability of mental health services (professionals and facilities) in the public health services.
e. Poor utilization of available services by the ill population and their families.
f. Problems in recovery and reintegration of persons with mental illnesses.

24.6 COMPONENTS OF MENTAL HEALTHCARE

The mental healthcare includes the following components:

i. **Promotive and preventive care**
   a. Promotive services include nutritional improvement, school mental health services (life skills education), counselling services in schools and colleges, suicide prevention services, promotion of activities like Yoga and Meditation for stress management at workplace. Besides, educating people regarding health, psychosexual behaviour and social welfare services, provision of job opportunities, social security and improvement in the standard of living are the steps towards promotive and preventive mental healthcare.
   b. Eugenic services, if developed properly, might be able to control the genetic factors in mental illnesses to some extent.
   c. Meditation and other techniques have recently been demonstrated to produce catharsis (emotional release), bring tranquility of mind and prepares individuals to face the crisis situations in life boldly. Some studies have been conducted on transcendental pattern of integrated response meditated by the CNS and are characterised by relaxation, hypometabolism and lowering of anxiety. If the values of relaxation, meditation, psychodrama and encounter groups are established, they should be integrated in our educational system to evolve emotionally adjusted groups.

ii. **Curative care**
   a. Early diagnosis and treatment of mental problems utilizing the services of community nurses, school teachers and voluntary workers. After initiation of treatment by a doctor at a health facility, the treatment and after care can be continued in the community by the community health nurses and trained peripheral health workers and volunteers.
   b. Community facilities can be organized for the mentally ill like day care, half way home (supervised hospital or hostel), foster homes and self-help groups.
   c. Organisation of mental health emergency services, helplines for suicide and violence, walk-in clinics, referral and consultation services.
   d. Strengthening of residential services like mental hospitals and psychiatric units for outdoor and indoor services in general hospitals.
   e. Organising and arranging services in certain special groups such as children, adolescents, old people, mentally retarded, juvenile delinquents, criminals, etc. that might require specialised mental care.

iii. **Rehabilitative care:** It includes arrangements for
   a. Resettlement of patients back into their family and society after their treatment is over.

b. Education and vocational training of mentally challenged and emotionally disturbed.

c. Supportive care such as drug suspension, resocialisation, family guidance.

d. Clubs for people with residual mental problems.

iv. Capacity building

a. Integration of mental health with primary healthcare through the National Mental Health Programme. Strengthening of tertiary care institutions for treatment of mental disorders by provision of additional manpower.

b. Provide appropriate task oriented training to the existing health staff and all the manpower recruited under the programme. To link health services with the existing community development programme.

c. Awareness and public education programmes to reduce stigma and generate awareness among masses regarding availability of services.

d. Optimum utilization of community nurses in planning and implementation of family and community-based interventions and evaluation.

Sample Question Paper

1. **A CMOS can maintain its configuration settings due to ....**
   - A. The BIOS
   - B. The system board
   - C. The power supply
   - D. A battery

2. **Your computer is showing incorrect time every time you restart the computer. This happens even after you have set the computer time several times. What needs to be done?**
   - A. The CPU needs to be replaced
   - B. The UPS needs to be replaced
   - C. The battery needs to be replaced
   - D. The operating system must be reloaded

3. **Which of the following helps in keeping our computer/CPU cool?**
   - A. A CPU fan
   - B. A heat sink
   - C. Move the computer to a well-ventilated location
   - D. All of these

4. **It is a computer bus which moves information between the internal hardware of a computer system (including the CPU and RAM) and peripheral devices:**
   - A. Information bus
   - B. Descend bus
   - C. Ascend bus
   - D. Expansion bus

5. **................................ is NOT a type of internal hard drive.**
   - A. IDE
   - B. SCSI
   - C. USB
   - D. EIDE

6. **Which of the following function key activates the speller?**
   - A. F5
   - B. F7
   - C. F9
   - D. Shift + F7

7. **Thesaurus tool in MS Word is used for:**
   - A. Spelling suggestions
   - B. Grammar options
   - C. Synonyms and antonyms words
   - D. All of the above

8. **A word processor would most likely be used to:**
   - A. Keep an account of money spent
   - B. Do a computer search in media center
   - C. Maintain an inventory
   - D. Type a biography

9. **After typing header text, how can you quickly enter footer text?**
   - A. Press Page Down key and type the text for footer
   - B. Click on Switch between Heder and Footer then type the text
   - C. Both of the above
   - D. None of the above

10. **It is possible to .... a data source before performing a merge.**
    - A. Create
    - B. Modify
    - C. Sort
    - D. All of the above

11. **When only one process may use a critical resource at a time while the others wait for it, the condition is called ....**
    - A. Circular wait
    - B. Pre-emption
    - C. Mutual exclusion
    - D. Hold and wait

12. **We usually measure efficiency of an operating system and overall performance of a computer system in terms of ....**
    - A. Throughput
    - B. Turnaround time
    - C. Response time
    - D. All of these

13. **What is the method of handling deadlocks?**
    - A. Use a protocol to ensure that the system will never enter a deadlock state
    - B. Allow the system to enter the deadlock state and then recover
    - C. Pretend that deadlocks never occur in the system.
    - D. All of the Above

14. **To delete a file without allowing it to store in recycle bin:**
    - A. Press Delete key
    - B. Press Shift + Delete key

C. Press Ctrl + Delete key

D. Press Alt + Delete key

15. User action such as keystroke or mouse click is referred to as:

A. Interrupt

B. Tasks

C. Processes

D. Event

16. What does the passive command provide to dynamic routing protocols?

A. Stops an interface from sending or receiving periodic dynamic updates

B. Stops an interface from sending periodic dynamic updates but not from receiving updates

C. Stops the router from receiving any dynamic updates

D. Stops the router from sending any dynamic updates

17. Which protocol is used to send a destination network unknown message back to originating hosts?

A. TCP

B. ARP

C. ICMP

D. BootP

18. How often are BPDUs sent from a layer 2 device?

A. Never

B. Every 2 seconds

C. Every 10 minutes

D. Every 30 seconds

19. How many broadcast domains are created when you segment a network with a 12-port switch?

A. 1

B. 2

C. 5

D. 12

20. What does the command router A (config)#line cons 0 allow you to perform next?

A. Set the Telnet password

B. Shut down the router

C. Set your console password

D. Disable console connections

21. Which attribute of the Anchor tag is used to specify the location of an internal reference in a document?

A. Href

B. Name

C. Title

D. Color

22. The following HTML tag indicates that ....

```
<table>
    <tr>
        <th>Month</th>
        <th>Savings</th>
    </tr>
    <tr>
```

```
        <td>January</td>
        <td>Rs 1000</td>
    </tr>
    <tr>
        <td>February</td>
        <td>Rs 800</td>
    </tr>
</table>
```

A. The table has no border

B. The table has border of default thickness

C. There is no table

D. The table has zero rows and zero columns

23. .... is a logical tag.

A. <big>

B. <b>

C. <cite>

D. <i>

24. Which of the following is NOT a type of hypertext link?

A. Internal hypertext link

B. Remote hypertext link

C. Local hypertext link

D. External hypertext link

25. Which of the following is NOT valid value for the align attribute of the <IMG> tag?

A. Top

B. Middle

C. Title

D. Colour

26. Which of the following statements describe streaming?

A. Playing audio files on the internet

B. Buffering online data received using a codec before playing a multimedia element usch that the multimedia can play uninterrupted

C. Reducing the load time of a webpage by caching online content on the disk

D. Breaking multimedia into packets before sending it to a web server such that the clients can view multimedia continuously

27. Planning the content and the flow of your multimedia presentation is known as it's ....

A. Design

B. Storyboard

C. Development

D. Layout

28. Which of the following statements is true?

A. MIDI files are usually larger than WAV files

B. Video files are much larger than audio files

C. Same format is used to create audio and video files

D. All video clips consume around 10 MB space

29. Which of the following best describes virtual reality?

A. A computer game involving graphics and multimedia

B. A 3D simulation of a real or imagined environment using computers

C. A simulator with a simulation suit and simulating goggles

D. Images created in five dimensions

30. Any clip of animation or film that spreads rapidly through online sharing is said to have become ....

A. Viral   B. Thermal

C. Promotional   D. Unintentional

31. The image here is displaying a ....

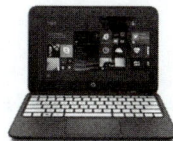

A. PDA   B. Smartphone

C. Notepad   D. Convertible laptop

32. Which of the following statements is incorrect for google glasses?

A. They are interactive and intelligent devices

B. They will be powered by Windows mobile

C. They are head mounted devices

D. They can be worn by users as eyewear

33. .... is a software for iPhone from Apple that provides user with a personal assistant that can perform various tasks based on the user's voice commands.

A. Pulse   B. Dragon

C. Siri   D. Safari

34. .... is NOT in iPhone 4.

A. 4G

B. Front facing camera

C. HD recording

D. Multitouch screen

35. The image shown here is the logo of ....

A. Bosch

B. Infrared connectivity

C. Wi-Fi

D. Viber

36. In the given figure, B is 300 km East ward of A and C is 400 km North of A. D is exactly in the middle of C and B. The distance between C and D is:

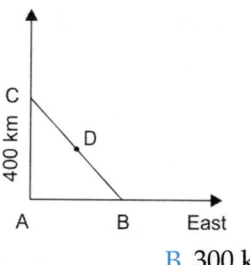

A. 250 km   B. 300 km

C. 250.2 km   D. 350 km

37. Ravi wants to go to the university. He starts from his home which is in the East and comes to a crossing. The road to the left ends in a theatre, straight ahead is the hospital. In which direction is the university?

A. North   B. South

C. East   D. West

38. BG, GC, HN, N ....

A. D   B. J

C. I   D. H

39. B, A, Z, D, C, Y, F, E, ...

A. W   B. X

C. U   D. G

40. Which number will complete the given series— 4, 8, 12, 16?

A. 18   B. 20

C. 22   D. 24

41. Find the odd one out:

A. PageMaker

B. CorelDRAW

C. Oracle

D. QuarkXPress

42. Which software has the punch line "Power of simplicity"?

A. WinZip

B. Lotus 1–2–3

C. Windows media player

D. Tally

43. The command Ctrl + X in MS-Word:

A. Print   B. Cut

C. Copy   D. Select All

44. The command Ctrl + P in MS-Word:

A. Print   B. Page up

C. Copy   D. Page down

45. **It is a memory management scheme. In this scheme the pages of the process are loaded when they are needed. This scheme is called ....**
   A. Fragmentation
   B. Segmentation
   C. Virtual paging
   D. Demand paging

46. **The Banker's algorithm is a ....**
   A. Deadlock avoidance algorithm
   B. Deadlock detection algorithm
   C. Deadlock rectification algorithm
   D. Deadlock manipulation algorithm

47. **A single packet on a data link is known as:**
   A. Path
   B. Frame
   C. Block
   D. Group

48. **The process of communicating with a file from a terminal is:**
   A. Interactive
   B. Interrogation
   C. Heuristic
   D. All of the above

DARKEN YOUR CHOICE WITH HB PENCIL

1	Ⓐ Ⓑ Ⓒ Ⓓ Ⓔ	11	Ⓐ Ⓑ Ⓒ Ⓓ Ⓔ	21
2	Ⓐ Ⓑ Ⓒ Ⓓ Ⓔ	12	Ⓐ Ⓑ Ⓒ Ⓓ Ⓔ	22
3	Ⓐ Ⓑ Ⓒ Ⓓ Ⓔ	13	Ⓐ Ⓑ Ⓒ Ⓓ Ⓔ	23
4	Ⓐ Ⓑ Ⓒ Ⓓ Ⓔ	14	Ⓐ Ⓑ Ⓒ Ⓓ Ⓔ	24
5	Ⓐ Ⓑ Ⓒ Ⓓ Ⓔ	15	Ⓐ Ⓑ Ⓒ Ⓓ Ⓔ	25
6	Ⓐ Ⓑ Ⓒ Ⓓ Ⓔ	16	Ⓐ Ⓑ Ⓒ Ⓓ Ⓔ	26
7	Ⓐ Ⓑ Ⓒ Ⓓ Ⓔ	17	Ⓐ Ⓑ Ⓒ Ⓓ Ⓔ	27
8	Ⓐ Ⓑ Ⓒ Ⓓ Ⓔ	18	Ⓐ Ⓑ Ⓒ Ⓓ Ⓔ	28
9	Ⓐ Ⓑ Ⓒ Ⓓ Ⓔ	19	Ⓐ Ⓑ Ⓒ Ⓓ Ⓔ	29
10	Ⓐ Ⓑ Ⓒ Ⓓ Ⓔ	20	Ⓐ Ⓑ Ⓒ Ⓓ Ⓔ	30

Bibliography

1. A-Post 2015 Global goal for water: synthesis of key finding and recommendations from UN water. Technical advice. UN water, 2014. Available from: www. unwater.org

2. Birendra Nath Ghosh. A Treatise on Hygiene and Public Health. 12th edn. Scientific Publishing Co. Calcutta, 1948.

3. CDC and the Safe Water System. Division of Foodborne, Waterborne, and Environmental Diseases. CDC, 2011. Available from: http://www.cdc.gov/safewater

4. Dilip Biswas. Pollution Control Act, Rules and Notification Issued thereunder. Pollution control law. 6th edn. PCB. Delhi, 2010.

5. Division of High-Consequence Pathogens and Pathology (DHCPP). Ebola (Ebola Virus Disease). National Center for Emerging and Zoonotic Infectious Diseases. Available form: http://www.cdc.gov/vhf/ebola/index.html.

6. Dr. DK Taneja. Health Policies and Programmes in India. 14th edn. New Delhi. The Health Sciences Publisher, 2016.

7. Dr. Joseph C. Boray. Revised by Dr GW Hutchinson and Stephen Love. Liver fluke disease in sheep and cattle, 2007. Available form: https://www.dpi.nsw.gov.a

8. Dr. Navpreet. Excreta disposal.pdf

9. Harvesting, Storing, and Treating Rainwater for Domestic Indoor Use. Texas Commission on Environmental Quality, 2007.

10. Household Water Treatment Ceramic Filtration. Division of Foodborne, Waterborne, and Environmental Diseases. CDC, 2011. Available from: https://www.cdc.gov

11. Household Water Treatment: Chlorination—the safe water system. Division of Foodborne, Waterborne, and Environmental Diseases. CDC, 2014.

12. Household Water Treatment: Flocculent/disinfectant powder. Division of Foodborne, Waterborne, and Environmental Diseases. CDC, 2011.

13. Household Water Treatment: slow sand filtration. Division of Foodborne, Waterborne, and Environmental Diseases. CDC, 2011.

14. Household Water Treatment: solar disinfection. Division of Foodborne, Waterborne, and Environmental Diseases. CDC, 2011.

15. Hygiene of water and water supply, 1999. Available from: http://intranet.tdmu.edu.ua

16. IJCM 2013 Jul–Sept; 38(3):185–6.

17. Iodine deficiency. American Thyroid Association, 2014. Available from: www.thyroid.org

18. Jacob Michael. Safe food handling. A training guide for managers of food service establishments. England. WHO Publications, 1989.

19. Judith F, Cundiff, John D. Malone, and Jeanne A. Pfeiffer. Bioterrorism Readiness Plan: A Template for Healthcare Facilities. 1999. CDC Hospital Infections Program Bioterrorism Working Group. Available from: https://emergency.cdc.gov/bioterrorism/pdf/13apr99APIC-CDCBioterrorism.pdf

20. K Park. Textbook on Preventive and Social Medicine. 23rd edn. Jabalpur. Bhanot Publications, 2015.

21. Kumar GS, Kar SS, Jain A. Health and environmental sanitation in India: Issues for prioritizing control strategies. Indian J Occup Environ Med 2011; 15(3): 93–96.

22. M. Adams, Y. Motarjemi. Basic Food Safety for Health Workers. Geneva. WHO Publications, 1999.

23. Manual of methods of analysis of foods (milk and milk products). Lab manual 1. Directorate General of Health Services. MoHFW, GOI. New Delhi, 2005.

24. Ministry of Health and Family Welfare. Food Safety and Standards Rules, 2011. New Delhi. Available from: www.cbec.gov.in

25. Module 2: System of Sanitation; Lecture 2: System of Sanitation. NPTEL, IIT Kharagpur Web Courses.

26. NN Basak. Environmental Engineering. Tata McGraw-Hill Education, 2003.

27. NFHS. IIPS Mumbai.

28. NHRM. School Health Programme. MoHFW. GOI.

29. NICEF/WHO. Diarrhoea: Why children are still dying and what can be done, 2009.

30. Nutrition Foundation of India. ICMR. Dietary guidelines for Indians—A Manual. 22nd edn. NIN: Hyderabad; 2011.

31. Pasteurization: Definition and Methods. IDFA, June; 2009.

32. S. Jeffery and W.H. van der Putten. Soil Borne Human Diseases. Luxembourg: Publications Office of the European Union, 2011.

33. Safe water for community. A Guide for Establishing a Community-based Safe Water System Program. 1st edn. CDC, 2008.

34. SDG guide.

35. Shaker, M. Arafat. Air Frying a New Technique for Produce of Healthy Fried Potato Strips. Journal of Food and Nutrition Sciences 2014; 2(4): 200–6.

36. Tefera Belachew, Kebede Faris, Tsegaye Asres. Acute and Chronic Malnutrition in Children. Jimma University. Ethiopia Public Health Training Initiative, 2005.

37. The Safe Water System: safe storage of drinking water. Division of Foodborne, Waterborne, and Environmental Diseases. CDC, 2011.

38. Water for the world. Testing the yield of wells. Program manual and policy perspectives.

39. Well Aware: A Guide for Well Owners. Well care. Green Communities Canada, 2003. Available from: www.greencommunitiescanada.org

40. WHO. Food Borne Disease Outbreak. Guidelines for Investigations and Control, 2008.

41. WHO Guidelines for drinking water quality. 4th edn. Geneva, 2011.

42. WHO. GPEI status report, 2015.

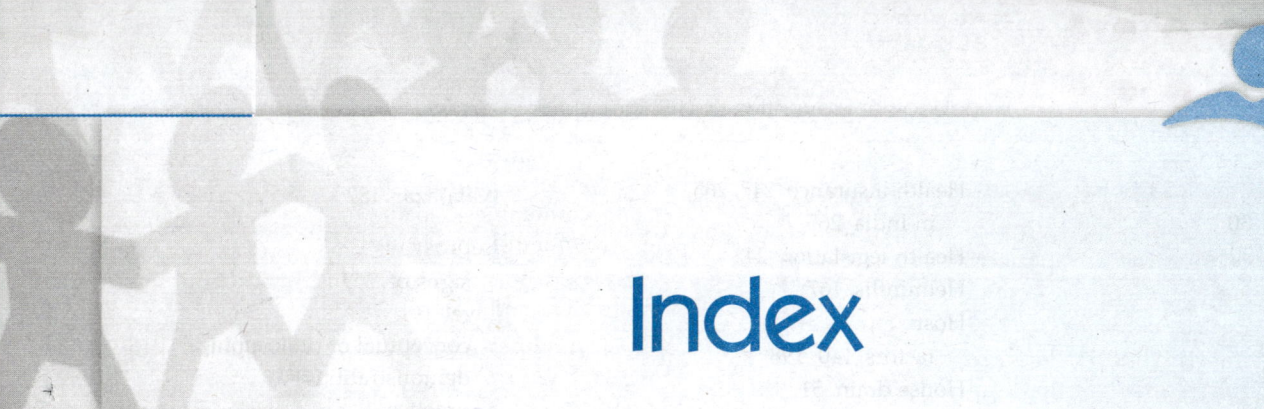
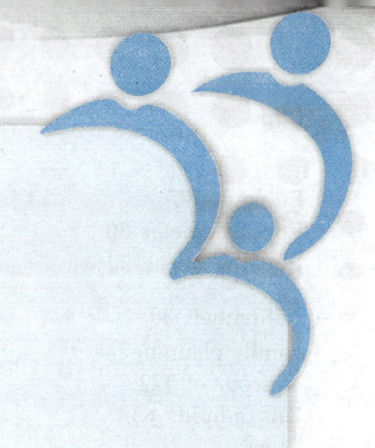

Index